PRINCIPLES & LABS FOR PHYSICAL FITNESS

Werner W. K. Hoeger
Boise State University

Sharon A. Hoeger

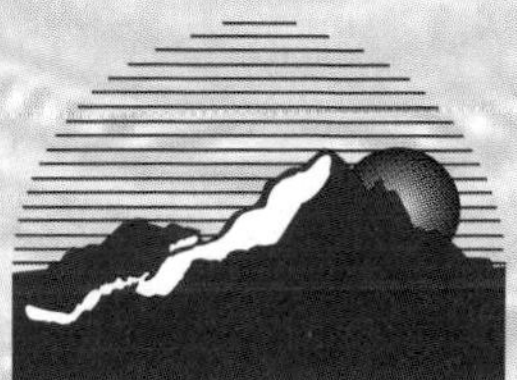

Morton Publishing Company

925 W. Kenyon Ave., Unit 12
Englewood, Colorado 80110

Book Team

Publisher	Ruth Horton
Designer	Joanne Saliger
Copy Editor	Carolyn Acheson
Illustrator	Jennifer Johnson
Cover Design	Bob Schram, Bookends
Typography	Ash Street Typecrafters, Inc.

Morton Publishing Company

CEO	Douglas N. Morton
President	Tom Doran

Printed in the United States of America
by Morton Publishing Company
925 W. Kenyon Ave., Unit 12, Englewood, CO 80110

10 9 8 7 6 5 4 3 2

ISBN: 0–89582–334-9

Recycled

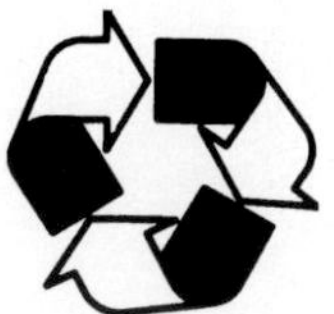

Paper

Preface

Most people go to college to learn how to make a living. Making a good living, however, won't help unless people live an active lifestyle that will allow them to enjoy what they have. Unfortunately, the current American way of life does not provide the human body with sufficient physical activity to maintain adequate health. Many present lifestyle patterns are such a serious threat to our health that they actually increase the deterioration rate of the human body and often lead to premature illness and mortality.

Several major research studies indicate that people who lead an active lifestyle live longer and enjoy a better quality of life. Furthermore, the U.S. Surgeon General has determined that lack of physical activity is detrimental to good health. As a result, the importance of sound fitness programs has assumed an entirely new dimension. From an initial fad in the early 1970s, fitness programs have become a trend that is now very much a part of the American way of life.

Because of the impressive scientific evidence on the benefits of physical activity, most people in North America are aware that physical fitness promotes a healthier, happier, and more productive life. Nevertheless, the great majority do not enjoy a better quality of life because they are either led astray by a multi-billion dollar "quick fix — fad" industry, or simply do not know how to implement a sound physical activity program that will yield positive results. Only in a fitness course will people learn sound principles of exercise prescription, that if implemented, will teach them how to live — that is, how to truly live life to its fullest potential.

Principles and Labs for Physical Fitness contains twelve chapters and twenty-five laboratories that serve as a guide to implement a comprehensive lifetime fitness program. Book contents are completely up to date to include the latest information reported in literature and at professional health, physical education, and sports medicine meetings. Students are also encouraged to adhere to a well-balanced diet and a healthy lifestyle to help them achieve total well-being. Furthermore, extensive information is provided on motivation and behavioral modification techniques to help students eliminate negative behaviors and implement a better way of life.

As students work through the various chapters and laboratories in this book, they will develop and regularly update their own lifetime program to improve fitness components. *The emphasis throughout the book is on teaching students how to take control of their own fitness and lifestyle habits so that they can make a constant and deliberate effort to stay healthy and achieve the highest potential for well-being.*

Key Features of Principles and Labs for Physical Fitness

- The book contains extensive information on the association between fitness and mortality, the relevance of initiating and adhering to a lifetime fitness program during youth, and the effects of a healthy lifestyle on quality of life and longevity. The U.S. Health Objectives for the Year 2000 are also included. These objectives emphasize the need for health promotion and disease prevention, personal responsibility, and health benefits for all people in the United States.
- Important terms appear in boldface type and, together with their definitions, appear in boxes within the text. The terms are also combined in a glossary at the end of the book.
- For the assessment of cardiorespiratory endurance, muscular strength, muscular flexibility, and body composition, several fitness tests are provided so that instructors may select a test according to the facilities, time, or equipment available and physical limitations of the participants.
- Both health fitness and physical fitness standards are provided for fitness components. Health fitness standards are the lowest fitness requirements for maintaining good health, decreasing the risk for chronic diseases, and lowering the incidence of muscular-skeletal injuries. Physical fitness standards are higher than the health fitness norms and require a more vigorous exercise program.
- The cardiorespiratory endurance chapter emphasizes the importance of strength conditioning prior to starting an aerobic exercise program to minimize the risk of exercise-related injuries. Guidelines for exercise during pregnancy have been included and information on exercise clothing is also given.
- All exercise prescriptions (cardiorespiratory endurance, muscular strength, and muscular flexibility) conform with the 1995 guidelines for exercise testing and prescription by the American College of Sports Medicine (ACSM).
- A comprehensive battery of skill-related fitness tests (agility, balance, coordination, reaction time, power, and speed) is provided in this book as well.
- A comprehensive nutrient analysis that allows students to compare their daily food intake against the Recommended Dietary Allowances (RDA) can be found in the nutrition chapter. Up to seven days may be analyzed if the software that accompanies this book is used. Extensive information on antioxidants, phytochemicals, new food labels, and daily values are given in this chapter.
- Based on some of the latest research, the importance of physical activity as a major factor, if not the most important one, in the prevention of obesity and maintenance of recommended body weight is extensively discussed in the weight control chapter. The terms obesity, overweight, recommended weight, and "tolerable" weight are thoroughly addressed. Such information helps students make an informed decision as to what constitutes a realistic target weight.
- A concise final chapter on the importance of an overall healthy lifestyle is included. This chapter presents an overview of cardiovascular and cancer risk reduction, substance abuse control (including cigarette smoking and tips for quitting smoking), prevention of sexually transmitted diseases (including HIV and AIDS), physical training in the older adult, guidelines for the prevention of consumer fraud, health/fitness club memberships, and issues related to the selection, purchase, and maintenance of exercise equipment.
- The book contains all color photography and some of the most outstanding graphs and illustrations provided with any fitness book.

Ancillaries

The following ancillaries are provided free of charge to all qualified Principles and Labs for Physical Fitness adopters:

- Profile Plus, one of the most comprehensive computer software packages available with any fitness book. The software includes a Fitness Profile, a Personalized Cardiorespiratory Exercise Prescription, a Nutrient Analysis, and a weekly and monthly Exercise Log. This software package helps provide a more meaningful experience to all participants and greatly decreases the workload of course instructors.

A unique feature of the software is the Nutrient Analysis Data Base Enhancer. This software allows instructors to add food items to the already existing data base available with the book.

- A video containing a detailed explanation of many of the fitness assessment test items used in the book. Instructors can use this video to help familiarize themselves with the proper test protocols for each fitness test. This audio-visual aid contains the following test items: 1.5-Mile Run Test, Step Test, Astrand-Ryhming Test, Muscular Strength and Endurance Test, Muscular Endurance Test, Strength-to-Body Weight Ratio Test, Modified Sit-and-Reach Test, Body Rotation Test, Shoulder Rotation Test, Skinfold Thickness Test, and Girth Measurements Test.
- Microtest, edited by Allan S. Cohen Consulting Services, a Fitness and Wellness Computerized Testbank contains the following options: (a) over 800 multiple choice questions, (b) capability to add/or edit test questions, (c) previously generated tests can be recalled — creating new exam versions because multiple choice answers can be rotated with each new test generated, and (d) capability to generate tests using a LaserJet printer.
- Over 60 color overhead transparency acetates of the book's most important illustrations and figures to facilitate class instruction and help explain key fitness and wellness concepts.
- An instructor's manual to aid with the implementation of your physical fitness and wellness course.

Student Supplement for the World Wide Web

The World Wide Web has emerged as a valuable educational resource, and visiting cyberspace can make for a unique teaching and learning experience. The problem is: How do students identify sites that are academically appropriate and begin to use WWW sites in an educational context?

To make use of the resources of the World Wide Web in a practical way, *JumpStart with WebLinks: A Guidebook for Fitness/Wellness/Personal Health* is a suggested supplement. Edited by Professor Eileen L. Daniel, Ph.D., this spiral-bound guidebook (approximately 168 pages) contains 36 topics on fitness, wellness, and personal health. For each topic (e.g., cardiovascular endurance, eating disorders), a topic introduction orients students to the topic and concludes with a mix of personal assessment and content-related questions.

Following the topic introduction is a directory of WebLinks: the addresses (URLs) of four to six relevant WWW sites and a brief description of each site. These sites are appropriate for students and faculty alike. Each site has been fully verified and approved by a WebAdvisory Board made up of academics from colleges and universities throughout the United States and Canada. A brief Instructor's Resource Guide provides general information on how to incorporate *JumpStart with WebLinks* into any classroom setting.

Morton Publishing Company
1-800-348-3777
Web Site
http://www.morton-pub.com

Acknowledgments

Special thanks to all of the following individuals who helped with the photography in this edition: Charles Scheer, Erin C. Caskey, David T. Aschenbrener, Julie Hammons, Brad Thompson, Jason Brooks Aberg, Heather Lloyd, Julie Wagner, Jennifer Blackman, Dr. Sherman Button, Nancy Button, Scott and Jamie Whiles, Neil Edwards, Bernhard Hoeger, Michelle Puetz, Amy Gibson, Phyllis Sawyer, Leland and Norma Hansen, Jim Moore, Brad Page, Eric Heinz, Monika Gangwer, Dan Barber, Cherianne Caulkins, Debra Cunningham, Michelle Jensen, and Sally O'Donnell.

Contents

Laboratories

Why Physical Fitness?

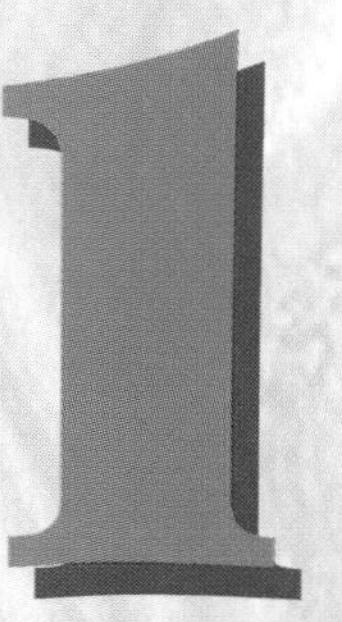

LABS

Widespread interest in health and preventive medicine has led to a tremendous increase in the number of people participating in physical fitness programs. From an initial fitness fad in the early 1970s, fitness activity programs became a trend that now is very much a part of the North American way of life. The growing number of participants is attributed primarily to scientific evidence linking regular physical activity and positive lifestyle habits to better health, longevity, quality of life, and total well-being.

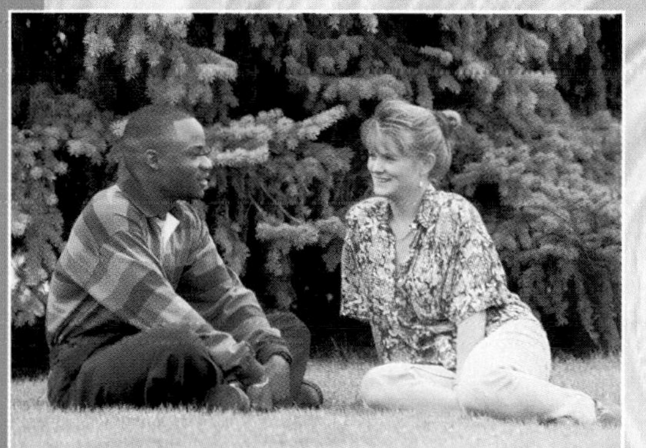

Research findings in the last few years have shown that physical inactivity and negative lifestyle seriously threaten our health and hasten the deterioration rate of the human body. Physically active people live longer than their inactive counterparts, even if activity is started later in life. Current U.S. estimates indicate that more than 250,000 yearly deaths in the United States are attributed to lack of regular physical activity.[1] Similar trends are found in most industrialized nations throughout the world.

Objectives

- Define physical fitness, and list the components of health-related and skill-related fitness.
- Become familiar with health-fitness standards and physical-fitness standards.
- Identify the major health problems in North America.
- Understand the benefits and the significance of participating in a lifetime fitness program.
- Learn motivation and behavior modification techniques to enhance compliance with a fitness program.
- Identify risk factors that may interfere with safe participation in exercise.

The human organism needs movement and activity to grow, develop, and maintain health. Advances in modern technology, however, have almost completely eliminated the necessity of physical exertion in daily life. The automated society in which we live no longer provides us with enough activity to ensure adequate health. Instead, it accelerates deterioration of the human body.

At the beginning of the 20th century, the most common health problems in the Western world were infectious diseases such as tuberculosis, diphtheria, influenza, kidney disease, polio, and other diseases of infancy. Progress in the field of medicine has largely eliminated these diseases. As the North American people started to enjoy the so-called good life (sedentary living, alcohol, fatty foods, excessive sweets, tobacco, drugs), though, we saw a parallel increase in the incidence of chronic diseases such as high blood pressure, coronary heart disease, atherosclerosis, strokes, diabetes, cancer, emphysema, and cirrhosis of the liver (see Figure 1.1).

As the incidence of **chronic diseases** climbed, we came to recognize prevention as the best medicine. Consequently, a new fitness movement developed gradually over the last three decades. People began to realize that good health is mostly self-controlled and that the leading causes of premature death and illness in North America could be prevented by adhering to positive lifestyle habits.

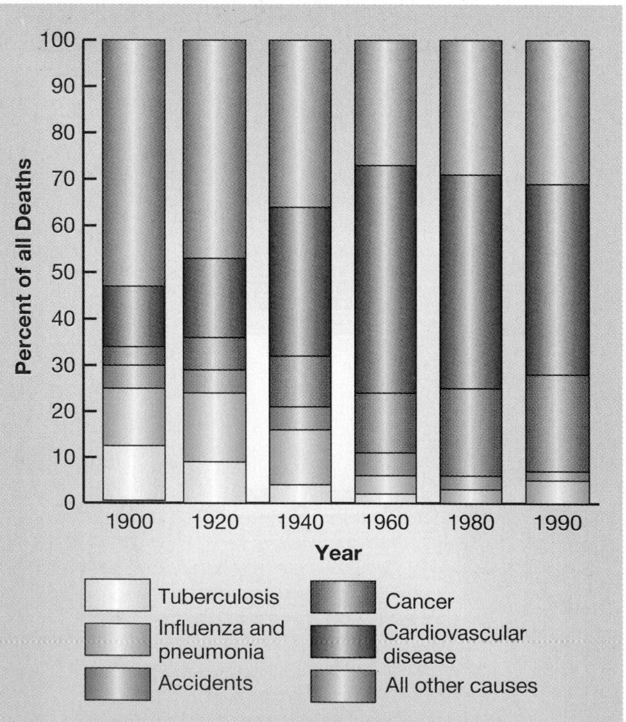

Based on the abundance of scientific research on physical activity and exercise, a clear distinction has been established between physical activity and exercise:

Physical activity is defined as "bodily movement produced by skeletal muscles that requires energy expenditure and produces progressive health benefits."[2] Examples of physical activity are walking to and from work and the store, taking stairs (instead of elevators and escalators), gardening, doing household chores, dancing, and washing the car by hand. Physical inactivity, on the other hand, implies a level of activity that is lower than that required to maintain good health.

Exercise is considered a type of physical activity that requires "planned, structured, and repetitive bodily movement done to improve or maintain one or more components of physical fitness."[3] Examples of exercise are a regular weekly program of walking, jogging, cycling, aerobics, swimming, strength training, or stretching exercises.

Source: National Center for Health Statistics, Division of Vital Statistics.

Figure 1.1 Causes of death in United States for selected years.

Surgeon General's Report on Physical Activity and Health

A landmark report on the influence of regular physical activity on health was released in July of 1996 by the U.S. Surgeon General. The significance of this historic document cannot be underestimated. Until 1996, only two previous reports had been released by the Surgeon General: One on smoking and health in 1964 and a second one on nutrition and health in 1988. Over 1,000 scientific studies from the fields of epidemiology, exercise physiology, medicine, and the behavioral sciences are summarized in this document on physical activity and health.

The report states that regular moderate physical activity provides substantial benefits in health and well-being for the vast majority of Americans who are not physically active. Among these benefits are a significant reduction in the risk of developing or dying from heart disease, diabetes, colon cancer, and high blood pressure. Regular physical activity also is important for health of muscles, bones, and joints; and it appears to reduce symptoms of depression and anxiety, improve mood, and enhance the ability to perform daily tasks throughout life. For individuals who are already moderately active, greater health benefits can be achieved by increasing the amount of physical activity.

According to the Surgeon General, improving health through physical activity is a serious public health challenge that we must meet head-on at once. More than 60% of adults do not achieve the recommended amount of physical activity, and 25% are not physically active at all. Further, almost half of all people between the ages of 12 and 21 are not vigorously active on a regular basis. This report has become a call to nationwide action. Regular moderate physical activity can prevent premature death, unnecessary illness, and disability. It can also help control health care costs and help to maintain a high quality of life into old age.

In the report, moderate physical activity has been defined as physical activity that uses 150 calories of energy per day, or 1,000 calories per week. People should strive to achieve at least 30 minutes of physical activity per day most days of the week. Examples of moderate physical activity include walking, cycling, playing basketball or volleyball, swimming, water aerobics, dancing fast, pushing a stroller, raking leaves, shoveling snow, washing or waxing a car, washing windows or floors, or even gardening.

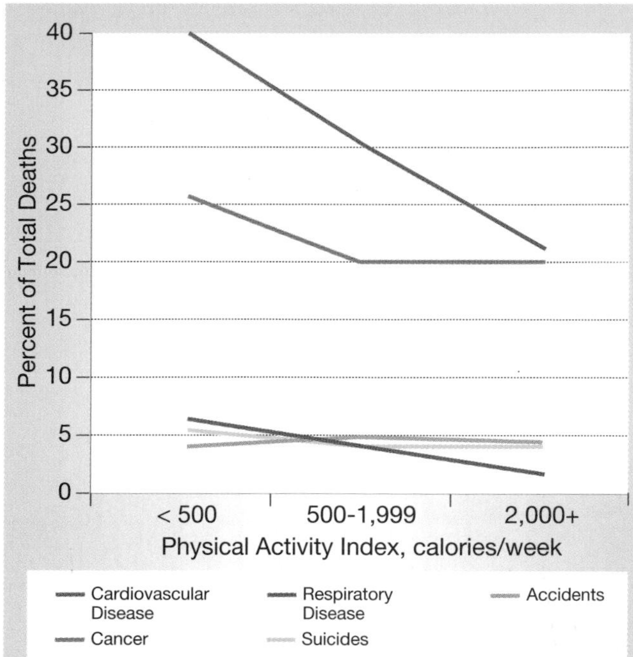

From "A Natural History of Athleticism on Cardiovascular Health," by R. S. Paffenbarger, R. T. Hyde, A. L. Wing,. and C. H. Steinmetz, *Journal of the American Medical Association*, 252 (1989), 491–495. Used by permission.

NOTE: The graph represents cause-specific death rates per 10,000 man-years of observation among 16,936 Harvard alumni, 1962–1978, by physical activity index; adjusted for differences in age, cigarette smoking, and hypertension.

Figure 1.2 Death rates by physical activity index.

Fitness and Longevity

During the late 1960s and in the 1970s we began to realize that good fitness is important in the fight against chronic diseases, particularly those of the cardiovascular system. Because of more participation in fitness programs in the last few years, cardiovascular mortality rates have dropped. The rate started to decline in about 1963, and between 1970 and 1988 the prevalence of heart disease dropped by 34%. This decrease is credited to healthier lifestyles and better health care in the United States. More than half of the decline is attributed to improvements in diet and fewer people smoking.

Furthermore, several studies have shown an inverse relationship between physical activity and premature cardiovascular mortality rates. In a study conducted among 16,936 Harvard alumni linking physical activity habits and mortality rates, as the amount of weekly physical activity increased, the risk of cardiovascular deaths decreased.[4] The largest decrease in cardiovascular deaths was observed among alumni who used up more than 2,000 calories per week through physical activity. Figure 1.2 illustrates the study results graphically.

Another major study upheld the findings of the Harvard alumni study.[5] Based on data from 13,344 people followed over an average of 8 years, the results confirmed that the level of cardiorespiratory fitness is related to mortality from all causes. The study revealed a graded and consistent inverse relationship between cardiorespiratory fitness and mortality, regardless of age and other risk factors. As illustrated in Figure 1.3, The higher the level of cardiorespiratory fitness, the longer the lifespan. Death

Chronic diseases Diseases that develop and last over a long time.

Physical activity Bodily movement produced by skeletal muscles that requires energy expenditure and produces progressive health benefits.

Exercise A type of physical activity that requires planned, structured, and repetitive bodily movement done to improve or maintain one or more components of physical fitness.

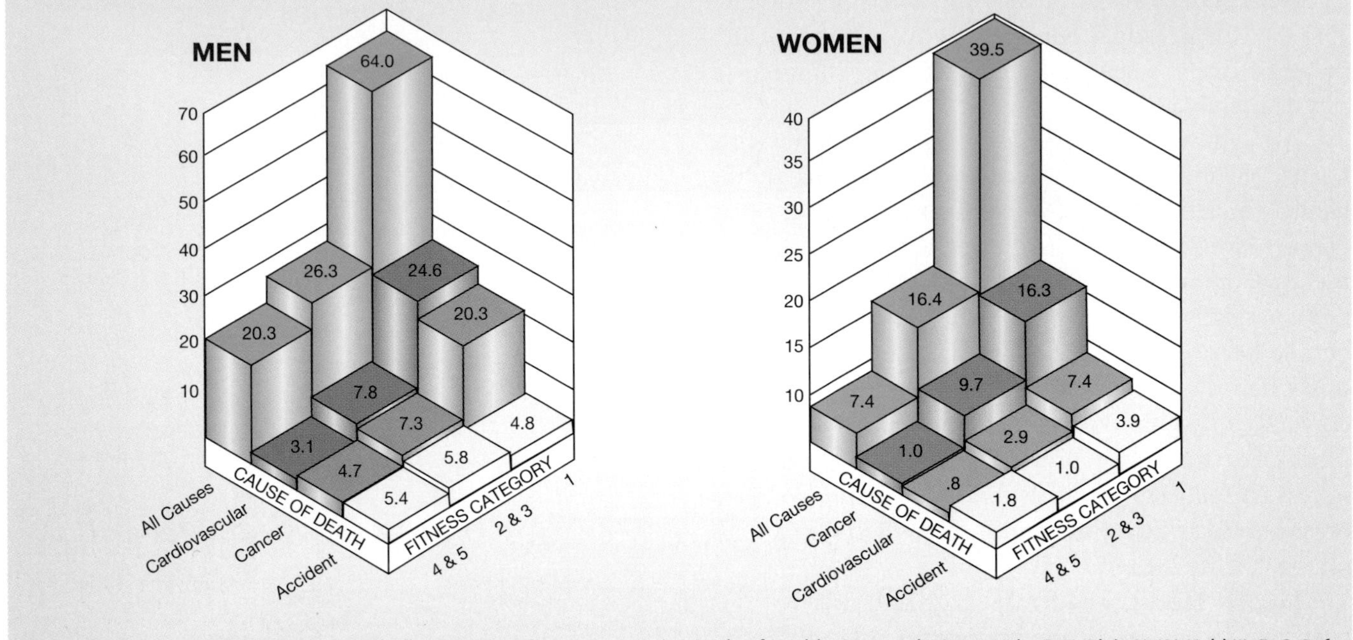

Figure 1.3 Death rates by physical fitness groups.

rates from all causes for the least-fit (group 1) men were 3.4 times higher than the most-fit men. For the least-fit women, the death rates were 4.6 times higher than the most fit women.

This study also reported a greatly reduced rate of premature death, even at moderate fitness levels that most adults can achieve easily. Even greater protection is attained when higher fitness levels are combined with reduction in other risk factors such as hypertension, serum cholesterol, cigarette smoking, and excessive body fat.

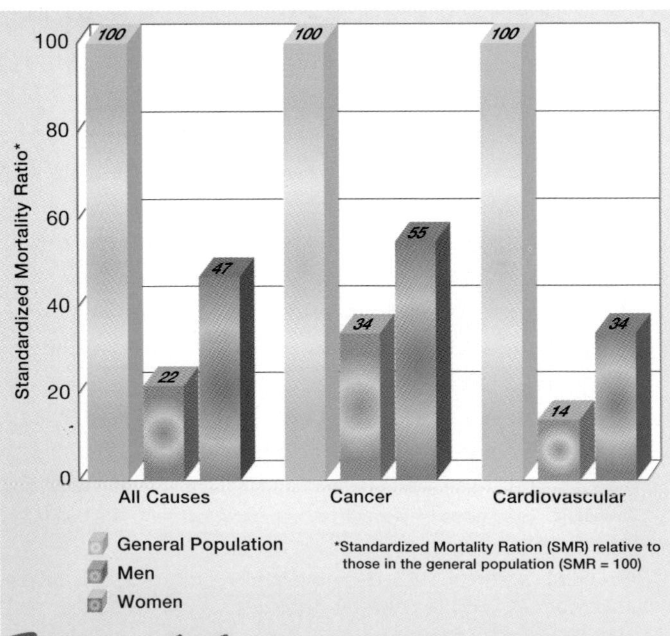

Figure 1.4 Effects of a healthy lifestyle on all causes, cancer, and cardiovascular death rates in White men and women.

In another major research study conducted in the 1980s, a healthy lifestyle was shown to contribute to some of the lowest mortality rates ever reported in the literature.[6] As illustrated in Figure 1.4, compared with the general White population, this group of 5,231 men and 4,631 women (wives) had much lower cancer, cardiovascular, and overall death rates.

Healthy lifestyle habits include abstaining from tobacco, alcohol, caffeine, and drugs, and adhering to a well-balanced diet, based on grains, fruits, and vegetables, and moderate consumption of poultry and red meat. The investigators in this study looked at three general health habits among the participants: lifetime abstinence from smoking, regular physical activity, and sleep.

Men in this study had one-third the death rate from cancer, one-seventh the death rate from cardiovascular disease, and one-fifth the rate of overall mortality. The wives had about half the rate of cancer and overall mortality and a third the death rate from cardiovascular disease. Life expectancy for

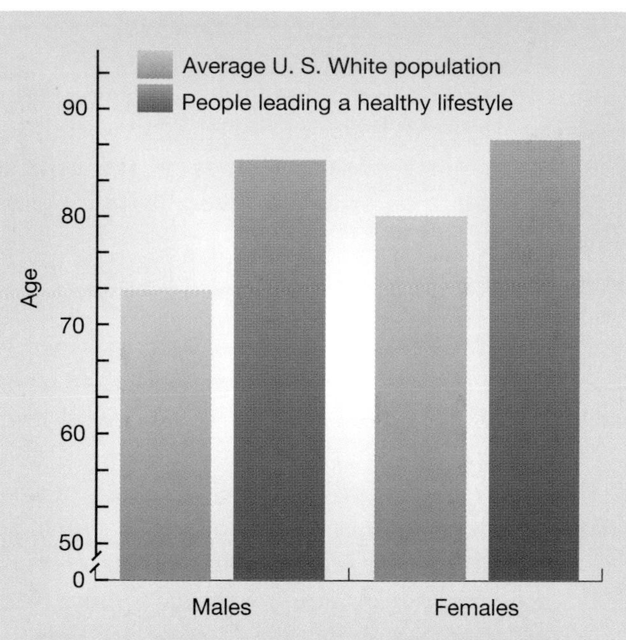

Figure 1.5 Life expectancy for 25-year-old individuals who adhere to a lifetime healthy lifestyle program.

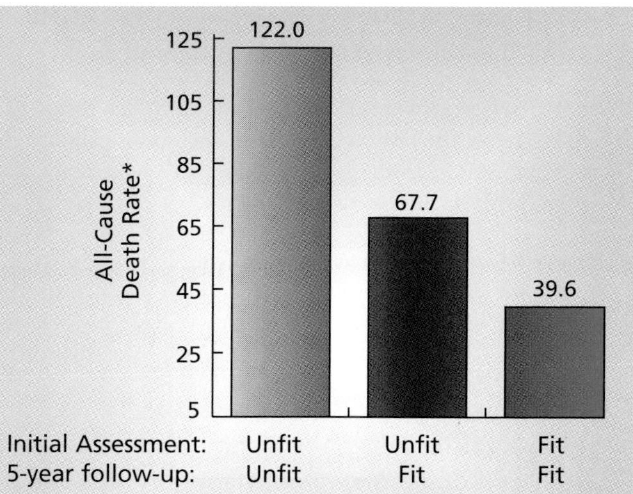

Figure 1.6 Five-year follow-up in mortality rates associated with maintenance and improvements in fitness.

25-year-olds who adhered to the three health habits were 85 and 86 years, respectively, as compared to 74 and 80 for the average U.S. White man and woman (see Figure 1.5).

From this study we can conclude that people who adhere to a lifetime healthy lifestyle indeed will reap healthy rewards. Better health leads to improvements in quality of life. The additional 6 to 11 years of "golden" life are precious to those who maintain a healthy lifetime program.

Additional research that looked at changes in fitness and mortality found a substantial (44%) reduction in mortality risk when people abandoned a sedentary lifestyle and become moderately fit.[7] The lowest death rate was found in people who were fit and remained fit. The highest rate was found in men who remained unfit (see Figure 1.6).

Subsequent research published in 1995 in the *Journal of the American Medical Association* substantiated the previous findings but also indicated that primarily vigorous activities are associated with greater longevity.[8] Vigorous activity was defined as activity that requires a **MET** level equal to or greater than 6 METs (21 ml/kg/min — see Health Fitness Standards below). Six or more METs represents exercising at an oxygen uptake (VO_2) equal to or greater than six times the resting energy requirement.

Examples of vigorous activities used in the previous study include brisk walking, jogging, swimming laps, squash, racquetball, tennis, and shoveling snow. Results also indicated that vigorous exercise is as important as not smoking and maintaining recommended weight.

The results of these studies clearly indicate that fitness improves health, quality of life, and longevity. If people are able to do this, vigorous exercise is preferable because it is best associated with longer life.

Ideally, healthy lifestyle habits should be taught and reinforced in early youth. Unfortunately, many young people are in such poor physical condition that they will add to national health concerns in years to come. Surveys conducted during the past decade have raised public concern regarding the fitness level of North American youth. As compared to the 1960s and 1970s, cardiorespiratory endurance and upper body strength have decreased and body fat has increased. These findings suggest that current physical education programs are not promoting lifetime physical fitness adequately.

Although the incidence of cardiovascular disease has declined remarkably, concern over youth fitness

MET The energy expenditure at rest, or approximately 3.5 ml/kg/min per MET.

led Dr. Kenneth Cooper, Director of the Aerobics Research Institute in Dallas, Texas to state:

> It's discouraging and I am afraid that as these kids grow up, we will see all the gains made against heart disease in the last twenty years wiped out in the next twenty years.[9]

1 Even 5- and 6-year-old children already have coronary heart disease risk factors such as high blood pressure, excessive body fat, and low fitness.[10]

Because of the unhealthy lifestyles that many young adults lead, physically they may be middle-aged or older! Healthy choices made today influence health a decade or two later. Many physical education programs do not emphasize the necessary skills for our youth to maintain a high level of fitness and health throughout life. That is the intent of this book: to provide the skills and help to prepare you for a lifetime of physical fitness. A healthy lifestyle is self-controlled, and people need to be taught how to be responsible for their own health and fitness.

What is Physical Fitness?

The most comprehensive definition of physical fitness is that of the American Medical Association, which has defined **physical fitness** as the general capacity to adapt and respond favorably to physical effort.

As the fitness concept grew during the 1970s, it became clear that no single test was sufficient to assess overall fitness. A battery of tests was necessary because several specific components have to be established to determine an individual's overall level of fitness.

Physical fitness can be classified into health-related and motor skill-related fitness. As shown in Figure 1.7, the four health-related fitness components are: cardiorespiratory (aerobic) endurance, muscular strength and endurance, muscular flexibility, and body composition. Skill-related fitness components consist of agility, balance, coordination, power, reaction time, and speed (Figure 1.8). The

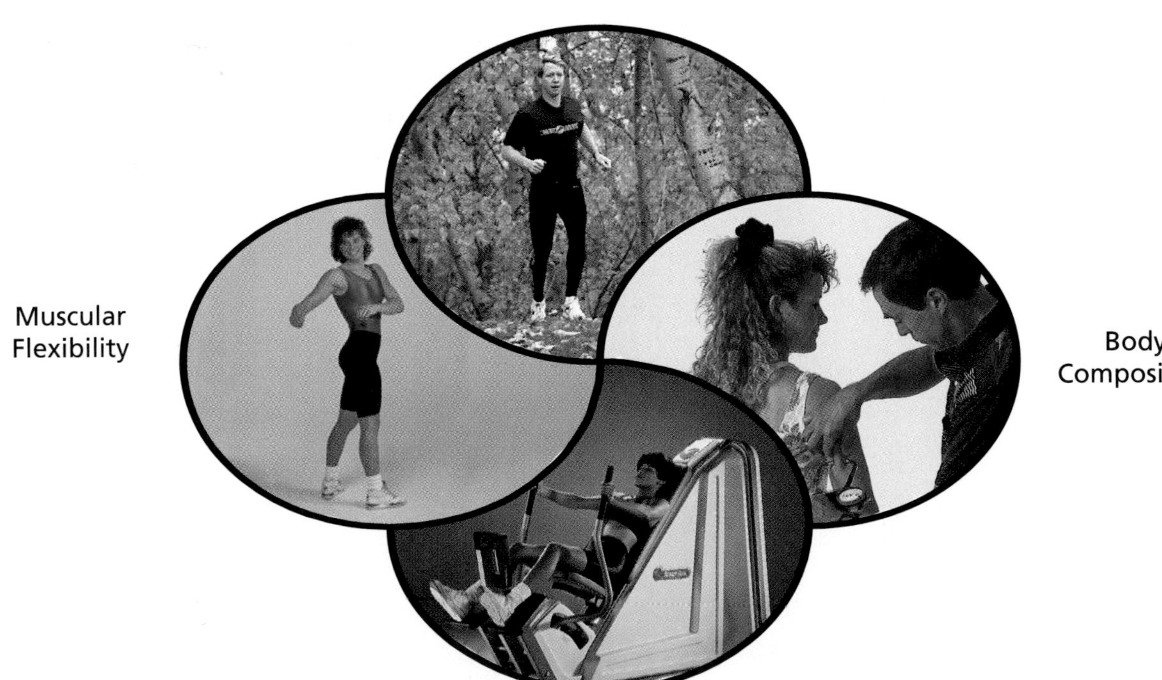

Figure 1.7 Health-related components of physical fitness.

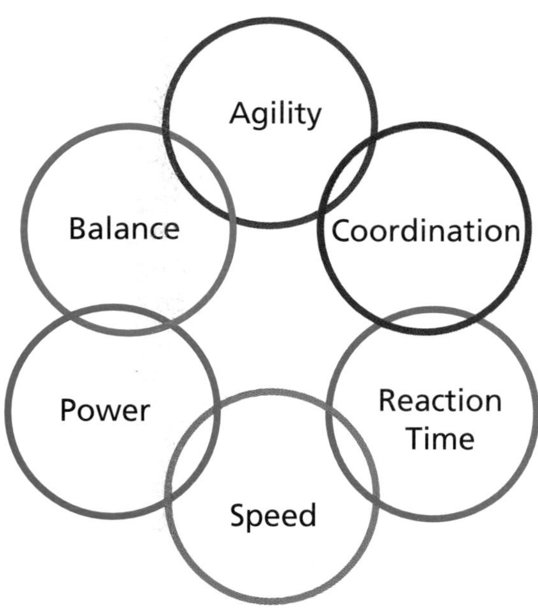

Figure 1.8 Motor-skill related components of physical fitness.

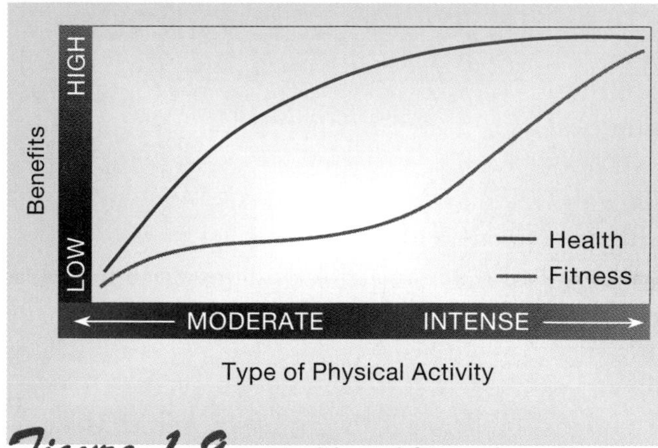

Figure 1.9 Health and fitness benefits based on type of aerobic fitness program.

latter are aimed primarily at succeeding in athletics and may not be as crucial in developing better health.

In terms of preventive medicine, the main emphasis of fitness programs should be on the health-related components. Nevertheless, total fitness is achieved by taking part in specific programs to improve both health-related and skill-related components.

Fitness Standards: Health versus Physical Fitness

Throughout the discussion of health-related fitness assessment in Chapters 3, 5, 7, and 9, several tests are identified to assess fitness. A meaningful debate regarding age- and gender-related fitness standards for the general population has resulted in the two standards: A health fitness standard (criterion-referenced) and a physical-fitness standard.

Health Fitness Standards

As illustrated in Figure 1.9, although fitness (VO_{2max} — see discussion below) improvements with a moderate aerobic activity program are not as notable, significant health benefits are reaped with such a program. These improvements are quite striking and only slightly greater health benefits are obtained with a more intense exercise program. These benefits include a reduction in blood lipids, lower blood pressure, decreased risk for diabetes, weight loss, stress release, and lower risk for disease and premature mortality.

The health fitness or criterion-referenced standards proposed here are based on **epidemiological** data linking minimum fitness values to disease prevention and health.

Attaining the health fitness standards requires only moderate amounts of physical activity. For example, a 2-mile walk in less than 30 minutes, five to six times per week, seems to be sufficient to achieve the **health-fitness standard** for cardiorespiratory endurance.

For instance, cardiorespiratory endurance is measured in terms of **maximal oxygen uptake or**

Physical fitness The ability to meet the ordinary as well as the unusual demands of daily life safely and effectively without being overly fatigued, and still have energy left for leisure and recreational activities.

Epidemiology Science that studies the relationship between diverse factors (lifestyle and environmental) and the occurrence of disease.

Health fitness standards The lowest fitness requirements for maintaining good health, decreasing the risk for chronic diseases, and lowering the incidence of muscular-skeletal injuries.

Maximal oxygen uptake (VO_{2max}) The maximum amount of oxygen the body is able to utilize per kilogram of body weight per minute (ml/kg/min).

VO_{2max}. Individual values can range from about 10 ml/kg/min in cardiac patients to approximately 80 to 90 ml/kg/min in world-class runners and cross-country skiers.

Data from the research study presented in Figure 1.3 indicate that VO_{2max} values of 35 and 32.5 ml/kg/min for men and women, respectively, may be sufficient to lower the risk for all-cause mortality significantly. Although greater improvements in fitness yield a slightly lower risk for premature death, the largest drop is seen between the least fit (group 1) and the moderately fit (groups 2 and 3). Therefore, the 35 and 32.5 ml/kg/min values could be selected as the health-fitness standards.

Physical Fitness Standards

Physical fitness standards are set higher than the health fitness norms and require a more vigorous exercise program. Many experts believe that people who meet the criteria of "good" physical fitness should be able to do moderate to vigorous physical activity without undue fatigue and to maintain this capability throughout life. In this context, physically fit people of all ages will have the freedom to enjoy most of life's daily and recreational activities to their fullest potential. Current health-fitness standards may not be enough to achieve these objectives.

Sound physical fitness gives the individual a degree of independence throughout life that many people in North America no longer enjoy. Most older people should be able to carry out activities similar to those conducted in their youth, though not with the same intensity.

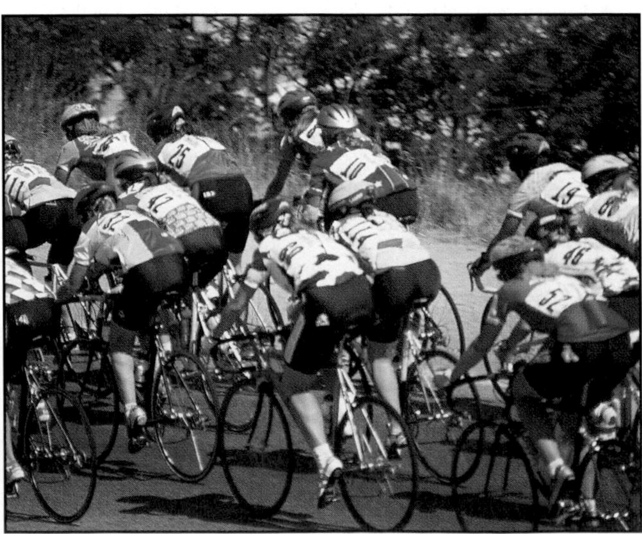

Vigorous exercise is required to achieve the high physical fitness standard.

Although a person does not have to be an elite athlete, activities such as changing a tire, chopping wood, climbing several flights of stairs, playing a vigorous game of basketball, mountain biking, playing soccer with grandchildren, walking several miles around a lake, and hiking through a national park require more than the current "average fitness" level of the American people.

If the main objective of the fitness program is to lower the risk for disease, attaining the health fitness standards may be enough to ensure better health. On the other hand, if the individual wants to participate in moderate to vigorous fitness activities, achieving a high physical fitness standard is recommended. For the purposes of this book, therefore, both health fitness and physical fitness standards are given for each fitness test. The individual then needs to decide the personal objectives for the fitness program.

Benefits of Fitness

A most inspiring story illustrating what fitness can do for a person's health and well-being is that of George Snell from Sandy, Utah. At age 45, Snell weighed approximately 400 pounds, his blood pressure was 220/180, he was blind because of diabetes he did not know he had, and his blood glucose level was 487.

Snell had determined to do something about his physical and medical condition, so he started a walking/jogging program. After about 8 months of conditioning, Snell had lost almost 200 pounds, his eyesight had returned, his glucose level was down to 67, and he was taken off medication. Two months later, less than 10 months after beginning his personal exercise program, he completed a marathon, a running course of 26.2 miles.

Health Benefits

Most people exercise because it improves their personal appearance and makes them feel good about themselves. Although many benefits accrue from participating in a regular fitness program and active people generally live longer, the greatest benefit of all is that physically fit individuals enjoy a better quality

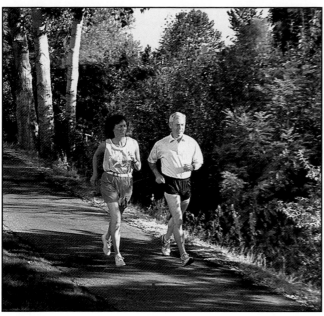

Regular participation in a lifetime physical activity program increases quality of life and longevity.

of life. These people live life to its fullest, with fewer health problems than inactive individuals who also may indulge in negative lifestyle patterns. Although compiling an all-inclusive list of the benefits reaped through a comprehensive fitness program is difficult, the following list provides a summary of many of these benefits.

1. Improves and strengthens the cardiorespiratory system (by facilitating oxygen supply to all parts of the body, including the heart, muscles, and brain).
2. Maintains better muscle tone, muscular strength and endurance.
3. Improves muscular flexibility.
4. Helps maintain recommended body weight.
5. Improves posture and physical appearance.
6. Lowers the risk for chronic diseases and illness (such as coronary heart disease, cancer, and strokes).
7. Decreases the mortality rate from chronic diseases.
8. Thins the blood so it is less likely to clot (decreasing the risk for coronary heart disease and strokes).
9. Lowers blood pressure.
10. Helps prevent diabetes.
11. Helps people sleep better.
12. Helps prevent chronic back pain.
13. Relieves tension and helps in coping with life stresses.
14. Raises levels of energy and job productivity.
15. Extends longevity and slows down the aging process.
16. Improves self-image and morale and helps fight depression.
17. Motivates toward positive changes in lifestyle (better nutrition, quitting smoking, alcohol and drug abuse control).
18. Speeds recovery time following physical exertion.
19. Speeds recovery following injury and disease.
20. Regulates and improves overall body functions.
21. Improves physical stamina and counteracts chronic fatigue.
22. Improves quality of life; makes people feel better and live a healthier and happier life.

1

Economic Benefits

The economic impact of sedentary living can leave a strong impression on a nation's economy. As the need for physical exertion in Western countries decreased steadily during the last century, health-care expenditures have increased dramatically. Health-care costs in the United States rose from $12 billion in 1950 to approximately $1 trillion in 1995 (Figure 1.10). At the present rate of escalation, health-care expenditures will reach $1.6 trillion by the year 2002. The 1995 figure represents about 14% of the gross national product (GNP). It is projected to reach about 18% by the year 2002 and 37% by 2030.

Unhealthy behaviors are contributing to the staggering U.S. health-care costs. Risk factors for disease carry a heavy price tag (see Figure 1.11). According to estimates, 1% of Americans account for 30% of these costs.[11] Half of the people use up about 97% of the health-care dollars. Furthermore, and as illustrated in Figure 1.12, the 1989 average health-care cost per person in the United States ($2,354) was almost twice as high as for most other industrialized nations.

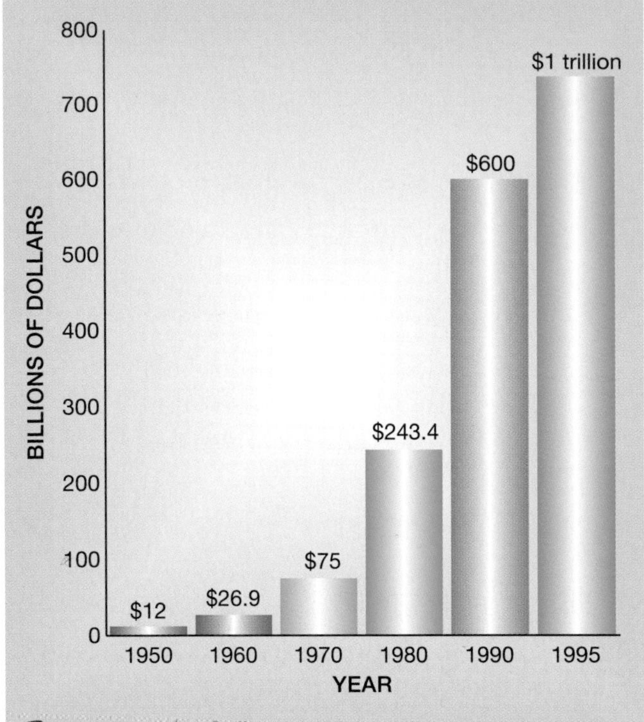

Figure 1.10 U.S. health-care cost increments since 1950.

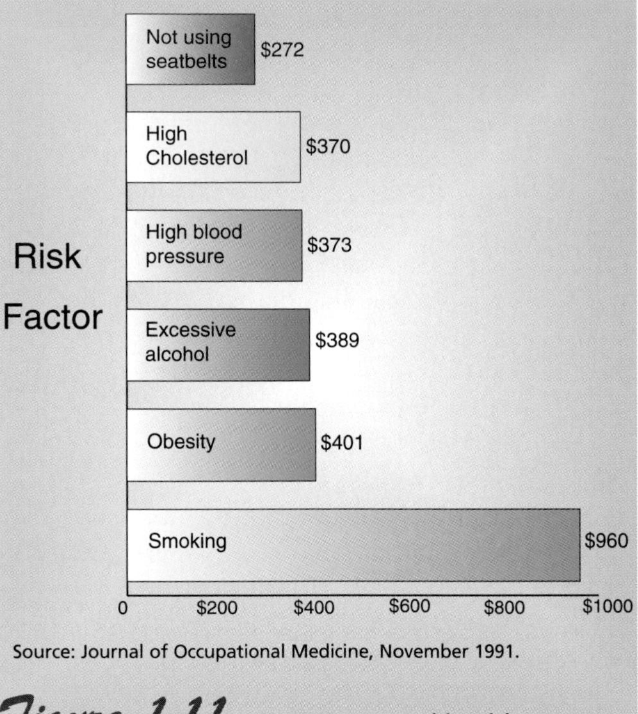

Figure 1.11 Average annual health-care costs for leading disease risk factors.

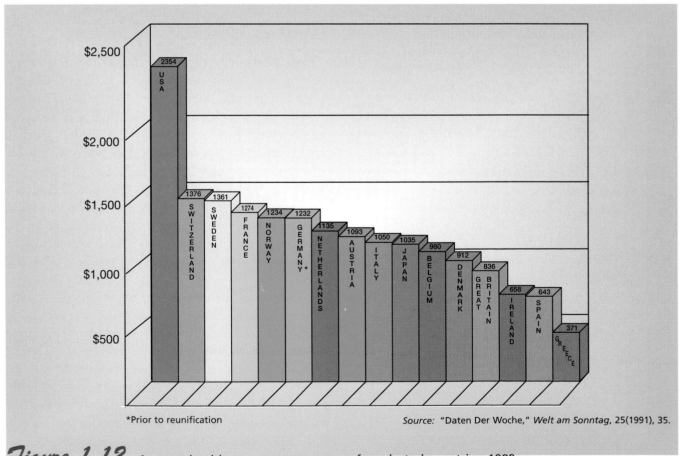

Figure 1.12 Average health-care costs per person for selected countries, 1989.

Strong scientific evidence now links participation in fitness programs not only to better health but also to lower medical costs and higher job productivity. Most of this research is being conducted and reported by organizations that already have implemented fitness programs. Approximately half of the health-care expenditures in the United States are being absorbed by American business and industry. In 1989, business spending on health insurance premiums and health care for employees and former employees was more than 100% of after-tax profits by all U.S. companies combined.

As a result of the recent staggering rise in medical costs, many organizations are beginning to realize that keeping employees healthy costs less than treating them once they are sick. A 1991 survey by the American Institute for Preventive Medicine found that large corporations are finding health-cost savings by implementing health promotion programs.[12] A sample return on investment per dollar spent is provided in Figure 1.13. Containing the costs of health care through fitness and health promotion programs has become a major issue for many organizations around North America. Let's examine the evidence.

The backache syndrome, usually the result of physical degeneration (inelastic and weak muscles), costs American industry more than $1 billion a year in lost productivity and services. An additional $250 million is spent in workers compensation. The Adolph Coors Company in Golden, Colorado, which offers a health promotion program for employees and their families, reported savings of more than $319,000 in 1983 alone through a preventive and rehabilitative back-injury program.

Strong scientific evidence links good fitness to better health, lower medical costs, and higher job productivity.

The Prudential Insurance Company of Houston, Texas, released the findings of a study conducted on its 1,386 employees. Those who participated for at least one year in the company's fitness program averaged 3.5 days of disability, compared to 8.6 days for nonparticipants. A further breakdown by level of fitness showed no disability days for those in the high-fitness group, 1.6 days for the good-fitness group, and 4.1 days for the fair-fitness group.

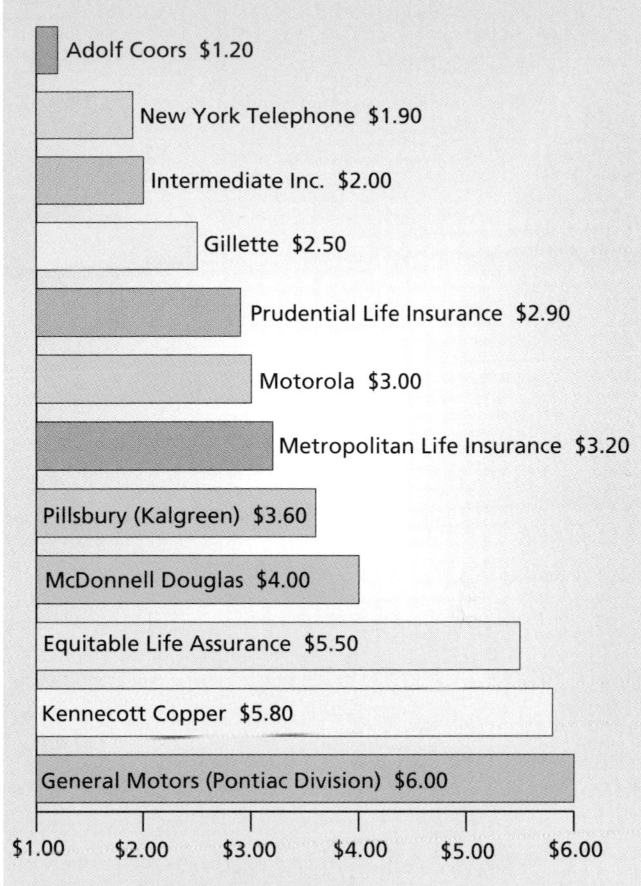

Figure 1.13 Returns on investment: Health-care cost savings by selected corporations.

Since 1979, the Mesa Petroleum Company in Amarillo, Texas, has offered an on-site fitness program to its employees and their family members. A 1982 company health-care analysis showed the average medical costs per person to be 150% higher for the nonparticipating than for the fitness-participating group. This represented a yearly reduction of $200,000 in medical expenses. Sick leave time also was significantly less for the physically active group — 27 hours per year, compared to 44 for the inactive group.

A similar study, conducted by Tenneco Incorporated in Houston, also showed a significant reduction in medical-care costs for men and women who participated in an exercise program. Annual medical care costs for male and female nonexercisers were 79% and 140% higher than the exercisers' (see Figure 1.14). Sick leave was reduced in the men and women participants.

Furthermore, a survey of the more than 3,000 employees at Tenneco found that job productivity is

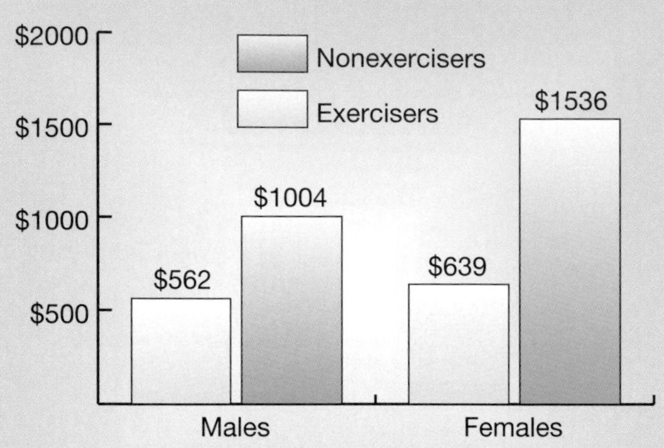

From "New Fitness Data Verifies: Employees Who Exercise Are Also More Productive." *Athletic Business*, 8:12 (1984), 24–30.

Figure 1.14 Annual medical care costs for Tenneco Inc., Houston, Texas, 1982–83.

related to fitness. The company reported that individuals with high job performance ratings also rated high in exercise participation.

Strong data also are coming in from Europe. Research in Germany reported 68.6% less absenteeism among workers with cardiovascular symptoms who participated in a fitness program. The law also mandates that corporations employing workers for sedentary jobs must provide an in-house facility for physical exercise.

The Goodyear Company in Norrkoping, Sweden, indicated a 50% reduction in absenteeism following implementation of a fitness program. Studies in the former Soviet Union report expanded physical work capacity and motor coordination, lower incidence of disease, shorter duration of illness, and fewer relapses among individuals participating in industrial fitness programs.

Another reason some organizations are offering fitness and health promotion programs to their employees — overlooked by many because it does not seem to affect the bottom line directly — is simply concern by top management for the physical well-being of employees. Whether the program lowers medical costs is not the main issue. The only reason that really matters to top management is that fitness and health promotion programs help individuals feel better about themselves and improve their quality of life.

Such is the case of Mannington Mills Corporation, which invested $1.8 million in an on-site fitness center. The return on investment is secondary to the company's interest in happier and healthier employees. The center also is open to dependents and retirees. As a result of this program, Mannington Mills believes the participants — about half of the 1,600 people who are eligible — can enjoy life to its fullest potential, and the employees most likely will be more productive simply because of the company's caring attitude.

In addition to the financial and physical benefits, some corporations are offering fitness and health promotion programs as an incentive to attract, hire, and retain employees. Many companies are taking a hard look at the fitness and health level of potential employees and are using this information in their screening process. Some organizations refuse to hire smokers or overweight individuals.

Other executives believe an on-site health promotion program is the best fringe benefit they can offer at their corporation. Young executives are looking for organizations such as these, not only for the added health benefits but also because the head corporate officers are showing an attitude of concern and care.

Thanks to current scientific data and the fitness movement, most North Americans now see a need to participate in programs that improve and maintain health. The "typical" American, however, is not a good role model when cardiorespiratory fitness is concerned. Almost 60% of U.S. adults engage in little or no leisure-time physical activity. In 1994, only 37% of the adults in the United States exercised strenuously three or more days per week.[13]

Aerobic activities are the most popular form of exercise, so even a lower percentage of the population probably engages in and derives benefits from strength and flexibility programs. In addition, an estimated half or more of the adult population in the United States has a weight problem and a third of all adults are considered obese (20% or more above recommended weight).

The "typical" American is not a good role model when cardiorespiratory fitness is concerned.

Even though people in the United States believe a positive lifestyle has a great impact on health and longevity, most do not reap the benefits because they don't know how to implement a safe and effective program. Others are exercising incorrectly and therefore are not reaping the full benefits of their program.

General Objectives

Most people go to college to learn how to make a living, but a fitness/wellness course can teach you how to live — how to truly live life to its fullest potential. Some people think that success in life is measured by how much money they make. Making a good living will not help you unless you live a **wellness** lifestyle that will allow you to enjoy what you have.

Everyone would like to enjoy good health and wellness, but most people don't know how to reach this objective. Lifestyle is the most important factor affecting our personal well-being. Although some people live long because of genetic factors, the quality of life during middle age and the "golden years" is related more often to wise choices initiated during youth and continued throughout life.

In a few short years, lack of health and fitness leads to a loss of vitality and gusto for life, as well as premature morbidity and mortality. Therefore, the information in the following chapters and the laboratory experiences in the back of the book set forth all of the necessary guidelines to develop a personal lifetime program to improve fitness and promote preventive health care. Because fitness needs vary significantly from one individual to the other, all exercise prescriptions in this book are based on your personal needs to obtain best results.

The laboratory experiences have been prepared on tear-out sheets so they can be turned in to class instructors. The corresponding labs for each chapter and any other information necessary to prepare for the labs are given at the end of the chapters. As you study this book and complete the respective laboratory experiences, you will learn to:

- Determine whether medical clearance is needed for your safe participation in exercise.
- Conduct nutritional analyses, and follow the recommendations for adequate nutrition.
- Write sound diet and weight-control programs.
- Assess the health-related components of fitness (cardiorespiratory endurance, muscular strength and endurance, muscular flexibility, and body composition).

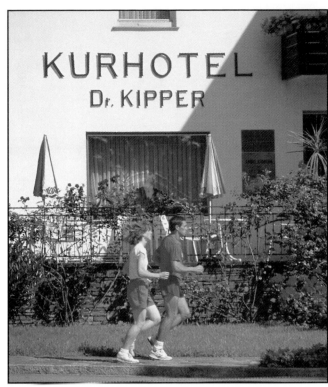

Good physical fitness enhances quality of life.

- Write exercise prescriptions for cardiorespiratory endurance, muscular strength and endurance, and muscular flexibility.
- Assess the various skill-related components of fitness (agility, balance, coordination, power, reaction time, and speed).
- Learn about positive lifestyle behaviors that will help you decrease your risk for chronic disease and attain better health and quality of life.
- Discover the relationship between fitness and aging.
- Write objectives to improve physical fitness and learn how to chart a healthy lifestyle program for the future.
- Discern between myths and facts of exercise and health-related concepts.

Lifestyle is the most important factor affecting our personal well-being.

Wellness The constant and deliberate effort to stay healthy and achieve the highest potential for well-being.

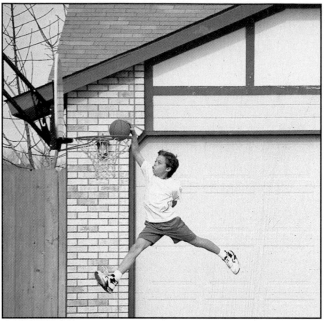

Physical activity and exercise habits are best established early in life.

U.S. Health Objectives for the Year 2000

Every 10 years the U.S. Department of Health and Human Services releases a list of objectives for disease prevention and health promotion. From its onset in 1980, this 10-year plan has helped instill a new sense of purpose and focus for public health and preventive medicine.

The Year 2000 objectives, published in the document *Healthy People 2000* address three important points:[14]

1. *Personal responsibility.* The need for individuals to become ever more health-conscious. Responsible and informed behaviors are the key to good health.
2. *Health benefits for all people.* Lower socioeconomic conditions and poor health often are interrelated. Extending the benefits of good health to all people is crucial to the health of the nation.
3. *Health promotion and disease prevention.* A shift from treatment to preventive techniques will cut health care costs drastically and help all Americans achieve a higher quality of life.

Development of the Year 2000 Health Objectives involved more than 10,000 people representing 300 national organizations, including the Institute of Medicine of the National Academy of Sciences, all state health departments, and the federal Office of Disease Prevention and Health Promotion. A summary of key objectives is provided in Figure 1.15. Living the fitness and healthy lifestyle principles provided in this book not only will enhance the quality of your life but also will allow you to be an active participant in achieving the Healthy People 2000 Objectives.

Motivation and Behavior Modification

Scientific evidence of the benefits derived from living a healthy lifestyle continues to mount each day. Although the data are impressive, most people still don't adhere to a healthy lifestyle. Understanding why people do not may help increase your readiness or motivation to do so. To answer this question, one has to examine what motivates people and what actions are required to make permanent changes in behavior.

Motivation is often used as an explanation as to why some people succeed and others don't. Although motivation comes from within, external factors are what trigger the inner desire to accomplish a given task. These external factors, then, control behavior.

When studying motivation, understanding **locus of control** is helpful. People who believe they have control over events in their lives are said to have an internal locus of control. People with an external locus of control believe that what happens to them is a result of chance, the environment, and is unrelated to their behavior.

People with an internal locus of control are healthier and have an easier time initiating and adhering to a fitness program. In contrast, those who perceive that they have no control think of themselves as powerless and vulnerable. Becoming motivated is often a challenge. These people are also at greater risk for illness. When illness strikes, restoring a sense of control is vital to regain health.

Motivation The desire and will to do something.

Locus of Control The extent to which a person believes he or she can influence the external environment.

HEALTHY PEOPLE 2000: SELECTED HEALTH OBJECTIVES FOR THE YEAR 2000

I. Physical Activity and Fitness

1. Increase the proportion of people who engage regularly, preferably daily, in *light* to *moderate* physical activity for at least 30 minutes per day.
2. Increase the proportion of people who engage in *vigorous* physical activity that promotes the development and maintenance of cardiorespiratory fitness 3 or more days per week for 20 or more minutes per occasion.
3. Increase the proportion of people who regularly perform physical activities that enhance and maintain muscular strength, muscular endurance, and flexibility.
4. Reduce the proportion of people who engage in no leisure-time physical activity.
5. Reduce overweight to a prevalence of no more than 20% among people aged 20 and older and no more than 15% among adolescents aged 12 through 19.
6. Increase to at least 50% the proportion of overweight people aged 12 and older who have adopted sound dietary practices combined with regular physical activity to attain an appropriate body weight.

II. Nutrition

1. Reduce dietary fat intake to an average of 30% of calories or less and average saturated fat intake to less than 10% of calories among people aged 2 and older.
2. Increase complex carbohydrate and fiber-containing foods in the diets of adults to 5 or more daily servings for vegetables and fruits, and to 6 or more daily servings for grain products.
3. Increase calcium consumption in the diet.
4. Reduce iron deficiency among children ages 1 through 4 and women of childbearing age.
5. Decrease salt and sodium intake in the diet.
6. Increase to at least 85% the proportion of people aged 18 and older who use food labels to make nutritious selections.

III. Chronic Diseases

1. Increase years of healthy life to at least 65 years.
2. Reduce coronary heart disease deaths.
3. Reduce the mean serum cholesterol level among adults to no more than 200 mg/dL.
4. Increase the proportion of adults with high blood cholesterol who are aware of their condition and are taking action to reduce their blood cholesterol to recommended levels.
5. Increase the proportion of people with high blood pressure whose blood pressure is under control.
6. Increase the proportion of people with high blood pressure who are taking action to help control their blood pressure.
7. Reverse the rise in cancer deaths.
8. Slow the rise in lung cancer deaths.
9. Reduce the rate of breast cancer deaths.
10. Reduce colorectal cancer deaths.
11. Reduce diabetes-related deaths.
12. Reduce the proportion of people with asthma who experience limitation in activity.
13. Reduce deaths from cirrhosis of the liver.
14. Reduce hip fractures among older adults.
15. Reduce limitation in activity because of chronic back conditions.
16. Reduce the proportion of people who experience a limitation in major activity because of chronic conditions.

IV. Mental Health and Disorders

1. Reduce the prevalence of mental disorders.
2. Reduce the suicide rate.
3. Reduce the proportion of people who experience adverse health effects from stress.
4. Decrease the proportion of people who experience stress who do not take steps to reduce or control their stress.

V. Tobacco

1. Reduce the incidence of cigarette smoking.
2. Reduce the initiation of cigarette smoking by children and youth.
3. Reduce the proportion of children who are exposed regularly to tobacco smoke at home.
4. Reduce use of smokeless tobacco.
5. Increase the proportion of worksites with a formal smoking policy that prohibits or severely restricts smoking at the workplace.

VI. Alcohol and Other Drugs

1. Reduce the proportion of young people who have used alcohol, marijuana, and cocaine.
2. Reduce the proportion of high school seniors and college students engaging in recent occasions of heavy drinking of alcoholic beverages.
3. Reduce alcohol consumption by people aged 14 and older to an annual average of no more than 2 gallons of ethanol per person.
4. Increase the proportion of high school seniors who associate risk of physical or psychological harm with the heavy use of alcohol, occasional use of marijuana, and experimentation with cocaine.
5. Reduce the proportion of male high school seniors who use anabolic steroids.
6. Reduce deaths caused by alcohol-related motor vehicle crashes.
7. Reduce drug-related deaths.
8. Increase the proportion of all intravenous drug abusers who are in drug abuse treatment programs.
9. Increase the proportion of intravenous drug abusers not in treatment who use only uncontaminated drug paraphernalia ("works").

VII. AIDS, HIV Infection, and Sexually Transmitted Diseases

1. Confine annual incidence of diagnosed AIDS cases to no more than 98,000 cases.
2. Confine the prevalence of HIV infection to no more than 800 per 100,000 people.
3. Increase the proportion of sexually active, unmarried people who used a condom at last sexual intercourse.
4. Reduce the incidence of gonorrhea.
5. Reduce the incidence of chlamydia.
6. Reduce the incidence of primary and secondary syphilis.
7. Reduce the incidence of genital herpes and genital warts.
8. Reduce the incidence of pelvic inflammatory disease.
9. Reduce the incidence of sexually transmitted hepatitis B infection.

VIII. Family Planning

1. Reduce the number of pregnancies that are unintended.
2. Reduce the proportion of adolescents who have engaged in sexual intercourse.
3. Increase the proportion of sexually active, unmarried people aged 19 and younger who use contraception, especially combined-method contraception that both effectively prevents pregnancy and provides barrier protection against disease.

IX. Unintentional Injuries

1. Reduce deaths caused by unintentional injuries.
2. Increase use of occupant protection systems, such as safety belts, inflatable safety restraints, and child safety seats among motor vehicle occupants.
3. Increase use of helmets among motorcyclists and bicyclists.

* Excerpted from *Healthy People 2000: National Health Promotion and Disease Prevention Objectives,* U.S. Department of Health and Human Services, Public Health Service, (Boston: Jones and Bartlett Publishers, 1992). Refer to this publication for further information on these objectives.

Figure 1.15

1

Few people have either a completely external or a completely internal locus of control. They fall somewhere along a continuum. Where a person is along the continuum relates to his or her health. Also, the more external, the greater is the challenge in adhering to exercise and other healthy lifestyle behaviors. Fortunately, developing a more internal locus of control can be accomplished. Understanding that most events in life are not controlled genetically or environmentally helps people pursue goals and gain control over their lives. Three impediments can keep people from taking action: competence, confidence, and motivation.[15]

When illness strikes, restoring a sense of control is vital to regain health.

1. *Problems of competence.* Lacking the skills to get a given task done leads to less competence. If your friends play basketball regularly but you don't know how to play, you might not be inclined to participate. The solution to this problem of competence is to master the skills needed to participate. Most people are not born with all-inclusive natural abilities, including playing sports.

   A college professor continuously watched a group of students play an entertaining game of basketball every Friday at noon. Having no basketball skills, he was reluctant to play. The desire to join in the fun was strong enough that he enrolled in a beginning course at the college so he would learn to play the game. To his surprise, most students were impressed that he was willing to do this. Now, with greater competence, he is able to join in on Friday's "pick-up" games.

   Another alternative is to select an activity in which you are skilled. It may not be basketball, but it well could be aerobics. Don't be afraid, however, to try new activities. If your body weight is a problem, for example, you could learn to cook low-fat meals. Try different recipes until you find dishes you like.

2. *Problems of confidence.* Problems with confidence arise when the skills are there but you don't believe you can do something. Fear and feelings of inadequacy often interfere with the ability to perform the task.

   You never should talk yourself out of something until you have given it a fair try. If the skills are there, the sky is the limit. Initially, try to visualize yourself doing the task and getting it done. Repeat this several times, then give it a try. You will surprise yourself.

   Sometimes lack of confidence develops when the task appears insurmountable. In these situations, dividing a goal into smaller realistic objectives helps to accomplish the task. You may know how to swim, but to swim a continuous mile may take several weeks to accomplish. Set up your training program so you swim a little farther each day until you are able to swim the entire mile. If on a particular day you don't meet your objective, try it again, reevaluate, cut back a little, and, most important, don't give up.

3. *Problems of motivation.* In problems of motivation, both the competence and the confidence are there, but the person is unwilling to change because the reasons for change are not important to him or her. For example, people begin contemplating a smoking cessation program when the reasons for quitting outweigh the reasons for smoking.

   When quality of life is concerned, lack of knowledge and lack of goals are the primary causes of unwillingness to change. Knowledge often determines goals, and goals determine motivation. How badly you want it dictates how hard you'll work at it. Many people are unaware of the magnitude of the benefits of a fitness and

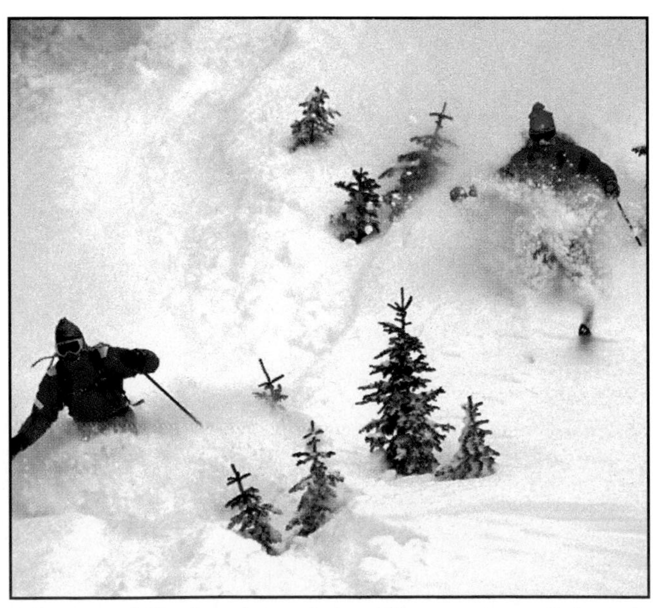

Adequate skill often determines willingness to participate in regular physical activity.

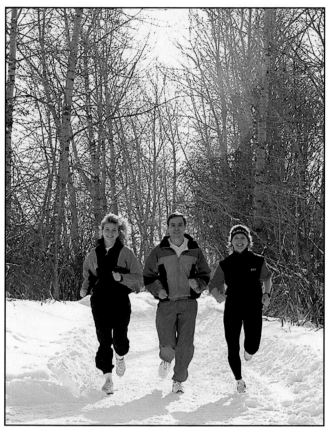
Good fitness enhances confidence and self-esteem.

healthy lifestyle program. Unfortunately, when it comes to a healthy lifestyle, there may not be a second chance. A stroke, a heart attack, or cancer can lead to irreparable or fatal consequences. Greater understanding of what leads to disease may be all that is needed to initiate change.

Also, feeling physically fit is difficult to explain unless you have experienced it yourself. Feelings of fitness, self-esteem, confidence, health, and quality of life cannot be conveyed to someone who is confined to sedentary living. In a way, living a healthy lifestyle is like reaching the top of a mountain. The quietness, the clean air, the lush vegetation, the flowing water in the river, the wildlife, and the majestic valley below are difficult to explain to someone who has spent a lifetime within city limits.

Behavior Modification

Over the course of many years, we all develop habits that at some point in time we would like to change; "old habits die hard." **Behavior modification** requires continual effort to achieve. When it comes to quality of life, the sooner we implement a healthy lifestyle program, the greater are the health benefits and quality of life that lie ahead. The following steps can be taken to help change behavior.

Self-analysis

The first step in behavior modification is a decisive desire to do so. If you have no interest in changing a behavior, you won't do it. A person who has no intention of quitting smoking will not quit, regardless of what anyone may say or how strong the evidence is against it. In your self-analysis you may want to prepare a list of reasons for continuing or discontinuing a certain behavior. As discussed earlier, when the reasons for change outweigh the reasons for not changing, you are ready for the next step.

Behavior Analysis

Determine the frequency, circumstances, and consequences of the behavior to be altered or implemented. If the desired outcome is to decrease fat consumption in the diet, you first must find out what foods in the diet are high in fat, when you eat them, and when you don't eat them. Knowing when you don't eat them points to circumstances under which you exert control of your diet and will help as you set goals.

> ***Knowledge often determines goals, and goals determine motivation.***

Goal Setting

Goals motivate change in behavior. The stronger the goal (desire), the more motivated you'll be to either change unwanted behaviors or to implement new healthy behaviors. The discussion on goal setting that follows will help you write goals and prepare an action plan to achieve those goals. The process will aid with behavior modification.

Social Support

You should surround yourself by people who either will work toward a common goal with you or will

Behavior modification The process to change destructive or negative behaviors permanently for positive behaviors that will lead to better health and well-being.

encourage you along the way. When attempting to quit smoking, it helps to do so with others who also are trying to quit. Or you may get help from friends who already have quit. Peer support is a strong incentive for behavioral change.

During this process, it's important to avoid people who will not support you. Friends who have no desire to quit smoking actually may tempt you to smoke and encourage relapse of unwanted behaviors. People who are beyond the goal you are trying to reach may not be supportive either. For instance, someone may say: "I can do 6 consecutive miles." Your response should be: "I'm proud that I can jog 3 consecutive miles."

Monitoring

Continuous behavior monitoring increases awareness of the desired outcome. Sometimes this principle by itself is sufficient to cause change. For example, keeping track of daily food intake reveals sources of fat in the diet. It can help you cut down gradually or completely eliminate high-fat foods prior to consuming them. If the goal is to increase daily intake of fruit and vegetables, keeping track of the number of servings consumed each day raises awareness and may help increase their intake.

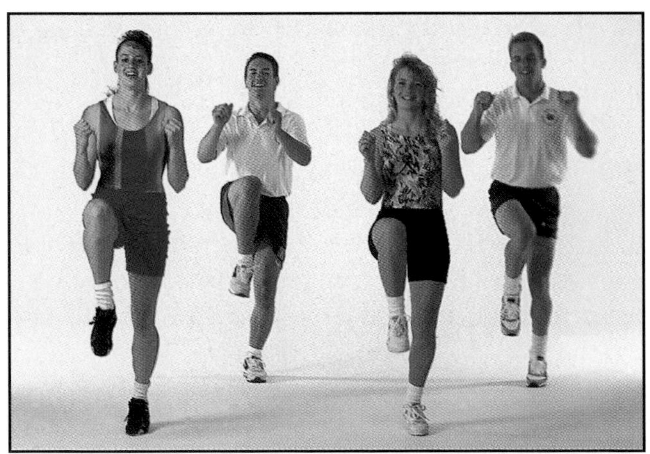

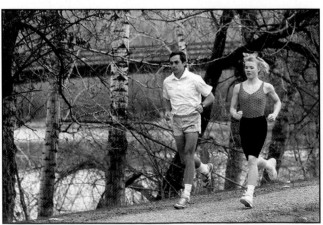

Social support enhances exercise participation.

Positive Outlook

From the beginning, you should take a positive approach and believe in yourself. Following the guidelines set out in this chapter will help you pace yourself so you can work toward change. Also look at the outcomes — how much healthier you will be, how much better you will look, or being able to jog a certain distance, for instance.

Reinforcement

People tend to repeat behaviors that are rewarded and disregard those that are not rewarded or are punished. If you have been successful in cutting down fat intake during the week, reward yourself by going to a show or buying a new pair of shoes. Do not reinforce yourself with destructive behaviors such as eating a high-fat dinner. If you fail to change a desired behavior (or implement a new one), you might put off buying those new shoes you planned for that week. When a positive behavior becomes habitual, give yourself an even better reward. Treat yourself to a weekend away from home or go on a short trip.

Goal Setting

Goals are critical to initiate change. Goals motivate behavioral change and provide a plan of action. Goals are most effective when they are:

1. *Well planned.* Only a well conceived action plan will help you attain your goal. The items below, as well as others discussed in different chapters, will help you design your plan of action. You also should write specific objectives to help you reach each goal.
2. *Personalized.* Goals that you set for yourself are more motivational than goals someone else sets for you.
3. *Written.* An unwritten goal is simply a wish. A written goal, in essence, becomes a contract with yourself. Show this goal to a friend or an in-

structor and have him or her witness, through a signature, the contract you made with yourself.

4. *Realistic.* Goals should be within reach. If you have not exercised regularly, it would be unrealistic to start a daily exercise program consisting of 45 minutes of step aerobics at a vigorous intensity level. Unattainable goals lead to discouragement and loss of interest. To set smaller, attainable goals is better.

   At times, problems arise even with realistic goals. Try to anticipate potential difficulties as much as possible, and plan for ways to deal with them. If your goal is to jog for 30 minutes on 6 consecutive days, what are the alternatives if the weather turns bad? Possible solutions are to jog in the rain, find an indoor track, jog at a different time of day when the weather improves, or participate in a different aerobic activity such as stationary cycling, swimming, or step aerobics.
5. *Measurable.* Write your goals so they are clear, and state specifically the objective to accomplish. "I will lose weight" is not clear enough and is not measurable. A better example is: "I will decrease my body fat to 17%."
6. *Time-specific.* A goal always should have a specific date for completion. This date should be realistic but not too distant in the future.
7. *Monitored.* Monitoring your progress as you move toward a goal reinforces behavior. Keeping a physical activity log or doing a body composition assessment periodically determines where you are at any given time.
8. *Evaluated.* Periodic reevaluations are vital for success. You may find that a given goal is unreachable. If so, reassess the goal. On the other hand, if a goal is too easy, you will lose interest and may stop working toward it. Once you achieve a goal, set a new one to improve upon or maintain what you have achieved. Goals keep you motivated.

Goals keep you motivated.

In addition to these guidelines, throughout this book you will find additional information on behavioral change. For example, tips for behavior modification and adherence to a lifetime weight management program on page 86, the Exercise Readiness Questionnaire on page 251, getting started and adhering to a lifetime exercise program on page 125, a six-step smoking cessation plan on page 200, and stress management techniques starting on page 200.

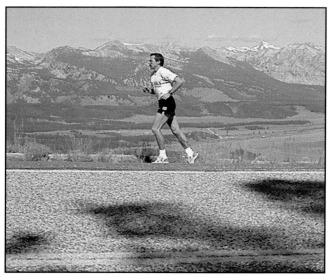

No current drug or medication provides as many health benefits as a regular physical activity program.

Safety of Exercise Participation

Even though exercise testing and participation is relatively safe for most apparently healthy individuals under age 45, the reaction of the cardiovascular system to higher levels of physical activity cannot be totally predicted. Consequently, a small but real risk exists for exercise-induced abnormalities in people with a history of cardiovascular problems and those who are at higher risk for disease.[16] These include abnormal blood pressure, irregular heart rhythm, fainting, and, in rare instances, a heart attack or cardiac arrest.

Before you engage in an exercise program or participate in any exercise testing, you should fill out the questionnaire in Lab 1A. If your answer to any of the questions is yes, you should see a physician before participating in a fitness program. Exercise testing and participation is not wise under some of the conditions listed in Lab 1A and may require a stress electrocardiogram (ECG) test. If you have any questions regarding your current health status, consult your doctor before initiating, continuing, or increasing your level of physical activity.

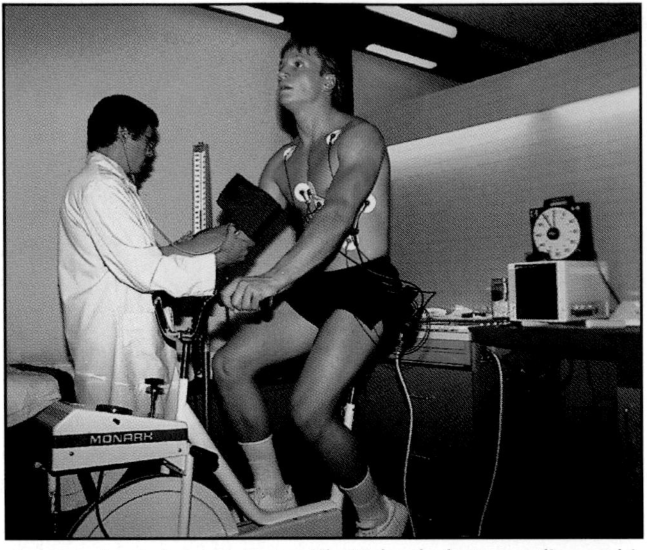

An exercise tolerance test with 12-lead electrocardiographic monitoring may be required of some individuals prior to initiating an exercise program.

Laboratory Experience

LAB 1A
Clearance for Exercise Participation

Lab Preparation
None required

Notes

1. U.S. Centers for Disease Control and Prevention and American College of Sports Medicine, Summary Statement: Workshop on Physical Activity and Public Health. *Sports Medicine Bulletin*, 28(4), 7.
2. National Institutes of Health, *Consensus Development Conference Statement: Physical Activity and Cardiovascular Health*, Washington, DC, December 18–20, 1995.
3. National Institutes of Health.
4. R. S. Paffenbarger, Jr., R. T. Hyde, A. L. Wing, and C. H. Steinmetz, "A Natural History of Athleticism and Cardiovascular Health," *Journal of the American Medical Association*, 252 (1984), 491–495.
5. S. N. Blair, H. W. Kohl III, R. S. Paffenbarger, Jr., D. G. Clark, K. H. Cooper, and L. W. Gibbons, "Physical Fitness and All-Cause Mortality: A Prospective Study of Healthy Men and Women," *Journal of the American Medical Association*, 262 (1989), 2395–2401.
6. J. E. Enstrom. "Health Practices and Cancer Mortality Among Active California Mormons," *Journal of the National Cancer Institute,* 81 (1989), 1807–1814.
7. S. N. Blair, H. W. Kohl III, C. E. Barlow, R. S. Paffenbarger, Jr., L. W. Gibbons, and C. A. Macera, "Changes in Physical Fitness and All-Cause Mortality: A Prospective Study of Healthy and Unhealthy Men," *Journal of the American Medical Association*, 273 (1995), 1193–1198.
8. I. Lee, C. Hsieh, and R. S. Paffenbarger, Jr., "Exercise Intensity and Longevity in Men: The Harvard Alumni Health Study," *Journal of the American Medical Association*, 273 (1995), 1179–1184.
9. P. E. Allsen, J. M. Harrison, and B. Vance, *Fitness for Life* (Madison, WI: Brown & Benchmark, 1993), p. 3.
10. In B. Gutin et al., "Blood Pressure, Fitness, and Fitness in 5- and 6-Year-Old Children," *Journal of the American Medical Association*, 264 (1990), 1123–1127.
11. "Wellness Facts," *University of California at Berkeley Wellness Letter*, April, 1995.
12. Robert C. Chadbourne, "Fit for Hire," *Fitness Management*, 12:2 (1996), 28–30.
13. Editors of Prevention Magazine, *The Prevention Index 1995: A Report Card on the Nation's Health* (Emmaus, PA: Rodale Press, 1995).
14. U. S. Department of Health and Human Services, Public Health Service, *Healthy People 2000: National Health Promotion and Disease Prevention Objectives* (Boston: Jones and Bartlett Publishers, 1992).
15. G. S. Howard, D. W. Nance, and P. Myers, *Adaptive Counseling and Therapy* (San Francisco: Jossey-Bass, 1987).
16. American College of Sports Medicine, *Guidelines for Exercise Testing and Prescription* (Baltimore: Williams & Wilkins, 1995).

Suggested Readings

American College of Sports Medicine. "The Recommended Quantity and Quality of Exercise for Developing and Maintaining Cardiorespiratory and Muscular Fitness in Healthy Adults." *Medicine and Science in Sports and Exercise,* 22 (1990), 265–274.

Davies, N. E., and L. H. Felder. "Applying Brakes to the Runaway American Health Care System." *Journal of the American Medical Association,* 263 (1990), 73–76.

Gettman, L. R. "Cost/Benefit Analysis of a Corporate Fitness Program." *Fitness in Business*, 1:1 (1986), 11–17.

Hatziandreu, E. L., J. P. Koplan, M. C. Weinstein, C. J. Caspersen, K. E. Warner. "A Cost-effectiveness Analysis of Exercise as a Health Promotion Activity." *American Journal of Public Health*, 78 (1988), 1417–1421.

Hoeger, W. W. K., and S. A. Hoeger. *Lifetime Physical Fitness & Wellness: A Personalized Program.* Englewood, CO: Morton Publishing, 1995.

Koplan, J. P., C. J. Caspersen, and K. E. Powell. "Physical Activity, Physical Fitness, and Health: Time to Act." *Journal of the American Medical Association*, 262 (1989), 2437.

Smith, L. K. "Cost-Effectiveness of Health Promotion Programs." *Fitness Management*, 2:3 (1986), 12–15.

"New Fitness Data Verifies: Employees Who Exercise are Also More Productive." *Athletic Business*, 8:12 (1984), 24–30.

Van Camp, S. P. "The Fixx Tragedy: A Cardiologist's Perspective." *Physician and Sportsmedicine*, 12:9 (1984), 153–155.

Wilmore, J. H. "Design Issues and Alternatives in Assessing Physical Fitness Among Apparently Healthy Adults in a Health Examination Survey of the General Population." In (Editor). *Assessing Physical Fitness and Activity in General Population Studies*, edited by F. Drury. (Washington, DC: U.S. Public Health Service, National Center for Health Statistics, 1988).

Principles of Nutrition for Wellness

2

LABS

*Although all the answers are not in yet, scientific evidence has long linked good **nutrition** to overall health and well-being. Proper nutrition means that a person's diet supplies all the essential nutrients to carry out normal tissue growth, repair, and maintenance. These **nutrients** should be obtained from a wide variety of sources. Figure 2.1 shows the basic food pyramid with the recommended number of servings from each food group for proper nutrition. The diet also should provide enough **substrates** to produce the energy necessary for work, physical activity, and relaxation.*

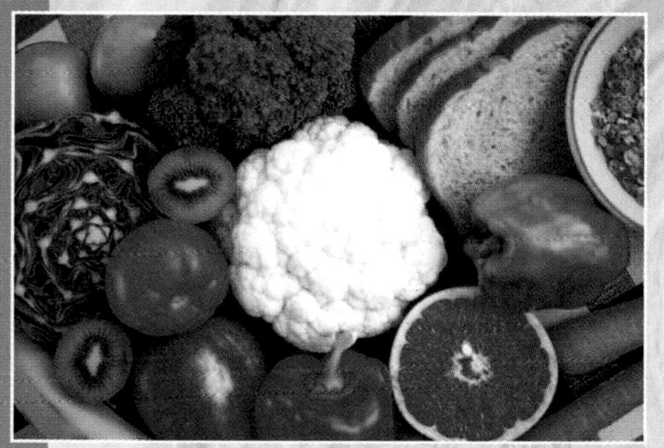

Too much or too little of any nutrient can precipitate serious health problems. The typical North American diet is too high in calories, sugar, fat, saturated fat, and sodium, and not high enough in fiber — factors that undermine good health. Food availability is not the problem. The problem is overconsumption.

According to a 1988 report on nutrition and health issued by the U. S. Surgeon General[1] — the first ever of its kind — diseases of dietary excess and imbalance are among the

Objectives

- Define nutrition and describe its relationship to health and well-being.
- Describe the functions of carbohydrates in the human body and be able to differentiate simple from complex carbohydrates.
- Describe the role and health benefits of adequate fiber in the diet.
- Describe the role of fats in the human body and be able to differentiate and characterize saturated, monounsaturated, and polyunsaturated fats.
- Describe the functions of proteins in the human body.
- Describe the role of vitamins and minerals in the human body.
- Learn to conduct a comprehensive nutrient analysis, be capable of recognizing areas of deficiencies, and be able to implement changes to improve overall nutrition.
- Become familiar with the five food groups and learn how to use them to achieve a balanced diet.
- Understand the role of antioxidants in preventing disease.
- Learn recommended guidelines for nutrient supplementation.
- Become familiar with the National Dietary Guidelines for Americans.
- Identify myths and fallacies regarding nutrition.

Fats, Oils, & Sweets
USE SPARINGLY

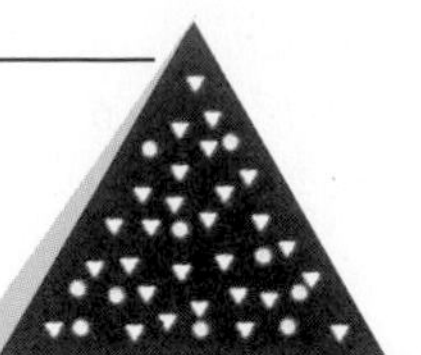

KEY
● Fat (naturally occurring and added) ▼ Sugars (added)
These symbols show fats, oils, and added sugars in foods.

Milk, Yogurt, & Cheese Group
2-3 SERVINGS

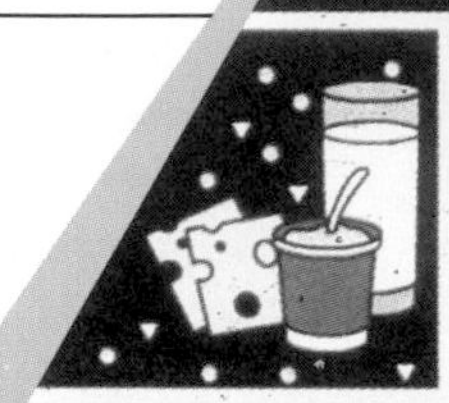

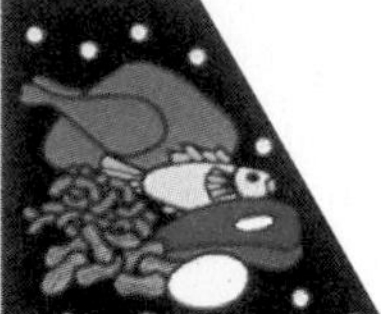

Meat, Poultry, Fish, Dry Beans, Eggs, & Nuts Group
2-3 SERVINGS

Vegetable Group
3-5 SERVINGS

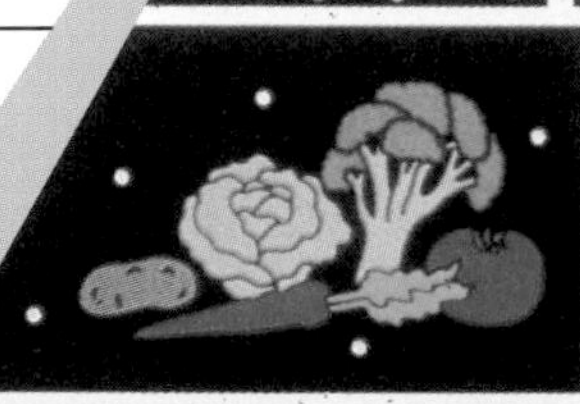

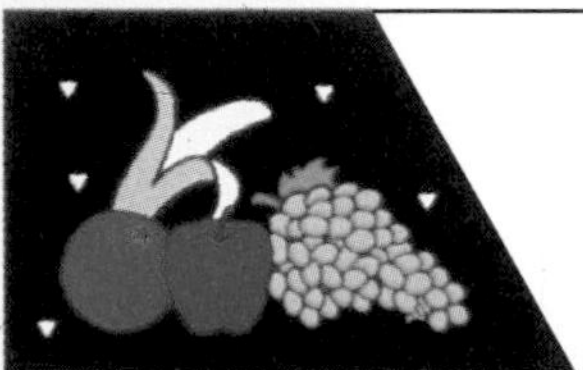

Fruit Group
2-4 SERVINGS

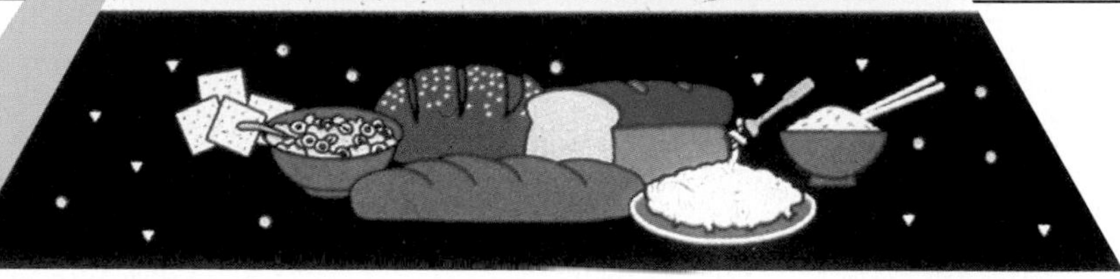

Bread, Cereal, Rice, & Pasta Group
6-11 SERVINGS

What counts as one serving?

Breads, Cereals, Rice, and Pasta
1 slice of bread
1/2 cup of cooked rice or pasta
1/2 cup of cooked cereal
1 ounce of ready-to-eat cereal

Vegetables
1/2 cup of chopped raw or cooked vegetables
1 cup of leafy raw vegetables

Fruits
1 piece of fruit or melon wedge
3/4 cup of juice
1/2 cup of canned fruit
1/4 cup of dried fruit

Milk, Yogurt, and Cheese
1 cup of milk or yogurt
1½ to 2 ounces of cheese

Meat, Poultry, Fish, Dry Beans, Eggs, and Nuts
2½ to 3 ounces of cooked lean meat, poultry, or fish
Count 1/2 cup of cooked beans, or 1 egg, or 2 tablespoons of peanut butter as 1 ounce of lean meat (about 1/3 serving)

Fats, Oils, and Sweets
LIMIT CALORIES FROM THESE
especially if you need to lose weight

The amount you eat may be more than one serving. For example, a dinner portion of spaghetti would count as two or three servings of pasta.

How many servings do you need each day?

	Women & some older adults	Children, teen girls, active women, most men	Teen boys & active men
Calorie level*	about 1,600	about 2,200	about 2,800
Bread group	6	9	11
Vegetable group	3	4	5
Fruit group	2	3	4
Milk group	2–3**	2–3**	**2–3
Meat group	2, for a total of 5 ounces	2, for a total of 6 ounces	3, for a total of 7 ounces

* These are the calorie levels if you choose lowfat, lean foods from the 5 major food groups and use foods from the fats, oils, and sweets group sparingly.
** Women who are pregnant or breastfeeding, teenagers, and young adults to age 24 need 3 servings.

A Closer Look at Fat and Added Sugars

The small tip of the Pyramid shows fats, oils, and sweets. These are foods such as salad dressings, cream, butter, margarine, sugars, soft drinks, candies, and sweet desserts. Alcoholic beverages are also part of this group. These foods provide calories but few vitamins and minerals. Most people should go easy on foods from this group.

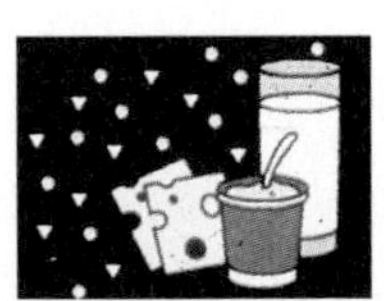

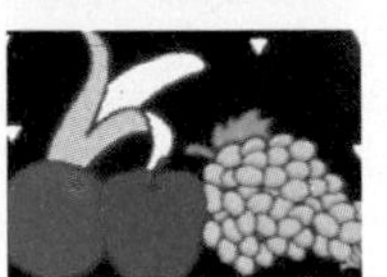

Some fat or sugar symbols are shown in the other food groups. That's to remind you that some foods in these groups can also be high in fat and added sugars, such as cheese or ice cream from the milk group, or french fries from the vegetable group. When choosing foods for a healthful diet, consider the fat and added sugars in your choices from all the food groups, not just fats, oils, and sweets from the Pyramid tip.

*Developed by the U.S. Department of Agriculture to promote a healthy diet for people in the United States.

Figure 2.1 Food Guide Pyramid: A Guide to Daily Food Choices.

leading causes of death in the United States. Similar trends are observed in developed countries throughout the world. Of the total 2.1 million deaths in the United States in 1987, an estimated 1.5 million people died of diseases associated with faulty nutrition. In the report, based on more than 2,000 scientific studies, the U.S. Surgeon General said dietary changes can bring better health to all Americans. Other surveys reveal that on a given day, nearly half of the American people eat no fruit and almost a fourth eat no vegetables.

An estimated 1.5 million people died in the United States in 1987 of diseases associated with faulty nutrition.

Studies also indicate that diet and nutrition often play a crucial role in the development and progression of chronic diseases. A diet high in saturated fat and cholesterol increases the risk for atherosclerosis and coronary heart disease. In sodium-sensitive individuals, high salt intake has been linked to high blood pressure. Some researchers believe that 30% to 50% of all cancers are diet-related. Obesity, diabetes, and osteoporosis also have been associated with faulty nutrition.

An effective wellness program must incorporate current dietary recommendations to lower the risk for chronic disease. A summary of guidelines for a healthful diet include:

- Eating a variety of foods.
- Avoiding too much fat, saturated fat, and cholesterol.
- Eating foods with adequate starch and fiber.
- Avoiding too much sugar and sodium.
- Maintaining adequate calcium intake.
- Maintaining recommended body weight.
- Drinking alcoholic beverages in moderation, if at all.

These guidelines will be discussed throughout this chapter and in later chapters of this book.

Nutrients

The essential nutrients the human body requires are carbohydrates, fat, protein, vitamins, minerals, and water. The first three are called fuel nutrients because they are the only substances the body uses to supply the energy (commonly measured in calories) needed for work and normal body functions. Vitamins, minerals, and water have no caloric value but still are necessary for a person to function normally and maintain good health. Many nutritionists add a seventh nutrient to this list, one that has received a great deal of attention recently: dietary fiber.

Carbohydrates, fats, proteins, and water are termed *macronutrients* because proportionately large amounts are needed daily. Vitamins and minerals are required only in small amounts. Therefore, nutritionists refer to them as *micronutrients*.

Depending on the amount of nutrients and calories, foods can be classified according to high nutrient density and low nutrient density. *High nutrient density* refers to foods that contain few or moderate calories but are packed with nutrients. Foods that have a lot of calories but few nutrients are of *low nutrient density* and commonly are called "junk food."

A **calorie** is the unit of measure indicating the energy value of food and the cost of physical activity. Technically, a kilocalorie (kcal) or large calorie is the amount of heat necessary to raise the temperature of 1 kilogram of water 1° Centigrade, but for simplification people call it a calorie rather than kcal. For example, if the caloric value of a food is 100 calories (kcal), the energy in this food would raise the temperature of 100 kilograms of water 1° Centigrade.

Carbohydrates

Carbohydrates constitute the major source of calories the body uses to provide energy for work, maintain cells, and generate heat. They also help digest and regulate fat and metabolize protein. Each gram of carbohydrates provides the human body with 4 calories.

The major sources of carbohydrates are breads, cereals, fruits, vegetables, and milk and other dairy products. Carbohydrates are classified into simple carbohydrates and complex carbohydrates (Figure 2.2).

Nutrition Science that studies the relationship of foods to optimal health and performance.

Nutrients Substances found in food that provide energy, regulate metabolism, and help with growth and repair of body tissues.

Substrate Substance acted upon by an enzyme (examples: carbohydrates and fats).

Calorie The amount of heat necessary to raise the temperature of one gram of water one degree Centigrade. Used to measure the energy value of food and cost of physical activity.

Carbohydrates Compounds containing carbon, hydrogen, and oxygen; the major source of energy for the human body.

2

2

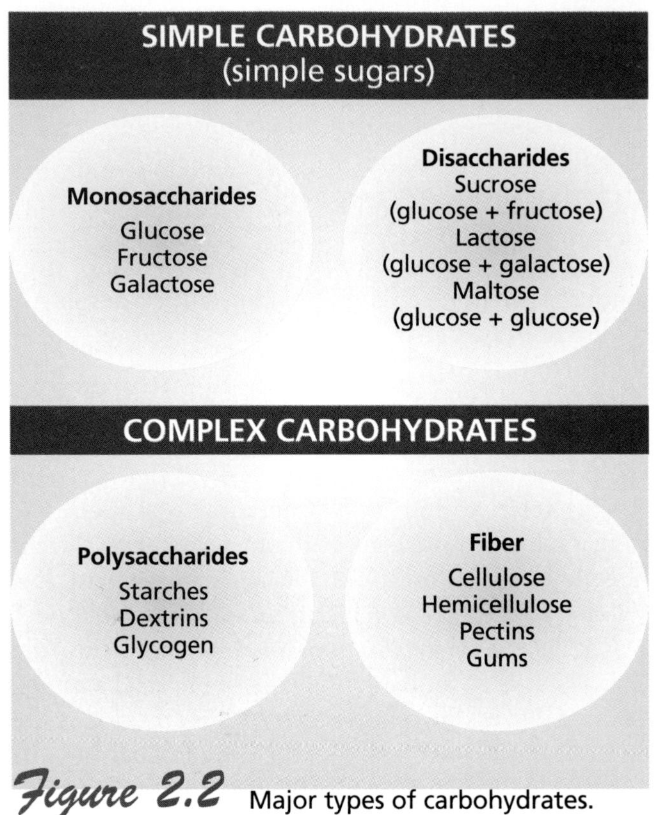

Figure 2.2 Major types of carbohydrates.

Simple Carbohydrates

Often called sugars, **simple carbohydrates** have little nutritive value (for example, candy, soda, cakes). Simple carbohydrates are divided into monosaccharides and disaccharides. These carbohydrates — with -ose endings — often take the place of more nutritive foods in the diet.

Monosaccharides

The simplest sugars are **monosaccharides.** The three most common monosaccharides are glucose, fructose, and galactose.

1. *Glucose* is a natural sugar found in food, but it also is produced in the body from other simple and complex carbohydrates.
2. *Fructose*, or fruit sugar, occurs naturally in fruits and honey.
3. *Galactose* is produced from milk sugar in the mammary glands of lactating animals.

Both fructose and galactose are converted readily to glucose in the body. Glucose is used as a source of energy, or it may be stored in the muscles and liver in the form of glycogen (a long chain of glucose molecules hooked together). Excess glucose in the blood is converted to fat and stored in **adipose tissue**. Some of it is eliminated by the kidneys through the urine.

Disaccharides

The three major **disaccharides** are:

1. *Sucrose* or table sugar (glucose + fructose).
2. *Lactose* (glucose + galactose).
3. *Maltose* (glucose + glucose).

Complex Carbohydrates

Complex carbohydrates are also called *polysaccharides*. Anywhere from about 10 to thousands of monosaccharide molecules can unite to form a single polysaccharide. Examples of complex carbohydrates are starches, dextrins, and glycogen.

1. *Starch* is the storage form of glucose in plants, needed to promote the earliest growth. Starch is found commonly in grains, seeds, corn, nuts, roots, potatoes, and legumes. Grains, the richest source of starch, should supply most of the energy in a healthful diet. Once eaten, starch is converted to glucose for the body's own energy use.
2. *Dextrins* are formed from the breakdown of large starch molecules exposed to dry heat, such as in baking bread or producing cold cereals. Complex carbohydrates of plant origin provide many valuable nutrients and can be an excellent source of fiber, or roughage.
3. *Glycogen* is the animal polysaccharide synthesized from glucose and found only in slight amounts in meats. Although it serves a function in humans similar to that of starch in plants, glycogen is not found in plants. Glycogen constitutes the body's reservoirs of glucose. Many hundreds to thousands of glucose molecules are linked together to be stored as glycogen in liver and muscle.

   When a surge of energy is needed, enzymes in the muscle and the liver break down glycogen and thus make glucose readily available for energy transformation. This is discussed later in the chapter, under Nutrition for Athletes.

Dietary Fiber

Dietary fiber is a type of complex carbohydrate present mainly in leaves, skins, roots, and seeds. Processing and refining foods remove almost all of the natural fiber. In our daily diets the main sources of dietary fiber are whole-grain cereals and breads, fruits, and vegetables.

The most common types of fiber are:

1. *Cellulose* and hemicellulose, found in plant cell walls.
2. *Pectins*, found in fruits.
3. *Gums*, also found in small amounts in foods of plant origin.

Cellulose and hemicellulose are water-insoluble fibers. Pectins and gums are water-soluble fibers.

Fiber is important in the diet because it binds water, causing a softer and bulkier stool that increases peristalsis (involuntary muscle contractions of intestinal walls that force the stool onward) and allows food residues to pass through the intestinal tract more quickly. Many researchers believe that speeding up passage of food residues through the intestines lowers the risk for colon cancer, mainly because cancer-causing agents are not in contact as long with the intestinal wall. Fiber also is thought to bind with carcinogens (cancer-producing substances), and more water in the stool may dilute the cancer-causing agents, lessening their potency.

Increased fiber intake also may lower the risk for coronary heart disease because: (a) saturated fats often take the place of fiber in the diet, increasing cholesterol formation or absorption, and (b) specific water-soluble fibers such as pectin and guar gum, found in beans, oat bran, corn, and fruits, seem to bind cholesterol in the intestines, preventing its absorption. In addition to heart disease, several health disorders, including constipation, diverticulitis, hemorrhoids, gallbladder disease, and obesity have been linked to low intake of fiber.

Determining the amount of fiber in your diet can be confusing at times because it can be measured either as crude fiber or as dietary fiber. Crude fiber is the smaller portion of the dietary fiber, which actually remains after chemical extraction in the digestive tract. The recommended amount of dietary fiber is 20 to 35 grams per day, the equivalent of 7 grams of crude fiber. Because most nutrition labels list the fiber content in terms of dietary fiber, the 20- to 35-gram guideline should be used (see Table 2.1).

This may be surprising, but too much fiber can be detrimental to health. It can produce loss of calcium, phosphorus, and iron, not to mention gastrointestinal discomfort. When eating more fiber, a person also should drink more water, as too little fluid can cause constipation and even dehydration.

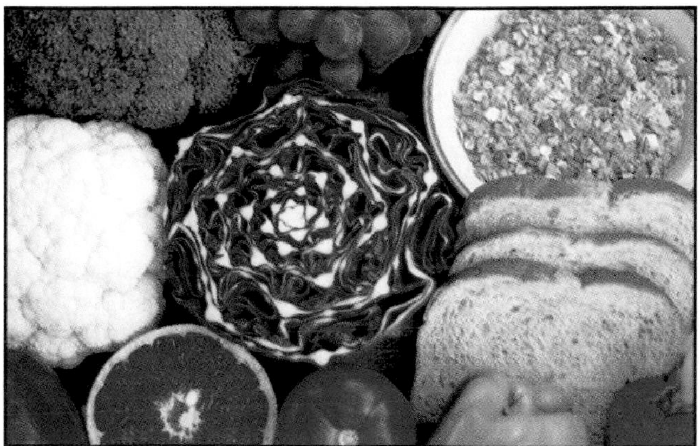

High-fiber foods are essential in a healthy diet.

Fat

The human body uses **fats**, or lipids, as a source of energy. Fats are the most concentrated energy source. Each gram of fat supplies 9 calories to the body. Fats are a part of the cell structure. They are used as stored energy and as an insulator to preserve body heat. They absorb shock, supply essential fatty acids, and carry the fat-soluble vitamins A, D, E, and K. Fats can be classified into three main groups: simple, compound, and derived (Figure 2.3). The basic sources of fat are milk and other dairy products, and meats and alternatives.

Simple Fats

A simple fat consists of a glyceride molecule linked to one, two, or three units of fatty acids. According to the number of fatty acids attached, simple fats are divided into monoglycerides (one fatty acid), diglycerides (two fatty acids), and triglycerides (three fatty acids). More than 90% of the weight of fat in foods and more than 95% of the stored fat in the human body are in the form of triglycerides.

The length of the carbon atom chain and the amount of hydrogen saturation in fatty acids vary.

Simple carbohydrates Formed by simple or double sugar units with little nutritive value; divided into monosaccharides and disaccharides.

Monosaccharides The simplest carbohydrates (sugars) formed by five- or six-carbon skeletons. The three most common monosaccharides are glucose, fructose, and galactose.

Adipose tissue Fat cells.

Disaccharides Simple carbohydrates formed by two monosaccharide units linked together, one of which is glucose. The major disaccharides are sucrose, lactose, and maltose.

Complex carbohydrates Carbohydrates formed by three or more simple sugar molecules linked together; also referred to as polysaccharides.

Dietary fiber A complex carbohydrate in plant foods that cannot be digested by the human body but is essential in the digestion process.

Fats Compounds made by a combination of triglycerides.

2

Table 2.1 Dietary Fiber Content of Selected Foods

Food	Serving Size	Dietary Fiber (gm)
Almonds	1 oz.	3.0
Apple	1 medium	4.3
Banana	1 medium	3.3
Beans — red, kidney	.5 cup	10.2
Blackberries	.5 cup	4.9
Beets (cooked)	.5 cup	2.0
Brazil nuts	1 oz.	2.5
Broccoli (cooked)	.5 cup	3.3
Brown rice (cooked)	.5 cup	2.0
Carrots (cooked)	.5 cup	2.9
Cauliflower (cooked)	.5 cup	1.7
Cereal		
All Bran	1 oz.	8.5
Cheerios	1 oz.	1.1
Cornflakes	1 oz.	0.5
Fruit and Fibre	1 oz.	4.0
Fruit Wheats	1 oz.	2.0
Just Right	1 oz.	2.0
Wheaties	1 oz.	2.0
Corn (cooked)	.5 cup	3.9
Eggplant (cooked)	.5 cup	3.0
Lettuce (chopped)	.5 cup	0.4
Orange	1 medium	3.0
Parsnips (cooked)	.5 cup	2.1
Pear	1 medium	5.0
Peas (cooked)	.5 cup	3.7
Popcorn (plain)	1 cup	1.5
Potato (baked)	1 medium	3.9
Strawberries	.5 cup	1.6
Summer squash (cooked)	.5 cup	1.6
Watermelon	1 cup	0.8

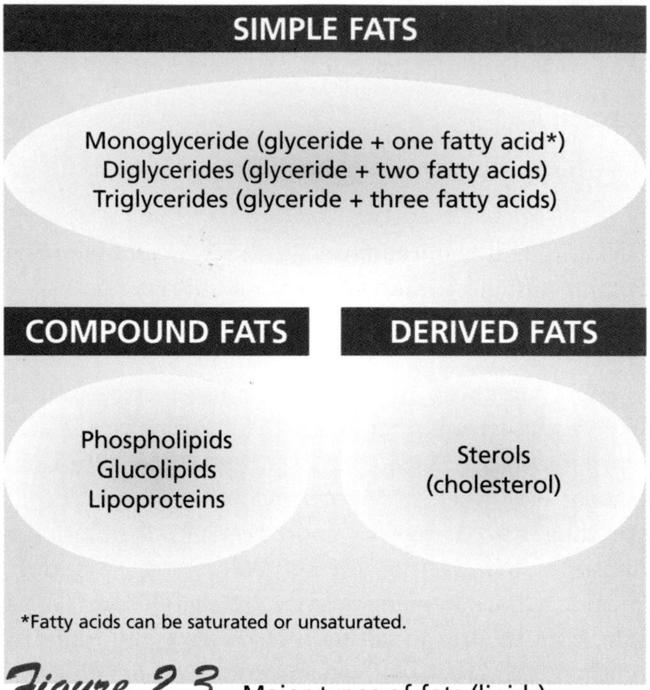

Figure 2.3 Major types of fats (lipids).

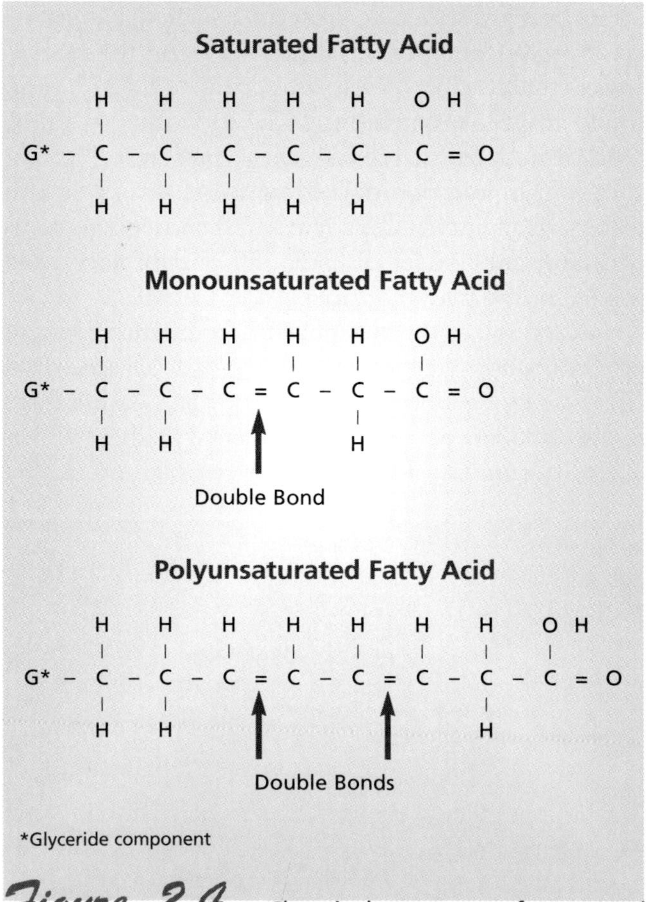

Figure 2.4 Chemical structure of saturated and unsaturated fats.

Based on the extent of saturation, fatty acids are said to be saturated or unsaturated. Unsaturated fatty acids are classified further into monounsaturated and polyunsaturated. Saturated fatty acids are mainly of animal origin. Unsaturated fats are found mostly in plant products.

In saturated fatty acids the carbon atoms are fully saturated with hydrogens; only single bonds link the carbon atoms on the chain (see Figure 2.4). These saturated fatty acids often are called saturated fats. Examples of foods high in saturated fatty acids are meats, meat fat, lard, whole milk, cream, butter, cheese, ice cream, hydrogenated oils (a process that makes oils saturated), coconut oil, and palm oils.

In unsaturated fatty acids (unsaturated fats), double bonds form between the unsaturated carbons. In monounsaturated fatty acids (MUFA), only one double bond is found along the chain. Olive, canola, rapeseed, peanut, and sesame oils are examples of monounsaturated fatty acids. Polyunsaturated fatty acids (PUFA) contain two or more double bonds between unsaturated carbon atoms along the chain. Corn, cottonseed, safflower, walnut, sunflower, and soybean oils are high in polyunsaturated fatty acids.

Saturated fats typically do not melt at room temperature. Unsaturated fats usually are liquid at room temperature. Coconut and palm oils are exceptions, as they are high in saturated fats. Shorter fatty acid chains also tend to be liquid at room temperature.

In general, saturated fats raise the blood cholesterol level, whereas polyunsaturated and monounsaturated fats tend to lower blood cholesterol. Polyunsaturated fats, nonetheless, also seem to cause reduction of the "good" (HDL) cholesterol, which may not really improve the cholesterol profile (high HDL-cholesterol levels help to decrease the risk of diseases of the cardiovascular system). Monounsaturated fats, on the other hand, seem to lower only the "bad" (LDL) cholesterol and not the good (HDL) cholesterol.

Hydrogen often is added to monounsaturated and polyunsaturated fats to increase shelf life and to solidify them so they are more spreadable. During this process of partial hydrogenation, the position of hydrogen atoms may be changed along the chain, transforming the fat into a **transfatty acid**.

Margarine and spreads, crackers, cookies, and french fries often contain transfatty acids. Intake of these types of fats should be minimized. Studies suggest that diets rich in transfatty acids elevate LDL cholesterol and lower HDL cholesterol to the same extent as saturated fats.[2] Paying attention to food labels is important because the words "partially hydrogenated" or "transfatty acids" may indicate that the product carries as high a health risk as consuming saturated fat (eating margarine is still a better choice because its total transfatty acid and saturated fat is about half the saturated fat in butter).

One type of polyunsaturated fatty acids that has gained attention in recent years are **omega-3 fatty acids**. These fatty acids seem to be effective in lowering triglycerides, which are a risk factor for coronary heart disease. Fish, especially fresh or frozen mackerel, herring, tuna, salmon, and lake trout, have omega-3 fatty acids. Canned fish is not recommended for this purpose because the canning process destroys most of the omega-3 oil. These fatty acids also are found, but to a lesser extent, in canola oil, walnuts, soybeans, and wheat germ.

Some data suggest that eating one or two servings of fish weekly lessens the risk for coronary heart disease. People with diabetes, a history of hemorrhaging or strokes, on aspirin, blood-thinning therapy, and presurgical patients should not consume fish oil except under a physician's instruction.

Compound Fats

Compound fats are a combination of simple fats and other chemicals. Examples are:

1. Phospholipids — similar to triglycerides except that phosphoric acid takes the place of one of the fatty acid units.
2. Glucolipids — a combination of carbohydrates, fatty acids, and nitrogen.
3. Lipoproteins — water-soluble aggregates of protein with triglycerides, phospholipids, or cholesterol.

Because lipids do not dissolve in water, lipoproteins transport fats in the blood.

The major forms of **lipoproteins** are high-density (HDL), low-density (LDL), and very-low-density (VLDL) lipoproteins. Lipoproteins play a large role in developing or in preventing heart disease. HDL is more than half protein and contains little cholesterol. High HDL levels have been associated with a lower risk for coronary heart disease. LDL is approximately a fourth protein and nearly half cholesterol. High LDL levels have been linked to increased risk for coronary heart disease. VLDL contains mostly (about half) triglycerides and only about 10% protein and 20% cholesterol.

Derived Fats

Derived fats combine simple and compound fats. **Sterols** are an example. Although sterols contain no fatty acids, they are considered fats because they do not dissolve in water. The most often mentioned sterol is cholesterol, which is found in many foods or can be manufactured from saturated fats in the body.

Transfatty acid Solidified fat formed by adding hydrogen to monosaturated and polyunsaturated fats to increase shelf life.

Omega-3 fatty acids Polyunsaturated fatty acids found primarily in cold-water seafood; thought to be effective in lowering blood cholesterol and triglycerides.

Lipoproteins Lipids covered by proteins; transport fats in the blood.

Sterols Derived fats, of which cholesterol is the best known example.

Protein

Proteins are the main substances the body uses to build and repair tissues such as muscles, blood, internal organs, skin, hair, nails, and bones. They are a part of hormones, antibodies, and enzymes. **Enzymes** play a key role in all of the body's processes. Because all enzymes are formed by proteins, this nutrient is necessary for normal functioning. Proteins also help maintain the normal balance of body fluids.

Proteins can be used as a source of energy, too, but only if not enough carbohydrates are available. Each gram of protein yields 4 calories of energy. The main sources of protein are meats and alternatives, and milk and other dairy products. Excess proteins may be converted to glucose or fat or even excreted in the urine.

The human body uses 20 **amino acids** to form different types of protein. Amino acids contain nitrogen, carbon, hydrogen, and oxygen. Nine of the 20 amino acids are called *essential amino acids* because the body cannot produce them. The other 11, termed *nonessential amino acids*, can be manufactured in the body if food proteins in the diet provide enough nitrogen (see Table 2.2). For the body to function normally, all amino acids must be present at the same time.

Proteins that contain all the essential amino acids are known as complete or higher-quality protein. These types of proteins usually are of animal origin. If one or more of the essential amino acids is missing, the proteins are termed incomplete or lower-quality protein. Individuals have to take in enough protein to ensure nitrogen for adequate amino acid production and also to get enough high-quality protein to obtain the essential amino acids.

Protein deficiency is not a problem in the usual American diet. Two glasses of skim milk combined with about 4 ounces of poultry or fish meet the daily protein requirement. Protein deficiency, however, could be a concern in some vegetarian diets. **Vegetarians** rely primarily on foods from the bread and cereal and fruit and vegetable groups and avoid most foods from animal sources found in the milk and meat groups. The four basic types of vegetarians are **vegans, ovovegetarians, lactovegetarians,** and **ovo-lactovegetarians**.

Vegans in particular must be careful to eat protein foods that provide a balanced distribution of essential amino acids, such as grain products and beans. Strict vegans also need a supplement of vitamin B_{12}. This vitamin is not found in plant foods, and its deficiency may lead to anemia.

Vegetarians who do not select their food combinations properly may develop nutritional deficiencies of protein, vitamins, minerals, and even calories. Vegetarian diets can be balanced, but this is a complicated issue that cannot be covered adequately in a few paragraphs. Those who are interested in vegetarian diets should consult other resources.

Too much animal protein can cause serious health problems as well. Some people eat twice as much protein as they need. Protein foods from animal sources often are high in fat, saturated fat, and cholesterol, which can lead to cardiovascular disease and cancer. Too much animal protein also decreases blood enzymes that prevent precancerous cells from developing into tumors.

As discussed later in this chapter, a well-balanced diet contains a variety of foods from all five basic food groups, including wise selection of foods from animal sources. Based on current nutrition data, meat (poultry and fish included) should be replaced by grains, legumes, vegetables, and fruits as main courses. Meats should be used more for flavoring than for substance. Daily consumption of beef, poultry, or fish should be limited to 3 to 6 ounces (about the size of a deck of cards).

Table 2.2 Amino Acids

Essential Amino Acids*	Nonessential Amino Acids
Histidine	Alanine
Isoleucine	Arginine
Leucine	Asparagine
Lysine	Aspartic acid
Methionine	Cysteine
Phenylalanine	Glutamic acid
Threonine	Glutamine
Tryptophan	Glycine
Valine	Proline
	Serine
	Tyrosine

*Must be provided in the diet as the body cannot manufacture them.

Vitamins

Vitamins are necessary for normal bodily metabolism, growth, and development. Vitamins are classified into two types based on their solubility: *fat-soluble vitamins* (A, D, E, and K), and *water-soluble* *vitamins* (B complex and C). In general, the body does not manufacture vitamins. Vitamins can be obtained only through a well-balanced diet. To decrease vitamin losses during cooking, natural foods should be microwaved or steamed rather than boiled in water that later is thrown out.

A few exceptions, such as A, D, and K, are formed in the body. Vitamin A is produced from **beta-carotene,** found in foods such as carrots, pumpkin, and sweet potatoes. Ultraviolet light from the sun changes a compound in the skin called 7-dehydrocholesterol into vitamin D. Vitamin K is created in the body by intestinal bacteria. The major functions of vitamins are outlined in Table 2.3.

Proteins Complex organic compounds containing nitrogen and formed by combinations of amino acids; the main substances used in the body to build and repair tissues.

Enzymes Catalysts that facilitate chemical reactions in the body.

Amino acids Chemical compounds that contain nitrogen, carbon, hydrogen, and oxygen; the basic building blocks the body uses to build different types of protein.

Vegetarians Individuals whose diet is of vegetable or plant origin.

Vegans Vegetarians who eat no animal products at all.

Ovovegetarians Vegetarians who allow eggs in the diet.

Lactovegetarians Vegetarians who eat foods from the milk group.

Ovolactovegetarians Vegetarians who include eggs and milk products in the diet.

Vitamins Organic substances essential for normal metabolism, growth, and development of the body.

Beta-carotene A precursor to vitamin A.

Table 2.3 Major Functions of Vitamins

Nutrient	Good Sources	Major Functions	Deficiency Symptoms
Vitamin A	Milk, cheese, eggs, liver, and yellow/dark green fruits and vegetables	Required for healthy bones, teeth, skin, gums, and hair; maintenance of inner mucous membranes, thus increasing resistance to infection; adequate vision in dim light.	Night blindness, decreased growth, decreased resistance to infection, rough-dry skin.
Vitamin D	Fortified milk, cod liver oil, salmon, tuna, egg yolk	Necessary for bones and teeth; needed for calcium and phosphorus absorption.	Rickets (bone softening), fractures, and muscle spasms
Vitamin E	Vegetable oils, yellow and green leafy vegetables, margarine, wheat germ, whole grain breads and cereals	Related to oxidation and normal muscle and red blood cell chemistry.	Leg cramps, red blood cell breakdown
Vitamin K	Green leafy vegetables, cauliflower, cabbage, eggs, peas, and potatoes	Essential for normal blood clotting.	Hemorrhaging
Vitamin B_1 (Thiamine)	Whole grain or enriched bread, lean meats and poultry, organ fish, liver, pork, poultry, organ meats, legumes, nuts, and dried yeast	Assists in proper use of carbohydrates; normal functioning of nervous system; maintenance of good appetite.	Loss of appetite, nausea, confusion, cardiac abnormalities, muscle spasms
Vitamin B_2 (Riboflavin)	Eggs, milk, leafy green vegetables, whole grains, lean meats, dried beans and peas	Contributes to energy release from carbohydrates, fats, and proteins; needed for normal growth and development, good vision, and healthy skin.	Cracking of the corners of the mouth, inflammation of the skin, impaired vision.
Vitamin B_6 (Pyridoxine)	Vegetables, meats, whole grain cereals, soybeans, peanuts, and potatoes	Necessary for protein and fatty acids metabolism, and normal red blood cell formation.	Depression, irritability, muscle spasms, nausea
Vitamin B_{12}	Meat, poultry, fish, liver, organ meats, eggs, shellfish, milk, and cheese	Required for normal growth, red blood cell formation, nervous system and digestive tract functioning.	Impaired balance, weakness, drop in red blood cell count
Niacin	Liver and organ meats, meat, fish, poultry, whole grains, enriched breads, nuts, green leafy vegetables, and dried beans and peas	Contributes to energy release from carbohydrates, fats, and proteins; normal growth and development, and formation of hormones and nerve-regulating substances.	Confusion, depression, weakness, weight loss
Biotin	Liver, kidney, eggs, yeast, legumes, milk, nuts, dark green vegetables	Essential for carbohydrate metabolism and fatty acid synthesis.	Inflamed skin, muscle pain, depression, weight loss
Folic Acid	Leafy green vegetables, organ meats, whole grains and cereals, and dried beans	Needed for cell growth and reproduction and red blood cell formation.	Decreased resistance to infection
Pantothenic Acid	All natural foods, especially liver, kidney, eggs, nuts, yeast, milk, dried peas and beans, and green leafy vegetables	Related to carbohydrate and fat metabolism.	Depression, low blood sugar, leg cramps, nausea, headaches
Vitamin C (Ascorbic Acid)	Fruits and vegetables	Helps protect against infection; formation of collagenous tissue; normal blood vessels, teeth, and bones.	Slow healing wounds, loose teeth, hemorrhaging, rough-scaly skin, irritability

Vitamins C, E, and beta-carotene also function as **antioxidants**, which are thought to play a key role in preventing chronic diseases.[3] The specific function of these antioxidant nutrients, along with the mineral selenium, also an antioxidant, are discussed later in this chapter.

Minerals

Approximately 25 **minerals** have important roles in body functioning. Minerals are contained in all cells, especially those in hard parts of the body (bones, nails, teeth). Minerals are crucial in maintaining water balance and the acid-base balance. They are essential components of respiratory pigments, enzymes, and enzyme systems, and they regulate muscular and nervous tissue excitability, blood clotting, and normal heart rhythm.

The three minerals mentioned most commonly are calcium, iron, and sodium. As pointed out later in this chapter, calcium deficiency may result in osteoporosis, and low iron intake can induce iron-deficiency anemia. High sodium intake may contribute to high blood pressure. The specific functions of some of the most important minerals are given in Table 2.4.

Water

Approximately 70% of total body weight is water. Water is the most important nutrient, involved in almost every vital body process: in digesting and absorbing food, in the circulatory process, in removing waste products, in building and rebuilding cells, and in transporting other nutrients.

Water is contained in almost all foods, but primarily in liquid foods, fruits, and vegetables. Besides the natural content in foods, every person should drink about eight glasses of fluids a day.

Energy (ATP) Production

The energy derived from food is not used directly by the cells. It is transferred to form **adenosine triphosphate (ATP)**. The subsequent breakdown of this compound provides the energy used by all energy-requiring processes of the body. ATP must be recycled continually to sustain life and work. ATP can be resynthesized in three ways (also see Figure 2.5):

1. **ATP and ATP-CP system**. The body stores small amounts of ATP and creatine phosphate (CP). These stores are used during all-out activities up

Table 2.4 Major Functions of Minerals

Nutrient	Good Sources	Major Functions	Deficiency Symptoms
Calcium	Milk, yogurt, cheese, green leafy vegetables, dried beans, sardines, and salmon	Required for strong teeth and bone formation; maintenance of good muscle tone, heartbeat, and nerve function.	Bone pain and fractures, periodontal disease, muscle cramps
Iron	Organ meats, lean meats, seafoods, eggs, dried peas and beans, nuts, whole and enriched grains, and green leafy vegetables	Major component of hemoglobin; aids in energy utilization.	Nutritional anemia, and overall weakness
Phosphorus	Meats, fish, milk, eggs, dried beans and peas, whole grains, and processed foods	Required for bone and teeth formation; energy release regulation.	Bone pain and fracture, weight loss, and weakness
Zinc	Milk, meat, seafood, whole grains, nuts, eggs, and dried beans	Essential component of hormones, insulin, and enzymes; used in normal growth and development.	Loss of appetite, slow-healing wounds, and skin problems
Magnesium	Green leafy vegetables, whole grains, nuts, soybeans, seafood, and legumes	Needed for bone growth and maintenance; carbohydrate and protein utilization; nerve function; temperature regulation.	Irregular heartbeat, weakness, muscle spasms, and sleeplessness
Sodium	Table salt, processed foods, and meat	Body fluid regulation; transmission of nerve impulses; heart action.	Rarely seen
Potassium	Legumes, whole grains, bananas, orange juice, dried fruits, and potatoes	Heart action; bone formation and maintenance; regulation of energy release; acid-base regulation.	Irregular heartbeat, nausea, weakness
Selenium	Seafood, meat, whole grains	Component of enzyme; functions in close association with vitamin E.	Muscle pain, possible heart muscle deterioration; possible hair and nail loss

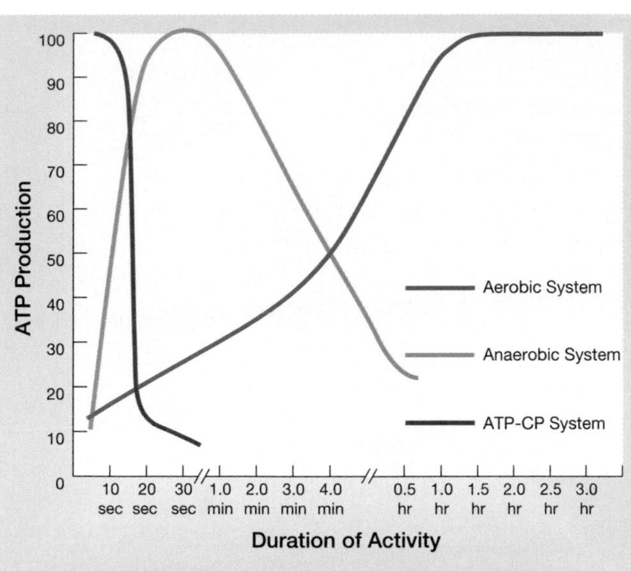

Figure 2.5 Contributions of energy formation mechanisms during various forms of physical activity.

to 10 seconds in duration, such as sprinting, long jumping, and power (weight) lifting. The amount of stored ATP provides energy for just a few seconds. With all-out efforts, ATP is resynthesized from CP, another high-energy phosphate compound. This is referred to as the ATP-CP or phosphagen system.

Depending on the amount of physical training, the concentration of CP stored in cells is sufficient to allow maximum exertion for about 10 seconds. Once the CP stores are depleted, the person is forced to slow down or rest to allow ATP to form through anaerobic and aerobic pathways.

2. *Anaerobic or lactic acid system.* During **anaerobic** exercise that is sustained between 10 and 180 seconds maximum, ATP is replenished from the breakdown of glucose through a series of chemical reactions that do not require oxygen. In the process, though, **lactic acid** is produced, which causes muscular fatigue.

   Because of the accumulation of lactic acid with high-intensity exercise, the formation of ATP during anaerobic activities is limited to about 3 minutes. A recovery period then is necessary to allow for the elimination of lactic acid. Formation of ATP through the anaerobic system is possible from glucose (carbohydrates) only.

3. *Aerobic system.* The production of energy during slow-sustained exercise is derived primarily through **aerobic** metabolism. Both glucose (carbohydrates) and fatty acids (fat) are used in this process. Oxygen is required to form ATP, and under steady-state exercise conditions lactic acid accumulation is minimal.

   Because oxygen is required, a person's capacity to utilize oxygen is crucial for successful athletic performance in aerobic events. The higher the maximal oxygen uptake (VO_{2max}), the greater is the capacity to generate ATP through the aerobic system.

Balancing the Diet

Most people would like to have good health and live life to its fullest. One of the fundamental ways to accomplish this is through a well-balanced diet. As illustrated in Figure 2.6, the generally recommended guideline states that daily caloric intake should be distributed so 58% of the total calories come from carbohydrates (48% complex carbohydrates and 10% sugar), less than 30% of the total calories from fat (equally divided [10% each] among saturated, monounsaturated, and polyunsaturated fats), and 12% of the total calories from protein (0.8 grams of protein per kilogram [2.2 pounds] of body weight). The diet also must include all of the essential vitamins, minerals, and water. To rate a diet accurately is difficult without a complete nutrient analysis.

A diet containing 20% or less fat calories might be necessary to significantly decrease cardiovascular and cancer risk.

The 30% fat guideline has been widely accepted and endorsed by most health organizations during the last two decades. More recently, however, nutritionists and preventive medicine specialists are beginning to point toward a daily fat intake much lower than

Antioxidants Compounds such as vitamins C, E, beta-carotene, and selenium that prevent oxygen from combining with other substances to which it may cause damage.

Minerals Inorganic elements found in the body and in food; essential for normal body functions.

Adenosine triphosphate (ATP) A high-energy chemical compound used for immediate energy by the body.

Anaerobic exercise Exercise that does not require oxygen to produce the necessary energy (ATP) to carry out the activity.

Lactic acid End product of anaerobic glycolysis (metabolism).

Aerobic exercise Exercise that requires oxygen to produce the necessary energy (ATP) to carry out the activity.

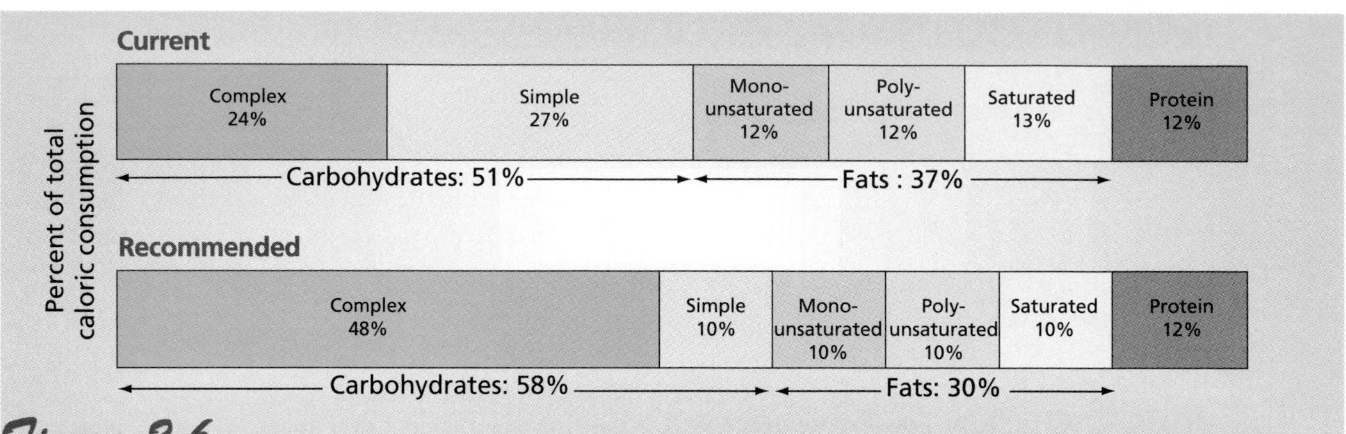

Figure 2.6 Current and recommended carbohydrate, fat, and protein intake.

the current 30% of total calories. In terms of reducing cardiovascular and cancer risk, limiting fat intake to 20% of calories or less might be necessary. Most scientific studies have shown little or no improvement in lowering cholesterol levels while on a 30%-fat diet.[4] The role of high fat intake in increasing cancer risk is undeniable, and the data suggest that an intake of about 20% is better for overall cancer risk reduction.[5] Although the 30% guideline is still valid, a gradual change to a lower value might take effect in the next few years.

Diets in most developed countries have changed significantly since the turn of the century. People in the 1990s eat more fat, fewer carbohydrates, and about the same amount of protein, but fewer calories. At the same time, people weigh more than they did in 1900, an indication that they are not as physically active as their grandparents were.

Diets also were much healthier at the turn of the century. In the United States in 1909, carbohydrates accounted for 57% of the total daily caloric intake, 67% of which were complex carbohydrates. Today, carbohydrate intake has decreased to 51%, and complex carbohydrates account for only 24% of the daily carbohydrate intake. The proportion of fat has risen from 32% to 37%. Protein intake has remained unchanged at about 12% of the total caloric intake.

Nutrient Analysis

The first step in evaluating your diet is to conduct a nutrient analysis. This can be quite educational because most people do not realize how harmful and non-nutritious many common foods are. The analysis covers calories, carbohydrates, fats, cholesterol, and sodium, as well as eight crucial nutrients: protein, calcium, iron, vitamin A, thiamine, riboflavin, niacin, and vitamin C. If the diet has enough of these eight nutrients, the foods consumed in natural form to provide these nutrients typically contain all the other nutrients the human body needs.

To do the nutrient analysis, keep a 3-day record of everything you eat, using the forms in Lab 2A, Figure 2A.1. At the end of each day, look up the nutrient content for those foods in the list of Nutritive Value of Selected Foods, in Appendix A. Record this information on your 3-day listing of foods in Figure 2A.1 (Lab 2A). If you do not find a food in the list given in Appendix A, the information often is stated on the food container itself, or you might refer to the references at the end of the list.

When you have recorded the nutritive values for each day, add up each column and write the totals at the bottom of the chart. After the third day, use Figure 2A.2 and compute an average for the 3 days. To rate your diet, compare your figures with those in the **recommended dietary allowances (RDA)** (Table 2.5). The results give a good indication of areas of strength and deficiency in your current diet.

Every 10 years or so, the National Academy of Sciences issues a new RDA based on a review of the most current research on nutrient needs of healthy people. The RDA provides daily nutrient intake recommendations, usually set high enough to encompass 97.5% of the healthy population in the United States. Stated another way, the RDA recommendation for any nutrient is well above almost everyone's actual requirement.

Between the late 1960s and the early 1990s, nutrient information on labels was expressed in terms of the U. S. RDA — a set of standard values for the average consumer — derived from the 1968 edition of the RDA. In 1993 the Food and Drug Administration (FDA) revised food labeling regulations

Table 2.5 Recommended Dietary Allowances (RDA)

	Calories	Protein	Fat	Sat. Fat	Choles-terol (mg)	Carbo-hydrates	Calcium (mg)	Iron (mg)	Sodium (mg)	Vit. A (I. U.)	Thiamin (Vit. B_1) (mg)	Riboflavin (Vit. B_2) (mg)	Niacin (mg)	Vit. C (mg)
Men 15–18 years	See below[a]	See below[b]	< 30%[c]	< 10%[c]	< 300	58% >[c]	1,200	12	2,400	5,000	1.5	1.8	20	60
Men 19–24 years			< 30%[c]	< 10%[c]	< 300	58% >[c]	1,200	10	2,400	5,000	1.5	1.7	19	60
Men 25–50 years			< 30%[c]	< 10%[c]	< 300	58% >[c]	800	10	2,400	5,000	1.5	1.7	19	60
Men 51 +			< 30%[c]	< 10%[c]	< 300	58% >[c]	800	10	2,400	5,000	1.2	1.4	15	60
Women 15–18 years			< 30%[c]	< 10%[c]	< 300	58% >[c]	1,200	15	2,400	4,000	1.1	1.3	15	60
Women 19–24 years			< 30%[c]	< 10%[c]	< 300	58% >[c]	1,200	15	2,400	4,000	1.1	1.3	15	60
Women 25–50 years			< 30%[c]	< 10%[c]	< 300	58% >[c]	800	15	2,400	4,000	1.1	1.3	15	60
Women 51 +			< 30%[c]	< 10%[c]	< 300	58% >[c]	800	10	2,400	4,000	1.0	1.2	13	60
Pregnant			< 30%[c]	< 10%[c]	< 300	58% >[c]	1,200	30	2,400	4,000	1.5	1.6	17	70
Lactating			< 30%[c]	< 10%[c]	< 300	58% >[c]	1,200	15	2,400	6,000	1.6	1.8	20	95

[a] Use Table 4.1 in Chapter 4 for all categories.
[b] Protein intake should be .8 grams per kilogram of body weight. Pregnant women should consume an additional 15 grams of daily protein; lactating women should have an extra 20 grams.
[c] Percentage of total calories based on recommendations by nutrition experts.
* Adapted from *Recommended Dietary Allowances*, © 1989, by National Academy of Sciences, National Academy Press, Washington DC.

and has replaced the U.S. RDA with **Daily Values** (see Figure 2.7). These daily values are based on a 2,000-calorie diet and may require adjustments depending on an individual's daily caloric needs.

In setting the Daily Values, the FDA first created two sets of standards: Reference Daily Intakes (RDI) and Daily Reference Values (DRV). For FDA purposes, these two sets of standards serve different functions. To avoid consumer confusion in food labeling, however, the FDA combined the RDI and DRV into the Daily Values.

The RDI are reference values for protein, vitamins, and minerals. These are similar in purpose to the old U.S. RDA, but they reflect average allowances based on the 1989 RDA. The DRV are standards for nutrients and food components that do not have an established RDA. The DRV include carbohydrate, fat, saturated fat, fiber, cholesterol, and sodium. These standards (computed in grams and milligrams based on a 2,000-calorie diet) represent dietary intakes to attain or restrict based on a consensus of critical values associated with health. For example, carbohydrate intake should be about 60% of total daily calories (300 grams), and fat intake should be limited to less than 30% (65 grams).

Both the RDA and the Daily Values apply only to healthy people. They are not intended for people who are ill and may require additional nutrients. If you are using the software available with this book, you need only record the foods by code and the number of servings based on the standard amounts given in the list of selected foods in Appendix A (the form provided in Figure 2A.3 of Lab 2A). A sample nutrient analysis printout is shown in Figures 2.8 and 2.9.

Some of the most revealing information learned in a nutrient analysis is the source of fat intake in the diet. The average daily fat consumption in the

Recommended dietary allowances (RDA) Daily suggested intakes of nutrients for normal, healthy people, as developed by National Academy of Sciences.

Daily values A set of standard nutritive values developed by the FDA (replaces the U.S. RDA).

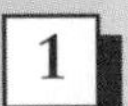

1 Better by Design

How to recognize the new food labels

The new food labels feature a revamped nutrition panel titled "Nutrition Facts," with nutrient listings that reflect current health concerns. Now you'll be able to find information on fat, fiber and other food components fundamental to lowering your risk of cancer and other chronic diseases. Listings for nutrients like thiamin and riboflavin will no longer be required, because Americans generally eat enough of them these days.

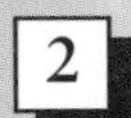

2 Size Up the Situation

All serving sizes are created equal

Now you can compare similar products and know that their serving sizes are basically identical. So when you realize how much fat is packed into that carton of double-dutch-chocolate-caramel-chew ice cream you're eyeing, you might opt for lowfat frozen yogurt instead. Serving sizes will also be standardized, so manufacturers can't make nutrition claims for unrealistically small portions. That means a chocolate cake, for example, must be divided into 8 servings sized to satisfy the average person — not 16 servings sized to satisfy the average munchkin.

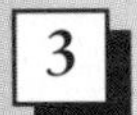

3 Look Before You Leap

Use the Daily Values

You will find the Daily Values on the bottom half of the "Nutrition Facts" panel. Some represent maximum levels of nutrients that should be consumed each day for a healthful diet (as with fat) while others refer to minimum levels that can be exceeded (as with carbohydrates). They are based on both a 2,000 and 2,500 calorie diet. Your own needs may be more or less, but these figures give you a point from which to compare. For example, the sample label indicates that someone with a 2,000 calorie diet should eat no more than 65 grams of fat per day. This is based on a diet getting 30% of calories as fat. If you normally eat less calories, or want to eat less than 30% of calories as fat, your daily fat consumption will be lower.

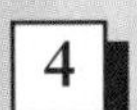

4 Rate It Right

Scan the % Daily Values

The % Daily Values make judging the nutritional quality of a food a snap. For instance, you can look at the % Daily Value column and find that a food has 25% of the Daily Value for fiber. This means the product will give you a substantial portion of the recommended amount of fiber for the day. You can also use this column to compare nutrients in similar products. The % Daily Values are based on a 2,000 calorie diet.

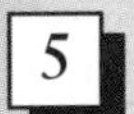

5 Trust Adjectives

Descriptors have legal definitions

Terms like "low," "high" and "free" have long been used on food labels. What these words actually mean, however, could vary. Thanks to the new labeling laws, such descriptions must now meet legal definitions. For example, you may be shopping for foods high in vitamin A, which has been linked to lower risk of certain cancers. Under the new label laws, a food described as "high" in a particular nutrient must contain 20% or more of the Daily Value for that nutrient. So if the bottle of juice you're thinking of buying says "high in vitamin A,'" you can now feel confident that it really is a good source of the vitamin.

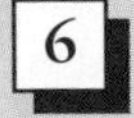

6 Read Health Claims with Confidence

The nutrient link to disease prevention

You can also expect to see food packages with health claims linking certain nutrients to reduced risk of cancer and other diseases. The federal government has approved three health claims dealing with cancer prevention: a low fat diet may reduce your risk for cancer; high fiber foods may reduce your risk for cancer; and fruits and vegetables may reduce your risk for cancer. A food may not make such a health claim for one nutrient if it contains other nutrients that undermine its health benefits. A high fiber, but high fat, jelly doughnut cannot carry a health claim!

1

2

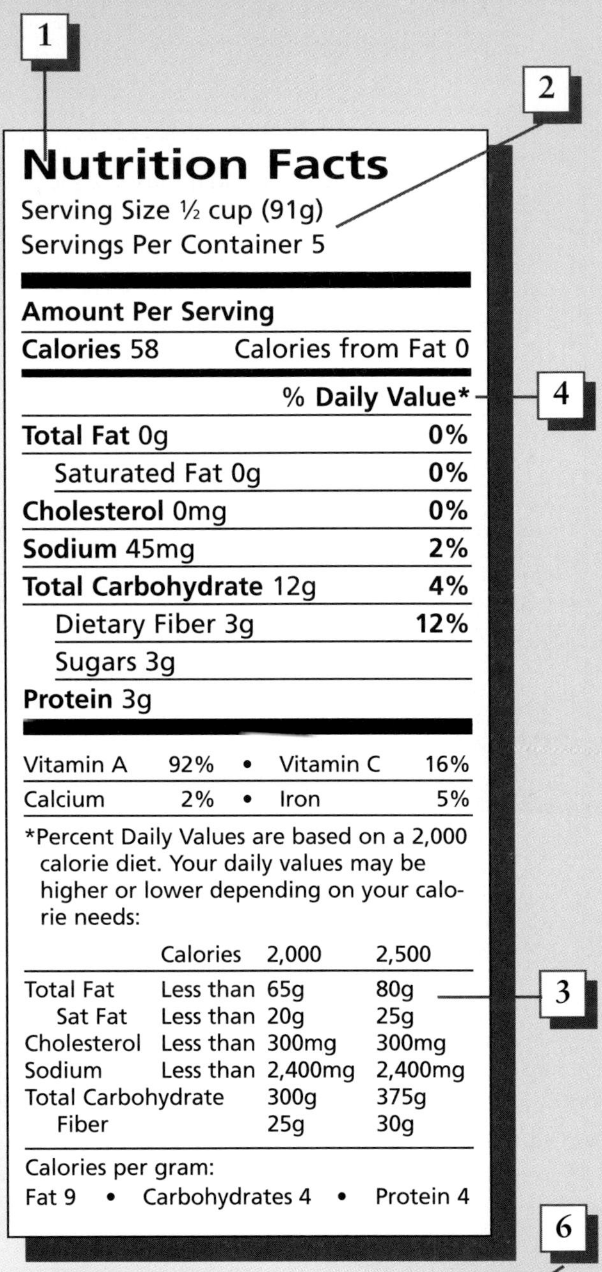

Nutrition Facts

Serving Size ½ cup (91g)
Servings Per Container 5

Amount Per Serving

Calories 58	Calories from Fat 0
	% Daily Value*
Total Fat 0g	**0%**
Saturated Fat 0g	**0%**
Cholesterol 0mg	**0%**
Sodium 45mg	**2%**
Total Carbohydrate 12g	**4%**
Dietary Fiber 3g	**12%**
Sugars 3g	
Protein 3g	

4

Vitamin A	92%	•	Vitamin C	16%
Calcium	2%	•	Iron	5%

*Percent Daily Values are based on a 2,000 calorie diet. Your daily values may be higher or lower depending on your calorie needs:

	Calories	2,000	2,500
Total Fat	Less than	65g	80g
Sat Fat	Less than	20g	25g
Cholesterol	Less than	300mg	300mg
Sodium	Less than	2,400mg	2,400mg
Total Carbohydrate		300g	375g
Fiber		25g	30g

3

Calories per gram:
Fat 9 • Carbohydrates 4 • Protein 4

6

Many factors affect cancer risk. Eating a diet low in fat and high in fiber may lower risk of this disease.

- GOOD SOURCE OF FIBER
- LOWFAT

5

Reprinted with permission from the American Institute for Cancer Research.

Figure 2.7 Food label with U.S. Recommended Daily Values.

NUTRIENT ANALYSIS
Fitness & Wellness Series - Ver 3.96
by Werner W.K. Hoeger & Sharon A. Hoeger
Morton Publishing Company -- Englewood, Colorado

Jane R. Moore Date: 09-12-1996
Age: 20
Body Weight: 141 lbs (64.0 kg)
Activity Rating: Moderate

Food Intake Day One

Food	Amount	Calories	Protein gm	Fat gm	Sat Fat gm	Cholesterol mg	Carbohydrate gm	Calcium mg	Iron mg	Sodium mg	Vit A I.U.	Thiamin mg	Riboflavin mg	Niacin mg	Vit C mg
Cocoa/hot/with whole milk	1 c	218	9.1	9	6.1	33	26	298	0.8	123	318	0.10	0.44	0.4	2
Egg/scrambled w/milk butter	1 egg(s)	95	6.0	7	3.0	244	1	54	0.9	176	510	0.04	0.18	0.0	0
Bread/white	2 slice(s)	136	4.4	2	0.4	0	26	42	1.2	254	0	0.12	0.10	1.2	0
Butter	2 tsp	72	0.0	8	0.8	24	0	2	0.0	92	320	0.00	0.00	0.0	0
Milk/whole	1 c	159	9.0	9	5.1	34	12	288	0.1	120	350	0.07	0.40	0.2	2
Bread/whole wheat	2 slice(s)	122	5.2	2	1.2	0	24	50	1.6	264	0	0.12	0.06	1.4	0
Tuna/canned/oil/drained	1.5 oz.	84	12.5	4	0.9	30	0	4	0.8	69	35	0.02	0.05	5.1	0
Mayonnaise	2 tsp.	72	0.0	8	1.4	6	0	2	0.0	56	26	0.00	0.00	0.0	0
Pickles/dill	1 large	15	0.9	0	0.0	0	3	35	1.4	1,928	140	0.00	0.03	0.0	8
Potato/French fried	20 strips	428	6.8	20	3.4	0	56	24	2.0	10	0	0.20	0.12	4.8	32
Tomato sauce (catsup)	1 tbsp.	16	0.3	0	0.0	0	4	3	0.1	156	105	0.01	0.01	0.2	2
Apple/raw	1 med	80	0.3	1	0.0	0	20	10	0.4	1	120	0.04	0.03	0.1	6
Soda pop/Root beer	12 oz.	140	0.0	0	0.0	0	36	17	0.2	45	0	0.00	0.00	0.0	0
Coleslaw	1 c	173	1.6	17	1.0	5	6	53	0.5	144	190	0.06	0.06	0.4	35
Spaghetti/meat balls/sauce	1 c	332	18.6	12	3.0	75	39	124	3.7	1,009	1,590	0.25	0.30	4.0	22
Pie/apple	1 pc. (3.5 in.)	302	2.6	13	3.5	120	45	9	0.4	355	40	0.02	0.02	0.5	1
Totals Day One		2,444	77.3	112	29.8	571	298	1,015	14.1	4,802	3,744	1.0	1.8	18.3	110

Figure 2.8 Computerized Nutrient Analysis: Sample food list.

2

Jane R. Moore

NUTRIENT ANALYSIS: DAILY ANALYSIS, AVERAGE, AND RECOMMENDED DIETARY ALLOWANCE (RDA) COMPARISON

	Calo-ries	Pro-tein gm	Fat %	Sat Fat %	Cho-les-terol mg	Car-bohy-drate %	Cal-cium mg	Iron mg	Sodium mg	Vit A I.U.	Thi-amin mg	Ribo-fla-vin mg	Nia-cin mg	Vit C mg
Day One	2,444	77.3	40	11	571	48	1,015	14.1	4,802	3,744	1.0	1.8	18.3	110
Day Two	2,139	99.7	43	11	258	38	611	19.7	5,606	1,582	1.1	1.6	21.6	60
Day Three	2,045	86.7	38	15	274	45	885	15.1	3,544	4,791	1.4	2.2	30.8	49
Three Day Average	2,209	87.9	41	12	368	44	837	16.3	4,651	3,372	1.2	1.9	23.6	73
RDA	1,904*	51.2	<30	<10	<300	58>	1,200	15.0	1,904	4,000	1.1	1.3	15.0	60

*Estimated caloric value based on gender, current body weight, and activity rating (does not include additional calories burned through a physical exercise program).

OBSERVATIONS

Daily caloric intake should be distributed in such a way that about 58 percent of the total calories come from carbohydrates and less than 30 percent of the total calories from fat. Protein intake should be about .8 to 1.5 grams per kilogram of body weight or about 12 percent of the total calories. Pregnant women need to consume an additional 15 grams of daily protein, while lactating women should have an extra 20 grams of daily protein (these additional grams of protein are already included in the RDA values for pregnant and lactating women). Saturated fats should constitute less than 10 percent of the total daily caloric intake.
Please note that the daily listings of food intake express the amount of carbohydrates, fat, saturated fat, and protein in grams. However, on the daily analysis and the RDA, only the amount of protein is given in grams. The amount of carbohydrates, fat, and saturated fat are expressed in percent of total calories. The final percentages are based on the total grams and total calories for all days analyzed, not from the average of the daily percentages.

If your average intake for protein, fat, saturated fat, cholesterol, or sodium is high, refer to the daily listings and decrease the intake of foods that are high in those nutrients. If your diet is deficient in carbohydrates, calcium, iron, vitamin A, thiamin, riboflavin, niacin, or vitamin C, refer to the statements below and increase your intake of the indicated foods or consult the list of selected foods in your textbook.

Caloric intake may be too high.

Total fat intake is too high.

Saturated fat intake is too high, which increases your risk for coronary heart disease.

Dietary cholesterol intake is too high. An average consumption of dietary cholesterol above 300 mg/day increases the risk for coronary heart disease. Do you know your blood cholesterol level?

Carbohydrate intake is low. Good sources of carbohydrates are whole grain breads and cereals, pasta, rice, fruits, and vegetables such as potatoes and peas.

Calcium intake is low. Good sources of calcium are milk, yogurt, cheese, green leafy vegetables, dried beans, sardines, and salmon.

Sodium intake is too high.

Vitamin A intake is low. Foods high in vitamin A include skim milk fortified with vit. A, cheese, butter, fortified margarine, eggs (yolk), liver, and dark green/yellow fruits and vegetables.

Figure 2.9 Computerized Nutritional Analysis: Sample daily analysis, average, and RDA comparison.

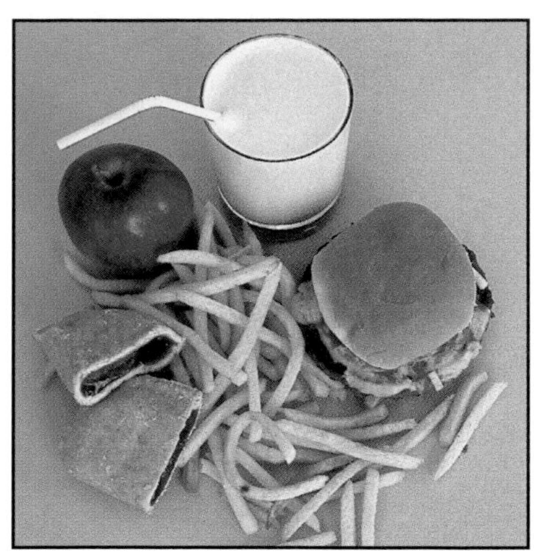

An apple a day will not keep the doctor away if most meals are high in fat content.

American diet is about 37% of the total caloric intake, which greatly increases the risk for chronic diseases such as cardiovascular disease, cancer, diabetes, and obesity. Less than 30% of total calories should come from fat.

As illustrated in Figure 2.10, each gram of carbohydrates and protein supplies the body with 4 calories, and fat provides 9 calories per gram consumed (alcohol yields 7 calories per gram). In this regard, just looking at the total grams consumed for each type of food can be misleading.

For example, a person who eats 160 grams of carbohydrates, 100 grams of fat, and 70 grams of protein has a total intake of 330 grams of food. This indicates that 30% of the total grams of food is in the form of fat (100 grams of fat ÷ 330 grams of total food × 100). In reality, almost half of that diet is fat calories.

In the sample diet, 640 calories are derived from carbohydrates (160 grams × 4 calories per gram), 280 calories from protein (70 grams × 4 calories per gram), and 900 calories from fat (100 grams × 9 calories per gram), for a total of 1,820 calories. If 900 calories are derived from fat, almost half of the total caloric intake is in the form of fat (900 ÷ 1,820 × 100 = 49.5%).

Each gram of fat provides 9 calories. When figuring out the fat content of individual foods, a useful guideline is given in Figure 2.11. Multiply the grams

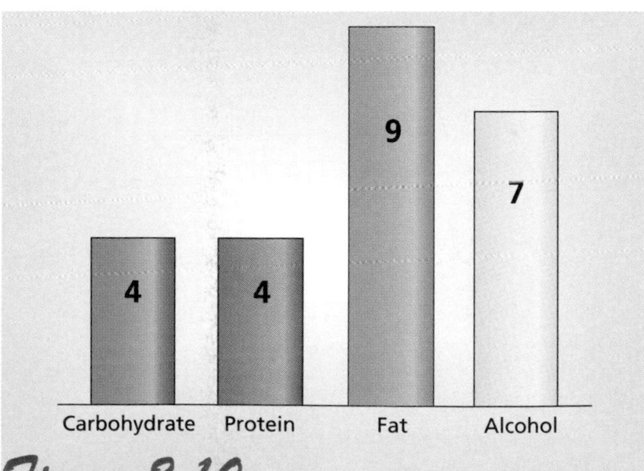

Figure 2.10 Caloric value of food (fuel nutrients).

Nutrition Facts

Serving Size 1 cup (240 ml)
Servings Per Container 4

Amount Per Serving

Calories 120 Calories from Fat 45

	% Daily Value*
Total Fat 5g	**8%**
Saturated Fat 3g	**15%**
Cholesterol 20mg	**7%**
Sodium 120mg	**5%**
Total Carbohydrate 12g	4%
Dietary Fiber 0g	**0%**
Sugars 12g	
Protein 8g	

Vitamin A	10%	Vitamin C	4%
Calcium	30%	Iron	0%

*Percent Daily Values are based on a 2,000 calorie diet. Your daily values may be higher or lower depending on your calorie needs:

	Calories	2,000	2,500
Total Fat	Less than	65g	80g
Sat Fat	Less than	20g	25g
Cholesterol	Less than	300mg	300mg
Sodium	Less than	2,400mg	2,400mg
Total Carbohydrate		300g	375g
Fiber		25g	30g

Calories per gram:
Fat 9 • Carbohydrate 4 • Protein 4

Percent fat calories = (grams of fat × 9) ÷ calories per serving × 100

5 grams of fat × 9 calories per grams of fat = 45 calories from fat

45 calories from fat ÷ 120 calories per serving × 100 = 38% fat

Figure 2.11 Computation for fat content in food.

of fat by 9 and divide by the total calories in that particular food (per serving). You then multiply that number by 100 to get the percentage. For example, if a food label lists a total of 100 calories and 7 grams of fat, the fat content is 63% of total calories. This simple guideline can help you decrease the fat in your diet. The fat content of selected foods, given in grams and as a percent of total calories, is presented in Figure 2.12. The percentage of fat is further subdivided into saturated, monounsaturated, polyunsaturated, and other fatty acids. Beware of products labeled "97% fat-free." These products use weight and not percent of total calories as a measure of fat. Many of these foods still are in the range of 30% fat calories.

Achieving a Balanced Diet

Anyone who has completed a nutrient analysis and has given careful attention to Tables 2.3 (vitamins) and 2.4 (minerals) probably will realize that a well-balanced diet entails eating a variety of foods and reducing daily intake of fats and sweets. The Healthy Eating Pyramid contained in Figure 2.13 provides simple and sound instructions for nutrition. The pyramid contains five major food groups, along with fats, oils, and sweets, which are to be used sparingly. The daily recommended number of servings of the five major food groups are:

1. Six to 11 servings of the bread, cereal, rice, and pasta group.
2. Three to five servings of the vegetable group.
3. Two to four servings of the fruit group.
4. Two to three servings of the milk, yogurt, and cheese group.
5. Two to three servings of the meat, poultry, fish, dry beans, eggs, and nuts group.

As illustrated in the Healthy Eating Pyramid, grains, vegetables, and fruits provide the nutritional base for a healthy diet. Daily fruits and vegetables should include as a minimum, one good source of vitamin A (apricots, cantaloupe, broccoli, carrots, pumpkin, dark leafy vegetables) and one good source of vitamin C (citrus fruit, kiwi fruit, cantaloupe, strawberries, broccoli, cabbage, cauliflower, green pepper).

An entirely new field of research with promising results in disease prevention, especially in the fight against cancer, is in the area of phytochemicals[6] ("phyto" comes from the Greek word for plant). These compounds, just recently discovered by scientists, are found in large quantities in fruits and vegetables.

The main function of phytochemicals in plants is to protect them from sunlight. In humans, they seem to have a powerful ability to block the formation of cancerous tumors. Their actions are so diverse that, at almost every stage of cancer, phytochemicals have the ability to block, disrupt, slow down, or even reverse the process. These compounds are not found in pills. The message here is to eat a diet with ample fruits and vegetables. The recommendation of five to nine servings of fruits and vegetables daily has absolutely no substitute. People can't expect to eat a poor diet, pop a few pills, and derive the same benefits.

Phytochemicals seem to have a powerful ability to block the formation of cancerous tumors.

Milk, poultry, fish, and meats are to be consumed in moderation. Milk should be skim, and milk products should be low-fat. Three ounces of poultry, fish, or meat and not to exceed 6 ounces daily is the recommendation. All visible fat and skin should be trimmed off meats and poultry before cooking. Egg consumption should be limited to no more than three eggs per week.

As an aid in balancing your diet, the form given in Figure 2B.1 in Lab 2B enables you to record your daily food intake. This record is much easier to keep than the complete dietary analysis. Make as many copies of this lab as the number of days you wish to record. Whenever you have something to eat, record, in Figure 2B.1, the food and the amount eaten. Record this information immediately after each meal so you will be able to keep track of your actual food intake more easily.

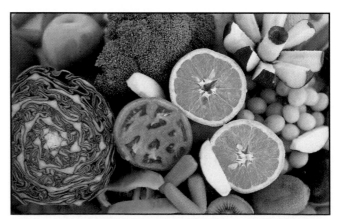

Fruits and vegetables in general contain large amounts of cancer-prevention phytochemicals.

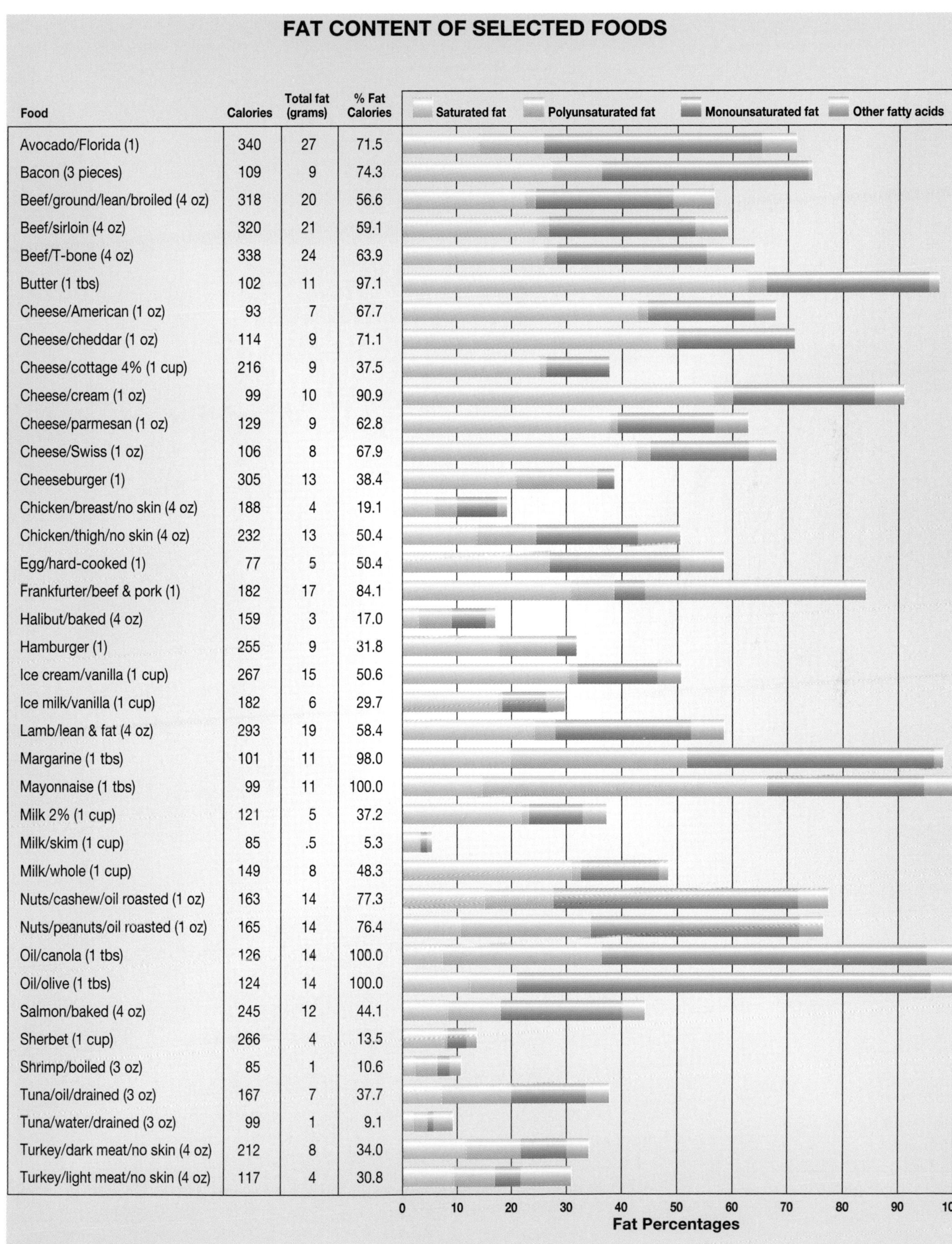

FAT CONTENT OF SELECTED FOODS

Food	Calories	Total fat (grams)	% Fat Calories
Avocado/Florida (1)	340	27	71.5
Bacon (3 pieces)	109	9	74.3
Beef/ground/lean/broiled (4 oz)	318	20	56.6
Beef/sirloin (4 oz)	320	21	59.1
Beef/T-bone (4 oz)	338	24	63.9
Butter (1 tbs)	102	11	97.1
Cheese/American (1 oz)	93	7	67.7
Cheese/cheddar (1 oz)	114	9	71.1
Cheese/cottage 4% (1 cup)	216	9	37.5
Cheese/cream (1 oz)	99	10	90.9
Cheese/parmesan (1 oz)	129	9	62.8
Cheese/Swiss (1 oz)	106	8	67.9
Cheeseburger (1)	305	13	38.4
Chicken/breast/no skin (4 oz)	188	4	19.1
Chicken/thigh/no skin (4 oz)	232	13	50.4
Egg/hard-cooked (1)	77	5	58.4
Frankfurter/beef & pork (1)	182	17	84.1
Halibut/baked (4 oz)	159	3	17.0
Hamburger (1)	255	9	31.8
Ice cream/vanilla (1 cup)	267	15	50.6
Ice milk/vanilla (1 cup)	182	6	29.7
Lamb/lean & fat (4 oz)	293	19	58.4
Margarine (1 tbs)	101	11	98.0
Mayonnaise (1 tbs)	99	11	100.0
Milk 2% (1 cup)	121	5	37.2
Milk/skim (1 cup)	85	.5	5.3
Milk/whole (1 cup)	149	8	48.3
Nuts/cashew/oil roasted (1 oz)	163	14	77.3
Nuts/peanuts/oil roasted (1 oz)	165	14	76.4
Oil/canola (1 tbs)	126	14	100.0
Oil/olive (1 tbs)	124	14	100.0
Salmon/baked (4 oz)	245	12	44.1
Sherbet (1 cup)	266	4	13.5
Shrimp/boiled (3 oz)	85	1	10.6
Tuna/oil/drained (3 oz)	167	7	37.7
Tuna/water/drained (3 oz)	99	1	9.1
Turkey/dark meat/no skin (4 oz)	212	8	34.0
Turkey/light meat/no skin (4 oz)	117	4	30.8

Figure 2.12 Fat content of selected foods.

2

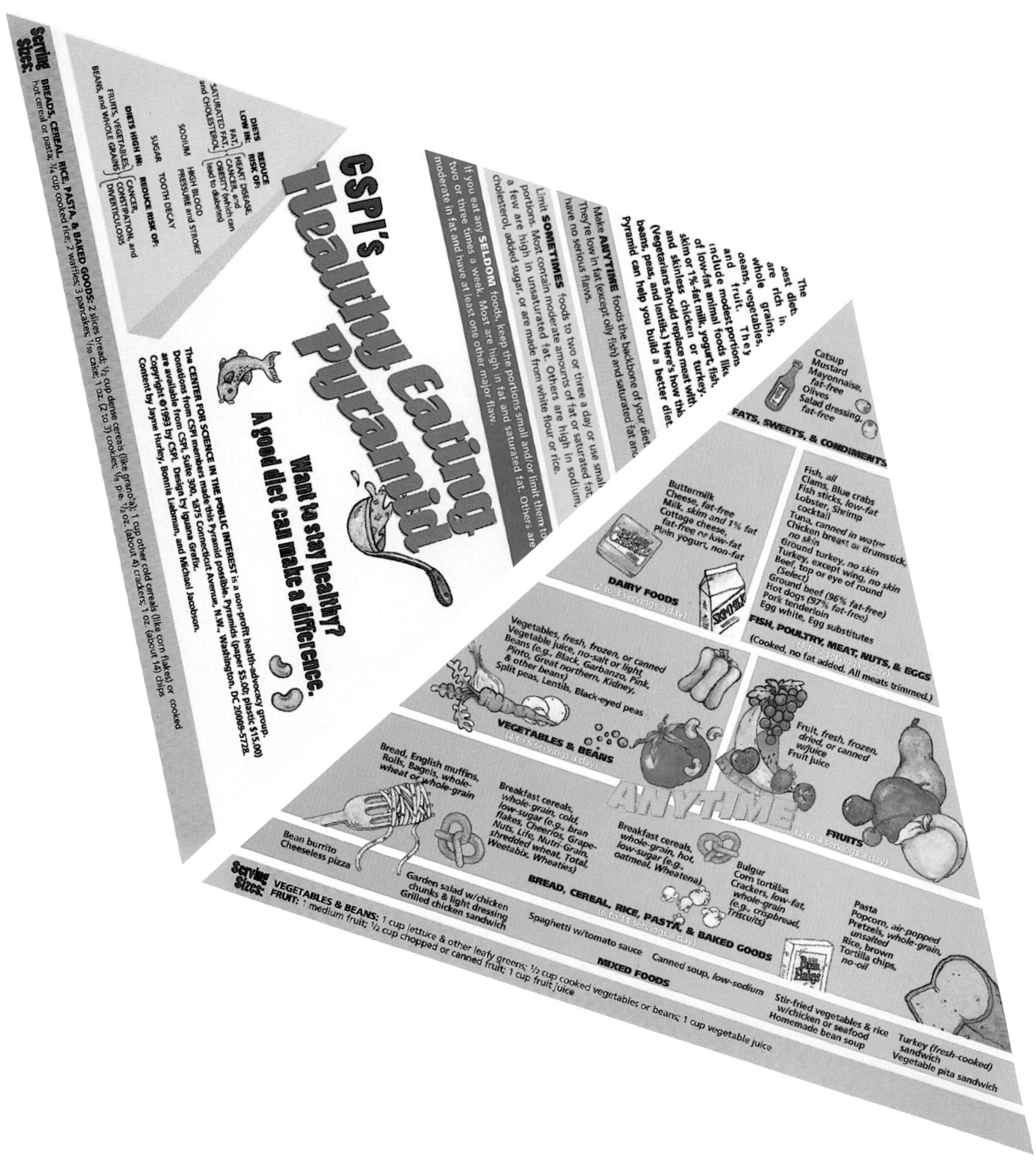

Reprinted with permission from the Center for Science in the Public Interest, 1875 Connecticut Avenue, N.W., Suite 300, Washington, DC, 20009. The Healthy Eating Pyramid can be obtained for $5.00 from the Center for Science in the Public Interest.

Figure 2.13 Healthy Eating Pyramid: A guide to daily food choices.

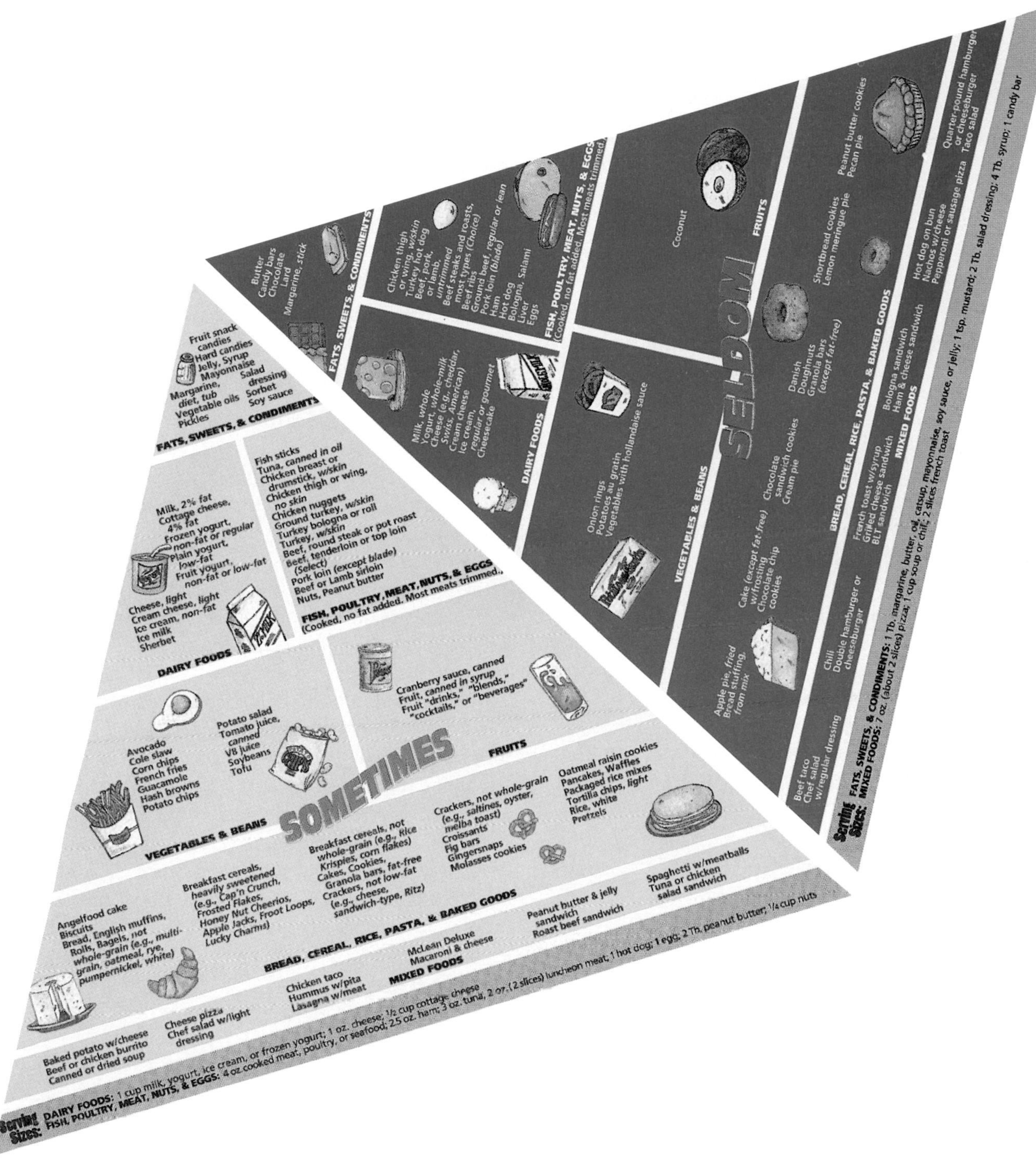
SOMETIMES
FATS, SWEETS, & CONDIMENTS
Fruit snack candies
Hard candies
Jelly, Syrup
Mayonnaise
Margarine, diet, tub
Salad dressing
Sorbet
Vegetable oils
Soy sauce
Pickles
DAIRY FOODS
Milk, 2% fat
Cottage cheese, 4% fat
Frozen yogurt, non-fat or regular
Plain yogurt, low-fat
Fruit yogurt, non-fat or low-fat
Cheese, light
Cream cheese, light
Ice cream, non-fat
Ice milk
Sherbet
FISH, POULTRY, MEAT, NUTS, & EGGS
(Cooked, no fat added. Most meats trimmed.)
Fish sticks
Tuna, canned in oil
Chicken breast or drumstick, w/skin
Chicken thigh or wing, no skin
Chicken nuggets
Ground turkey, w/skin
Turkey bologna or roll
Turkey, w/skin
Beef, round steak or pot roast
Beef, tenderloin or top loin (Select)
Pork loin (except blade)
Beef or Lamb sirloin
Nuts, Peanut butter
VEGETABLES & BEANS
Avocado
Cole slaw
Corn chips
French fries
Guacamole
Hash browns
Potato chips
Potato salad
Tomato juice, canned
V8 juice
Soybeans
Tofu
FRUITS
Cranberry sauce, canned
Fruit, canned in syrup
Fruit "drinks," "blends," "cocktails," or "beverages"
BREAD, CEREAL, RICE, PASTA, & BAKED GOODS
Angelfood cake
Biscuits
Bread, English muffins, Rolls, Bagels, not whole-grain (e.g., multi-grain, oatmeal, rye, pumpernickel, white)
Breakfast cereals, heavily sweetened (e.g., Cap'n Crunch, Frosted Flakes, Honey Nut Cheerios, Apple Jacks, Froot Loops, Lucky Charms)
Breakfast cereals, not whole-grain (e.g., Rice Krispies, corn flakes)
Cakes, Cookies, Granola bars, fat-free
Crackers, not low-fat (e.g., cheese, sandwich-type, Ritz)
Crackers, not whole-grain (e.g., saltines, oyster, melba toast)
Croissants
Fig bars
Gingersnaps
Molasses cookies
Oatmeal raisin cookies
Pancakes, Waffles
Packaged rice mixes
Tortilla chips, light
Rice, white
Pretzels
MIXED FOODS
Baked potato w/cheese
Beef or chicken burrito
Canned or dried soup
Cheese pizza
Chef salad w/light dressing
Chicken taco
Hummus w/pita
Lasagna w/meat
McLean Deluxe
Macaroni & cheese
Peanut butter & jelly sandwich
Roast beef sandwich
Spaghetti w/meatballs
Tuna or chicken salad sandwich
Serving Sizes: DAIRY FOODS: 1 cup milk, yogurt, ice cream, or frozen yogurt; 1 oz. cheese; ½ cup cottage cheese
FISH, POULTRY, MEAT, NUTS, & EGGS: 4 oz cooked meat, poultry, or seafood; 2.5 oz. ham; 3 oz. tuna, 2 oz. (2 slices) luncheon meat; 1 hot dog; 1 egg; 2 Tb. peanut butter; ¼ cup nuts
SELDOM
FATS, SWEETS, & CONDIMENTS
Butter
Candy bars
Chocolate
Lard
Margarine, stick
FISH, POULTRY, MEAT, NUTS, & EGGS
(Cooked, no fat added. Most meats trimmed.)
Chicken thigh or wing, w/skin
Turkey hot dog
Beef, pork, or lamb, untrimmed
Beef steaks and roasts, most types (Choice)
Beef ribs
Ground beef, regular or lean
Pork loin (blade)
Ham
Hot dog
Bologna, Salami
Liver
Eggs
DAIRY FOODS
Milk, whole
Yogurt, whole-milk
Cheese (e.g., cheddar, Swiss, American)
Cream cheese
Ice cream, regular or gourmet
Cheesecake
FRUITS
Coconut
VEGETABLES & BEANS
Onion rings
Potatoes au gratin
Vegetables with hollandaise sauce
BREAD, CEREAL, RICE, PASTA, & BAKED GOODS
Apple pie, fried
Bread stuffing, from mix
Cake (except fat-free) w/frosting
Chocolate chip cookies
Chocolate sandwich cookies
Cream pie
Danish
Doughnuts
Granola bars (except fat-free)
Shortbread cookies
Lemon meringue pie
Peanut butter cookies
Pecan pie
MIXED FOODS
Beef taco
Chef salad w/regular dressing
Chili
Double hamburger or cheeseburger
French toast w/syrup
Grilled cheese sandwich
BLT sandwich
Bologna sandwich
Ham & cheese sandwich
Hot dog on bun
Nachos w/cheese
Pepperoni or sausage pizza
Quarter-pound hamburger or cheeseburger
Taco salad
Serving Sizes: FATS, SWEETS, & CONDIMENTS: 1 Tb. margarine, butter, oil, catsup, mayonnaise, soy sauce, or jelly; 1 tsp. mustard; 2 Tb. salad dressing; 4 Tb. syrup; 1 candy bar
MIXED FOODS: 7 oz. (about 2 slices) pizza; 1 cup soup or chili; 2 slices french toast

Figure 2.13 Continued.

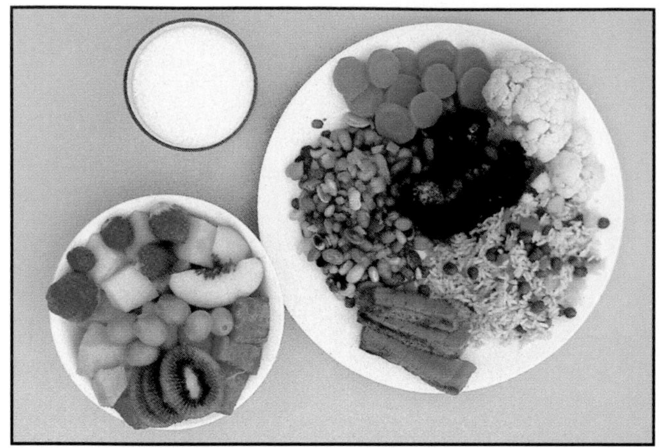

Contemporary Nutrition Concept: Restructuring your meals so rice, pasta, beans, breads, and vegetables are the main course; if meats are used, they should be used as a side dish or added primarily for flavoring; fruits should be used for desserts and low or nonfat milk products are used.

If you eat twice the amount of a standard serving, double the number of servings. Evaluate your diet by checking whether you ate the minimum required servings for each food group. If you meet the minimum required servings at the end of each day, you are doing well in balancing your diet.

Restructure your meals on the plate so rice, pasta, beans, breads, and vegetables are in the center, meats are on the side and are added primarily for flavoring, and desserts consist of fruits. Substitute lowfat or nonfat milk and milk products. This is another strategy to help you enjoy a healthy diet, prevent disease, and improve your overall quality of life.

Nutrient Supplementation

According to the Food and Drug Administration, four of every 10 adults in the United States take nutrient supplements daily, and one in every seven has a nutrient intake almost eight times the RDA. With some exceptions, vitamin and mineral requirements for the body can be met by consuming as few as 1200 calories per day, as long as the diet contains the recommended servings from the five food groups.

Water-soluble vitamins cannot be stored as long as fat-soluble vitamins. The body excretes excessive intakes readily. Small amounts, however, can be retained for weeks or months in various organs and tissues of the body. Fat-soluble vitamins, on the other hand, are stored in fatty tissue. Therefore, daily intake of these vitamins is not as crucial. Too much vitamin A and vitamin D actually can be detrimental to health.

People should not take **megadoses** of vitamins. Mineral doses should not exceed three times the RDA.

Presently, no standard percentage above the RDA is available to guide us in determining the level at which a high dose of a given nutrient may cause health problems. For some nutrients, a dose of five times the RDA taken over several months may create problems. For others, it may not pose any threat to human health.

Iron deficiency (determined through blood testing) is common in women. Iron supplementation frequently is recommended for these women who have heavy menstrual flow. Some pregnant and lactating women also may require supplements. According to 1990 guidelines by the National Academy of Science, the average pregnant woman who eats an adequate amount of a variety of foods needs only to take a low dose of iron supplement daily. Women who are pregnant with more than one baby may need additional supplements. In the above instances, supplements should be taken under a physician's supervision.

Other people who may benefit from supplementation are alcoholics and street-drug users who do not have a balanced diet, smokers, strict vegetarians, individuals on extremely low-calorie diets, elderly people who don't eat balanced meals regularly, and newborn infants (usually given a single dose of vitamin K to prevent abnormal bleeding). While some supplements are encouraged (see discussion that follows), for healthy people with a balanced diet, most supplements do not seem to provide additional benefits. They do not help people run faster, jump higher, relieve stress, improve sexual prowess, cure a common cold, or boost energy levels.

Antioxidants: Free Radical Combatants

Much research currently is being done to study the effects of antioxidant supplements in thwarting several chronic diseases. Vitamins C, E, beta-carotene (a precursor to vitamin A), and the mineral selenium serve as antioxidants, preventing oxygen from combining with other substances it may damage (see Table 2.6). Oxygen is utilized during metabolism to change carbohydrates and fats into energy. During this process oxygen is transformed into stable forms of water and carbon dioxide. A small amount of oxygen, however, ends up in an unstable form, referred to as **oxygen free radicals**.

Table 2.6 Antioxidant Nutrients, Sources, and Functions

Nutrient	Good Sources	Antioxidant Effect
Vitamin C	Citrus fruit, kiwi fruit, cantaloupe, strawberries, broccoli, green or red peppers, cauliflower, cabbage	Appears to inactivate oxygen-free radicals
Vitamin E	Vegetable oils, yellow and green leafy vegetables, margarine, wheat germ, oatmeal, almonds, and whole grain breads, cereals	Protects lipids from oxidation.
Beta-carotene	Carrots, squash, pumpkin, sweet potatoes, broccoli, green leafy vegetables	Soaks up oxygen-free radicals
Selenium	Seafood, meat, whole grains	Helps prevent damage to cell structures

A free radical molecule has a normal proton nucleus with a single unpaired electron. Having only one electron makes the free radical extremely reactive, and it constantly looks to pair the electron up with one from another molecule. When a free radical steals the second electron from another molecule, that other molecule in turn becomes a free radical. This chain reaction goes on until two free radicals meet to form a stable molecule. Antioxidants help stabilize free radicals so they will not be as reactive until a match can be found.

Free radicals attack and damage proteins and lipids, in particular the cell membrane and DNA. This damage is thought to contribute to the development of conditions such as cardiovascular disease, cancer, emphysema, cataracts, Parkinson's disease, and premature aging. Solar radiation, cigarette smoke, radiation, and other environmental factors also seem to encourage the formation of free radicals. Antioxidants are thought to offer protection by absorbing free radicals before they can cause damage and also by interrupting the sequence of reactions once damage has begun, thwarting certain chronic diseases (see Figure 2.14).

Antioxidants are found abundantly in food, especially in fruits and vegetables. Unfortunately, only 9% of Americans eat the minimum five daily servings of fruits and vegetables[7] (five to nine are recommended). In a departure from past recommendations, in 1994 the editorial board of the *University of California at Berkeley Wellness Letter* issued the following antioxidant supplementation guidelines for people who eat at least five daily servings of antioxidant-rich fruits and vegetables:[8]

- 250 to 500 mg of vitamin C.
- 200 to 800 IU of vitamin E.
- 10,000 to 25,000 IU of beta-carotene.

Megadoses For most vitamins, 10 times the RDA or more. For A and D, five and two times the RDA, respectively.

Oxygen free radicals Substances formed during metabolism which attack and damage proteins and lipids, in particular the cell membrane and DNA, leading to the development of diseases such as heart disease, cancer, and emphysema.

IU International units, for measuring nutrients.

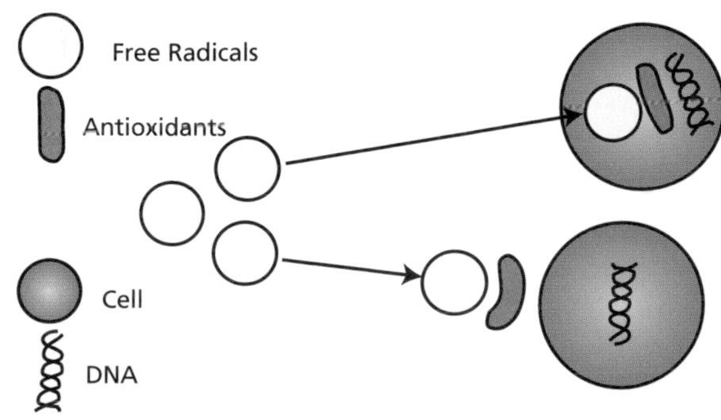

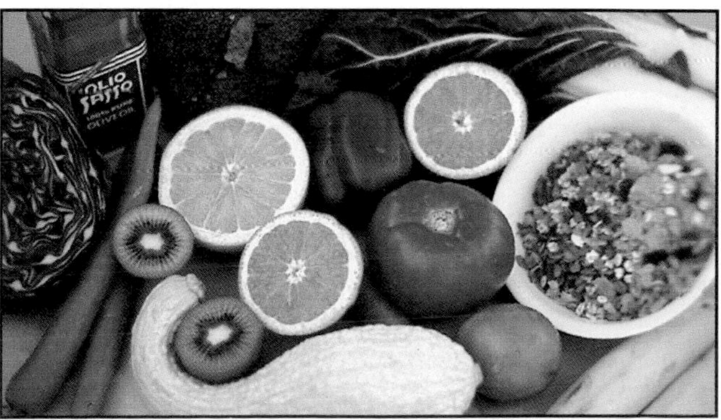

Figure 2.14 Antioxidant protection: blocking and absorbing oxygen-free radicals to prevent chronic diseases.

2

In a special report, the editorial board also issued the following statement:[9]

> The editorial board of the Wellness Letter has been reluctant to recommend supplementary vitamins on a broad scale for healthy people eating healthy diets. But the accumulation of research in recent years has caused us to change our minds.

Based on these recommendations, people who consume nine ample amounts of fresh fruits and vegetables daily could get their daily beta-carotene and vitamin C requirements through the diet. To obtain the recommended guideline for vitamin E through diet alone, however, is practically impossible. As shown in Table 2.7, vitamin E is not easily found in large quantities in foods typically consumed in the diet. Thus, supplements are encouraged. When supplements (in general) are taken, they should be taken with meals and split in two to three doses per day.[10]

Based on newly released evidence in 1996, the editorial board of *University of California at Berkeley Wellness Letter* has indicated that it is better to obtain your daily dose of beta-carotene from natural sources (food) and not from supplements (pills).[11]

Two separate clinical trials found that beta-carotene supplements offered no protection against heart disease and cancer. One of these studies actually found a higher lung cancer and mortality rate in smokers who took beta-carotene supplements. For former smokers and nonsmokers, these supplements do not cause any harm but offer no additional health benefits either. It is therefore recommended that you "skip the pill and eat the carrot." One medium raw carrot contains about 20,000 IU of beta-carotene (the recommended daily dose). Supplements of vitamin E and C are still encouraged as they offer several potential health benefits.

Supplements of the mineral selenium are not recommended at this point, although one Brazil nut per day seems to provide the necessary amount of antioxidant for this nutrient. Five or more Brazil nuts per day can lead to toxic levels of this mineral in the body.[12]

Although not an antioxidant, folacin (a B vitamin) also is recommended (400 mcg) for all premenopausal women.[13] Folacin helps prevent certain birth defects and seems to offer protection against colon and cervical cancers.

Toxic effects with antioxidant supplementation are rare when taken in the previously recommended amounts. Generally, up to 4,000 mg of vitamin C, 3,200 IU of vitamin E, and 50,000 IU of beta-carotene seem safe. If any of the following side effects arise, stop supplementation and check with your physician:

- Vitamin E: gastrointestinal disturbances; increase in blood lipids (determined through blood tests).

Table 2.7 Antioxidant Content of Selected Foods

Beta-Carotene		IU
Apricot (1 medium)		675
Broccoli (½ cup, frozen)		1,740
Broccoli (½ cup, raw)		680
Cantaloupe (1 cup)		5,160
Carrot (1 medium, raw)		20,255
Green peas (½ cup, frozen)		535
Mango (1 medium)		8,060
Mustard greens (½ cup, frozen)		3,350
Papaya (1 medium)		6,120
Spinach (½ cup, frozen)		7,395
Sweet potato (1 medium, baked)		24,875
Tomato (1 medium)		1,395
Turnip greens (½ cup, boiled)		3,960
Vitamin C		**mg**
Acerola (1 cup, raw)		1,640
Acerola juice (8 oz)		3,864
Cantaloupe (½ melon, medium)		90
Cranberry juice (8 oz)		90
Grapefruit (½, medium, white)		52
Grapefruit juice (8 oz)		92
Guava (1 medium)		165
Kiwi (1 medium)		75
Lemon juice (8 oz)		110
Orange (1 medium)		66
Orange juice (8 oz)		120
Papaya (1 medium)		85
Pepper (½ cup, red, chopped, raw)		95
Strawberries (1 cup, raw)		88
Vitamin E	**IU**	**mg***
Almond oil (1 tbsp)		5.3
Almonds (1 oz)	10.1	
Canola oil (1 tbsp)		9.0
Cottonseed oil (1 tbsp)		5.2
Hazelnuts (1 oz)	4.4	
Kale (1 cup)	15.0	
Margarine (1 tbsp)		2.0
Peanuts (1 oz)	3.0	
Shrimp (3 oz, boiled)	3.1	
Sunflower seeds (1 oz, dry)	14.2	
Sunflower seed oil (1 tbsp)		6.9
Sweet potato (1 medium, baked)	7.2	
Wheat germ oil (1 tbsp)		20.0

* Vitamin E values for oils are commonly expressed in milligrams (mg). One mg is almost equal to 1 IU (international unit).

- Vitamin C: nausea, diarrhea, abdominal cramps, kidney stones, liver problems.
- Beta-carotene: although not harmful, yellow pigmentation of the skin.
- Selenium: vomiting, diarrhea, irritability, fatigue, lesions of the skin and nervous tissue, loss of hair and nails.

Large supplements of vitamin E are not recommended for individuals on **anticoagulant** therapy. Vitamin E is an anticoagulant in itself. If you are on such therapy, check with your physician. Pregnant women need a physician's approval prior to beta-carotene supplementation. It also may be unsafe if taken with alcohol and by people who drink more than 4 ounces of pure alcohol per day (the equivalent of eight beers).

A few researchers are expressing concern for people who participate regularly in high-intensity exercise (above 70% of heart rate reserve — see Chapter 6) or prolonged exercise (more than 5 hours per week). Overtraining increases the production of free radicals and well may exceed the body's antioxidant defense mechanism. This high amount of free radicals may increase the risk for chronic diseases, including cancer.[14]

Scientists, therefore, are examining a possible link between "heavy" exercise and disease in people who otherwise lead a healthy lifestyle. Although the research is scarce, Dr. Kenneth Cooper, in his book *Antioxidant Revolution*, recommends higher doses of antioxidants for athletes and heavy exercisers: 3000 mg of vitamin C, 1200 IU of vitamin E, and 50,000 IU of beta-carotene.[15] Awareness of side effects is important if these higher amounts are taken.

Many people who regularly eat foods high in fat content or too many sweets think they need supplementation to balance their diet. This is another fallacy about nutrition. The problem in these cases is not necessarily a lack of vitamins and minerals but, instead, a diet too high in calories, fat, and sodium. Vitamin, mineral, and fiber supplements do not supply all of the nutrients and other beneficial substances present in food and needed for good health. Supplements are no substitute for a well-balanced diet.

Wholesome foods contain vitamins, minerals, carbohydrates, fiber, proteins, fats, phytochemicals, and others not yet discovered. Researchers do not know if the protective effects are caused by the antioxidants themselves, in combination with other nutrients (such as phytochemicals), or actually by some other nutrients in food that have not been investigated yet. Many nutrients work in **synergy**, enhancing chemical processes in the body. Supplementation will not offset poor eating habits. Pills are no substitute for common sense.

If you think your diet is not balanced, you first need to conduct a nutrient analysis to determine which nutrients are missing. Use the Healthy Eating Pyramid and the vitamin and mineral tables in this chapter, and eat more of the foods high in antioxidants and phytochemicals, and those with nutrients that are deficient in your diet.

Specific Nutrition Considerations

Nutrition for Athletes

The two main fuels that supply energy for physical activity are glucose and fat (fatty acids). The body uses amino acids, derived from proteins, as an energy substrate when glucose is low, such as during fasting, prolonged aerobic exercise, or a low carbohydrate diet.

Glucose is derived from foods high in carbohydrates such as breads, cereals, grains, pasta, beans, fruits, vegetables, and sweets in general. Glucose is stored as **glycogen** in muscles and the liver. As noted earlier in the chapter, fatty acids are derived from the breakdown of fats. Unlike glucose, an almost unlimited supply of fatty acids, stored as fat in the body, can be used during exercise.

During resting conditions fat supplies about two-thirds of the energy to sustain the vital processes. During exercise the body uses both glucose and fat in combination to supply the energy demands. The proportion of fat to glucose changes with the intensity of exercise. When exercising below 60% to 70% of the individual's maximal work capacity, fat is used as the primary energy substrate. As the intensity of exercise increases, so does the percentage of glucose utilization, up to 100% during maximal work sustained for 2 to 3 minutes.

In general, athletes do not require special supplementation or any other special type of diet. Unless

Anticoagulant Any substance that inhibits blood clotting.

Synergy A reaction in which the result is greater than the sum of its two parts.

Glycogen Form in which glucose is stored in muscle.

the diet is deficient in basic nutrients, no special, secret, or magic diet will help people perform better or develop faster as a result of what they eat. As long as the diet is balanced, based on a large variety of nutrients from the basic food groups, athletes do not require supplements. Even in strength training and body building, protein in excess of 20% of total daily caloric intake is not necessary.

The main difference between a sedentary person and a highly active individual is in the total number of calories required daily and the amount of carbohydrate intake during bouts of prolonged physical activity. During training, people consume more calories because of the greater energy expenditure required as a result of intense physical training.

Carbohydrate Loading

While on a regular diet, the body is able to store between 1,500 and 2,000 calories in the form of glycogen. About 75% of this glycogen is stored in muscle tissue. This amount, however, can be increased greatly through **carbohydrate loading**.

A regular diet should be altered during several days of heavy aerobic training or when a person is going to participate in a long-distance event of more than 90 minutes (for example, marathon, triathlon, road cycling). For events shorter than 90 minutes, carbohydrate loading does not seem to enhance performance.

During prolonged exercise, glycogen is broken down into glucose, which then is readily available to the muscle for energy production. In comparison to fat, glucose frequently is referred to as the "high-octane fuel" because it provides about 6% more energy per unit of oxygen consumed.

Heavy training over several consecutive days leads to glycogen depletion faster than it can be replaced through the diet. Glycogen depletion with heavy training is common in athletes. Signs of depletion include chronic fatigue, difficulty in maintaining accustomed exercise intensity, and lower performance.

On consecutive days of exhaustive physical training (several hours daily), a carbohydrate-rich diet, 70% of total daily caloric intake or 8 grams of carbohydrate per 2.2 pounds of body weight, is recommended. This diet often restores glycogen levels in 24 hours. Along with the high-carbohydrate diet, a day of rest often is needed to allow the muscles to recover from glycogen depletion following days of intense training. For people who exercise less than an hour a day, a 60% carbohydrate diet or 6 grams of carbohydrate per 2.2 pounds (1 kilogram) of body weight is enough to restore glycogen stores.

Following an exhaustive workout, eating a combination of carbohydrates and protein (tuna sandwich) within 30 minutes of exercise seems to speed up glycogen storage at an even faster rate.[16] Protein intake increases insulin activity, thus enhancing glycogen replenishment. A 70% carbohydrate intake then should be maintained throughout the rest of the day.

By following a special diet/exercise regimen 5 days before a long-distance event, highly trained (aerobically) individuals are capable of storing two to three times the amount of glycogen found in the average person. Athletic performance may be enhanced for long-distance events of more than 90 minutes by eating a regular balanced diet along with intensive physical training the fifth and fourth days before the event, followed by a diet high in carbohydrates (about 70%) and a gradual decrease in training intensity the 3 days before the event.

The amount of glycogen stored as a result of a carbohydrate-rich diet does not seem to be related to the proportion of complex and simple carbohydrates. Intake of simple carbohydrate (sugar) can be raised while on a 70% carbohydrate diet, as long as 48% of the total calories are derived from complex carbohydrates. The latter provide more nutrients and fiber, making them a better choice for a healthier diet.

On the day of the long-distance event, high carbohydrates are still the recommended choice of substrate. But high sugar intake 30 minutes prior to the event might be counterproductive. A "sugar shock" shortly before the event can cause **hypoglycemia**. The pancreas responds to high sugar intake with a large production of insulin. **Insulin** in turn lowers blood glucose. Further, the muscles draw glucose from the blood at the start of exercise, exacerbating the condition.

As a rule of thumb, individuals should consume 1 gram of carbohydrate for each 2.2 pounds of body weight 1 hour prior to exercise. The amount of carbohydrate can be increased to 2, 3, or 4 grams per 2.2 pounds of weight 2, 3, or 4 hours, respectively, before exercise.

During the long-distance event, researchers recommend that 50 to 60 grams of carbohydrate (200 to 240 calories) be consumed every hour. This is best accomplished by drinking 8 ounces of a 6% to 8% carbohydrate sports drink every 15 minutes. This also lessens the chance of dehydration during exercise, which hinders performance and endangers health.

The percentage of the carbohydrate drink is determined by dividing the amount of carbohydrate in grams by the amount of fluid, in ml, and multiplying by 100. For example, 18 grams of carbohydrate in 240 ml (8 oz) of fluid yields a drink at 7.5% ($18 \div 240 \times 100$).

Amino Acid Supplements

A myth regarding athletic performance is that protein (amino acid) supplements will increase muscle mass. The claims and safety of these products have not been proven scientifically. The RDA for protein is .8 grams per kilogram of body weight.

Most athletes, including weight lifters and body builders, increase their caloric intake automatically during intense training. As caloric intake increases, so does the intake of protein, approaching in many instances 2 or more grams per kilogram of body weight. This amount is more than enough to build and repair muscle tissue. Athletes in strength training typically consume between 3 and 4 grams per kilogram of body weight.

People who take costly free-amino acid supplements are led to believe that this contributes to the development of muscle mass. The human body cannot distinguish between amino acids obtained from food or through supplements. Excess protein either is used for energy or is turned into fat. With amino acid supplements, each capsule provides up to 500 milligrams of amino acids and no additional nutrients. Three ounces of meat or fish provide more than 20,000 milligrams of amino acids, along with other essential nutrients such as iron, niacin, and thiamin.

Proponents of free-amino acid supplements further claim that only a small amount of amino acids in food is absorbed and that free-amino acids are absorbed more readily than protein food. Neither claim is correct. The human body absorbs and utilizes between 85% and 99% of all protein from food intake. The body handles whole proteins better than single amino acids predigested in the laboratory setting.

Amino acid supplementation can even be dangerous to the body. Supplementation of a group of chemically similar amino acids often prevents the absorption of other amino acids, potentially causing critical imbalances and toxicities. Long-term risks associated with amino acid supplementation have not been determined.

The rate of absorption provides no additional benefit because building muscle takes hours, not minutes. Muscle overload through heavy training, not supplementation, builds muscle. Expensive protein supplements benefit only those who stand to gain financial benefits from selling them.

Bone Health and Osteoporosis

In **osteoporosis,** bones, primarily of the hip, wrist, and spine, become so weak and brittle that they fracture readily. Osteoporosis is preventable. The process begins slowly in the third and fourth decades of life. Women are especially susceptible after menopause because of the accompanying **estrogen** loss, which increases the rate at which bone mass is broken down.

Approximately 15 to 20 million women in the United States have osteoporosis, and about 1.5 million fractures are attributed to this condition each year. An estimated 30,000 to 60,000 of the 200,000 women with hip fractures die of complications resulting from these fractures. According to Dr. Barbara Drinkwater, a leading researcher in this area, "Shocking as these figures are, they cannot adequately convey the pain and deterioration in the quality of life of women who suffer the crippling effects of osteoporotic fractures."[17]

In maximizing bone density in young women and decreasing the rate of bone loss later in life, the importance of normal estrogen levels, adequate calcium intake, and physical activity cannot be overemphasized (see Figure 2.15). All three factors are crucial in preventing osteoporosis. The absence of any one of these three factors leads to bone loss for which the other two factors never completely compensate.

Prevention of osteoporosis begins early in life by having enough calcium in the diet (the RDA is 800 to 1200 mg per day) and by participating in exercise. The calcium RDA can be met easily through diet alone. Some experts, however, recommend calcium supplements for children before puberty. Along with adequate calcium intake, an additional amount of vitamin D may be needed for optimal calcium

Carbohydrate loading Increasing intake of carbohydrates during heavy aerobic training or prior to aerobic endurance events lasting longer than 90 minutes.

Hypoglycemia Low blood sugar (glucose).

Insulin Hormone secreted by the pancreas used in the absorption and utilization of glucose by the body.

Osteoporosis The softening, deterioration, or loss of total body bone.

Estrogen Female sex hormone; essential for bone formation and bone density conservation.

2

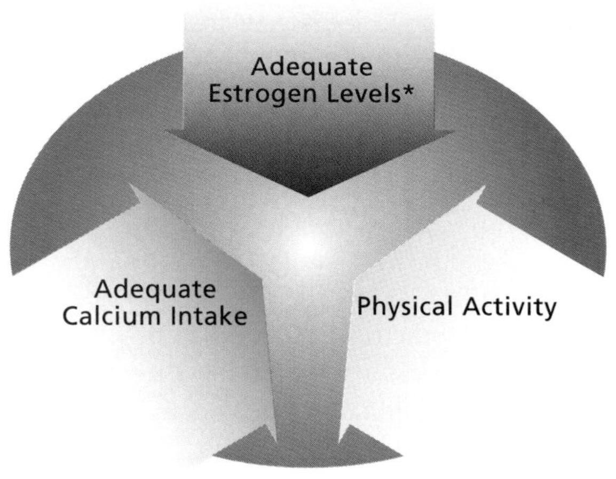

*Most important factor in the prevention of osteoporosis.

Figure 2.15 Factors that impact the prevention of osteoporosis.

absorption. Table 2.8 provides a list of selected foods with their calcium content. A common recommendation is that women after age 45 get 1,500 mg of calcium per day and men, 1,000 mg.

Also, high protein intake may affect calcium absorption by the body. The more protein eaten, the higher the calcium content in the urine. This might be the reason why countries with a high protein intake, including the United States, also have the highest rates of osteoporosis.

The key role of exercise in preventing osteoporosis seems to be related to the decrease in rate of bone density loss following menopause. Active people are able to maintain bone density much more effectively than their inactive counterparts, helping to prevent osteoporosis. A combination of weight-bearing exercises, such as walking or jogging and weight training, is especially helpful. The benefits of exercise go beyond maintaining bone density. Exercise strengthens muscles, ligaments, and tendons — all of which provide support to the bones (skeleton). Exercise also improves balance and coordination, which can help prevent falls and injuries.

Current studies indicate that people who are active have denser bone mineral than inactive people do. Similar to other benefits of participating in exercise, there is no such thing as "bone in the bank." To have good bone health, people need to participate in a regular lifetime exercise program.

Estrogen is the most important factor in preventing bone loss.

Prevailing research also tells us that estrogen is the most important factor in preventing bone loss. In one study, lumbar bone density in women who had always had regular menstrual cycles exceeded that of women with a history of oligomenorrhea (irregular cycles) and amenorrhea (cessation of menstruation) interspaced with regular cycles. Furthermore, the lumbar density of these two groups of women was higher than that of women who had never had regular menstrual cycles.

Following menopause, every woman should consider hormone replacement therapy and discuss it

Table 2.8 Low-Fat Calcium-Rich Foods

Food	Amount	Calcium (mg)	Calories	Calories From Fat
Beans, red kidney, cooked	1 cup	70	218	4%
Beet, greens, cooked	1/2 cup	72	13	—
Broccoli, cooked, drained	1 sm stalk	123	36	—
Burrito, bean	1	173	307	28%
Cottage cheese, 2% low-fat	1/2 cup	78	103	18%
Milk, nonfat, powdered	1 tbsp	52	27	1%
Milk, skim	1 cup	296	88	3%
Ice milk (vanilla)	1/2 cup	102	100	27%
Instant breakfast, whole milk	1 cup	301	280	26%
Kale, cooked, drained	1/2 cup	103	22	—
Okra, cooked, drained	1/2 cup	74	23	—
Shrimp, boiled	3 oz.	99	99	9%
Spinach, raw	1 cup	51	14	—
Yogurt, fruit	1 cup	345	231	8%
Yogurt, low-fat, plain	1 cup	271	160	20%

with her physician. Women who have estrogen therapy do not lose bone mineral density at the rate of women who do not have estrogen therapy. Neither exercise nor calcium supplementation will offset the damaging effects of lower estrogen levels. Hormone replacement therapy seems to be the only reasonable therapy that post-menopausal women have to prevent osteoporosis in future years.

For instance, athletes with **amenorrhea** (who have lower estrogen levels) have lower bone mineral density than even nonathletes with normal estrogen levels. One study[18] showed that amenorrheic athletes at age 25 have the bones of 52-year-old women. Other research[19] showed four amenorrheic athletes with a bone density equivalent to that of 70- to 80-year-old women. Over the last few years, it has become clear that sedentary women with normal estrogen levels have better bone mineral density than active amenorrheic athletes. Many experts believe the best predictor of bone mineral content is the history of menstrual regularity.

Iron Deficiency

Iron is a key element of **hemoglobin** in blood. The RDA of iron for adult women is 15 mg per day (10 mg for men). According to a survey by the U.S. Department of Agriculture, 19- to 50-year-old women in the United States consumed only 60% of the RDA for iron. People who do not have enough iron in the body can develop iron-deficiency anemia, in which the concentration of hemoglobin in the red blood cells is less than it should be.

Physically active women also may have a greater than average need for iron. Heavy training creates a demand for iron that is higher than the recommended intake because small amounts of iron are lost through sweat, urine, and stools. Mechanical trauma, caused by the pounding of the feet on the pavement during extensive jogging, also may lead to the destruction of iron-containing red blood cells.

A large percentage of female endurance athletes is reported to have iron deficiency. Blood **ferritin** levels should be checked frequently in women who participate in intense physical training.

The rates of iron absorption and iron loss vary from person to person. In most cases, though, people can get enough iron by eating more iron-rich foods such as beans, peas, green leafy vegetables, enriched grain products, egg yolk, fish, and lean meats. Although organ meats, such as liver, are especially good sources, they also are high in cholesterol. A list of foods high in iron content is given in Table 2.9.

Dietary Guidelines for North Americans

Based on the available scientific research on nutrition and health and the current dietary habits of the American people, in 1995 the Scientific Committee

Amenorrhea Cessation of regular menstrual flow.

Hemoglobin Protein-iron compound in red blood cells that transports oxygen in the blood.

Ferritin Iron stored in the body.

Table 2.9 Iron-Rich Foods

Food	Amount	Iron (mg)	Calories	Cholesterol	Calories From Fat
Beans, red kidney, cooked	1 cup	4.4	218	0	4%
Beef, ground lean	3 oz.	3.0	186	81	48%
Beef, sirloin	3 oz.	2.5	329	77	74%
Beef, liver, fried	3 oz.	7.5	195	345	42%
Beet, greens, cooked	1/2 cup	1.4	13	0	—
Broccoli, cooked, drained	1 sm stalk	1.1	36	0	—
Burrito, bean	1	2.4	307	14	28%
Egg, hard-cooked	1	1.0	72	250	63%
Farina (Cream of Wheat), cooked	1/2 cup	6.0	51	0	—
Instant breakfast, whole milk	1 cup	8.0	280	33	26%
Peas, frozen, cooked, drained	1/2 cup	1.5	55	0	—
Shrimp, boiled	3 oz.	2.7	99	128	9%
Spinach, raw	1 cup	1.7	14	0	—
Vegetables, mixed, cooked	1 cup	2.4	116	0	—

of the U. S. Department of Health and Human Services and the U.S. Department of Agriculture on diet and health issued the fourth edition of the Dietary Guidelines for healthy American adults and children. These guidelines potentially can reduce the risk of developing certain chronic diseases. The committee's recommendations are:[20]

- Eat a variety of food. No single food can provide all of the necessary nutrients and other beneficial substances in the amounts the body needs. For good nutrition, you should meet the recommended number of daily servings from each of the five food groups in the Food Guide Pyramid. Within each food group, choose a variety of foods. Food items vary, and each item provides different combinations of nutrients and other substances needed for good health.
- Balance the food you eat with physical activity to maintain or improve your weight. Excessive body weight increases the risk for diseases including heart disease, stroke, diabetes, high blood pressure, and certain cancers. Many people gain weight as adults, and this does not have to be the case. To maintain body weight, you need to balance food intake with the amount of calories the body uses. In ensuing chapters you will find extensive information on weight management and exercise programs to help you balance your energy requirements according to your personal needs.
- Choose a diet with plenty of grain products, vegetables, and fruits. Most of your daily calories should come from these food products. They contain ample amounts of vitamins, minerals, complex carbohydrates, and other substances important for good health.
- Choose a diet low in fat, saturated fat, and cholesterol. Reduce fat intake to 30% or less of total calories. Reduce saturated fatty acid intake to less than 10% of total calories and intake of cholesterol to no more than 300 mg daily. Intake of fat and cholesterol can be lowered by substituting fish, poultry without skin, lean meats, and low or nonfat dairy products for fatty meats and whole-milk dairy products; by choosing more vegetables, fruits, cereals, and legumes; and by limiting oils, fats, egg yolks, and fried and other fatty foods.
- Choose a diet moderate in sugars. Excessive sugar and starch intake can contribute to weight gain and tooth decay. This guideline advises against frequent and large consumption of food items and snacks high in sugar that provide unnecessary calories and few nutrients. The more often that high sugar foods are consumed, and the longer before brushing the teeth following their consumption, the greater is the risk for tooth decay.
- Choose a diet moderate in salt and sodium. Limit total daily intake of salt (sodium chloride) to 6 grams or less. This amount represents the equivalent of 2,400 mg of sodium listed in the Daily Value of the Nutrition Label. To decrease your daily sodium intake, limit the use of salt in cooking and do not add it to food at the table. Sparingly consume salty, highly processed salty, salt-preserved, and salt-pickled foods.
- If you drink alcoholic beverages, do so in moderation. Alcoholic beverages provide calories but few or no nutrients. Moderate drinking has been linked to a decreased risk for coronary heart disease in some people. High levels of alcohol consumption lead to an increased risk for heart disease, stroke, high blood pressure, certain cancers, cirrhosis of the liver, inflammation of the pancreas, brain damage, birth defects, accidents, violence, suicides, and malnutrition. Limit consumption to the equivalent of less than an ounce of pure alcohol in a single day. This translates into two cans of beer, two small glasses of wine, or two average cocktails. If pregnant, avoid alcoholic beverages altogether.

Proper Nutrition: A Lifetime Prescription for Healthy Living

Proper nutrition, a sound exercise program, and quitting smoking (for those who smoke) are the

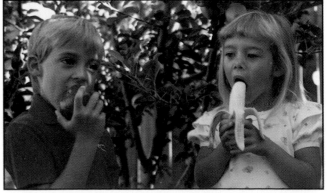

Positive nutrition habits should be taught and reinforced in early youth.

three factors that do the most for health, longevity, and quality of life. Achieving and maintaining a balanced diet is not as difficult as most people would think. If parents were to do a better job of teaching and reinforcing proper nutrition habits in early youth, we would not have the magnitude of nutrition-related health problems that we do. Although the treatment of obesity is important, we should place far greater emphasis in preventing obesity in youth and adults alike.

Children tend to eat the way their parents do. If parents adopt a healthy diet, children most likely will follow. The difficult part for most people is retraining themselves to follow a lifetime healthy nutrition plan — a diet that includes lots of grains, legumes, fruits, vegetables, and low-fat dairy products, with moderate use of animal protein, junk food, sodium, and alcohol.

In spite of the ample scientific evidence linking poor dietary habits to early disease and mortality rates, most people are not willing to change their eating patterns. Even when faced with obesity, elevated blood lipids, hypertension, and other nutrition-related conditions, people do not change. The motivating factor to change one's eating habits seems to be a major health breakdown, such as a heart attack, a stroke, or cancer. By this time the damage already has been done. In many cases it is irreversible and, for some, fatal.

An ounce of prevention is worth a pound of cure. The sooner you implement the dietary guidelines presented in this chapter, the better will be your chances of preventing chronic diseases and reaching a higher state of wellness.

Laboratory Experience

LAB 2A
Nutrient analysis

Lab Preparation
Prior to your lab, keep a 3-day record of all food you consume using Figure 2A.1 from Lab 2. You also should record all of the nutrients from the Nutritive Values of Selected Foods listing in Appendix A. Please note that if your serving is twice the standard amount, you need to double all of the nutrient contents. If you have only half a serving, record only half of the contents, and so forth. You also should total your nutrient intake for each day before the lab session. If the computer software available with this book is used, you will need only to record the codes and the number of servings eaten (use Figure 2A.3) prior to your lab session.

LAB 2B
Achieving a balanced diet

Lab Preparation
None required. This lab will be given as homework to follow up the nutrient analysis (see Lab 2A).

2

Notes

1. *Surgeon General's Report on Nutrition and Health: Summary and Recommendations*, DHHS (PHS) publication no. 88-50211 (Washington, D.C.: U.S. Government Printing Office, 1988).
2. D. J. Mela and D. A. Sacchetti. "Sensory Preferences for Fat: Relationships with Diet and Body Composition." *American Journal of Clinical Nutrition*, 53 (1991), 908–915.
3. J. M. Gaziano and C. H. Hennekens. "A New Look at What Can Unclog Your Arteries." *Executive Health Report*, 27:8 (1991), 16.
4. R. J. Barnard, "Effects of Lifestyle Modification on Serum Lipids," *Archives of Internal Medicine*, 151 (1991), 1389–1394.
5. J. H. Weisburger and G. M. Williams, "Causes of Cancer," in *Textbook of Clinical Oncology* (Atlanta: American Cancer Society, 1995).
6. S. Begley. "Beyond Vitamins," *Newsweek*, April 25, 1994, pp. 45–49.
7. "Vitamin Report," *University of California at Berkeley Wellness Letter* (Palm Coast, FL: The Editors, October, 1994).
8. "Antioxidants: Never Too Late," *University of California at Berkeley Wellness Letter*, 10:8 (1994), 2.
9. "Vitamin Report."
10. S. Kalish, "The Free Radical Radical: Kenneth Cooper, M.D., on Antioxidants and the Dangers of Hard Running," *Running Times*, March 1995, pp. 16–17.
11. "Beta Carotene Pills: Should You Take Them?" *University of California at Berkeley Wellness Letter*, 12:7 (1996), 1–2.
12. J. Carper, "Say 'Nuts' to Heart Disease," *USA Weekend*, December 2–4, 1994, pp. 8–9.
13. "Vitamin Report."
14. K. H. Cooper, *Antioxidant Revolution* (Nashville, TN: Thomas Nelson Publishers, 1994).
15. Cooper.
16. K. M. Zawadzki, B. B. Yaspelkis III, and J. L. Ivy, "Carbohydrate-Protein Complex Increases the Rate of Muscle Glycogen Storage After Exercise," *Journal of Applied Physiology*, 72 (1992), 1854–1859.
17. "Nutrition, Exercise, and Bone Health" (Seattle, WA: Pacific Medical Center, 1990).
18. B. L. Drinkwater, "Osteoporosis and the Female Masters Athlete," *Sports Medicine for the Mature Athlete*, edited by J. R. Sutton and R. M. Brock, Benchmark Press: 353-359, 1986.
19. K. H. Myburgh, L. K. Bachrach, B. Lewis, K. Kent, and R. Marcus, "Low Bone Mineral Density at Axial and Appendicular Sites in Amenorrheic Athletes," *Medicine and Science in Sports and Exercise*, 25:11(1993), 1197–1202.
20. U. S. Department of Agriculture and U. S. Department of Health and Human Services, "Nutrition and Your Health: Dietary Guidelines for Americans," *Home and Garden Bulletin No. 232*, December 1995.

Suggested Readings

American Medical Association: Council on Scientific Affairs. "Dietary Fiber and Health." *Journal of the American Medical Association*, 262 (1989), 542–546.

Brownell, K., and J. P. Forey. *Handbook of Eating Disorders*. New York: Basic Books, 1986.

Cristian, J. L., and J. L. Greger. *Nutrition for Living*. Menlo Park, CA: Benjamin/Cummings Publishing, 1991.

Coleman, E. *Eating for Endurance*. Palo Alto, CA: Bull Publishing, 1992.

Drinkwater, B. L.. "Does Physical Activity Play a Role in Preventing Osteoporosis?" *Research Quarterly for Exercise and Sport*, 65 (1994), 197–206.

Drinkwater, B. L., B. Bruemner, and C. H. III Chestnut. "Menstrual History as a Determinant of Current Bone Density in Young Athletes." *Journal of the American Medical Association*, 263 (1990), 545–548.

Girdano, D. A., D. Dusek, and G. S. Everly. *Experiencing Health*. Englewood Cliffs, NJ: Prentice-Hall, 1985.

"How to Balance Your Diet." *Fitness*: April 1983, pp. 46–47.

Hoeger, W. W. K., and S. A. Hoeger. *Lifetime Physical Fitness and Wellness*. Englewood, CO: Morton Publishing, 1995.

Kanders, B., D. W. Demster, and R. Lindsay. "Interaction of Calcium Nutrition and Physical Activity on Bone Mass in Young Women." *Journal of Bone Mineral Research*, 3 (1988), 145–149.

Kirschmann, J. D. *Nutrition Almanac*. New York: McGraw-Hill Book Company, 1989.

Kleiner, S. M. "Seafood and Your Heart." *The Physician and Sportsmedicine*, 18:4 (1990), 19–20.

Morgan, B. L. G. *The Lifelong Nutrition Guide*. Englewood Cliffs, NJ: Prentice Hall, 1983.

National Academy of Sciences, Institute of Medicine. *Eat for Life: the Food and Nutrition Board's Guide to Reducing Your Risk of Chronic Disease*, edited by C. E. Woteki and P. R. Thomas. Washington, DC: National Academy Press, 1992.

Thornton, J. S. "Feast or Famine: Eating Disorders in Athletes." *The Physician and Sportsmedicine*, 18:4 (1990), 116–122.

Whitney, E. N., and S. R. Rolfes. *Understanding Nutrition*. St. Paul: West Publishing, 1996.

Body Composition Assessment

3

LABS

*B**ody composition** consists of fat and nonfat components. The fat component usually is called fat mass or **percent body fat**. The nonfat component is termed **lean body mass**.*

For many years people relied on height/weight charts to determine recommended body weight. We now know, that these tables can be highly inaccurate for many people, and they fail to identify critical fat values associated with higher risk for disease. The proper way to determine recommended weight is through body composition by finding out what percent of total body weight is fat and what amount is lean tissue.

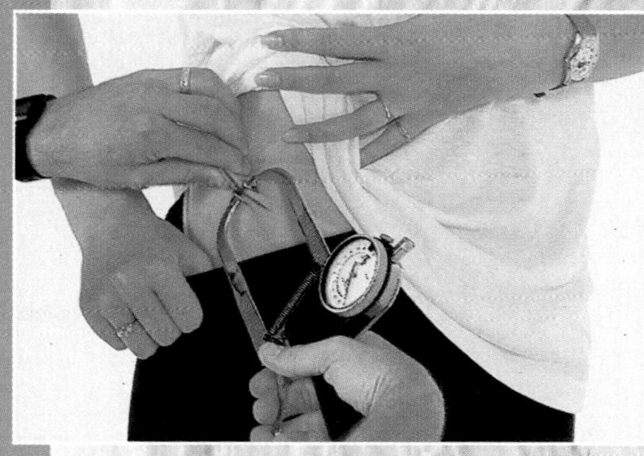

*Once the fat percentage is known, **recommended body weight** can be calculated from recommended body fat. Recommended body weight is described as "healthy weight." It implies the absence of any medical condition that would improve with weight loss and a fat distribution pattern that is not associated with increased risk for illness.*

Although various techniques for determining percent body fat were developed several years ago, many people still are unaware of these procedures and continue to depend on height/weight charts to find out their recommended body weight. The standard height/weight tables were first published in 1912. They were based on average weights (including shoes and clothing) for men and women who obtained life insurance policies between 1888 and 1905. The recommended body weight on these tables is obtained according to gender,

Objectives

- Define body composition and its relationship to recommended body weight assessment.
- Learn the difference between essential fat and storage fat.
- Understand the methodology used to assess body composition according to hydrostatic weighing, skinfold thickness, and girth measurements.
- Understand the importance of waist-to-hip ratio and body mass index.
- Be able to determine recommended weight according to recommended percent body fat values.

height, and frame size. Because no scientific guidelines are given to determine frame size, most people choose their frame size based on the column in which the weight comes closest to their own!

To determine whether people are truly obese or falsely at recommended body weight, body composition must be established. Obesity is related to an excess of body fat. If body weight is the only criterion, an individual easily can be overweight, according to height/weight charts, yet not have any excess body fat. Football players, body builders, weight lifters, and other athletes with large muscle size are typical examples. Some of these athletes who appear to be 20 or 30 pounds overweight really have little body fat.

The inaccuracy of height/weight charts was illustrated clearly when a young man who weighed about 225 pounds applied to join a city police force but was turned down without having been granted an interview. The reason? He was "too fat," according to the height/weight charts. When this young man's body composition was assessed later at a preventive medicine clinic, he was shocked to find out that only 5% of his total body weight was in the form of fat — considerably lower than the recommended standard. In the words of the technical director of the clinic, "The only way this fellow could come down to the chart's target weight would have been through surgical removal of a large amount of his muscle tissue."

At the other end of the spectrum, some people who weigh very little and are viewed by many as skinny or underweight actually can be classified as obese because of their high body fat content. People who weigh as little as 100 pounds but are more than 30% fat (about one-third of their total body weight) are not uncommon. These cases are found more readily in sedentary people and those who are always dieting. Physical inactivity and constant negative caloric balance both lead to a loss in lean body mass (see Chapter 4). From these examples, body weight alone clearly does not always tell the true story.

Essential and Storage Fat

Total fat in the human body is classified into two types: essential fat and storage fat. **Essential fat** is needed for normal physiological functions, and without it, human health deteriorates. This essential fat constitutes about 3% of the total weight in men and 12% in women. The percentage is higher in women because it includes sex-specific fat, such as that found in the breast tissue, the uterus, and other sex-related fat deposits.

Storage fat is stored mostly beneath the skin (subcutaneous fat) and around major organs in the body. This fat serves three basic functions:

1. As an insulator to retain body heat.
2. As energy substrate for metabolism.
3. As padding against physical trauma to the body.

The amount of storage fat does not differ between men and women, except that men tend to store fat around the waist and women more so around the hips and thighs.

Techniques for Assessing Body Composition

Body composition can be determined through several different procedures. The most common techniques are: (a) hydrostatic or underwater weighing, (b) skinfold thickness, (c) girth measurements, and (d) bioelectrical impedance. When using the different techniques, slightly different values are obtained. Therefore, when assessing body composition, the same technique should be used for pre- and post-test comparisons.

Hydrostatic Weighing

Hydrostatic weighing has been considered by many as the "gold standard" of body composition. Almost all other techniques to determine body composition are validated against hydrostatic weighing. It seems to be the most accurate technique available if it is administered properly and if the individual is able to perform the test adequately.

The procedure for hydrostatic weighing, as outlined in Figure 3.1, requires a considerable amount

---

Body composition Refers to the fat and nonfat components of the human body. Important in assessing recommended body weight.

Percent body fat Total amount of fat in the body based on the person's weight, includes both essential and storage fat.

Lean body mass Body weight without body fat.

Recommended body weight Body weight at which there seems to be no harm to human health.

Essential fat Minimal amount of body fat needed for normal physiological functions; constitutes about 3% of the total weight in men and 12% in women.

Storage fat Body fat in excess of the essential fat; stored in adipose tissue.

Hydrostatic weighing Underwater technique to assess body composition, including percent body fat.

HYDROSTATIC WEIGHING

A small tank or pool, an autopsy scale, and a submergible chair are needed. The scale should measure up to about 10 kilograms (kg) and should be readable to the nearest 100th of a kilogram. The chair is suspended from the scale and submerged in a tank of water or pool measuring at least 5 × 5 × 5 feet. A swimming pool can be used in place of the tank.

The procedure for the technician is:

1. Ask the person to be weighed to fast for approximately 6 to 8 hours and to have a bladder and bowel movement prior to underwater weighing.
2. Measure the individual's residual lung volume (RV or amount of air left in the lungs following complete exhalation). If no equipment (spirometer) is available to measure the residual volume, estimate it using the following predicting equations* (to convert inches to centimeters, multiply inches by 2.54):

   Men: $RV = [(0.027 \times \text{height in centimeters}) + (0.017 \times \text{age})] - 3.447$

   Women: $RV = [(0.032 \times \text{height in centimeters}) + (0.009 \times \text{age})] - 3.9$

3. Have the person remove all jewelry prior to weighing or testing. Weigh the person on land in a swimsuit, and subtract the weight of the suit. Convert the weight from pounds to kilograms (divide pounds by 2.2046).
4. Record the water temperature in the tank in degrees Centigrade. Use that temperature to obtain the water density factor provided below, which is required in the formula to compute body density.

Temp (°C)	Water Density (gr/ml)	Temp (°C)	Water Density (gr/ml)
28	0.99626	35	0.99406
29	0.99595	36	0.99371
30	0.99567	37	0.99336
31	0.99537	38	0.99299
32	0.99505	39	0.99262
33	0.99473	40	0.99224
34	0.99440		

5. Ask the person, dressed in the swimsuit, to enter the tank and completely wipe off all air clinging to the skin and hair. Have the person sit in the chair with the water at chin level (raise or lower the chair as needed). Make sure the water and scale remain as still as possible during the entire procedure, as this allows for a better underwater reading. (During underwater weighing, you can decrease scale movement by holding and slowly releasing the neck of the scale until the subject is floating freely in the water.)
6. Place a clip on the person's nose and have him or her forcefully exhale all of the air out of the lungs. The individual then totally submerges underwater. (Make sure that all the air is exhaled from the lungs prior to submerging. Record the reading on the scale. Repeat this procedure 8 to 10 times, as practice and experience increases the accuracy of the underwater weight. Use the average of the three heaviest underwater weights as the gross underwater weight.
7. Because tare weight (the weight of the chair and chain or rope used to suspend the chair) accounts for part of the gross underwater weight, subtract this weight to obtain the person's net underwater weight. To determine tare weight, place a clothes pin on the chain or rope at the water level when the person is submerged completely. After the person comes out of the water, lower the chair into the water to the pin level. Now record tare weight. Determine the net underwater weight by subtracting the tare weight from the gross underwater weight.
8. Compute body density and percent fat using the following equations:

$$\text{Body density} = \frac{BW}{\frac{BW - UW}{WD} - RV - .1}$$

$$\text{Percent fat**} = \frac{495}{BD} - 450$$

Where:

BW = body weight in kg
UW = net underwater weight
WD = water density (determined by water temperature)
RV = residual volume
BD = body density

A sample computation for body fat assessment according to hydrostatic weighing is provided in Lab 3A.

*From: "Respiratory Function Tests: Normal Values at Medium Altitudes and the Prediction of Normal Results," by H. L. Goldman and M. R. Becklake, in *American Review of Tuberculosis,* 79 (1959), 457–467.

**From *Body Composition from Fluid Spaces and Density*, by W. E. Siri (Berkeley, CA: University of California, Donner Laboratory of Medical Physics, March 19, 1956).

Figure 3.1 Hydrostatic weighing procedure for body composition assessment.

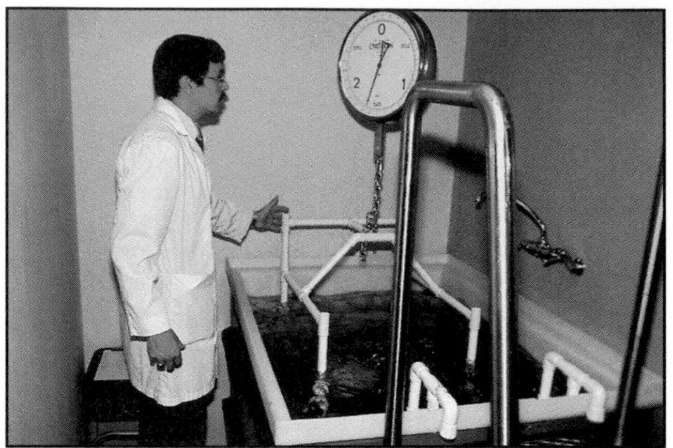

Hydrostatic weighing is used in the assessment of body composition.

of time, skill, space, and equipment. An experienced instructor must train all technicians who will administer this test.

Because each individual assessment can take as long as 30 minutes, hydrostatic weighing is not feasible when testing large numbers of people. Furthermore, the person's residual lung volume (amount of air left in the lungs following complete forceful exhalation) has to be measured prior to testing. If residual volume cannot be measured, as is the case in many laboratories and health/fitness centers, it can be estimated using the predicting equations in Figure 3.1. Estimating residual volume, however, may decrease the accuracy of hydrostatic weighing.

A major concern during hydrostatic weighing is the person's ability to follow the test procedure. Also, the psychological variables in being weighed while submerged underwater makes hydrostatic weighing difficult to administer to **aquaphobic** people. For each underwater weighing trial, the person has to: (a) force out all of the air in the lungs, (b) lean forward and completely submerge underwater in a sitting position for about 5 to 10 seconds (long enough to take a reading on the scale), and (c) remain as calm as possible (chair movement makes reading the scale difficult). This procedure has to be repeated 8 to 10 times.

Forcing all of the air out of the lungs is not easy for everyone. Leaving additional air (beyond residual volume) in the lungs makes a person more buoyant. Because fat is less dense than water, overweight individuals weigh less in water. Additional air in the lungs makes a person lighter in water, yielding a false higher body fat percentage.

Because of the cost, time, and complexity of hydrostatic weighing, most health and fitness programs prefer **anthropometric measurement techniques**, which correlate quite well with hydrostatic weighing. These techniques, primarily skinfold thickness and girth measurements, allow a quick, simple, and inexpensive estimate of body composition.

Skinfold Thickness

Assessing body composition using **skinfold thickness** is based on the principle that approximately half of the body's fatty tissue is directly beneath the skin. Valid and reliable estimates of this tissue give a good indication of percent body fat.

The skinfold test is done with the aid of pressure calipers. Several sites must be measured to reflect the total percentage of fat: triceps, suprailium, and thigh skinfolds for women; and chest, abdomen, and thigh for men (Figure 3.2). All measurements should be taken on the right side of the body.

Even with the skinfold technique, some training is necessary to obtain accurate measurements. Also, different technicians may produce slightly different measurements from the same person. Therefore, the same technician should take pre- and post-measurements.

Measurements should be done at the same time of the day, preferably in the morning, as changes in

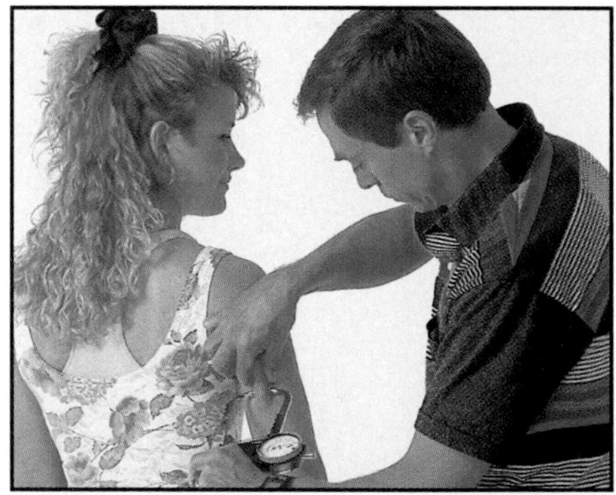

Skinfold thickness technique used to assess body composition.

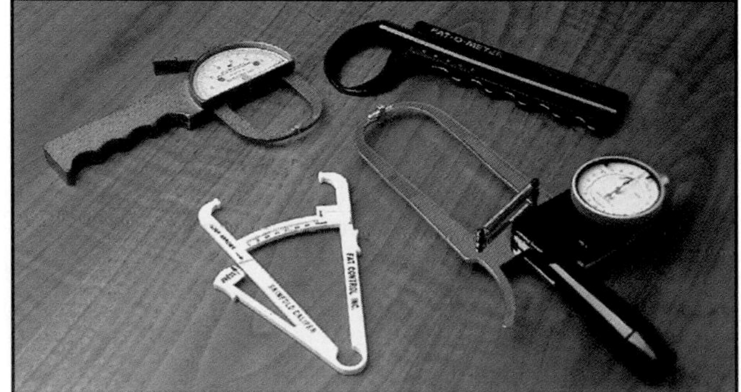

Various types of skinfold calipers can be used to assess skinfold thickness.

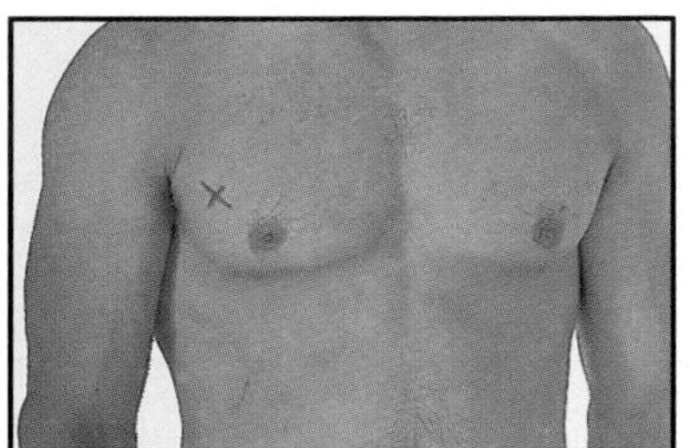
Chest (men)

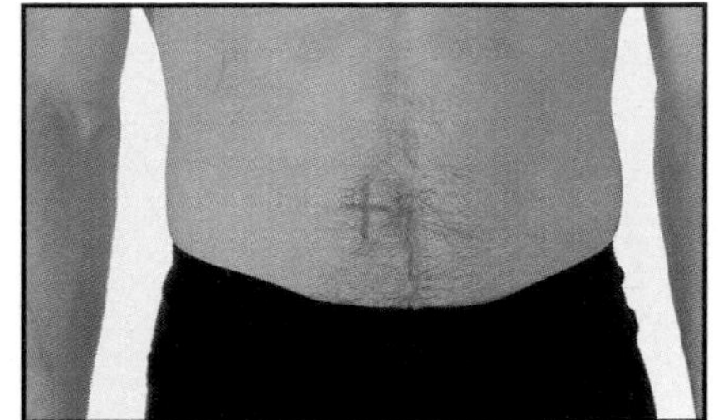
Abdominal (men)

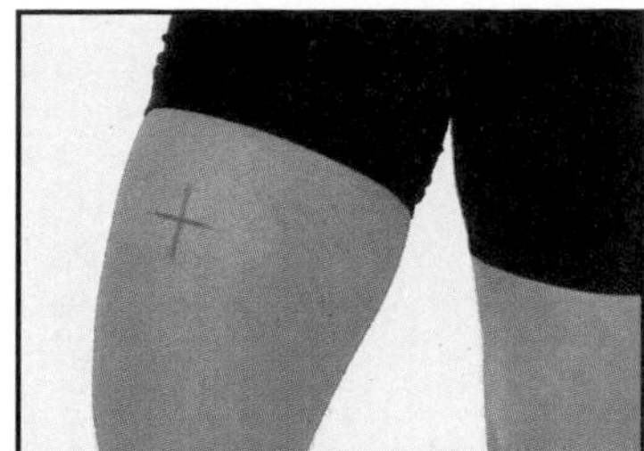
Thigh (men and women)

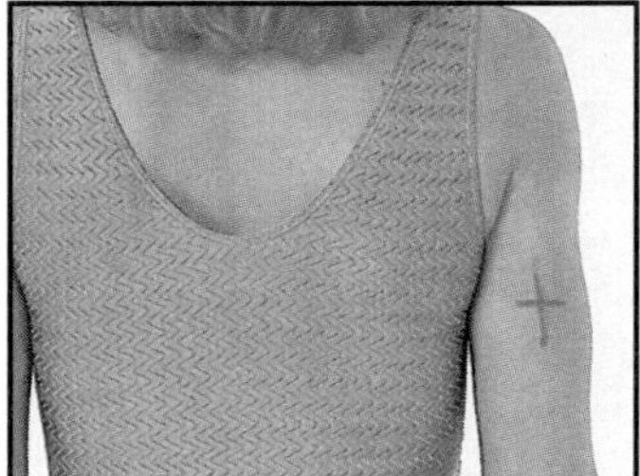
Triceps (women)

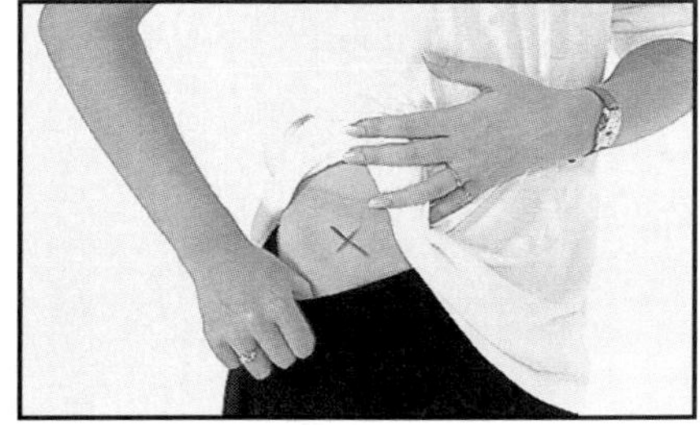
Suprailium (women)

Figure 3.2
Anatomical landmarks for skinfold measurements.

water hydration from activity and exercise can increase skinfold girth. The procedure for assessing percent body fat using skinfold thickness is given in Figure 3.3. If skinfold calipers* are available to you, you may proceed to assess your percent body fat with the help of your instructor or an experienced technician.

* This instrument is available at most colleges and universities. If unavailable, you can purchase an inexpensive, yet reliable skinfold caliper from: Fat Control Inc., P. O. Box 10117, Towson, MD 21204, Phone 301/296–1993.

Aquaphobic Having a fear of water.

Anthropometric measurement techniques Measurement of body girths at different sites.

Skinfold thickness Technique to assess body composition, including percent body fat, by measuring the thickness of a double fold of skin at different body sites.

BODY FAT ASSESSMENT ACCORDING TO SKINFOLD THICKNESS TECHNIQUE

1. Select the proper anatomical sites. For men, use chest, abdomen, and thigh skinfolds. For women, use triceps, suprailium, and thigh skinfolds. Take all measurements on the right side of the body with the person standing. The correct anatomical landmarks for skinfolds are:

   Chest: a diagonal fold halfway between the shoulder crease and the nipple.

   Abdomen: a vertical fold taken about one inch to the right of the umbilicus.

   Triceps: a vertical fold on the back of the upper arm, halfway between the shoulder and the elbow.

   Thigh: a vertical fold on the front of the thigh, midway between the knee and the hip.

   Suprailium: a diagonal fold above the crest of the ilium (on the side of the hip).

2. Measure each site by grasping a double thickness of skin firmly with the thumb and forefinger, pulling the fold slightly away from the muscular tissue. Hold the calipers perpendicular to the fold, and take the measurement ½ inch below the finger hold. Measure each site three times and read the values to the nearest .1 to .5 mm. Record the average of the two closest readings as the final value. Take the readings without delay to avoid excessive compression of the skinfold. Releasing and refolding the skinfold is required between readings.

3. When doing pre- and post-assessments, conduct the measurement at the same time of day. The best time is early in the morning to avoid water hydration changes resulting from activity or exercise.

4. Obtain percent fat by adding the three skinfold measurements and looking up the respective values on Table 3.1 for women, Table 3.2 for men under age 40, and Table 3.3 for men over 40.

5. For example, if the skinfold measurements for an 18-year-old female are: (a) triceps = 16, (b) suprailium = 4, and (c) thigh = 30 (total = 50), the percent body fat would be 20.6%

Figure 3.3 Procedure for assessing body fat according to skinfold thickness technique.

Table 3.1 Percent Fat Estimates for Women Calculated From Triceps, Suprailium, and Thigh Skinfold Thickness

	Age to the Last Year								
Sum of 3 Skinfolds	**22 or Under**	**23 to 27**	**28 to 32**	**33 to 37**	**38 to 42**	**43 to 47**	**48 to 52**	**53 to 57**	**58 and Over**
23- 25	9.7	9.9	10.2	10.4	10.7	10.9	11.2	11.4	11.7
26- 28	11.0	11.2	11.5	11.7	12.0	12.3	12.5	12.7	13.0
29- 31	12.3	12.5	12.8	13.0	13.3	13.5	13.8	14.0	14.3
32- 34	13.6	13.8	14.0	14.3	14.5	14.8	15.0	15.3	15.5
35- 37	14.8	15.0	15.3	15.5	15.8	16.0	16.3	16.5	16.8
38- 40	16.0	16.3	16.5	16.7	17.0	17.2	17.5	17.7	18.0
41- 43	17.2	17.4	17.7	17.9	18.2	18.4	18.7	18.9	19.2
44- 46	18.3	18.6	18.8	19.1	19.3	19.6	19.8	20.1	20.3
47- 49	19.5	19.7	20.0	20.2	20.5	20.7	21.0	21.2	21.5
50- 52	20.6	20.8	21.1	21.3	21.6	21.8	22.1	22.3	22.6
53- 55	21.7	21.9	22.1	22.4	22.6	22.9	23.1	23.4	23.6
56- 58	22.7	23.0	23.2	23.4	23.7	23.9	24.2	24.4	24.7
59- 61	23.7	24.0	24.2	24.5	24.7	25.0	25.2	25.5	25.7
62- 64	24.7	25.0	25.2	25.5	25.7	26.0	26.2	26.4	26.7
65- 67	25.7	25.9	26.2	26.4	26.7	26.9	27.2	27.4	27.7
68- 70	26.6	26.9	27.1	27.4	27.6	27.9	28.1	28.4	28.6
71- 73	27.5	27.8	28.0	28.3	28.5	28.8	29.0	29.3	29.5
74- 76	28.4	28.7	28.9	29.2	29.4	29.7	29.9	30.2	30.4
77- 79	29.3	29.5	29.8	30.0	30.3	30.5	30.8	31.0	31.3
80- 82	30.1	30.4	30.6	30.9	31.1	31.4	31.6	31.9	32.1
83- 85	30.9	31.2	31.4	31.7	31.9	32.2	32.4	32.7	32.9
86- 88	31.7	32.0	32.2	32.5	32.7	32.9	33.2	33.4	33.7
89- 91	32.5	32.7	33.0	33.2	33.5	33.7	33.9	34.2	34.4
92- 94	33.2	33.4	33.7	33.9	34.2	34.4	34.7	34.9	35.2
95- 97	33.9	34.1	34.4	34.6	34.9	35.1	35.4	35.6	35.9
98-100	34.6	34.8	35.1	35.3	35.5	35.8	36.0	36.3	36.5
101-103	35.2	35.4	35.7	35.9	36.2	36.4	36.7	36.9	37.2
104-106	35.8	36.1	36.3	36.6	36.8	37.1	37.3	37.5	37.8
107-109	36.4	36.7	36.9	37.1	37.4	37.6	37.9	38.1	38.4
110-112	37.0	37.2	37.5	37.7	38.0	38.2	38.5	38.7	38.9
113-115	37.5	37.8	38.0	38.2	38.5	38.7	39.0	39.2	39.5
116-118	38.0	38.3	38.5	38.8	39.0	39.3	39.5	39.7	40.0
119-121	38.5	38.7	39.0	39.2	39.5	39.7	40.0	40.2	40.5
122-124	39.0	39.2	39.4	39.7	39.9	40.2	40.4	40.7	40.9
125-127	39.4	39.6	39.9	40.1	40.4	40.6	40.9	41.1	41.4
128-130	39.8	40.0	40.3	40.5	40.8	41.0	41.3	41.5	41.8

Body density is calculated based on the generalized equation for predicting body density of women developed by A. S. Jackson, M. L. Pollock, and A. Ward and published in *Medicine and Science in Sports and Exercise,* 12 (1980), 175–182. Percent body fat is determined from the calculated body density using the Siri formula.

Table 3.2 Percent Fat Estimates for Men 40 and Under Calculated From Chest, Abdomen, and Thigh Skinfold Thickness

	Age to the Last Year							
Sum of 3 Skinfolds	19 or Under	20 to 22	23 to 25	26 to 28	29 to 31	32 to 34	35 to 37	38 to 40
8- 10	.9	1.3	1.6	2.0	2.3	2.7	3.0	3.3
11- 13	1.9	2.3	2.6	3.0	3.3	3.7	4.0	4.3
14- 16	2.9	3.3	3.6	3.9	4.3	4.6	5.0	5.3
17- 19	3.9	4.2	4.6	4.9	5.3	5.6	6.0	6.3
20- 22	4.8	5.2	5.5	5.9	6.2	6.6	6.9	7.3
23- 25	5.8	6.2	6.5	6.8	7.2	7.5	7.9	8.2
26- 28	6.8	7.1	7.5	7.8	8.1	8.5	8.8	9.2
29- 31	7.7	8.0	8.4	8.7	9.1	9.4	9.8	10.1
32- 34	8.6	9.0	9.3	9.7	10.0	10.4	10.7	11.1
35- 37	9.5	9.9	10.2	10.6	10.9	11.3	11.6	12.0
38- 40	10.5	10.8	11.2	11.5	11.8	12.2	12.5	12.9
41- 43	11.4	11.7	12.1	12.4	12.7	13.1	13.4	13.8
44- 46	12.2	12.6	12.9	13.3	13.6	14.0	14.3	14.7
47- 49	13.1	13.5	13.8	14.2	14.5	14.9	15.2	15.5
50- 52	14.0	14.3	14.7	15.0	15.4	15.7	16.1	16.4
53- 55	14.8	15.2	15.5	15.9	16.2	16.6	16.9	17.3
56- 58	15.7	16.0	16.4	16.7	17.1	17.4	17.8	18.1
59- 61	16.5	16.9	17.2	17.6	17.9	18.3	18.6	19.0
62- 64	17.4	17.7	18.1	18.4	18.8	19.1	19.4	19.8
65- 67	18.2	18.5	18.9	19.2	19.6	19.9	20.3	20.6
68- 70	19.0	19.3	19.7	20.0	20.4	20.7	21.1	21.4
71- 73	19.8	20.1	20.5	20.8	21.2	21.5	21.9	22.2
74- 76	20.6	20.9	21.3	21.6	22.0	22.2	22.7	23.0
77- 79	21.4	21.7	22.1	22.4	22.8	23.1	23.4	23.8
80- 82	22.1	22.5	22.8	23.2	23.5	23.9	24.2	24.6
83- 85	22.9	23.2	23.6	23.9	24.3	24.6	25.0	25.3
86- 88	23.6	24.0	24.3	24.7	25.0	25.4	25.7	26.1
89- 91	24.4	24.7	25.1	25.4	25.8	26.1	26.5	26.8
92- 94	25.1	25.5	25.8	26.2	26.5	26.9	27.2	27.5
95- 97	25.8	26.2	26.5	26.9	27.2	27.6	27.9	28.3
98-100	26.6	26.9	27.3	27.6	27.9	28.3	28.6	29.0
101-103	27.3	27.6	28.0	28.3	28.6	29.0	29.3	29.7
104-106	27.9	28.3	28.6	29.0	29.3	29.7	30.0	30.4
107-109	28.6	29.0	29.3	29.7	30.0	30.4	30.7	31.1
110-112	29.3	29.6	30.0	30.3	30.7	31.0	31.4	31.7
113-115	30.0	30.3	30.7	31.0	31.3	31.7	32.0	32.4
116-118	30.6	31.0	31.3	31.6	32.0	32.3	32.7	33.0
119-121	31.3	31.6	32.0	32.3	32.6	33.0	33.3	33.7
122-124	31.9	32.2	32.6	32.9	33.3	33.6	34.0	34.3
125-127	32.5	32.9	33.2	33.5	33.9	34.2	34.6	34.9
128-130	33.1	33.5	33.8	34.2	34.5	34.9	35.2	35.5

Body density is calculated based on the generalized equation for predicting body density of men developed by A. S. Jackson,and M. L. Pollock and published in the *British Journal of Nutrition,* 40 (1978), 497-504. Percent body fat is determined from the calculated body density using the Siri formula.

3

3

Table 3.3 Percent Fat Estimates for Men Over 40 Calculated From Chest, Abdomen, and Thigh Skinfold Thickness

Sum of 3 Skinfolds	Age to the Last Year: 41 to 43	44 to 46	47 to 49	50 to 52	53 to 55	56 to 58	59 to 61	62 and Over
8- 10	3.7	4.0	4.4	4.7	5.1	5.4	5.8	6.1
11- 13	4.7	5.0	5.4	5.7	6.1	6.4	6.8	7.1
14- 16	5.7	6.0	6.4	6.7	7.1	7.4	7.8	8.1
17- 19	6.7	7.0	7.4	7.7	8.1	8.4	8.7	9.1
20- 22	7.6	8.0	8.3	8.7	9.0	9.4	9.7	10.1
23- 25	8.6	8.9	9.3	9.6	10.0	10.3	10.7	11.0
26- 28	9.5	9.9	10.2	10.6	10.9	11.3	11.6	12.0
29- 31	10.5	10.8	11.2	11.5	11.9	12.2	12.6	12.9
32- 34	11.4	11.8	12.1	12.4	12.8	13.1	13.5	13.8
35- 37	12.3	12.7	13.0	13.4	13.7	14.1	14.4	14.8
38- 40	13.2	13.6	13.9	14.3	14.6	15.0	15.3	15.7
41- 43	14.1	14.5	14.8	15.2	15.5	15.9	16.2	16.6
44- 46	15.0	15.4	15.7	16.1	16.4	16.8	17.1	17.5
47- 49	15.9	16.2	16.6	16.9	17.3	17.6	18.0	18.3
50- 52	16.8	17.1	17.5	17.8	18.2	18.5	18.8	19.2
53- 55	17.6	18.0	18.3	18.7	19.0	19.4	19.7	20.1
56- 58	18.5	18.8	19.2	19.5	19.9	20.2	20.6	20.9
59- 61	19.3	19.7	20.0	20.4	20.7	21.0	21.4	21.7
62- 64	20.1	20.5	20.8	21.2	21.5	21.9	22.2	22.6
65- 67	21.0	21.3	21.7	22.0	22.4	22.7	23.0	23.4
68- 70	21.8	22.1	22.5	22.8	23.2	23.5	23.9	24.2
71- 73	22.6	22.9	23.3	23.6	24.0	24.3	24.7	25.0
74- 76	23.4	23.7	24.1	24.4	24.8	25.1	25.4	25.8
77- 79	24.1	24.5	24.8	25.2	25.5	25.9	26.2	26.6
80- 82	24.9	25.3	25.6	26.0	26.3	26.6	27.0	27.3
83- 85	25.7	26.0	26.4	26.7	27.1	27.4	27.8	28.1
86- 88	26.4	26.8	27.1	27.5	27.8	28.2	28.5	28.9
89- 91	27.2	27.5	27.9	28.2	28.6	28.9	29.2	29.6
92- 94	27.9	28.2	28.6	28.9	29.3	29.6	30.0	30.3
95- 97	28.6	29.0	29.3	29.7	30.0	30.4	30.7	31.1
98-100	29.3	29.7	30.0	30.4	30.7	31.1	31.4	31.8
101-103	30.0	30.4	30.7	31.1	31.4	31.8	32.1	32.5
104-106	30.7	31.1	31.4	31.8	32.1	32.5	32.8	33.2
107-109	31.4	31.8	32.1	32.4	32.8	33.1	33.5	33.8
110-112	32.1	32.4	32.8	33.1	33.5	33.8	34.2	34.5
113-115	32.7	33.1	33.4	33.8	34.1	34.5	34.8	35.2
116-118	33.4	33.7	34.1	34.4	34.8	35.1	35.5	35.8
119-121	34.0	34.4	34.7	35.1	35.4	35.8	36.1	36.5
122-124	34.7	35.0	35.4	35.7	36.1	36.4	36.7	37.1
125-127	35.3	35.6	36.0	36.3	36.7	37.0	37.4	37.7
128-130	35.9	36.2	36.6	36.9	37.3	37.6	38.0	38.5

Body density is calculated based on the generalized equation for predicting body density of men developed by A. S. Jackson and M. L. Pollock and published in the *British Journal of Nutrition*, 40 (1978), 497-504. Percent body fat is determined from the calculated body density using the Siri formula.

Girth Measurements

A simpler method to determine body fat is by measuring circumferences at various body sites. All this technique requires is a standard measuring tape, and good accuracy can be achieved with little practice. The limitation is that it may not be valid for athletic individuals (men or women) who participate actively in strenuous physical activity or people who can be classified visually as thin or obese.

The required procedure for **girth measurements** is given in Figure 3.4. Measurements for women include the upper arm, hip, and wrist; for men, the waist and wrist.

Girth measurements Technique to assess body composition, including percent body fat, by measuring circumferences at various body sites.

3

GIRTH MEASUREMENTS

Girth Measurements for Women*

1. Using a regular tape measure, determine the following girth measurements in centimeters (cm):

   Upper arm: Take the measure halfway between the shoulder and the elbow.
   Hip: Measure at the point of largest circumference.
   Wrist: Take the girth in front of the bones where the wrist bends.

2. Obtain the person's age.
3. Using Table 3.4, find the girth measurement for each site and age in the lefthand column below. Look up the constant values in the righthand column. These values will allow you to derive body density (BD) by substituting the constants in the following formula:

   BD = A – B – C + D

4. Using the derived body density, calculate percent body fat (%F) according to the following equation:

   %F = (495 ÷ BD) – 450**

5. Example: Jane is 20 years old, and the following girth measurements were taken: biceps = 27 cm, hip = 99.5 cm, wrist = 15.4 cm.

Data	Constant
Upper arm = 27 cm	A = 1.0813
Age = 20	B = .0102
Hip = 99.5 cm	C = .1206
Wrist = 15.4 cm	D = .0971

BD = A – B – C + D
BD = 1.0813 – .0102 – .1206 + .0971 = 1.0476

%F = (495 ÷ BD) – 450
%F = (495 ÷ 1.0476) – 450 = 22.5

Girth Measurements for Men***

1. Using a regular tape measure, determine the following girth measurements in inches (the men's measurements are taken in inches, as opposed to centimeters for women):

   Waist: measure at the umbilicus (belly button)
   Wrist: measure in front of the bones where the wrist bends.

2. Subtract the wrist from the waist measurement.
3. Obtain the weight of the subject in pounds.
4. Look up the percent body fat (%F) in Table 3.5 by using the difference obtained in number 2 above and the person's body weight.
5. Example: John weighs 160 pounds, and his waist and wrist girth measurements are 36.5 and 7.5 inches, respectively.

   Waist girth = 36.5 inches
   Wrist girth = 7.5 inches
   Difference = 29.0 inches
   Body weight = 160.0 lbs.
   %F = 22

* From "Generalized Body Density Prediction Equations for Women Using Simple Anthropometric Measurements." by R. B. Lambson, unpublished doctoral dissertation, Brigham Young University, Provo, UT August 1987. Reproduced by permission.

** From *Body Composition from Fluid Spaces and Density.* by W. E. Siri (Berkeley, CA: University of California, Donner Laboratory of Medical Physics, 1956).

*** From *Jogging,* by A. G. Fisher and P. E. Allsen, Dubuque, IA: Wm. C. Brown, 1987. This table was developed according to the generalized body composition equation for men using simple measurement techniques by K. W. Penrouse, A. G Nelson, and A G. Fisher. Medicine and Science in Sports and Exercise 17(2):189, 1985. © American College of Sports Medicine 1985..

Figure 3.4 Procedure for assessing body fat according to girth measurements.

Table 3.4 Conversion Constants from Girth Measurements (Centimeters) to Calculate Body Density for Women

Upper Arm (cm)	Constant A	Age	Constant B	Hip (cm)	Constant C	Hip (cm)	Constant C	Wrist (cm)	Constant D
20.5	1.0966	17	.0086	79	.0957	114.5	.1388	13.0	.0819
21	1.0954	18	.0091	79.5	.0963	115	.1394	13.2	.0832
21.5	1.0942	19	.0096	80	.0970	115.5	.1400	13.4	.0845
22	1.0930	20	.0102	80.5	.0976	116	.1406	13.6	.0857
22.5	1.0919	21	.0107	81	.0982	116.5	.1412	13.8	.0807
23	1.0907	22	.0112	81.5	.0988	117	.1418	14.0	.0882
23.5	1.0895	23	.0117	82	.0994	117.5	.1424	14.2	.0895
24	1.0883	24	.0122	82.5	.1000	118	.1430	14.4	.0908
24.5	1.0871	25	.0127	83	.1006	118.5	.1436	14.6	.0920
25	1.0860	26	.0132	83.5	.1012	119	.1442	14.8	.0933
25.5	1.0848	27	.0137	84	.1018	119.5	.1448	15.0	.0946
26	1.0836	28	.0142	84.5	.1024	120	.1454	15.2	.0958
26.5	1.0824	29	.0147	85	.1030	120.5	.1460	15.4	.0971
27	1.0813	30	.0152	85.5	.1036	121	.1466	15.6	.0983
27.5	1.0801	31	.0157	86	.1042	121.5	.1472	15.8	.0996
28	1.0789	32	.0162	86.5	.1048	122	.1479	16.0	.1009
28.5	1.0777	33	,0168	87	.1054	122.5	.1485	16.2	.1021
29	1.0775	34	.0173	87.5	.1060	123	.1491	16.4	.1034
29.5	1.0754	35	.0178	88	.1066	123.5	.1497	16.6	.1046
30	1.0742	36	.0183	88.5	.1072	124	.1503	16.8	.1059
30.5	1.0730	37	.0188	89	.1079	124.5	.1509	17.0	.1072
31	1.0718	38	.0193	89.5	.1085	125	.1515	17.2	.1084
31.5	1.0707	39	.0198	90	.1091	125.5	.1521	17.4	.1097
32	1.0695	40	,0203	90.5	.1097	126	.1527	17.6	.1109
32.5	1.0683	41	.0208	91	.1103	126.5	.1533	17.8	.1122
33	1.0671	42	.0213	91.5	.1109	127	.1539	18.0	.1135
33.5	1.0666	43	.0218	92	.1115	127.5	.1545	18.2	.1147
34	1.0648	44	.0223	92.5	.1121	128	.1551	18.4	.1160
34.5	1.0636	45	.0228	93	.1127	128.5	.1558	18.6	.1172
35	1.0624	46	.0234	93.5	.1133	129	.1563		
35.5	1.0612	47	.0239	94	.1139	129.5	.1569		
36	1.0601	48	,0244	94.5	.1145	130	.1575		
36.5	1.0589	49	.0249	95	.1151	130.5	.1581		
37	1.0577	50	.0254	95.5	.1157	131	.1587		
37.5	1.0565	51	.0259	96	.1163	131.5	.1593		
38	1.0554	52	.0264	96.5	.1169	132	.1600		
38.5	1.0542	53	.0269	97	.1176	132.5	.1606		
39	1.0530	54	.0274	97.5	.1182	133	.1612		
39.5	1.0518	55	.0279	98	.1188	133.5	.1618		
40	1.0506	56	.0284	98.5	.1194	134	.1624		
40.5	1.0495	57	.0289	99	.1200	134.5	.1630		
41	1.0483	58	.0294	99.5	.1206	135	.1636		
41.5	1.0471	59	.0300	100	.1212	135.5	.1642		
42	1.0459	60	.0305	100.5	.1218	136	.1648		
42.5	1.0448	61	.0310	101	.1224	136.5	.1654		
43	1.0434	62	.0315	101.5	.1230	137	.1660		
43.5	1.0424	63	.0320	102	.1236	137.5	.1666		
44	1.0412	64	.0325	102.5	.1242	138	.1672		

(continued)

Table 3.4 Continued.

Upper Arm (cm)	Constant A	Age	Constant B	Hip (cm)	Constant C	Hip (cm)	Constant C	Wrist (cm)	Constant D
		65	.0330	103	.1248	138.5	.1678		
		66	.0335	103.5	.1254	139	.1685		
		67	.0340	104	.1260	139.5	.1691		
		68	.0345	104.5	.1266	140	.1697		
		69	.0350	105	.1272	140.5	.1703		
		70	.0355	105.5	.1278	141	.1709		
		71	.0360	106	.1285	141.5	.1715		
		72	.0366	106.5	.1291	142	.1721		
		73	.0371	107	.1297	142.5	.1728		
		74	.0376	107.5	.1303	143	.1733		
		75	.0381	108	.1309	143.5	.1739		
				108.5	.1315	144	.1745		
				109	.1321	144.5	.1751		
				109.5	.1327	145	.1757		
				110	.1333	145.5	.1763		
				110.5	.1339	146	.1769		
				111	.1345	146.5	.1775		
				111.5	.1351	147	.1781		
				112	.1357	147.5	.1787		
				112.5	.1363	148	.1794		
				113	.1369	148.5	.1800		
				113.5	.1375	149	.1806		
				114	.1382	149.5	.1812		
						150	.1818		

Bioelectrical Impedance

The **bioelectrical impedance** technique is much simpler to administer, but it does require costly equipment. In this technique, the individual is hooked up to a machine and a weak electrical current (totally painless) is run through the body to analyze body composition (body fat, lean body mass, and body water). The technique is based on the principle that fat tissue is not as good a conductor of an electrical current as lean tissue is. The easier the conductance, the leaner the individual.

The accuracy of current equations used in estimating percent body fat with this technique is still questionable. More research is required before the equations approach the accuracy of hydrostatic weighing, skinfolds, or girth measurements.

An advantage of bioelectrical impedance is that results are highly reproducible. Unlike other techniques, in which experienced technicians are necessary to obtain valid results, almost anyone can administer bioelectrical impedance. And, although the test results may not be completely accurate, this instrument is valuable in assessing body composition changes over time.

If this instrument or some other type of equipment for body composition assessment is available to you, you can use it to determine your percent body fat. You may want to compare the results with other techniques. Following all manufacturer's instructions will ensure the best possible result.

Waist-to-Hip Ratio

Scientific evidence suggests that the way people store fat affects the risk for disease. Some individuals tend to store fat in the abdominal area (called the "apple" shape). Others store it primarily around the hips and thighs (gluteal femoral fat, the "pear" shape).

Bioelectrical impedance Technique to assess body composition, including percent body fat, by running a weak electrical current through the body.

Table 3.5 Estimated Percent Body Fat for Men Obtained from Waist Minus Wrist Girth Measurements (Inches) and Body Weight

	22	22.5	23	23.5	24	24.5	25	25.5	26	26.5	27	27.5	28	28.5	29	29.5	30	30.5	31	31.5	32	32.5	33	33.5	34	34.5	35	35.5	36	36.5	37	37.5	38	38.5	39	39.5	40	40.5	41	41.5	42	42.5	43	43.5	44	44.5	45	45.5	46	46.5	47	47.5	48	48.5	49	49.5	50
120	4	6	8	10	12	14	16	18	20	21	23	25	27	29	31	33	35	37	39	41	43	45	47	49	50	52	54	56	58
125	4	6	7	9	11	13	15	17	19	20	22	24	26	28	30	32	33	35	37	39	41	43	45	46	48	50	52	54	56	58
130	3	5	7	9	11	12	14	16	18	20	21	23	25	27	28	30	32	34	36	37	39	41	43	44	46	48	50	52	53	55	57
135	3	5	7	8	10	12	13	15	17	19	20	22	24	26	27	29	31	32	34	36	38	39	41	43	44	46	48	50	51	53	55	56
140	3	5	6	8	10	11	13	15	16	18	19	21	23	24	26	28	29	31	33	34	36	38	39	41	43	44	46	48	49	51	53	54	56
145	3	4	6	7	9	11	12	14	15	17	19	20	22	23	25	27	28	30	31	33	35	36	38	39	41	43	44	46	47	49	51	52	54	55
150	2	4	6	7	9	10	12	13	15	16	18	19	21	23	24	26	27	29	30	32	33	35	36	38	40	41	43	44	46	47	49	50	52	53	55
155	2	4	5	7	8	10	11	13	14	16	17	19	20	22	23	25	26	28	29	31	32	34	35	37	38	40	41	43	44	46	47	49	50	52	53	55
160	2	4	5	6	8	9	11	12	14	15	17	18	19	21	22	24	25	27	28	30	31	33	34	35	37	38	40	41	43	44	46	47	48	50	51	53	54
165	2	3	5	6	8	9	10	12	13	15	16	17	19	20	22	23	24	26	27	29	30	31	33	34	36	37	38	40	41	43	44	45	47	48	50	51	52	54
170	2	3	4	6	7	9	10	11	13	14	15	17	18	19	21	22	24	25	26	28	29	30	32	33	34	36	37	39	40	41	43	44	45	47	48	49	51	52	54
175	2	3	4	6	7	8	10	11	12	13	15	16	17	19	20	21	23	24	25	27	28	29	31	32	33	35	36	37	39	40	41	43	44	45	47	48	49	51	52	53
180		3	4	5	7	8	9	10	12	13	14	16	17	18	19	21	22	23	25	26	27	28	30	31	32	34	35	36	37	39	40	41	43	44	45	47	48	49	50	52	53
185		3	4	5	6	8	9	10	11	13	14	15	16	18	19	20	21	23	24	25	26	28	29	30	31	33	34	35	36	38	39	40	41	43	44	45	46	48	49	50	51	53
190		2	4	5	6	7	8	10	11	12	13	15	16	17	18	19	21	22	23	24	26	27	28	29	30	32	33	34	35	37	38	39	40	41	43	44	45	46	48	49	50	51	52
195		2	3	5	6	7	8	9	11	12	13	14	15	16	18	19	20	21	22	24	25	26	27	28	30	31	32	33	34	35	37	38	39	40	41	43	44	45	46	47	49	50	51	52
200		2	3	4	6	7	8	9	10	11	12	14	15	16	17	18	19	21	22	23	24	25	26	28	29	30	31	32	33	35	36	37	38	39	40	41	43	44	45	46	47	48	50	51	52
205		2	3	4	5	6	8	9	10	11	12	13	14	15	17	18	19	20	21	22	23	25	26	27	28	29	30	31	32	34	35	36	37	38	39	40	41	43	44	45	46	47	48	49	51	52
210		2	3	4	5	6	7	8	9	11	12	13	14	15	16	17	18	19	21	22	23	24	25	26	27	28	29	30	32	33	34	35	36	37	38	39	40	42	43	44	45	46	47	48	49	50	51
215		2	3	4	5	6	7	8	9	10	11	12	13	15	16	17	18	19	20	21	22	23	24	25	26	28	29	30	31	32	33	34	35	36	37	38	39	40	42	43	44	45	46	47	48	49	50	51
220			2	3	4	6	7	8	9	10	11	12	13	14	15	16	17	18	19	20	22	23	24	25	26	27	28	29	30	31	32	33	34	35	36	37	38	39	41	42	43	44	45	46	47	48	49	50	51
225			2	3	4	6	7	8	9	10	11	12	13	14	15	16	17	18	19	20	21	22	23	24	25	26	27	28	29	30	31	32	33	34	35	36	37	38	40	41	42	43	44	45	46	47	48	49	50	51
230			2	3	4	5	6	7	8	9	10	11	12	13	14	15	16	17	18	19	20	21	22	23	24	25	26	27	28	30	31	32	33	34	35	36	37	38	39	40	41	42	43	44	45	46	47	48	49	50	51
235			2	3	4	5	6	7	8	9	10	11	12	13	14	15	16	17	18	19	20	21	22	23	24	25	26	27	28	29	30	31	32	33	34	35	36	37	38	39	40	41	42	43	44	45	46	47	48	49	50	51
240			2	3	4	5	6	7	8	9	10	11	12	13	14	15	16	17	17	18	19	20	21	22	23	24	25	26	27	28	29	30	31	32	33	34	35	36	37	38	39	40	41	42	43	44	45	46	46	47	48	49	50
245			2	3	4	5	6	7	8	9	9	10	11	12	13	14	15	16	17	18	19	20	21	22	23	24	25	26	27	27	28	29	30	31	32	33	34	35	36	37	38	39	40	41	42	43	44	44	45	46	47	48	49	50
250			2	3	4	5	6	6	7	8	9	10	11	12	13	14	15	16	17	18	18	19	20	21	22	23	24	25	26	27	28	29	30	31	31	32	33	34	35	36	37	38	39	40	41	42	43	44	44	45	46	47	48	49	50
255			2	3	3	4	5	6	7	8	9	10	11	12	13	14	14	15	16	17	18	19	20	21	22	23	24	24	25	26	27	28	29	30	31	32	33	34	34	35	36	37	38	39	40	41	42	43	44	44	45	46	47	48	49	50
260			2	2	3	4	5	6	7	8	9	10	10	11	12	13	14	15	16	17	18	19	19	20	21	22	23	24	25	26	27	27	28	29	30	31	32	33	34	35	35	36	37	38	39	40	41	42	43	43	44	45	46	47	48	49	50
265				2	3	4	5	6	7	8	8	9	10	11	12	13	14	15	15	16	17	18	19	20	21	22	22	23	24	25	26	27	28	29	29	30	31	32	33	34	35	36	36	37	38	39	40	41	42	43	43	44	45	46	47	48	49
270				2	3	4	5	6	7	7	8	9	10	11	12	13	13	14	15	16	17	18	19	19	20	21	22	23	24	25	25	26	27	28	29	30	31	31	32	33	34	35	36	37	37	38	39	40	41	42	43	43	44	45	46	47	48
275				2	3	4	5	5	6	7	8	9	10	11	11	12	13	14	15	16	16	17	18	19	20	21	22	22	23	24	25	26	27	27	28	29	30	31	32	32	33	34	35	36	37	38	38	39	40	41	42	43	43	44	45	46	47
280				2	3	4	4	5	6	7	8	9	9	10	11	12	13	14	14	15	16	17	18	19	19	20	21	22	23	24	24	25	26	27	28	29	29	30	31	32	33	33	34	35	36	37	38	38	39	40	41	42	43	43	44	45	46
285				2	3	4	4	5	6	7	8	8	9	10	11	12	12	13	14	15	16	17	17	18	19	20	21	21	22	23	24	25	26	26	27	28	29	30	30	31	32	33	34	34	35	36	37	38	39	39	40	41	42	43	43	44	45
290				2	3	3	4	5	6	7	7	8	9	10	11	11	12	13	14	15	15	16	17	18	19	19	20	21	22	23	23	24	25	26	27	27	28	29	30	31	31	32	33	34	35	35	36	37	38	39	39	40	41	42	43	43	44
295				2	2	3	4	5	6	6	7	8	9	10	10	11	12	13	14	14	15	16	17	17	18	19	20	21	21	22	23	24	25	25	26	27	28	28	29	30	31	32	32	33	34	35	36	36	37	38	39	39	40	41	42	43	43
300				2	2	3	4	5	5	6	7	8	9	9	10	11	12	12	13	14	15	16	16	17	18	19	19	20	21	22	22	23	24	25	26	26	27	28	29	29	30	31	32	33	33	34	35	36	36	37	38	39	39	40	41	42	43

Obese individuals with a lot of abdominal fat clearly are at higher risk for coronary heart disease, congestive heart failure, hypertension, adult-onset (Type II) diabetes, and strokes than are obese people with similar amounts of total body fat that is stored primarily in the hips and thighs. Relatively new evidence also indicates that, among individuals with high abdominal fat, those whose fat deposits are around internal organs (visceral fat) are at even greater risk for disease than those whose abdominal fat is primarily beneath the skin (subcutaneous fat).[1]

Because of the higher risk for disease in individuals who tend to store a lot of fat in the abdominal area, as contrasted with the hips and thighs, a **waist-to-hip ratio test** was designed by a panel of scientists appointed by the National Academy of Sciences and the Dietary Guidelines Advisory Council for the U.S. Departments of Agriculture and Health and Human Services. The waist measurement is taken at the point of smallest circumference, and the hip measurement is taken at the point of greatest circumference.

The waist-to-hip ratio differentiates the "apples" from the "pears." More men are apples, and more women are pears. The panel recommends that men need to lose weight if the waist-to-hip ratio is 1.0 or higher. Women need to lose weight if the ratio is .85 or higher. More conservative estimates indicate that the risk starts to increase when the ratio exceeds .95 and .80 for men and women, respectively. For example, the waist-to-hip ratio for a man with a 40-inch waist and a 38-inch hip would be 1.05 (40 ÷ 38). This ratio may indicate higher risk for disease.

Body Mass Index

Another technique scientists use to determine thinness and excessive fatness is the **Body Mass Index (BMI)**. This index incorporates height and weight to estimate critical fat values at which the risk for disease increases. BMI is calculated by dividing the weight in kilograms by the square of the height in meters or multiplying your weight in pounds by 705, dividing this figure by your height in inches, and then dividing by the same height again. For example, the BMI for an individual who weighs 172 pounds (78 kg) and is 67 inches (1.7 mts) tall would be 27 [$78 \div (1.7)^2$] or ($172 \times 705 \div 67 \div 67$).

According to BMI, the lowest risk for chronic disease is in the 22 to 25 range (see Table 3.6).

Table 3.6 Disease Risk According to Body Mass Index (BMI)

BMI	Disease Risk	Classification
<20.00	Moderate to Very High	Underweight
20.00 to 21.99	Low	Acceptable
22.00 to 24.99	Very Low	
25.00 to 29.99	Low	Overweight
30.00 to 34.99	Moderate	Obese
35.00 to 39.99	High	
≥40.00	Very High	

Individuals are classified as overweight between 25 and 30. BMIs above 30 are defined as obesity and below 20 as underweight.

BMI is a useful tool to screen the general population, but, similar to height/weight charts, it fails to differentiate fat from lean body mass or where most of the fat is located (see waist-to-hip ratio). Using BMI, athletes with a large amount of muscle mass (body builders, football players) easily can fall in the moderate or even high-risk categories. Therefore, body composition and waist-to-hip ratios are better procedures to determine health risk and recommended body weight.

Determining Recommended Body Weight

After finding out your percent body fat, you can determine your current body composition classification according to Table 3.7. In this table you will find the health fitness and the high physical fitness percent fat standards.

For example, the recommended health fitness fat percentage for a 20-year-old female is 28% or less. The health fitness standard is established at the point at which there seems to be no harm to health in terms of percent body fat. A high physical fitness range for this same woman would be between 18% and 23%.

The high physical fitness standard does not mean you cannot be somewhat below this number. Many highly trained male athletes are as low as 3%, and some female distance runners have been measured at 6% body fat (which may not be healthy).

Waist-to-hip ratio A test to assess potential risk for diseases associated with obesity.

Body mass index (BMI) Ratio of weight to height, used to determine thinness and fatness.

3

Table 3.7 Body Composition Classification According to Percent Body Fat

		MEN			
Age	**Excellent**	**Good**	**Moderate**	**Overweight**	**Significantly Overweight**
≤19	12.0	12.1–17.0	17.1–22.0	22.1–27.0	≥ 27.1
20–29	13.0	13.1–18.0	18.1–23.0	23.1–28.0	≥ 28.1
30–39	14.0	14.1–19.0	19.1–24.0	24.1–29.0	≥ 29.1
40–49	15.0	15.1–20.0	20.1–25.0	25.1–30.0	≥ 30.1
≥ 50	16.0	16.1–21.5	21.1–26.0	26.1–31.0	≥ 31.1
		WOMEN			
Age	**Excellent**	**Good**	**Moderate**	**Overweight**	**Significantly Overweight**
≤19	17.0	17.1–22.0	22.1–27.0	27.1–32.0	≥ 32.1
20–29	18.0	18.1–23.0	23.1–28.0	28.1–33.0	≥ 33.1
30–39	19.0	19.1–24.0	24.1–29.0	29.1–34.0	≥ 34.1
40–49	20.0	20.1–25.0	25.1–30.0	30.1–35.0	≥ 35.1
≥ 50	21.0	21.1–26.5	26.1–31.0	31.1–36.0	≥ 36.1

High physical fitness standard

Health fitness standard

See Chapter 1, Fitness Standards: Health versus Physical Fitness, page 7.

Although people generally agree that the mortality rate is greater for obese people, some evidence indicates that the same is true for underweight people. "Underweight" and "thin" do not necessarily mean the same thing. A healthy thin person has total body fat around the high physical fitness standard, whereas an underweight person has extremely low body fat, even to the point of compromising the essential fat.

The 3% essential fat for men and 12% for women seem to be the lower limits for people to maintain good health. Below these percentages, normal physiologic functions can be seriously impaired. Some experts point out that a little storage fat (over the essential fat) is better than none at all. As a result, the health and high fitness standards for percent fat in Table 3.7 are set higher than the minimum essential fat requirements, at a point beneficial to optimal health and well-being. Finally, because lean tissue decreases with age, one extra percentage point is allowed for every additional decade of life.

Your recommended body weight is computed based on the selected health or high fitness fat percentage for your age and gender. Your decision to select a "desired" fat percentage should be based on your current percent body fat and your personal health/fitness objectives. To compute your own recommended body weight:

1. Determine the pounds of body weight in fat (FW). Multiply body weight (BW) by the current percent fat (%F) expressed in decimal form (FW = BW × %F).
2. Determine lean body mass (LBM) by subtracting the weight in fat from the total body weight (LBM = BW − FW). (Anything that is not fat must be part of the lean component.)
3. Select a desired body fat percentage (DFP) based on the health or high fitness standards given in Table 3.7.
4. Compute recommended body weight (RBW) according to the formula: RBW = LBM ÷ (1.0 – DFP).

As an example of these computations, a 19-year-old female who weighs 160 pounds and is 30% fat would like to know what her recommended body weight would be at 22%:

Gender: female
Age: 19
BW: 160 lbs.
%F: 30% (.30 in decimal form)

1. FW = BW × %F
   FW = 160 × .30 = 48 lbs.
2. LBM = BW – FW
   LBM = 160 – 48 = 112 lbs.
3. DFP: 22% (.22 in decimal form)
4. RBW = LBM ÷ (1.0 – DFP)
   RBW = 112 ÷ (1.0 – .22)
   RBW = 112 ÷ (.78) = 143.6 lbs.

In Labs 3A and 3B you will have the opportunity to determine your own body composition and recommended body weight using the procedures outlined in this chapter. In Lab 3C you can determine your disease risk according to waist-to-hip ratio and BMI.

Other than hydrostatic weighing, skinfold thickness seems to be the most practical and valid technique to estimate body fat. If skinfold calipers are available, use this technique to assess percent body fat. If calipers are unavailable, you can estimate your percent fat according to the girth measurements technique or another technique available to you. (You may wish to use several techniques and compare the results.)

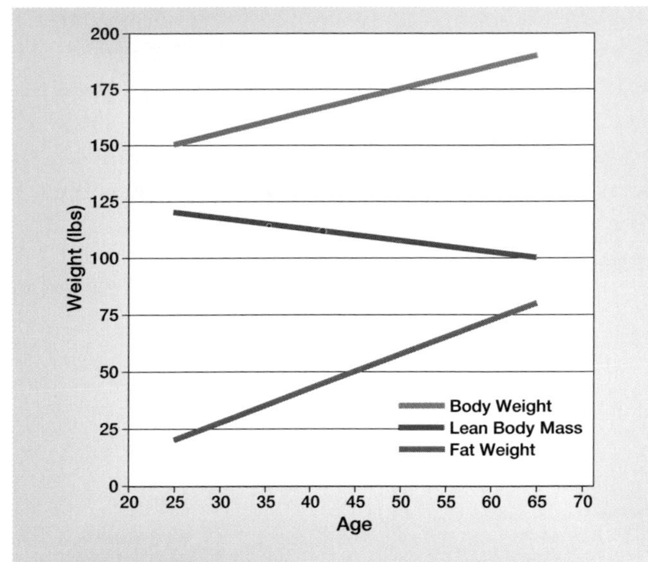

Figure 3.5 Typical body composition changes for adults in the United States.

Importance of Regular Body Composition Assessment

Children do not start with a weight problem. Although a small group struggles with weight throughout life, most are not overweight when they reach age 20.

Current trends indicate that starting at age 25, the average man and woman in the United States gains 1 pound of weight per year. Thus, by age 65, the average American will have gained 40 pounds of weight. Because of the typical reduction in physical activity in our society, however, the average person also loses a half a pound of lean tissue each year. Therefore, over this span of 40 years, there has been an actual fat gain of 60 pounds accompanied by a 20-pound loss of lean body mass[2] (see Figure 3.5). These changes cannot be detected unless body composition is assessed periodically.

If you are on a diet/exercise program, you should repeat the computations about once a month to monitor changes in your body composition. This is important because lean body mass is affected by weight reduction programs and amount of physical activity. As lean body mass changes, so will your recommended body weight. To make valid comparisons, the same technique should be used between pre- and post-assessments.

Changes in body composition resulting from a weight control/exercise program were illustrated in a co-ed aerobic dance course taught during a 6-week summer term. Students participated in aerobic dance routines four times a week, 60 minutes each time. On the first and last days of class, several physiological parameters, including body composition, were assessed. Students also were given information on diet and nutrition, and they basically followed their own weight control program.

At the end of the 6 weeks, the average weight loss for the entire class was 3 pounds (see Figure 3.6). Because body composition was assessed, however, class members were surprised to find that the average fat loss was actually 6 pounds, accompanied by a 3-pound increase in lean body mass.

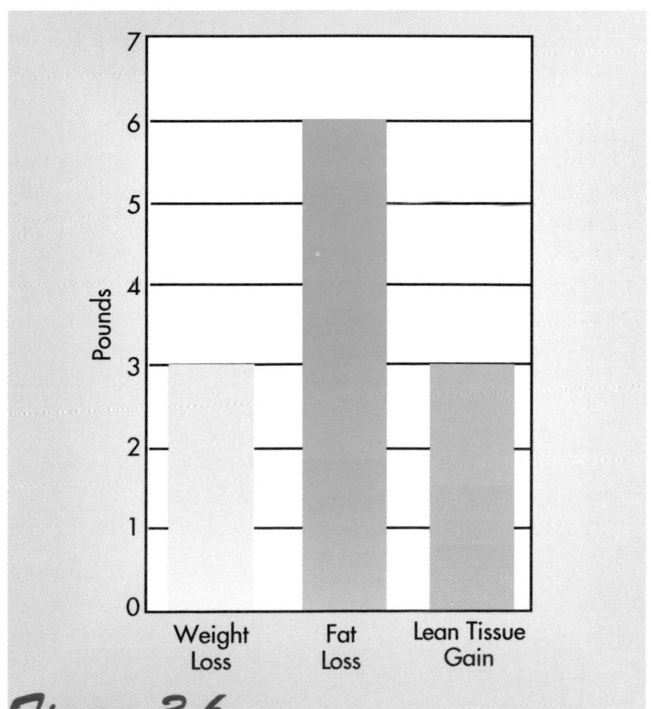

Figure 3.6 Effects of a 6-week aerobics program on body composition.

When dieting, body composition should be reassessed periodically because of the effects of negative caloric balance on lean body mass. As is discussed in Chapter 4, dieting does decrease lean body mass. This lean body mass loss can be reduced or eliminated by combining a sensible diet with physical exercise.

Laboratory Experience

LAB 3A
Hydrostatic Weighing for Body Composition Assessment

Lab Preparation
Bring a swimsuit and towel to this lab. A 6- to 8-hour fast and bladder and bowel movements are recommended prior to underwater weighing. If pulmonary function equipment is available, measure residual lung volume before going into the water.

LAB 3B
Anthropometric Measurements for Body Comparison Assessment and Recommended Body Weight Determination

Lab Preparation
Wear shorts and a loose-fitting t-shirt (no leotards). Do not use lotion on your skin the day of this lab.

LAB 3C
Weight and Health: Disease Risk Assessment

Lab Preparation
None required.

3

Notes

1. C. Bouchard, and F. E. Johnson, editors, *Fat Distribution During Growth and Later Health Outcomes* (New York: Alan R. Liss, 1988).
2. J. H. Wilmore, "Exercise and Weight Control: Myths, Misconceptions, and Quackery," lecture given at annual meeting of the American College of Sports Medicine, Indianapolis, June 1994.

Suggested Readings

C. Bouchard, G. A. Bray, and V. S. Hubbard, "Basic and Clinical Aspects of Regional Fat Distribution," *American Journal of Clinical Nutrition,* 52 (1990), 946–950.

G. A. Bray, "Pathophysiology of Obesity." *American Journal of Clinical Nutrition,* 55 (1992): 488S–494S.

Fisher, A. G., and P. E. Allsen. *Jogging.* Dubuque, IA: Wm. C. Brown, 1987.

Goldman, H. L., and M. R. Becklake. "Respiratory Function Tests: Normal Values at Medium Altitudes and the Prediction of Normal Results." *American Review of Tuberculosis,* 79 (1959), 457–467.

Hoeger, W. W. K., and S. A. Hoeger. *Lifetime Physical Fitness & Wellness: A Personalized Program.* Englewood, CO: Morton Publishing, 1995.

Jackson, A. S., and M. L. Pollock. "Generalized Equations for Predicting Body Density of Men." *British Journal of Nutrition*, 40 (1978), 497–504.

Jackson, A. S., M. L. Pollock, and A. Ward. "Generalized Equations for Predicting Body Density of Women." *Medicine and Science in Sports and Exercise,* 3 (1980), 175–182.

Lambson, R. B. *Generalized Body Density Prediction Equations for Women Using Simple Anthropometric Measurements.* Unpublished doctoral dissertation, Brigham Young University, Provo, Utah, August 1987.

Penrouse, K. W., A. G. Nelson, and A. G. Fisher. "Generalized Body Composition Equation for Men Using Simple Measurement Techniques." *Medicine and Science in Sports and Exercise,* 17:2 (1985), 189.

W. E. Siri, *Body Composition from Fluid Spaces and Density* (Berkeley, CA: Donner Laboratory of Medical Physics, University of California, 1956).

Stensland, S. H., and S. Margolis. "Simplifying the Calculation of Body Mass Index for Quick Reference." *Journal of the American Dietetic Association*, 90 (1990):856.

Principles of Weight Management

4

LABS

Two terms commonly are used in reference to people who weigh more than recommended are overweight and obesity. Obesity levels are established at a point at which the excess body fat can lead to serious health problems.

***Obesity** is a health hazard of epidemic proportions in most developed countries around the world. An estimated 35% of the adult population in industrialized nations is obese.*

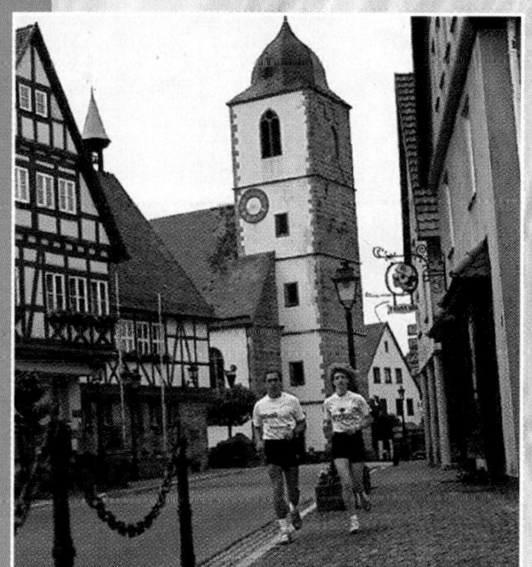

When Yankee Stadium in New York was renovated several years ago, total seating capacity had to be reduced to accommodate the wider bodies of the spectators. During the last decade, the average weight of American adults increased by about 15 pounds. In 1991, 33% of adults were at least 10% above recommended body weight. In 1993, that percentage of adults grew to 40%.

Obesity by itself has been associated with several serious health problems and accounts for 15% to 20% of the annual mortality rate in the United States. Obesity is a major risk factor for diseases of the cardiovascular system, including coronary heart disease, hypertension, congestive heart failure, high levels of blood lipids, atherosclerosis, strokes, thromboembolitic disease, osteoarthritis, and varicose veins.

Objectives

- Understand the health consequences of obesity.
- Learn about fad diets and other myths and fallacies regarding weight control.
- Become familiar with eating disorders and their associated medical problems and behavior patterns, and understand the need for professional help in treating these conditions.
- Understand the physiology of weight loss, including setpoint theory and the effects of diet on basal metabolic rate.
- Recognize the role of a lifetime exercise program as the key to a successful weight loss and maintenance program.
- Learn how to implement a physiologically sound weight reduction and weight maintenance program.
- Learn behavior modification techniques that help a person adhere to a lifetime weight maintenance program.

Other research points toward a possible link between obesity and cancer of the colon, rectum, prostate, gallbladder, breast, uterus, and ovaries. In addition, obesity has been associated with diabetes, ruptured intervertebral discs, gallstones, gout, respiratory insufficiency, and complications during pregnancy and delivery. Furthermore, it is implicated in psychological maladjustment and increased accidental death rate.

Achieving and maintaining recommended body weight is a major objective of a good physical fitness and wellness program. The assessment of recommended body weight was discussed in detail in Chapter 3. Next to poor cardiovascular fitness, obesity is the problem encountered most commonly in fitness and wellness assessments.

The health consequences of obesity apply primarily to the severely overweight individual.

4

Approximately 65 million Americans are **overweight** or consider themselves to be overweight. Of these, 30 million are obese. About 50% of all women and 25% of all men are on a diet at any given moment. People spend about $40 billion yearly attempting to lose weight. More than $10 billion goes to memberships in weight-reduction centers and another $30 billion to diet food sales.

Overweight and obesity are not the same thing. Most overweight people (an excess of 10 to 15 pounds) are not obese. The health consequences of obesity apply primarily to severely overweight individuals.

Granted, genetic differences exist. Some moderately overweight people do have health problems, but this is not the case for most. Moderately overweight people with diabetes and other cardiovascular risk factors benefit from weight loss.

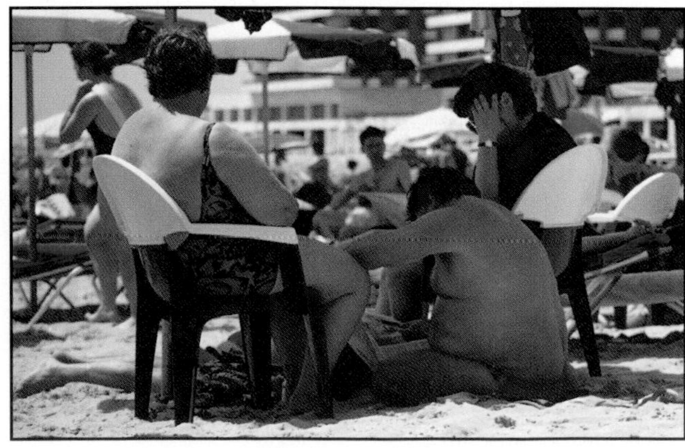

Obesity: A health hazard of epidemic proportions in developed countries.

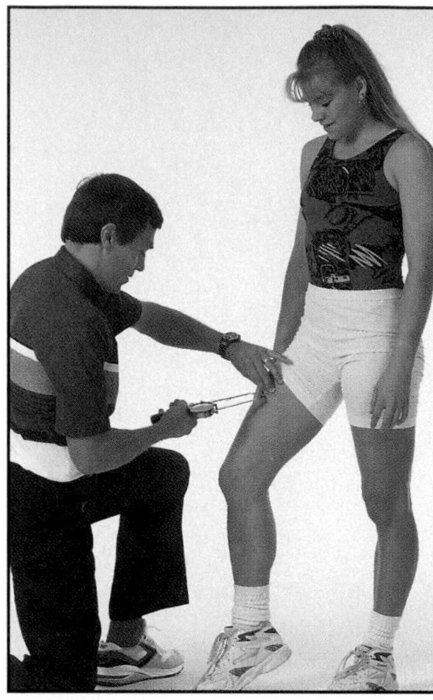

Recommended body weight is best determined through the assessment of body composition.

Scientific evidence also recognizes problems with being underweight. The social pressure to be thin has decreased slightly in recent years, but the pressure to attain model-like thinness is still with us and contributes to the gradual increase in the number of people who develop eating disorders (anorexia nervosa and bulimia, discussed later in this chapter).

Extreme weight loss can lead to medical conditions such as heart damage, gastrointestinal problems, shrinkage of internal organs, immune system abnormalities, disorders of the reproductive system, loss of muscle tissue, damage to the nervous system, and even death. About 14% of the American people are underweight.

Tolerable Weight

Many people want to lose weight so they will look better. That's a noteworthy goal. The problem, however, is that they have a distorted image of what they would really look like if they were to reduce to what they think is their ideal weight. Hereditary factors play a big role, and only a small fraction of the population has the genes for a "perfect body."

As people set their own target weight, they should be realistic. Attaining the excellent percent body fat figure in Table 3.7, page 68, is extremely difficult for some. It is even more difficult to maintain, unless they are willing to make a commitment to a vigorous lifetime exercise program and permanent dietary changes. Few people are willing to do that. The moderate percent body fat category may be more realistic for many people.

A question you should ask yourself is: Are you happy with your weight? Part of enjoying a higher quality of life is being happy with yourself. If you are not, you either need to do something about it or learn to live with it!

If you are above the moderate percent body fat category, you should try to come down and stay in this category, for health reasons. This is the category in which there appears to be no detriment to health.

If you are in the moderate category but would like to be lower, you need to ask yourself a second question: How badly do I want it? Do I want it badly enough to implement lifetime exercise and dietary changes? If you are not willing to change, you should stop worrying about your weight and deem the moderate category as "tolerable" for you.

The Weight Loss Dilemma

Yo-yo dieting carries as great a health risk as being overweight and remaining overweight in the first place. Epidemiological data are beginning to show that frequent fluctuations in weight (up or down) markedly increase the risk of dying of cardiovascular disease.

Based on the findings that constant losses and regains can be hazardous to health, quick-fix diets should be replaced by a slow but permanent weight loss program, as described in this chapter. Individuals reap the benefits of recommended body weight when they get to their recommended body weight and stay there throughout life.

Unfortunately, only about 10% of all people who begin a traditional weight loss program without exercise are able to lose the desired weight. Worse, only one in 200 is able to keep the weight off. The body is highly resistant to permanent weight changes through caloric restrictions alone.

Traditional diets have failed because few of them incorporate lifetime changes in food selection and exercise as fundamental to successful weight loss. When the diet stops, weight gain begins. The $40 billion diet industry tries to capitalize on the idea that weight can be lost quickly without taking into consideration the consequences of fast weight loss or the importance of lifetime behavioral changes to ensure proper weight loss and maintenance.

In addition, various studies indicate that most people, especially obese people, underestimate their energy intake. Those who try to lose weight but apparently fail to do so are often described as "diet-resistant." A study published by Dr. Steven Lichtman and colleagues[1] found that, while on a "diet," a group of obese individuals with a self-reported history of diet resistance underreported their average daily caloric intake by almost 50% (1028 self-reported versus 2081 actual — see Figure 4.1). These individuals also overestimated their amount of daily physical activity by about 25% (1022 calories self-reported versus 771 actual calories). These differences represent an additional 1304 calories of energy unaccounted for by the subjects in the study. These findings indicate that failing to lose weight often is related to misreports of actual food intake and level of physical activity.

Fad diets continue to appeal to people. These diets deceive people and claim the person will lose weight by following all instructions. Most fad diets are very low in calories and deprive the body of certain nutrients, generating a metabolic imbalance. Under these conditions, a lot of the weight lost is in the form of water and protein, and not fat.

4

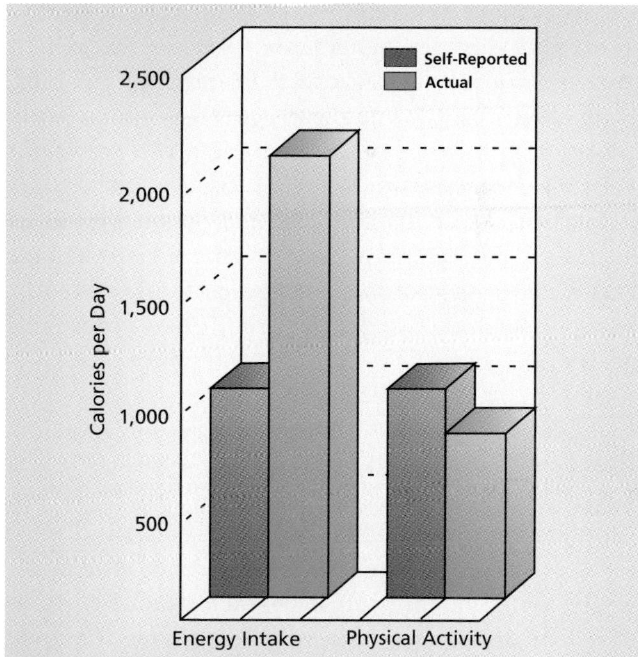

Source: "Discrepancy Between Self-Reported and Actual Caloric Intake and Exercise in Obese Subjects" by S. W. Lichtman et al., in *New England Journal of Medicine*, 327 (1992), 1893-1898.

Figure 4.1 Differences between self-reported and actual daily caloric intake and exercise in obese individuals attempting to lose weight.

Obesity A chronic disease characterized by an excessively high amount of body fat in relation to lean body mass.

Overweight An excess amount of weight against a given standard such as height or recommended percent body fat.

Yo-yo dieting Constantly losing and gaining weight.

On a crash diet, close to half the weight loss is in lean (protein) tissue. When the body uses protein instead of a combination of fats and carbohydrates as a source of energy, weight is lost as much as 10 times faster.[2] A gram of protein produces half the amount of energy that fat does. In the case of muscle protein, one-fifth of protein is mixed with four-fifths water. Each pound of muscle yields only one-tenth the amount of energy of a pound of fat. As a result, most of the weight loss is in the form of water, which on the scale, of course, looks good.

Some diets allow only certain specialized foods. If people would realize that no magic foods will provide all of the necessary nutrients, and that a person has to eat a variety of foods to be well-nourished, the diet industry would not be as successful. Most of these diets create a nutritional deficiency, which at times can be fatal.

The reason some of these diets succeed is that people eventually get tired of eating the same thing day in and day out and start eating less. If they happen to achieve the lower weight but do not make permanent dietary changes, they regain the weight quickly once they go back to their old eating habits.

A few diets recommend exercise along with caloric restrictions — the best method for weight reduction, of course. A lot of the weight lost is because of the exercise, so the diet has achieved its purpose. Unfortunately, if the people do not change their food selection and activity level permanently, they gain back the weight once they discontinue dieting and exercise.

Eating Disorders

Anorexia nervosa and bulimia are physical and emotional problems, thought to develop from individual, family, or social pressures, characterized by an intense fear of becoming fat, which does not disappear even when losing extreme amounts of weight. These medical disorders are increasing steadily in most industrialized nations where society encourages low-calorie diets and thinness.

Anorexia Nervosa

Approximately 19 of every 20 anorexics are young women. An estimated 1% of the female population in the United States is anorexic. Anorexic individuals seem to fear weight gain more than death from starvation. Furthermore, they have a distorted image of their body and think of themselves as being fat even when they are emaciated.

Although a genetic predisposition may contribute, the anorexic person often comes from a mother-dominated home, with possible drug addictions in the family. The syndrome may emerge following a stressful life event and uncertainty about the ability to cope efficiently.

Anorexic individuals seem to fear weight gain more than death from starvation.

Because the female role in society is changing more rapidly, women seem to be especially susceptible. Life experiences such as gaining weight, starting menstrual periods, beginning college, losing a boyfriend, having poor self-esteem, being socially rejected, starting a professional career, or becoming a wife or mother may trigger the syndrome.

These individuals typically begin a diet and at first feel in control and happy about the weight loss, even if they are not overweight. To speed up the weight loss, they frequently combine extreme dieting with exhaustive exercise and overuse of laxatives and diuretics.

Diagnostic Criteria for Anorexia Nervosa

- Refusal to maintain body weight over a minimal normal weight for age and height, e.g., weight loss leading to maintenance of body weight 15% below that expected; or failure to make expected weight gain during period of growth, leading to body weight 15% below that expected.
- Intense fear of gaining weight or becoming fat, even though underweight.
- Disturbance in the way in which one's body weight, size, or shape is experienced; e.g., the person claims to "feel fat" even when emaciated or believes that one area of the body is "too fat" even when obviously underweight.
- In females, absence of at least three consecutive menstrual cycles when otherwise expected to occur (primary or secondary amenorrhea). (A woman is considered to have amenorrhea if her periods occur only following hormone, e.g., estrogen, administration.)

Source: American Psychiatric Association, *Diagnostic and Statistical Manual of Mental Disorders* (Washington, DC, Association, 1987), p. 67.

Anorexics commonly develop obsessive and compulsive behaviors and emphatically deny their condition. They are preoccupied with food, meal planning, grocery shopping, and unusual eating habits. As they lose weight and their health begins to deteriorate, anorexics feel weak and tired and may realize they have a problem but will not stop the starvation and refuse to consider the behavior as abnormal.

Once they have lost a lot of weight and malnutrition sets in, physical changes become more visible. Some typical changes are amenorrhea (stopping menstruation), digestive problems, extreme sensitivity to cold, hair and skin problems, fluid and electrolyte abnormalities (which may lead to an irregular heartbeat and sudden stopping of the heart), injuries to nerves and tendons, abnormalities of immune function, anemia, growth of fine body hair, mental confusion, inability to concentrate, lethargy, depression, skin dryness, lower skin and body temperature, and osteoporosis.

Many of the changes of anorexia nervosa can be reversed, but treatment almost always requires professional help. The sooner it is started, the better the chances for reversibility and cure. Therapy consists of a combination of medical and psychological techniques to restore proper nutrition, prevent medical complications, and modify the environment or events that triggered the syndrome.

Unfortunately, anorexics strongly deny their condition. They are able to hide it and deceive friends and relatives quite effectively. Based on their behavior, many of them meet all of the characteristics of anorexia nervosa, but it goes undetected because both thinness and dieting are socially acceptable. Only a well-trained clinician is able to make a positive diagnosis.

Diagnostic Criteria for Bulimia

- Recurrent episodes of binge eating (rapid consumption of a large amount of food in a discrete period of time).
- A feeling of lack of control over eating behavior during the eating binges.
- Regular practice of either self-induced vomiting, use of laxatives or diuretics, strict dieting or fasting, or vigorous exercise to prevent weight gain.
- A minimum average of two binge eating episodes a week for at least three months.
- Persistent overconcern with body shape and weight.

Source: American Psychiatric Association, *Diagnostic and Statistical Manual of Mental Disorders* (Washington, DC, Association, 1987), p. 68-69.

Bulimia

A pattern of binge eating and purging, **bulimia** is more prevalent than anorexia nervosa. For many years it was thought to be a variant of anorexia nervosa, but now it is identified as a separate condition. It afflicts mainly young people. As many as one in every five women on college campuses may be bulimic, according to some estimates. Bulimia also is more prevalent than anorexia nervosa in males.

Bulimics usually are healthy-looking people, well-educated, near recommended body weight, who enjoy food and often socialize around it. In actuality, they are emotionally insecure, rely on others, and lack self-confidence and esteem. Recommended weight and food are important to them.

The binge-purge cycle usually occurs in stages. As a result of stressful life events or the simple compulsion to eat, bulimics periodically engage in binge eating that may last an hour or longer.

With some apprehension, bulimics anticipate and plan the cycle. Then they feel an urgency to begin. First they consume a large amount of food — several thousand calories and up to 10,000 calories in extreme cases — in a short amount of time. A brief period of relief and satisfaction is followed by feelings of deep guilt, shame, and intense fear of gaining weight. Purging seems to be an easy answer, as the binging cycle can continue without fear of gaining weight.

The most common form of purging is self-induced vomiting. Bulimics might ingest strong laxatives and emetics. They often go on near-fasting diets and strenuous bouts of exercise. Medical problems associated with bulimia include cardiac arrhythmias, amenorrhea, kidney and bladder damage, ulcers, colitis, tearing of the esophagus or stomach, tooth erosion, gum damage, and general muscular weakness.

Anorexia nervosa An eating disorder characterized by self-imposed starvation to lose and maintain very low body weight.

Bulimia An eating disorder characterized by a pattern of binge eating and purging to attempt to lose and maintain low body weight.

Unlike anorexics, bulimics realize their behavior is abnormal and feel great shame about it. Fearing social rejection, they pursue the binge-purge cycle in secrecy and at unusual times of the day.

Bulimia can be treated successfully when the person realizes this destructive behavior is not the solution to life's problems. A change in attitude can prevent permanent damage or death. Treatment is available on most school campuses through the school's counseling center or the health center. Local hospitals also offer treatment for eating disorders. Many communities have support groups, frequently led by professional personnel and usually free of charge.

The sooner treatment for eating disorders is initiated, the better the chances for recovery.

4

Physiology of Weight Loss

Only a few years ago the principles governing a weight loss and maintenance program seemed to be fairly clear, but now we know the final answers are not yet in. Traditional concepts related to weight control have centered on three assumptions: (a) that balancing food intake against output allows a person to achieve recommended weight, (b) that all fat people just eat too much, and (c) that the human body doesn't care how much (or little) fat it stores. Although these statements have some truth, they still are open to much debate and research.

Energy-Balancing Equation

The principle embodied in the **energy-balancing equation** is simple: If daily energy requirements could be determined accurately, caloric intake could be balanced against output. This is not always the case, though, because genetic and lifestyle-related individual differences determine the number of calories required to maintain or lose body weight.

Table 4.1 offers some general guidelines for estimating daily caloric intake according to lifestyle patterns. This is only an estimated figure and, as discussed later in the chapter, it serves only as a starting point from which individual adjustments have to be made.

One pound of fat equals 3,500 calories. Assuming that a person's basic daily caloric expenditure is 2,500 calories, if this person were to decrease the daily intake by 500 calories per day, it should result in a loss of one pound of fat in 7 days ($500 \times 7 = 3{,}500$). But research has shown — and many dieters probably have experienced — that even when they carefully balance caloric input against caloric output, weight loss does not always happen as predicted. Furthermore, two people with similar measured caloric intake and output seldom lose weight at the same rate.

The most common explanation regarding individual differences in weight loss and weight gain has been the variation in human metabolism from one person to another. We are all familiar with people who can eat "all day long" and not gain an ounce of weight, while others cannot even "dream about food" without gaining weight. Because experts did not believe that human metabolism alone could account for such extreme differences, they developed several theories that may better explain these individual variations.

Setpoint Theory

Results of several research studies point toward a **weight-regulating mechanism (WRM)** that has a setpoint for controlling both appetite and the amount of fat stored. **Setpoint** is hypothesized to work like a thermostat for body fat, maintaining fairly constant body weight, because it knows at all times the exact amount of adipose tissue stored in the fat cells. Some people have high settings; others have low settings.

If body weight decreases (as in dieting), the setpoint senses this change and triggers the WRM to increase the person's appetite or make the body conserve energy to maintain the "set" weight. The opposite also may be true. Some people have a hard time gaining weight. In this case, the WRM decreases appetite or causes the body to waste energy to maintain the lower weight.

Setpoint and Caloric Input

Every person has his or her own certain body fat percentage (as established by the setpoint) that the body attempts to maintain. The genetic instinct to survive tells the body that fat storage is vital, and therefore it sets an acceptable fat level. This level remains somewhat constant or may climb gradually because of poor lifestyle habits.

For instance, under strict calorie reduction, the body may make extreme metabolic adjustments in an effort to maintain its setpoint for fat. The **basal**

metabolic rate may drop dramatically against a consistent negative caloric balance, and a person may be on a plateau for days or even weeks without losing much weight. A low metabolic rate compounds a person's problems in maintaining recommended body weight.

These findings were substantiated by research conducted at Rockefeller University in New York.[3] The authors showed that the body resists maintaining altered weight. Obese and lifetime nonobese individuals were used in the investigation. Following a 10% weight loss, in an attempt to regain the lost weight, the body compensated by burning up to 15% fewer calories than were expected for the new reduced weight (after accounting for the 10% loss). The effects were similar in the obese and nonobese participants. These results imply that after a 10% weight loss, a person would have to eat less or exercise more to account for the estimated deficit of about 200 to 300 calories.

In this same study, when the participants were allowed to increase their weight to 10% above their "normal" body weight (pre-weight loss), the body burned 10% to 15% more calories than expected — an attempt by the body to waste energy and return to the pre-set weight. This is another indication that the body is highly resistant to weight changes unless additional lifestyle changes are incorporated to ensure successful weight management. These methods will be discussed in this chapter.

Dietary restriction alone will not lower the setpoint, even though the person may lose weight and fat. When the dieter goes back to the normal or even below-normal caloric intake, at which the weight may have been stable for a long time, he or she quickly regains the fat loss as the body strives to regain a comfortable fat store.

Let's use a practical illustration. A person would like to lose some body fat and assumes that a stable body weight has been reached at an average daily caloric intake of 1,800 calories (no weight gain or loss occurs at this daily intake). In an attempt to lose weight rapidly, this person now goes on a strict low-calorie diet, or even worse, a near-fasting diet. Immediately the body activates its survival mechanism and readjusts its metabolism to a lower caloric balance. After a few weeks of dieting at fewer than 400 to 600 calories per day, the body now can maintain its normal functions at 1,000 calories per day.

Having lost the desired weight, the person terminates the diet but realizes the original intake of 1,800 calories per day will have to be lower to maintain the new lower weight. To adjust to the new lower body weight, the intake is restricted to about 1,500 calories per day. The individual is surprised to find that, even at this lower daily intake (300 fewer calories), weight comes back at a rate of one pound every one to two weeks. After ending the diet, this new lowered metabolic rate may take several months to kick back up to its normal level.

From this explanation, individuals clearly should never go on very low-calorie diets. Not only will this slow down resting metabolic rate, but it also will deprive the body of basic daily nutrients required for normal function.

Daily caloric intakes of 1,200 to 1,500 calories provide the necessary nutrients if they are distributed properly over the five basic food groups (meeting the daily required servings from each group). Of course, the individual will have to learn which foods meet the requirements and yet are low in fat and sugar.

4

Under no circumstances should a person go on a diet that calls for below 1,200 and 1,500 calories for women and men, respectively. Weight (fat) is gained over months and years, not overnight. Likewise, weight loss should be gradual, not abrupt.

Lowering the Setpoint

A second way in which the setpoint may work is by keeping track of the nutrients and calories consumed daily. It is thought that the body, like a cash register, records the daily food intake and the brain will not feel satisfied until the calories and nutrients have been "registered."

This setpoint for calories and nutrients seems to work for some people, even when they participate in moderately intense exercise. Some studies have shown that people do not become hungrier with moderate physical activity. Therefore, people can choose to lose weight either by going hungry or by stepping up their daily physical activity. A greater number of

---

Energy-balancing equation A principle holding that as long as caloric input equals caloric out put, the person will not gain or lose weight. If caloric intake exceeds output, the person gains weight; when output exceeds input, the person loses weight.

Weight-regulating mechanism (WRM) A feature of the hypothalamus of the brain that controls how much the body should weigh (*also see* Setpoint theory).

Setpoint The weight control theory that indicates the body has an established weight and strongly attempts to maintain that weight.

Basal metabolic rate The lowest level of oxygen consumption necessary to sustain life.

calories burned through physical activity helps to lower body fat.

The most common question regarding the setpoint is how it can be lowered so the body will feel comfortable at a lesser fat percentage. Several factors seem to affect the setpoint directly by lowering the fat thermostat:

1. Aerobic exercise.
2. A diet high in complex carbohydrates.
3. Nicotine.
4. Amphetamines.

The last two are more destructive than the overfatness, so they are not reasonable alternatives (as far as the extra strain on the heart is concerned, smoking one pack of cigarettes per day is said to be the equivalent of carrying 50 to 75 pounds of excess body fat).

On the other hand, a diet high in fats and refined carbohydrates, near-fasting diets, and perhaps even artificial sweeteners seem to raise the setpoint. Therefore, the only practical and sensible way to lower the setpoint and lose fat weight is a combination of aerobic exercise and a diet high in complex carbohydrates and low in fat.

Because of the effects of proper food management on the body's setpoint, many nutritionists believe the total number of calories should not be the main concern in a weight-control program. Rather, it should be the source of those calories. In this regard, most of the effort is spent in retraining eating habits, increasing the intake of complex carbohydrates and high-fiber foods, and decreasing the consumption of refined carbohydrates (sugars) and fats. In most cases, this change in eating habits will bring about a decrease in total daily caloric intake.

In 1996 a new fat substitute, **olestra**, was approved by the FDA for use in "savory snacks." According to the *University of California at Berkeley Wellness Letter*[4] consumers should "just say no" to olestra and not buy products that contain this fat substitute.

Olestra can cause diarrhea and cramping, and it can deplete the body of fat-soluble vitamins, including A, D, E, and K. Vitamin E is a strong antioxidant, and low levels of vitamin K pose a risk for people with bleeding disorders and those on blood-thinning medication. Additionally, potential cancer-causing liver-cell changes have been found in animal studies. Although the fat and caloric content of olestra-containing foods is lower than that of foods cooked with natural fats, consuming snacks using this fat substitute may not only pose a risk to good health but also may reinforce unhealthy eating habits.

A "diet" no longer is viewed as a temporary tool to aid in weight loss but, instead, as a permanent change in eating behaviors to ensure weight management and better health. The role of increased physical activity also must be considered, because successful weight loss, maintenance, and recommended body composition seldom are attained without a moderate reduction in caloric intake combined with a regular exercise program.

Diet and Metabolism

Fat can be lost by selecting the proper foods, exercising, or restricting calories. When a person tries to lose weight by dietary restrictions alone, lean body mass (muscle protein, along with vital organ protein) always decreases. The amount of lean body mass lost depends entirely on caloric limitation.

When obese people go on a near-fasting diet, up to half of the weight loss is lean body mass and the other half is actual fat loss (see Figure 4.2).[5] When diet is combined with exercise, close to 100% of the weight loss is in the form of fat, and lean tissue actually may increase.

Loss of lean body mass is never good, because it weakens the organs and muscles and slows down metabolism. Large losses in lean tissue can cause disturbances in heart function and damage to other organs. Equally important is not to overindulge (binge) following very-low-calorie diets. This may cause

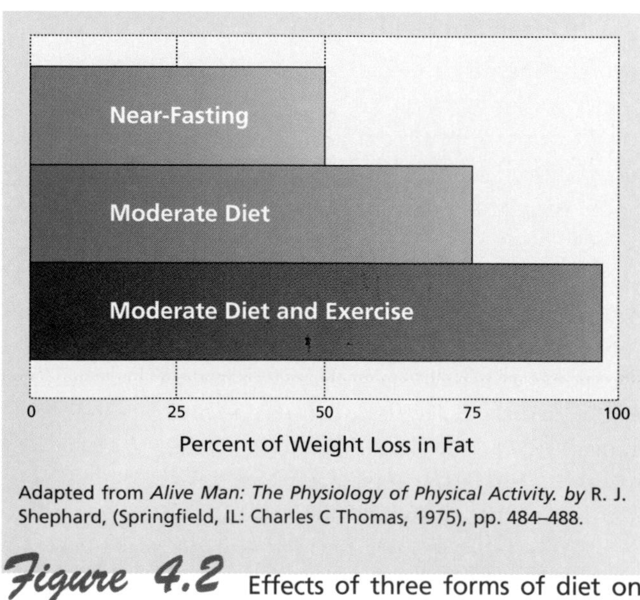

Adapted from *Alive Man: The Physiology of Physical Activity.* by R. J. Shephard, (Springfield, IL: Charles C Thomas, 1975), pp. 484–488.

Figure 4.2 Effects of three forms of diet on fat loss.

changes in metabolic rate and electrolyte balance, which could trigger fatal cardiac arrhythmias.

Contrary to some beliefs, aging is not the main reason for the lower metabolic rate. It is not so much that metabolism slows down as that people slow down. As people age, they tend to rely more on the amenities of life (remote controls, cellular telephones, intercoms, single-level homes, riding lawnmowers) that lull a person into sedentary living.

Basal metabolism is related directly to lean body weight. The more the lean tissue, the higher the metabolic rate. As a consequence of sedentary living and less physical activity, the lean component decreases and fat tissue increases. The human body requires a certain amount of oxygen per pound of lean body mass. As fat is considered metabolically inert from the point of view of caloric use, the lean tissue uses most of the oxygen, even at rest. As muscle and organ mass (lean body mass) decreases, so do the energy requirements at rest.

Reductions in lean body mass are common in aging people (because of physical inactivity) and those on severely restricted diets. The loss of lean body mass also may account for a lower metabolic rate (described earlier) and the longer time it takes to kick back up.

Diets with caloric intakes below 1,200 to 1,500 calories cannot guarantee the retention of lean body mass. Even at this intake level, some loss is inevitable unless the diet is combined with exercise. Despite the claims of many diets that they do not alter the lean component, the simple truth is that, regardless of what nutrients may be added to the diet, severe caloric restrictions always prompt a loss of lean tissue. Too many people go on low-calorie diets constantly. Every time they do, the metabolic rate slows down as more lean tissue is lost.

Many people in their 40s or older who weigh the same as they did when they were 20 think they are at recommended body weight. During this span of 20 years or more, these people may have dieted many times without participating in an exercise program. They regain the weight shortly after they terminate each diet, but most of that gain is in fat. Maybe at age 20 they weighed 150 pounds, of which only 15% was fat. Now at age 40, even though they still weigh 150 pounds, they might be 30% fat (see Figure 4.3 and also Figure 3.5 on page 69). At recommended body weight, they wonder why they are eating very little and still having trouble staying at that weight.

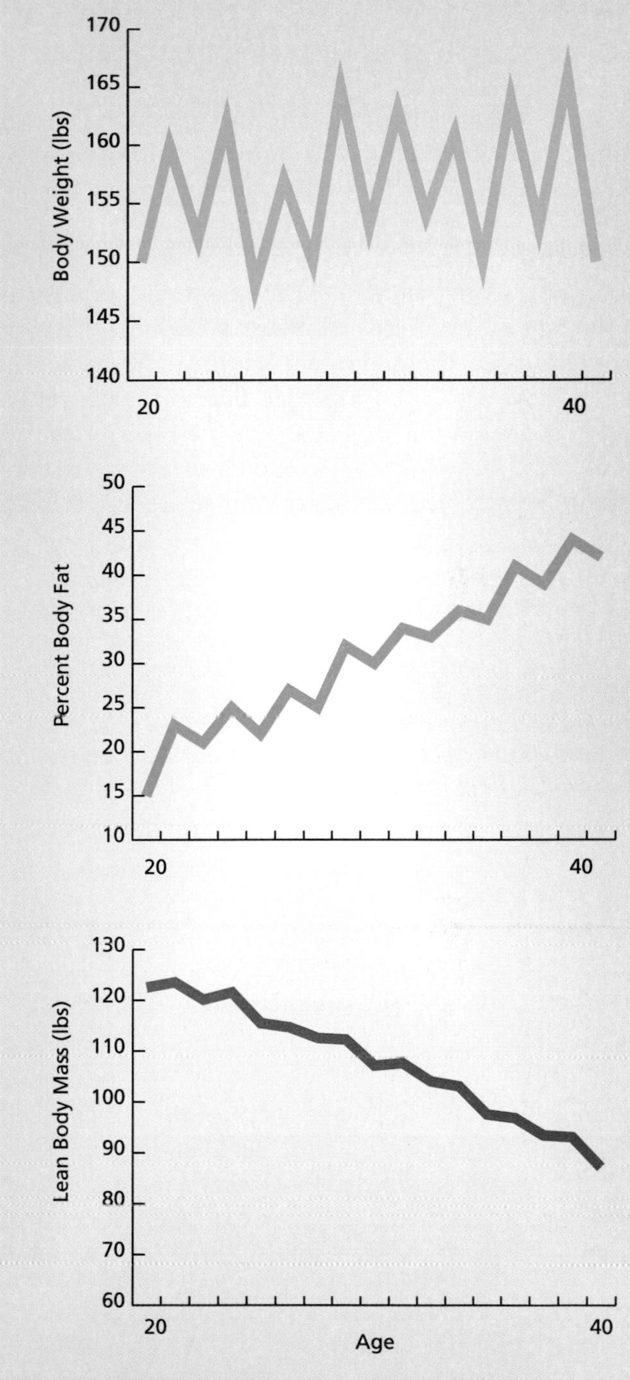

Figure 4.3 Effects of frequent dieting without exercise on lean body mass, percent body fat, and body weight.

Olestra Fat substitute made from sugar and fatty acids; provides no calories to the body because it passes through the digestive system without being absorbed.

4

Exercise: The Key to Weight Loss and Weight Maintenance

A more effective way to tilt the energy-balancing equation in your favor is by burning calories through physical activity. Exercise also appears to exert control over how much a person weighs.

Starting at age 25, the typical American gains 1 pound of weight per year. This weight gain represents a simple energy surplus of under 10 calories per day. In most cases, the additional weight accumulated in middle age comes from people becoming less physically active and not as a result of increases in caloric intake. Dr. Jack Wilmore, a leading exercise physiologist and expert weight management researcher, stated:[6]

> *Physical inactivity is certainly a major, if not the primary, cause of obesity in the United States today. A certain minimal level of activity might be necessary for us to accurately balance our caloric intake to our caloric expenditure. With too little activity, we appear to lose the fine control we normally have to maintain this incredible balance. This fine balance amounts to less than 10 calories per day, or the equivalent of one potato chip.*

Exercise is crucial to losing weight and maintaining weight. Not only will exercise maintain lean tissue, but advocates of the setpoint theory say that exercise resets the fat thermostat to a new, lower level. This change may be rapid, or it may take time. A few overweight individuals have exercised faithfully almost daily, 60 minutes at a time, for a whole year before seeing significant weight change. People with a "sticky" setpoint have to be patient and persistent.

If a person is trying to lose weight, a combination of aerobic and strength-training exercises works best. Aerobic exercise is the best to offset the setpoint, and the continuity and duration of these types of activities cause many calories to be burned in the process. The role of aerobic exercise in successful lifetime weight management cannot be overestimated.

As illustrated in Figure 4.4, greater weight loss is achieved by combining a diet with an aerobic exercise program.[7] Of even greater significance, only the individuals who participated in an 18-month post-diet aerobic exercise program were able to keep the weight off. Those who discontinued exercise gained weight. Furthermore, all those who initiated or resumed exercise during the 18-month follow-up were able to lose weight again. Individuals who only dieted and never exercised regained 60% and 92% of their weight loss at the 6- and 18-month follow-up, respectively.

Weight loss may come more rapidly when aerobic exercise is combined with a strength-training program.[8] Two exercise groups — a 30-minute aerobic group and a 15-minute aerobic plus 15-minute strength-training (30-minutes total) group — participated in an 8-week, 3-days-per-week study. Both groups followed a dietary plan consisting of approximately 60% carbohydrates, 20% fats, and 20% proteins.

The aerobic group lost an average of 3½ pounds, 3 of which were fat and the remaining half-pound lean tissue. The combined aerobic and strength-training group lost an average of 8 pounds. Changes in body composition, however, indicated that the latter group actually lost 10 pounds of fat and gained 2 pounds of lean tissue (see Figure 4.5). These findings suggest that a sensible strength-training program is better to lose weight and to maintain or increase muscle mass and metabolic rate.

Another point of interest is that each additional pound of muscle tissue can raise the basal metabolic

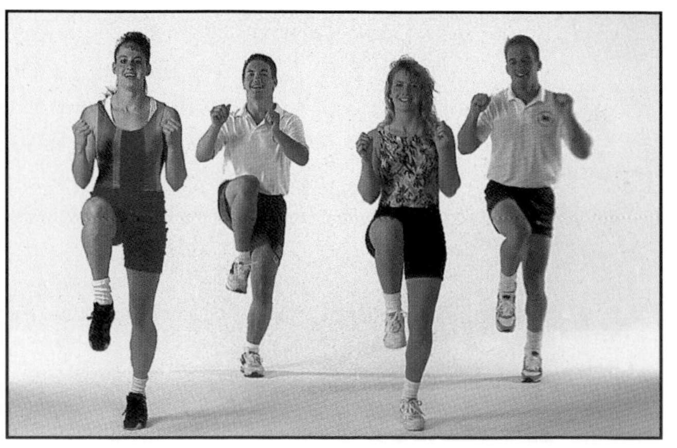

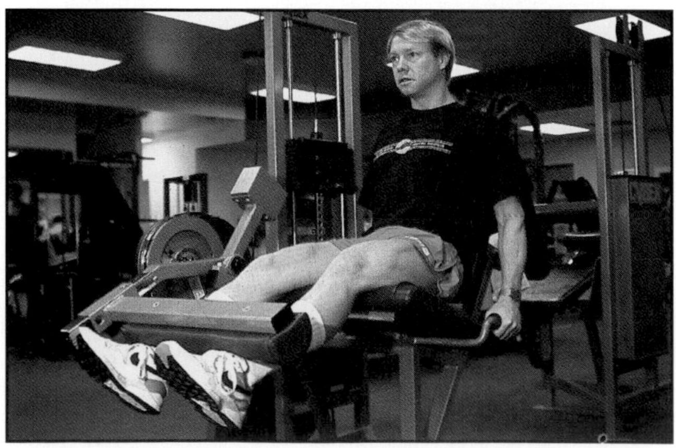

Regular participation in a combined aerobic and strength-training exercise program is the key to successful weight management.

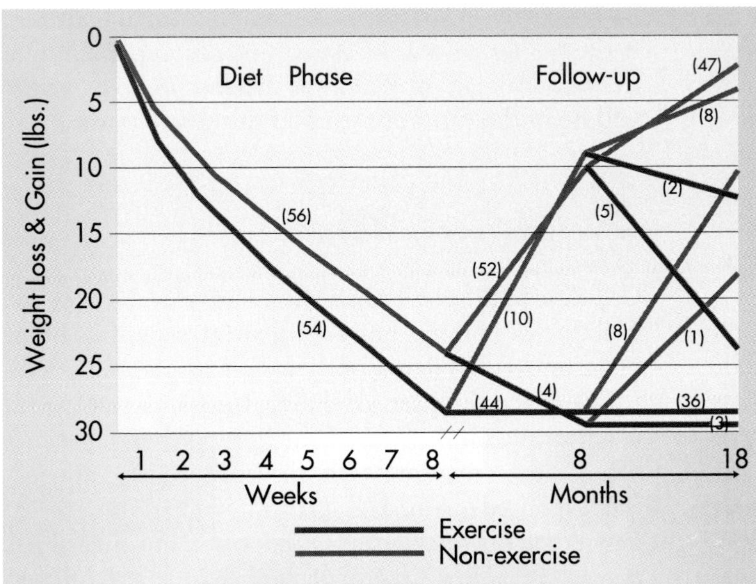

Note: Numbers in parenthesis indicate number of participants).

Source: "Exercise as an Adjunct to Weight Loss and Maintenance in Moderately Obese Subjects," K. N., Pavlou, S. Krey, and W. P. Steffe, *American Journal of Clinical Nutrition,* 49 (1989), 1115-1123.

Figure 4.4 Aerobic exercise and weight loss and maintenance in moderately obese individuals.

body weight, yet their body fat percentage is higher than recommended. The number of calories burned during a typical hour-long strength-training session is much less than during an hour of aerobic exercise. Because of the high intensity of strength training, the person needs frequent rest intervals to recover from each set of exercise. The average person actually lifts weights only 10 to 12 minutes in each hour of exercise. In the long run, however, the person enjoys the benefits of gains in lean tissue. Guidelines for developing aerobic and strength-training programs are given in Chapters 6 and 8.

Because exercise results in more lean body mass, body weight often remains the same or even increases after beginning an exercise program, while inches and percent body fat decrease. More lean tissue means a higher functional capacity of the human body. With exercise, most of the weight loss becomes apparent after a few weeks of training, after the lean component has stabilized.

rate by about 35 calories per day.[9] Thus, an individual who adds 5 pounds of muscle tissue as a result of strength training increases the basal metabolic rate by 175 calories per day (35 × 5), which equals 63,875 calories per year (175 × 365) or the equivalent of 18.25 pounds of fat (63,875 ÷ 3,500).

Strength training is suggested especially for people who think they are at their recommended

Although we now know that a negative caloric balance of 3,500 calories does not always result in a loss of exactly one pound of fat, the role of exercise in achieving a negative balance by burning additional calories is significant in weight reduction and maintenance programs.

Sadly, some individuals claim that the amount of calories burned during exercise is hardly worth the effort. They think that cutting their daily intake by some 300 calories is easier than participating in some sort of exercise that would burn the same amount of calories. The problem is that the willpower to cut those 300 calories lasts only a few weeks, and then the person goes right back to the old eating patterns.

If a person gets into the habit of exercising regularly, say three times a week, running 3 miles per exercise session (about 300 calories burned), this represents 900 calories in one week, about 3,600 in one month, or 46,800 calories per year. This minimal amount of exercise could mean as many as 13.5 extra pounds of fat in one year, 27 in two, and so on.

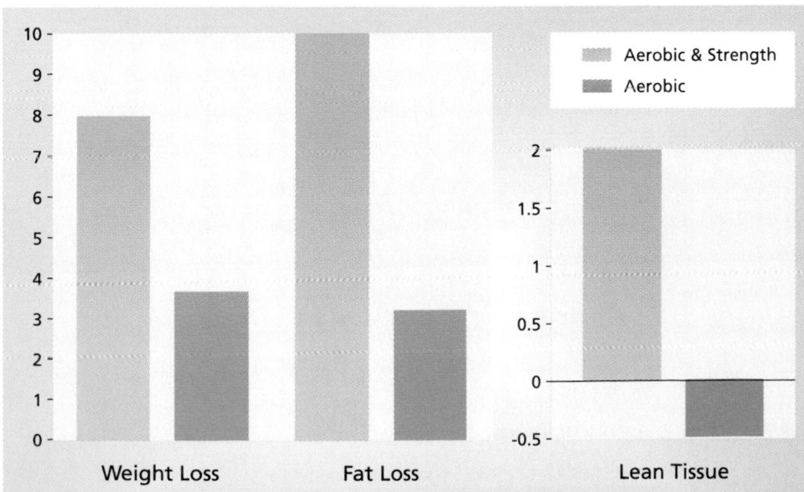

Source: "You Can Sell Exercise for Weight Loss," by W. L. Wescott, *Fitness Management,* 7:12 (1991), 33–34.

Figure 4.5 Changes in body composition through aerobic exercise and aerobic/strength-training exercise.

We tend to forget that our weight creeps up gradually over the years, not just overnight. Hardly worth the effort? And we have not even taken into consideration the increase in lean tissue, possible resetting of the setpoint, the benefits to the cardiovascular system, and most important, the improved quality of life. The fundamental reasons for overfatness and obesity, few could argue, are lack of physical activity and sedentary living.

In terms of preventing disease, many of the health benefits people try to achieve by losing weight are reaped through exercise alone, even without weight loss. Exercise offers protection against premature morbidity and mortality for everyone, including people who already have risk factors for disease (see Chapter 12). *The lack of exercise, not the weight problem itself, possibly is the cause of many of the health risks associated with obesity.*

Healthy Weight Gain

"Skinny" people, too, should realize that the only healthy way to gain weight is through exercise (mainly strength-training exercises) and a slight increase in caloric intake. Attempting to gain weight just by overeating will raise the fat component and not the lean component — which is not the path to better health. Exercise is the best solution to weight (fat) reduction and weight (lean) gain.

A strength-training program such as the one outlined in Chapter 8 is the best approach to add body weight. The training program should include at least two exercises of three sets for each major body part (see Principles of Strength Training, Chapter 8). Each set should consist of about 10 repetitions maximum.

The lack of exercise, not the weight problem itself, possibly is the cause of many of the health risks associated with obesity.

Even though the metabolic cost of synthesizing a pound of muscle tissue is still unclear, an estimated 500 additional calories daily, including 15 grams of protein above the RDA, are recommended to gain an average of 1 pound of muscle tissue per week. Based on the typical American diet, the extra 15 grams of protein are not necessary. Each day, the average American already consumes 30 to 60 grams of protein above the RDA. The extra 500 calories should be primarily in the form of complex carbohydrates. If the higher caloric intake is not accompanied by a strength-training program, the increase in body weight will be in the form of fat and not muscle tissue.

Weight-loss Myths

Cellulite and **spot reducing** are mythical concepts. Cellulite is nothing but enlarged fat cells that bulge out from accumulated body fat.

Doing several sets of daily sit-ups will not get rid of fat in the midsection of the body. When fat comes off, it does so throughout the entire body, not just the exercised area. The greatest proportion of fat may come off the biggest fat deposits, but the caloric output of a few sets of sit-ups has practically no effect on reducing total body fat. A person has to exercise much longer to really see results.

Other touted means toward quick weight loss — rubberized sweatsuits, steam baths, mechanical vibrators — are misleading. When a person wears a sweatsuit or steps into a sauna, the weight lost is not fat but merely a significant amount of water. Sure, it looks nice when you step on the scale immediately afterward, but this represents a false loss of weight. As soon as you replace body fluids, you gain back the weight quickly.

Wearing rubberized sweatsuits not only hastens the rate of body fluid loss — fluid that is vital during prolonged exercise — but it raises core temperature at the same time. This combination puts a person in danger of dehydration, which impairs cellular function and in extreme cases can even cause death.

Similarly, mechanical vibrators are worthless in a weight-control program. Vibrating belts and turning rollers may feel good, but they require no effort whatsoever. Fat cannot be shaken off; it is lost primarily by burning it in muscle tissue.

Losing Weight the Sound and Sensible Way

Dieting never has been fun and never will be. People who are overweight and are serious about losing weight, however, have to include regular exercise in their life along with proper food management and a sensible reduction in caloric intake.

Some precautions are in order, as excessive body fat is a risk factor for cardiovascular disease.

Depending on the extent of the weight problem, a medical examination and possibly a stress ECG (see Abnormal Electrocardiogram in Chapter 12, page 195) may be a good idea before undertaking the exercise program. A physician should be consulted in this regard.

Significantly overweight individuals also may have to choose activities in which they will not have to support their own body weight but that still will be effective in burning calories. Joint and muscle injuries are common in overweight individuals who participate in weight-bearing exercises such as walking, jogging, and aerobics.

Swimming may not be a good exercise either. More body fat makes a person more buoyant, and most people are not at the skill level to swim fast enough to get the best training effect. They tend to just float along, limiting the amount of calories burned as well as the benefits to the cardiovascular system.

Some better alternatives are riding a bicycle (either road or stationary), walking in a shallow pool, doing water aerobics,[10] or running in place in deep water (treading water). The latter forms of water exercise are gaining popularity and have proven to be effective in weight reduction without the "pain" and fear of injuries. Through the caloric expenditure of selected physical activities given in Table 4.2, you will be able to determine your own daily caloric requirement in Lab 4A.

How long should each exercise session last? To develop and maintain cardiorespiratory fitness, 20 to 30 minutes of exercise at the recommended target rate, three to five times per week, is suggested (see Chapter 6). For weight-loss purposes, many experts recommend exercising at least 45 minutes at a time, five to six times a week.

A person should not try to do too much too fast. Unconditioned beginners should start with about 15 minutes of aerobic exercise three times a week, gradually increasing the duration by approximately 5 minutes per week and the frequency by one day per week during the next three to four weeks.

One final benefit of exercise for weight control is that it allows fat to be burned more efficiently. Both carbohydrates and fats are sources of energy. When the glucose levels begin to drop during prolonged exercise, more fat is used as energy substrate.

Equally important is that fat-burning enzymes increase with aerobic training. Fat is lost primarily by burning it in muscle. Therefore, as the concentration of the enzymes increases, so does the ability to burn fat.[11]

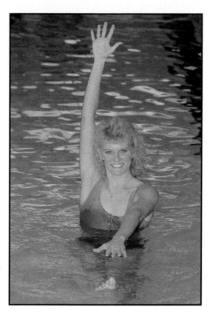

Body fat can be lost through water aerobics.

4

In addition to exercise and adequate food management, sensible adjustments in caloric intake are recommended. Most research finds that a negative caloric balance is required to lose weight. Perhaps the only exception is in people who are eating too few calories. A nutrient analysis (see Chapter 2) often reveals that faithful dieters are not consuming enough calories. These people actually need to increase their daily caloric intake (combined with an exercise program) to get their metabolism to kick back up to a normal level.

The reasons for prescribing a lower caloric figure to lose weight are:

1. Most people underestimate their caloric intake and are eating more than they should be eating.
2. Developing new behaviors takes time, and some people have trouble changing and adjusting to new eating habits.
3. Many individuals are in such poor physical condition that they take a long time to increase their activity level enough to offset the setpoint and burn enough calories to aid in loss of body fat.
4. Some dieters have difficulty succeeding unless they can count calories.

Cellulite Term frequently used in reference to fat deposits that "bulge out." These deposits are nothing but enlarged fat cells from excessive accumulation of body fat.

Spot reducing Fallacious theory that claims that exercising a specific body part will result in significant fat reduction in that area.

5. A few people simply will not alter their food selection. For those who will not change their food selection (which will still increase the risk for chronic diseases), a large increase in physical activity, a negative caloric balance, or a combination of the two is the only solution to lose weight successfully.

The daily caloric requirement can be estimated by consulting Tables 4.1 and 4.2. This activity is conducted in Lab 4A. As this is only an estimated value, individual adjustments related to many of the factors discussed in this chapter may be necessary to establish a more precise value. Nevertheless, the estimated value does offer a beginning guideline for weight control or reduction.

Table 4.1 Average Caloric Requirement Per Pound of Body Weight Based on Lifestyle Patterns and Gender

	Calories Per Pound	
	Men	Women*
Sedentary — limited physical activity	13.0	12.0
Moderate physical activity	15.0	13.5
Hard Labor — strenuous physical effort	17.0	15.0

*Pregnant or lactating women add 3 calories to these values.

4

Table 4.2 Caloric Expenditure of Selected Physical Activities

Activity*	Cal/lb/min	Activity*	Cal/lb/min	Activity*	Cal/lb/min
Aero-belt Exercise		Dance		Stairmaster	
Aero-belt Jogging/6 mph	0.098	Moderate	0.030	Moderate	0.070
Aero-belt Step-Aerobics/8"	0.105	Vigorous	0.055	Vigorous	0.090
Aero-belt Walking/4 mph	0.073	Golf	0.030	Stationary Cycling	
Aerobics		Gymnastics		Moderate	0.055
Moderate	0.065	Light	0.030	Vigorous	0.070
Vigorous	0.095	Heavy	0.056	Strength Training	0.050
Step-Aerobics	0.070	Handball	0.064	Swimming (crawl)	
Archery	0.030	Hiking	0.040	20 yds/min	0.031
Badminton		Judo/Karate	0.086	25 yds/min	0.040
Recreation	0.038	Racquetball	0.065	45 yds/min	0.057
Competition	0.065	Rope Jumping	0.060	50 yds/min	0.070
Baseball	0.031	Rowing (vigorous)	0.090	Table Tennis	0.030
Basketball		Running		Tennis	
Moderate	0.046	11.0 min/mile	0.070	Moderate	0.045
Competition	0.063	8.5 min/mile	0.090	Competition	0.064
Bowling	0.030	7.0 min/mile	0.102	Volleyball	0.030
Calisthenics	0.033	6.0 min/mile	0.114	Walking	
Cycling (level)		Deep water**	0.100	4.5 mph	0.045
5.5 mph	0.033	Skating (moderate)	0.038	Shallow pool	0.090
10.0 mph	0.050	Skiing		Water Aerobics	
13.0 mph	0.071	Downhill	0.060	Moderate	0.050
		Level (5 mph)	0.078	Vigorous	0.070
		Soccer	0.059	Wrestling	0.085

*Values are for actual time engaged in the activity. **Treading water

Adapted from:
Allsen, P. E., J. M. Harrison, and B. Vance. *Fitness for Life: An Individualized Approach* (Dubuque, IA: Wm. C. Brown, 1989).
Bucher, C. A., and W. E. Prentice, *Fitness for College and Life* (St. Louis: Times Mirror/Mosby College Publishing, 1989).
Consolazio, C. F., R. E. Johnson, and L. J. Pecora. *Physiological Measurements of Metabolic Functions in Man* (New York: McGraw-Hill, 1963).
Hockey, R. V. *Physical Fitness: The Pathway to Healthful Living* (St. Louis: Times Mirror/Mosby College Publishing, 1989).
Hoeger, W. W. K., et al. Research conducted at Boise State University, 1986-1993.

The average daily caloric requirement without exercise is based on typical lifestyle patterns, total body weight, and gender. Individuals who hold jobs that require heavy manual labor burn more calories during the day than those who have sedentary jobs such as working behind a desk. To find your activity level, refer to Table 4.1 and rate yourself accordingly. The number given in Table 4.1 is per pound of body weight, so you should multiply your current weight by that number. For example, the typical caloric requirement to maintain body weight for a moderately active male who weighs 160 pounds is 2,400 calories (160 lbs × 15 calories per pound).

The second step is to determine the average number of calories you use daily as a result of exercise. To get this number, figure out the total number of minutes you exercise weekly, and then figure the daily average exercise time. For instance, a person cycling at 13 miles per hour, five times a week, 30 minutes each time, exercises 150 minutes per week (5 × 30). The average daily exercise time is 21 minutes (150 ÷ 7). Round off to the lowest unit.

Next, from Table 4.2, find the energy requirement for the activity (or activities) chosen for the exercise program. In the case of cycling (13 miles per hour), the requirement is .071 calories per pound of body weight per minute of activity (cal/lb/min). With a body weight of 160 pounds, this man uses 11.4 calories each minute (body weight × .071, or 160 × .071). In 21 minutes, he uses approximately 240 calories (21 × 11.4).

The fourth step is to obtain the estimated total caloric requirement, with exercise, needed to maintain body weight. To do this, add the typical daily requirement (without exercise) and the average calories used through exercise. In our example, it is 2,640 calories (2,400 + 240).

If a negative caloric balance is recommended to lose weight, this person has to consume fewer than 2,640 daily calories to achieve the objective. Because of the many factors that play a role in weight control, the previous value is only an estimated daily requirement. Furthermore, to lose weight, a person can't predict that exactly one pound of fat will be lost in one week by reducing daily intake by 500 calories (500 × 7 = 3,500 calories, or the equivalent of one pound of fat).

The estimated daily caloric figure provides only a target guideline for weight control. Periodic readjustments are necessary because individuals differ, and the estimated daily cost changes as you lose weight and modify your exercise habits.

The recommended number of calories to be subtracted from the daily intake to obtain a negative caloric balance depends on the typical daily requirement. At this point, the best recommendation is to decrease the daily intake moderately, never below 1,200 calories for women and 1,500 for men.

A good rule to follow is to restrict the intake by no more than 500 calories if the daily requirement is below 3,000 calories. For caloric requirements in excess of 3,000, as many as 1,000 calories per day may be subtracted from the total intake. The daily distribution should be approximately 60% carbohydrates (mostly complex carbohydrates), less than 30% fat, and about 12% protein.

Many experts believe a person may take off weight more efficiently by reducing the amount of daily fat intake to 10% to 20% of the total daily caloric intake. Because 1 gram of fat supplies more than twice the amount of calories that carbohydrates and protein do, the general tendency is not to overeat.

Further, it takes only 3% to 5% of ingested calories to store fat as fat, whereas it takes approximately 25% of ingested calories to convert carbohydrates to fat. Other research points to the fact that if people eat the same amount of calories as carbohydrate or fat, those on the fat diet will store more fat. Successful weight-loss programs allow only small amounts of fat in the diet.

Many people have trouble adhering to a 10%- to 20%-fat-calorie diet. During weight loss periods, however, you are strongly encouraged to do so. Start with a 20% fat-calorie diet. Refer to Table 4.3 to aid you in determining the grams of fat at 10%, 20%, and 30% of the total calories for selected energy intakes. Also, use the form provided in Lab 2B to monitor your daily fat intake.

The time of day when food is consumed also may play a part in weight reduction. A study conducted at the Aerobics Research Center in Dallas, Texas, indicated that, when a person is on a diet, weight is lost most effectively if most of the calories are consumed before one o'clock and not during the evening meal. This center recommends that, when a person is attempting to lose weight, intake should consist of a minimum of 25% of the total daily calories for breakfast, 50% for lunch, and 25% or less at dinner.

Other experts have reported that if most of the daily calories are consumed during one meal, the body may perceive that something is wrong and will slow down the metabolism so it can store a greater amount of calories in the form of fat. Eating most of

Table 4.3 Grams of Fat as a Percentage of Total Calories for Selected Energy Intakes

Caloric Intake	Grams of Fat 10%	20%	30%
1,200	13	27	40
1,300	14	29	43
1,400	16	31	47
1,500	17	33	50
1,600	18	36	53
1,700	19	38	57
1,800	20	40	60
1,900	21	42	63
2,000	22	44	67
2,100	23	47	70
2,200	24	49	73
2,300	26	51	77
2,400	27	53	80
2,500	28	56	83
2,600	29	58	87
2,700	30	60	90
2,800	31	62	93
2,900	32	64	97
3,000	33	67	100

the calories in one meal also causes a person to go hungry the rest of the day, making the diet more difficult to follow.

Consuming most of the calories earlier in the day seems helpful in losing weight, and also in managing atherosclerosis. The time of day when most of the fats and cholesterol are consumed can influence blood lipids and coronary heart disease. Peak digestion time following a heavy meal is about 7 hours after that meal. If most lipids are consumed during the evening meal, digestion peaks while the person is sound asleep, when the metabolism is at its lowest rate. Consequently, the body may not metabolize fats and cholesterol as well, leading to a higher blood lipid count and increasing the risk for atherosclerosis and coronary heart disease.

To monitor daily progress, you may use a form such as the one given in Figure 2B.1 (Lab 2B). Meeting the basic requirements from each food group should get top priority. The caloric content for each food is given in the Nutritive Value of Selected Foods list, Appendix A. For a more precise record, the information should be recorded immediately after each meal. According to the person's progress, adjustments can be made in the typical daily requirement or the exercise program, or both.

Tips for Behavior Modification and Adherence to a Weight Management Program

Achieving and maintaining recommended body composition is by no means impossible, but this does require desire and commitment. If weight management is to become a priority in life, people must realize they have to retrain behavior to some extent.

Modifying old habits and developing new positive behaviors take time. Individuals have applied the following management techniques to change detrimental behavior successfully and adhere to a positive lifetime weight-control program. In developing a retraining program, people are not expected to incorporate all of the strategies listed but should note the ones that apply to them. The form provided in Lab 4C will allow you to evaluate and monitor your own weight-management behaviors.

1. *Make a commitment to change.* The first ingredient to modify behavior is the desire to do so. The reasons for change must be more compelling than those for continuing present lifestyle patterns. You must accept the fact that you have a problem and decide by yourself whether you really want to change. If you have a sincere commitment, your chances for success are enhanced already.
2. *Set realistic goals.* Most people with a weight problem would like to lose weight in a relatively short time but fail to realize that the weight problem developed over a span of several years. A sound weight reduction and maintenance program can be accomplished only by establishing new lifetime eating and exercise habits, both of which take time to develop. In setting a realistic long-term goal, you should also plan short-term objectives. The long-term goal may be to decrease body fat to 20% of total body weight. The short-term objective may be to decrease body fat 1% each month. Objectives like these allow for regular evaluation and help maintain motivation and renewed commitment to attain the long-term goal.
3. *Incorporate exercise into the program.* Choose enjoyable activities, places, times, equipment, and people to exercise with. This will help you adhere to an exercise program. Details on developing a complete exercise program are found in

Chapters 6 (cardiorespiratory), 8 (strength), and 10 (flexibility).

4. *Develop healthy eating patterns.* Plan to eat three regular meals per day consistent with the body's nutritional requirements. Learn to differentiate hunger from appetite. Hunger is the actual physical need for food. Appetite is a desire for food, usually triggered by factors such as stress, habit, boredom, depression, food availability, or just the thought of food itself. Eat only when you have a physical need. In this regard, developing and sticking to a regular meal pattern helps control hunger.
5. *Avoid automatic eating.* Many people associate certain daily activities with eating. For example, people eat while cooking, watching television, reading, talking on the telephone, or visiting with neighbors. Most of the time, the foods consumed in these situations lack nutritional value or are high in sugar and fat.
6. *Stay busy.* People tend to eat more when they sit around and do nothing. Occupying the mind and body with activities not associated with eating helps take away the desire to eat. Try walking, cycling, playing sports, gardening, sewing, or visiting a library, a museum, a park. Develop other skills and interests, or try something new and exciting to break the routine.
7. *Plan your meals ahead of time.* Sensible shopping is required to accomplish this objective (by the way, shop on a full stomach, because hungry shoppers tend to buy unhealthy foods impulsively, and then snack on the way home). Include whole-grain breads and cereals, fruits and vegetables, low-fat milk and dairy products, lean meats, fish, and poultry.
8. *Cook wisely.* Use less fat and refined foods in food preparation. Trim all visible fat off meats, and remove skin from poultry before cooking. Skim the fat off gravies and soups. Bake, broil, and boil instead of frying. Sparingly use butter, cream, mayonnaise, and salad dressings. Avoid coconut oil, palm oil, and cocoa butter. Prepare plenty of bulky foods. Add whole-grain breads and cereals, vegetables, and legumes to most meals. Try fruits for dessert. Beware of soda pop, fruit juices, and fruit-flavored drinks. In addition to sugar, cut down on other refined carbohydrates such as corn syrup, malt sugar, dextrose, and fructose. Drink plenty of water — at least eight glasses a day.
9. *Do not serve more food than you should eat.* Measure the food portions and keep serving dishes away from the table. This means you will eat less, have a harder time getting seconds, and have less appetite because food is not visible. People should not be forced to eat when they are satisfied (including children after they have already had a healthy, nutritious serving).
10. *Learn to eat slowly and at the table only.* Eating is one of the pleasures of life, and we need to take time to enjoy it. Eating on the run is not good because the body doesn't have enough time to "register" nutritive and caloric consumption and people overeat before the body perceives the signal of fullness. Always eating at the table also forces people to take time out to eat, and it deters snacking between meals, primarily because of the extra time and effort required to sit down and eat. When done eating, do not sit around the table. Clean up and put away the food to keep from unnecessary snacking.

Successful weight management is accomplished by making a lifetime commitment to physical activity and proper food selection.

11. *Avoid social binges.* Social gatherings commonly entice self-defeating behavior. Plan ahead and visualize yourself in that gathering. Do not feel pressured to eat or drink, and don't rationalize in these situations. Choose low-calorie foods, and entertain yourself with other activities such as dancing and talking.
12. *Beware of raids on the refrigerator and the cookie jar.* When you find yourself in these tempting situations, take control. Stop and think what is happening. If you have the propensity for raids, try environmental management. Do not bring high-calorie, high-sugar, or high-fat foods into the house. If they are already in the house, store them where they are hard to get to or see. If they are out of sight or not readily available, the temptation is less. Keeping food in places such as the garage and the basement tends to discourage people from taking the time and effort to get them. By no means should you have to eliminate treats completely. Do all things in moderation.

13. *Avoid eating out.* Most meals served at restaurants (especially fast-food restaurants) are high in calories and fat. People who eat out regularly often have a difficult time managing their weight. When eating out, plan your choices by selecting low-fat and low-calorie meals, or go to a restaurant noted for healthful menus.
14. *Practice stress management techniques.* Many people snack and increase food consumption in stressful situations. Eating is not a stress-releasing activity and actually can aggravate the problem if weight control is an issue. Several stress-management techniques are set forth in Chapter 14.
15. *Monitor changes and reward accomplishments.* Feedback on fat loss, lean tissue gain, and weight loss is a reward in itself. Awareness of changes in body composition also helps reinforce new behaviors. Being able to exercise without interruption for 15, 20, 30, 60 minutes, cycling a certain distance, running a mile — all these accomplishments deserve recognition. Meeting objectives calls for rewards, but not related to eating. Buy new clothing, a tennis racquet, a bicycle, exercise shoes, or something else that is special and you would not have acquired otherwise.
16. *Think positive.* Avoid negative thoughts on how difficult changing your past behaviors might be. Instead, think of the benefits you will reap, such as feeling, looking, and functioning better, plus enjoying better health and improving your quality of life. Attempt to stay away from negative environments and people who will not be supportive. Avoid those who do not have the same desires and who encourage self-defeating behaviors.

4

In Conclusion

There is no simple and quick way to take off excessive body fat and keep it off for good. Weight management is accomplished by making a lifetime commitment to physical activity and proper food selection. When taking part in a weight (fat) reduction program, people also have to decrease their caloric intake moderately and implement strategies to modify unhealthy eating behaviors.

During the process, relapses into past negative behaviors are almost inevitable. The three most common reasons for relapse are:

1. Stress-related factors (major life changes, depression, job changes, illness).
2. Social reasons (entertaining, eating out, business travel).
3. Self-enticing behaviors (placing yourself in a situation to see how much you can get away with ("One small taste won't hurt," leading to "I'll eat just one slice," and finally, "I haven't done so well so I might as well eat some more").

Making mistakes is human and does not necessarily mean failure. Failure comes to those who give up and do not use previous experiences to build upon and, in turn, develop skills that will prevent self-defeating behaviors in the future. Where there's a will, there's a way, and those who persist will reap the rewards.

Laboratory Experience

LAB 4A
Estimation of Daily Caloric Requirement

Lab Preparation
None required.

LAB 4B
Behavioral Objectives for Exercise, Nutrition, Weight Management

Lab Preparation
Read Chapters 2, 3, and 4 of this textbook.

LAB 4C
Weight Management: Behavior Modification Progress Form

Lab Preparation
Read the section on tips for behavior modification and adherence to a lifetime weight management program.

Notes

1. Lichtman, S. "Discrepancy Between Self-Reported and Actual Caloric Intake and Exercise in Obese Subjects," *New England Journal of Medicine,* 327(1992), 1893–1898.
2. D. Remington, A. G. Fisher, and E. A. Parent, *How to Lower Your Fat Thermostat* (Provo, UT: Vitality House International, 1983).
3. R. L. Leibel, M. Rosenbaum, and J. Hirsh. "Changes in Energy Expenditure Resulting from Altered Body Weight," *New England Journal of Medicine,* 332 (1995), 621–628.
4. "Olestra: Just Say No," *University of California at Berkeley Wellness Letter* (Palm Coast, FL: The Editors, February, 1996).
5. R. J. Shepard. *Alive Man: The Physiology of Physical Activity* (Springfield, IL: Charles C Thomas, 1975), pp. 484–488.
6. Wilmore, J. "Exercise, Obesity, and Weight Control," *Physical Activity and Fitness Research Digest* (Washington DC: President's Council on Physical Fitness & Sports, May 1994).
7. K. N. Pavlou, S. Krey, and W. P. Steffe. "Exercise as an Adjunct to Weight Loss and Maintenance in Moderately Obese Subjects," *American Journal of Clinical Nutrition*, 49 (1898), 1115–1123.
8. W. L. Wescott. "You Can Sell Exercise for Weight Loss," *Fitness Management*, 7:12 (1991), 33–34.
9. W. W. Campbell, M. C. Crim, V. R. Young, and W. J. Evans, "Increased Energy Requirements and Changes in Body Composition with Resistance Training in Older Adults," *American Journal of Clinical Nutrition*, 60 (1994), 167–175.
10. W. W. K. Hoeger, T. Spitzer-Gibson, J. R. Moore, and D. R. Hopkins, "A Comparison of Selected Training Responses to Water Aerobics and Low-Impact Aerobic Dance," *National Aquatics Journal*, 9 (1993), 13–16.
11. Remington.

4

Suggested Readings

American Diabetes Association and American Dietetic Association. *Exchange Lists for Meal Planning.* Chicago: American Dietetic Association and American Diabetes Association, 1986.

Anderson, A. J., et. al. "Body Fat Distribution, Plasma Lipids and Lipoproteins." *Arteriosclerosis*, 8 (1988), 88–94.

Bouchard, C. "Heredity and the Path to Overweight and Obesity." *Medicine and Science in Sports and Exercise*, 23 (1991), 285–291.

Bouchard, C., et al. "The Response to Long-term Overfeeding in Identical Twins." *New England Journal of Medicine*, 322 (1990), 1477–1482.

Bouchard, C., et al. *Physical Activity, Fitness, and Health.* Champaign, IL: Human Kinetics, 1994.

Bray, G. "The Nutrient Balance Approach to Obesity." *Nutrition Today*, 28 (1993, May/June), 13–18.

Broeder, C. E., K. A. Burrhus, L. S. Svanevick, and J. H. Wilmore. "The Effects of Either High-Intensity Resistance or Endurance Training on Resting Metabolic Rate." *American Journal of Clinical Nutrition,* 55(1992), 802–810.

Broeder, C. E., et al. "The Metabolic Consequences of Low and Moderate Intensity Exercise With or Without Feeding in Lean and Borderline Obese Males." *International Journal of Obesity,* 15(1990), 95–104.

Brownell, K., and F. Kramer. "Behavioral Management of Obesity." *Medical Clinics of North America*, 73 (1989), 185–202.

Brownell, K., et al. "Matching Weight Control Programs to Individuals." *Weight Control Digest*, 1 (1991), 65.

Clark, N. "How to Gain Weight Healthfully." *Physician and Sportsmedicine*, 19 (1991), 53.

Health Implications of Obesity: National Institutes of Health Consensus Development Conference. *Annals of Internal Medicine*, 103 (1985), 977–1077.

Jenkins, D. J. A., et al. "Nibbling Versus Gorging: Metabolic Advantages of Increased Meal Frequency." *New England Journal of Medicine*, 321 (1989), 929–934.

Miller, W., et al. "Clinical Symposium: Obesity: Diet Composition, Energy Expenditure, and Treatment of the Obese Patient." *Medicine and Science in Sports and Exercise*, 23 (1991), 273–297.

National Academy of Sciences: Committee on Diet and Health, Food and Nutrition Board. "Diet and Health: Implications for Reducing Chronic Disease Risk." Washington, DC: National Academy Press, 1989.

Prentice, A., et al. "Effects of Weight Cycling on Body Composition." *American Journal of Clinical Nutrition*, 56 (1992), 209S–216S.

Robison, J., et al. "Obesity, Weight Loss, and Health." *Journal of the American Dietetic Association* 93 (1993), 445–449.

Rolls, B., and D. Shide. "The Influence of Dietary Fat on Food Intake and Body Weight." *Nutrition Reviews*, 50 (1992), 283–290.

Sims, E. A. H. "Obesity is Hazardous to Your Health: Affirmative." *Debates in Medicine*, 2 (1989), 103–137.

Sjödin, A. M., et al. "The Influence of Physical Activity on BMR." *Medicine and Science in Sports and Exercise,* 28 (1996), 85–91.

Stefanick, M. "Exercise and Weight Control." Exercise and Sport Sciences Review, 21 (1993), 363–396.

Stunkard, A. J., et al. "An Adoption Study of Human Obesity." *New England Journal of Medicine,* 314 (1986), 193–198.

Tremblay, A., J. A. Simoneau, and C. Bouchard. "Impact of Exercise on Body Fatness and Skeletal Muscle Metabolism." *Metabolism*, 43 (1994) 814–818.

Wadden, T. A., T. B. Van Itallie, and G. L. Blackburn. "Responsible and Irresponsible Use of Very-Low-Calorie Diets in the Treatment of Obesity." *Journal of the American Medical Association*, 263 (1990), 83–85.

Wilmore, J. Body Weight and Body Composition. In *Eating, Body Weight, and Performance in Athletes: Disorders of Modern Society*, edited by K. Brownell, et al. Philadelphia: Lea & Febiger.

Wilmore, J. "Exercise, Obesity, and Weight Control." *Physical Activity and Fitness Research Digest,* 1 (1994, May), 1–8.

Cardiorespiratory Endurance Assessment

5

LABS

*The most important component of physical fitness and best indicator of overall health is **cardiorespiratory endurance**. Physical activity is no longer a natural part of our existence. We live in an automated world, one in which most of the activities that used to require strenuous physical exertion can be done by machines with the simple pull of a handle or push of a button. For instance, if there is a need to go to a store only a couple of blocks away, most people drive their automobiles and then spend a couple of minutes driving around the parking lot to find a spot 10 yards closer to the store's entrance. They do not even have to carry out the groceries any more. A youngster working at the store usually takes them out in a cart and places them in the vehicle.*

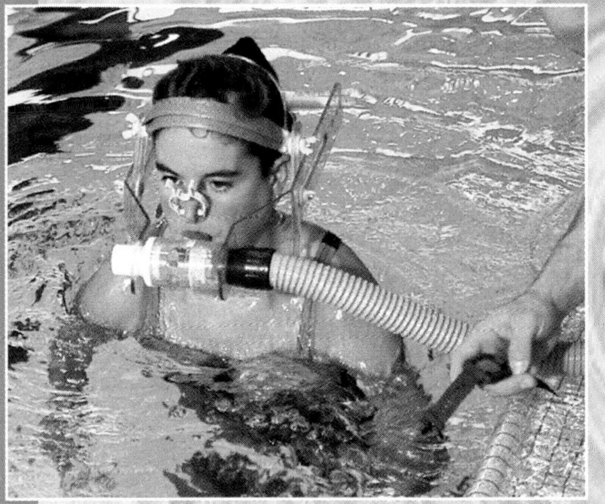

Similarly, during a visit to a multi-level shopping mall, almost everyone chooses to ride the escalators instead of taking the stairs. Automobiles, elevators, escalators, telephones, intercoms, remote controls, electric garage door openers — all are modern-day commodities that minimize the amount of movement and effort required of the human body.

One of the most harmful effects of modern-day technology is an increase in chronic conditions related to a lack of physical activity. These include hypertension, heart disease,

Objectives

- Understand the importance of adequate cardiorespiratory endurance in maintaining good health and well-being.
- Define cardiorespiratory endurance and the benefits of cardiorespiratory endurance training.
- Define aerobic and anaerobic exercise.
- Be able to assess cardiorespiratory fitness through six different test protocols (1.5-Mile Run Test, 1.0-Mile Walk Test, Step Test, Astrand-Ryhming Test, 12-Minute Swim Test, and Houston Non-Exercise Test).
- Learn to interpret cardiorespiratory endurance assessment test results according to health fitness and physical fitness standards.

chronic low-back pain, and obesity. They are referred to as **hypokinetic diseases.** The term "hypo" means low or little, and "kinetic" implies motion. Lack of adequate physical activity is a fact of modern life that most people can avoid no longer. To enjoy modern-day commodities and still expect to live life to its fullest, however, a personalized lifetime exercise program must become a part of daily living.

For most people around the world, modern-day technology has led to a lower level of cardiorespiratory endurance. As a person breathes, part of the oxygen in the air is taken up in the lungs and transported in the blood to the heart. The heart then is responsible for pumping the oxygenated blood through the circulatory system to all organs and tissues of the body. At the cellular level, oxygen is used to convert food substrates, primarily carbohydrates and fats, into energy necessary to conduct body functions and maintain constant internal equilibrium. During physical exertion, more energy is needed to perform the activity. As a result, the heart, lungs, and blood vessels have to deliver more oxygen to the cells to supply the required energy.

Modern-day commodities have reduced the amount of daily physical activity, thus enhancing the deterioration rate of the human body.

During prolonged exercise, an individual with a high level of cardiorespiratory endurance is able to deliver the required amount of oxygen to the tissues with relative ease. The cardiorespiratory system of a person with a low level of endurance has to work much harder, as the heart has to pump more often to supply the same amount of oxygen to the tissues and, consequently, fatigues faster. Hence, a higher capacity to deliver and utilize oxygen (oxygen uptake) indicates a more efficient cardiorespiratory system.

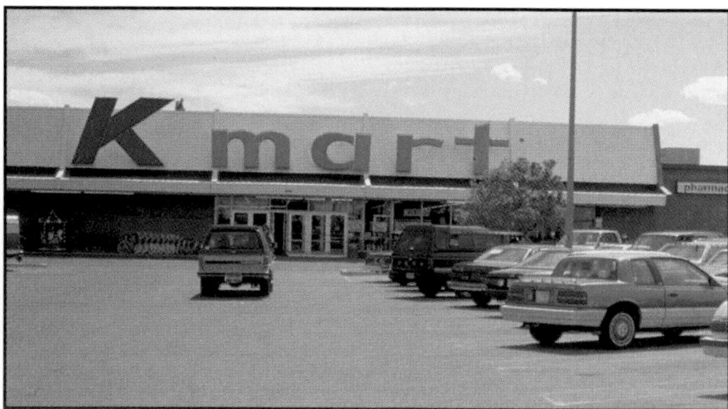

The epitome of physical inactivity: driving around a parking lot for several minutes in search of a parking spot 10 to 20 yards closer to the store's entrance.

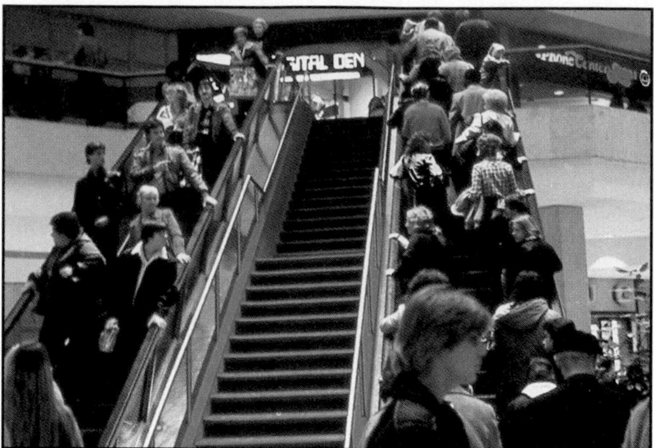
Advances in modern technology have almost completely eliminated the need for physical activity, significantly contributing to the deterioration of the human body.

Aerobic and Anaerobic Exercise

Cardiorespiratory endurance activities often are called **aerobic** exercises. Examples of cardiorespiratory or aerobic exercises are walking, jogging, swimming, cycling, cross-country skiing, water aerobics, rope skipping, and aerobics.

The intensity of **anaerobic** exercise is so high that oxygen cannot be delivered and utilized to produce energy. Because energy production is limited in the absence of oxygen, these activities can be carried

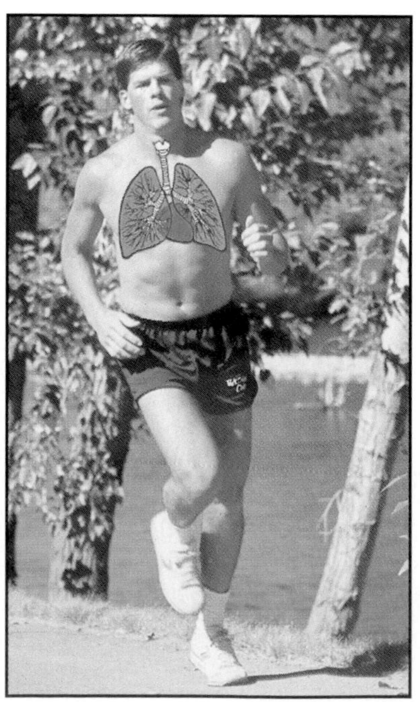
Cardiorespiratory endurance is the ability of the lungs, heart, and blood vessels to deliver adequate amounts of oxygen to the cells to meet the demands of prolonged physical activity.

5

out for only short periods (2 to 3 minutes). The higher the intensity of the activity, the shorter the duration.

Good aerobic or cardiorespiratory fitness implies an efficient system to deliver and utilize oxygen.

Activities such as the 100, 200, and 400 meters in track and field, the 100 meters in swimming, gymnastics routines, and strength training are good examples of anaerobic activities. Anaerobic activities do not contribute much to development of the cardiorespiratory system. Only aerobic activities will help increase cardiorespiratory endurance. The basic guidelines for cardiorespiratory exercise prescription are set forth in Chapter 6.

Benefits of Cardiorespiratory Endurance Training

Everyone who participates in a cardiorespiratory or aerobic exercise program can expect a number of physiological adaptations from training. Among these benefits are:

1. *A higher* ***maximal oxygen uptake.*** The amount of oxygen the body is able to use during physical activity increases significantly. This allows the individual to exercise longer and at a higher rate before becoming fatigued. Depending on the initial fitness level, maximal oxygen uptake may increase as much as 30%, although higher increases have been reported in people with very low initial levels of fitness.

Cardiorespiratory endurance The ability of the lungs, heart, and blood vessels to deliver adequate amounts of oxygen to the cells to meet the demands of prolonged physical activity.

Hypokinetic diseases Diseases associated with a lack of physical activity.

Aerobic Exercise that requires oxygen to produce the necessary energy (ATP) to carry out the activity.

Anaerobic Exercise that does not require oxygen to produce the necessary energy (ATP) to carry out the activity.

Maximal oxygen uptake (VO_{2max}) The maximum amount of oxygen the body is able to utilize per minute of physical activity, commonly expressed in ml/kg/min. The best indicator of cardiorespiratory or aerobic fitness.

5

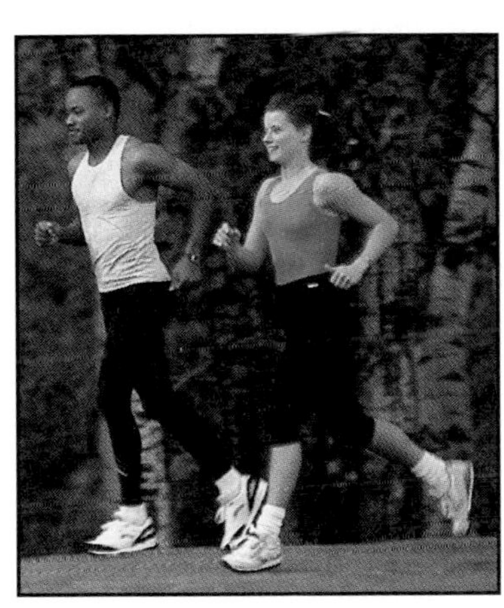

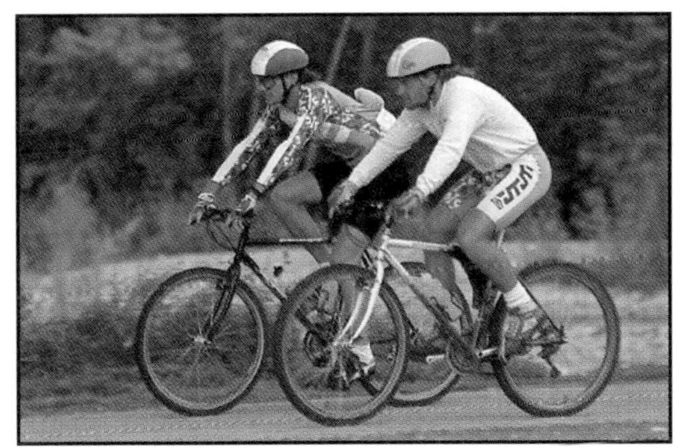

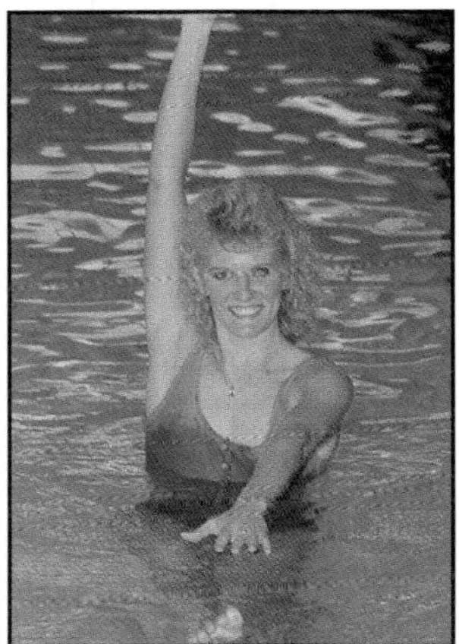

AEROBIC ACTIVITIES

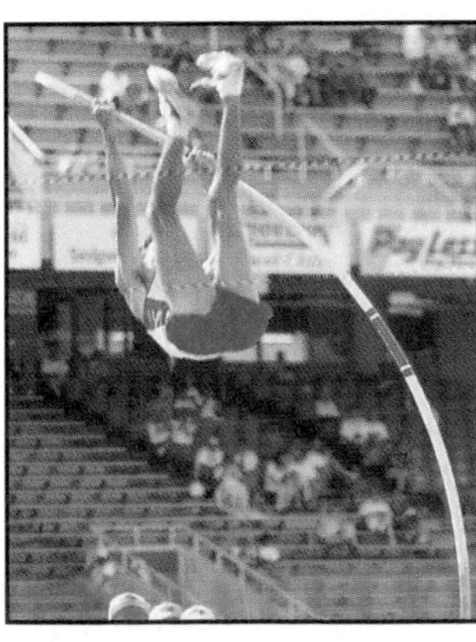

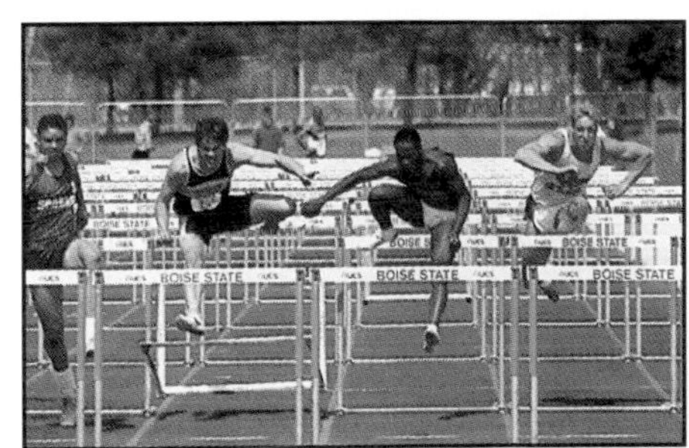

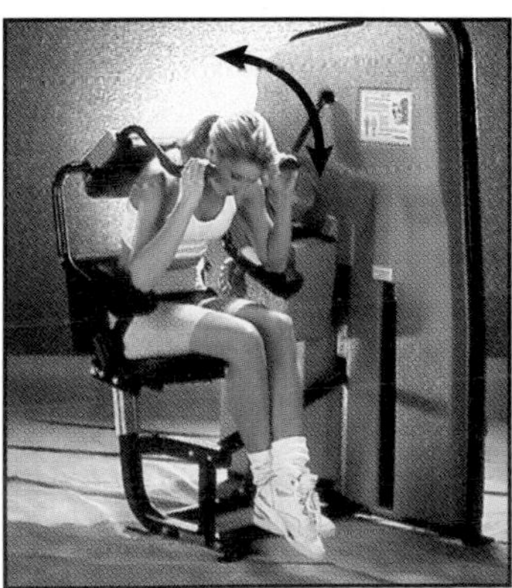

ANAEROBIC ACTIVITIES

2. *An increase in the oxygen-carrying capacity of the blood.* As a result of training, the red blood cell count goes up. Red blood cells contain hemoglobin, which transports oxygen in the blood.

3. *A decrease in resting heart rate and an increase in cardiac muscle strength.* During resting conditions, the heart ejects between 5 and 6 liters of blood per minute (a liter is slightly larger than a quart). This amount of blood, also referred to as **cardiac output**, meets the body's energy demands in the resting state.

   Like any other muscle, the heart responds to training by increasing in strength and size. As the heart gets stronger, the muscle can produce a more forceful contraction, which causes the heart to eject more blood with each beat. This **stroke volume** yields a lower heart rate. The lower heart rate also allows the heart to rest longer between beats. Average resting and maximal cardiac outputs, stroke volumes, and heart rates for sedentary, trained, and highly trained (elite) individuals are shown in Table 5.1.

   Resting heart rates frequently decrease by 10 to 20 beats per minute (bpm) after only 6 to 8 weeks of training. A reduction of 20 bpm saves the heart about 10,483,200 beats per year. The average heart beats between 70 and 80 bpm. As seen in Table 5.1, resting heart rates in highly trained athletes are often around 45 bpm.

4. *A lower heart rate at given* ***workloads***. When compared with untrained individuals, a trained person has a lower heart rate response to a given task. This is because of the greater efficiency of the cardiorespiratory system. Individuals also are surprised to find that, following several weeks of training, a given workload (let's say a 10-minute mile) elicits a much lower heart rate response as compared to the response when training first started.

5. *An increase in the number and size of the* ***mitochondria***. All energy necessary for cell function is produced in the mitochondria. As the size and number increase, so does the potential to produce energy for muscular work.

6. *An increase in the number of functional* ***capillaries***. These smaller vessels allow for the exchange of oxygen and carbon dioxide between the blood and the cells. As more vessels open up, more gas exchange can take place, delaying the onset of fatigue during prolonged exercise. This increase in capillaries also speeds up the rate at which waste products of cell metabolism can be removed. Increased capillarization also is seen in the heart, which enhances the oxygen delivery capacity to the heart muscle itself.

7. *Faster* ***recovery time***. Trained individuals recover more rapidly after exercising. A fit system is able to restore more quickly any internal equilibrium disrupted during exercise.

8. *Lower blood pressure and blood lipids.* A regular aerobic exercise program leads to lower blood pressure and fats such as cholesterol and triglycerides, all of which have been linked to the formation of atherosclerotic plaque, which obstructs the arteries. This decreases the risk of coronary heart disease (see Chapter 12). High blood pressure also is a leading risk factor for strokes.

9. *An increase in fat-burning enzymes.* The role of fat-burning enzymes is significant because fat is lost primarily by burning it in muscle. As the concentration of the enzymes increases, so does the ability to burn fat.

Table 5.1 Average Resting and Maximal Cardiac Output, Stroke Volume, and Heart Rate, for Sedentary, Trained, and Highly Trained Males

	RESTING			MAXIMAL		
	$\dot{Q}$ (l/min)	SV (ml)	HR (bpm)	$\dot{Q}$ L/min)	SV (ml)	HR (bpm)
Sedentary	5	68	74	20	100	200
Trained	5	90	56	30	150	200
Highly Trained	5	110	45	35	175	200

$\dot{Q}$ = cardiac output
SV = stroke volume
HR = heart rate

Assessment of Cardiorespiratory Endurance

The level of cardiorespiratory endurance, cardiorespiratory fitness, or aerobic capacity is determined by the maximal amount of oxygen the human body is able to utilize per minute of physical activity. This value can be expressed in liters per minute (l/min) or milliliters per kilogram per minute (ml/kg/min). The relative value in ml/kg/min is used most often because it considers total body mass (weight). When comparing two individuals with the same absolute value, the one with the lesser body mass will have a higher relative value, indicating that more oxygen is available to each kilogram (2.2 pounds) of body weight. Because all tissues and organs of the body need oxygen to function, higher oxygen consumption indicates a more efficient cardiorespiratory system.

The most precise way to determine maximal oxygen uptake (VO_{2max}) is through direct gas analysis. This is done by using a metabolic cart through which the amount of oxygen consumption can be measured directly. This type of equipment is not available in most health/fitness centers. Therefore, several alternative methods of estimating maximal oxygen uptake have been developed using limited equipment.

Even though most cardiorespiratory endurance tests probably are safe to administer to apparently healthy individuals (those with no major coronary risk factors or symptoms), the American College of Sports Medicine recommends that a physician be present for all maximal exercise tests on apparently healthy men over age 40 and women over age 50. A maximal test is any test that requires the participant's all-out or nearly all-out effort. For submaximal exercise tests, a physician should be present when testing higher risk/symptomatic individuals or diseased people, regardless of the participant's current age.

Five exercise tests used to assess cardiorespiratory fitness are introduced in this chapter: the 1.5-Mile Run Test, 1.0-Mile Walk Test, Step Test, Astrand-Ryhming Test, and 12-Minute Swim Test. The test procedures are explained in detail in Figures 5.1, 5.2, 5.3, 5.4, and 5.5, respectively.

Depending on time, equipment, and individual physical limitations, you may perform one or more of these tests. For example, people who can't jog or walk could take the bike or swim test. Because these are different tests, they will not necessarily yield the exact same results. Therefore, to make valid comparisons, you should take the same test when doing pre- and post-assessments.

A sixth test, the University of Houston Non-Exercise Test, also is presented, at the end of this chapter (Figure 5.6). This non-exercise test is a valuable tool for making initial estimates of maximal oxygen uptake, hopefully to motivate people to exercise. The test is also valuable for mass screening, because the required information is collected through a self-reported method.

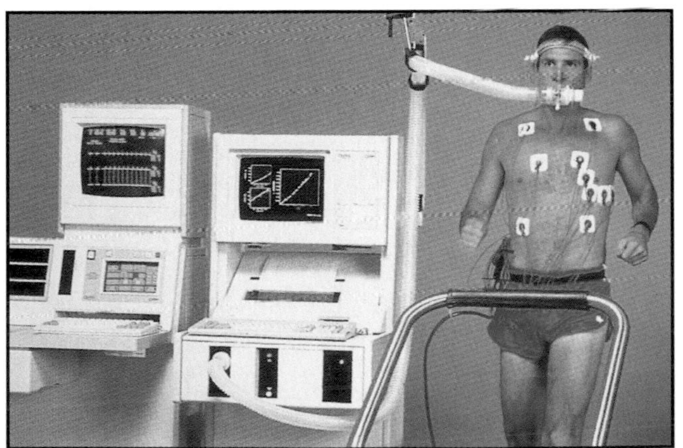

Maximal oxygen uptake (cardiorespiratory fitness) as determined through direct gas analysis.

Photo Courtesy of Quinton Instrument Co., 2121 Terry Ave., Seattle, WA 98121-2791.

1.5-Mile Run Test

This test is used most frequently to predict cardiorespiratory fitness according to the time the person takes to run or walk a 1.5-mile course (see Figure 5.1). Maximal oxygen uptake is estimated based on the time the person takes to cover the distance (see Table 5.2).

The only equipment necessary to conduct this test is a stopwatch and a track or premeasured 1.5-mile course. This perhaps is the easiest test to administer, but a note of caution is in order when conducting the test. As the objective is to cover the distance in the shortest time, it is considered a maximal exercise test. The 1.5-Mile Run Test should be limited to conditioned individuals who have been cleared for exercise. The test is not recommended for unconditioned beginners, men over age 40, and women over age 50 without proper medical clearance, symptomatic individuals, and those with known disease or coronary heart disease risk factors. A program of at least 6 weeks of aerobic training is recommended before unconditioned individuals take this test.

Cardiac output Amount of blood pumped by the heart in one minute.

Stroke volume Amount of blood pumped by the heart in one beat.

Workload Load (or intensity) placed on the body during physical activity.

Mitochondria Structures within the cells where energy transformations take place.

Capillaries Smallest blood vessels carrying oxygenated blood to the tissues in the body.

Recovery time Amount of time the heart takes to return to resting heart rate after exercise.

5

1.5 MILE RUN TEST

1. Make sure you qualify for this test. This test is contraindicated for unconditioned beginners, individuals with symptoms of heart disease, and those with known heart disease or risk factors.
2. Select the testing site. Find a school track (each lap is one-fourth of a mile) or a premeasured 1.5-mile course.
3. Have a stopwatch available to determine your time.
4. Conduct a few warm-up exercises prior to the test. Do some stretching exercises, some walking, and slow jogging.
5. Initiate the test and try to cover the distance in the fastest time possible (walking or jogging). Time yourself during the run to see how fast you have covered the distance. If any unusual symptoms arise during the test, do not continue. Stop immediately and retake the test after another 6 weeks of aerobic training.
6. At the end of the test, cool down by walking or jogging slowly for another 3 to 5 minutes. Do not sit or lie down after the test.
7. According to your performance time, look up your estimated maximal oxygen uptake(VO_{2max}) in Table 5.2.
8. Example: A 20-year-old female runs the 1.5-mile course in 12 minutes and 40 seconds. Table 5.2 shows a VO_{2max} of 39.8 ml/kg/min for a time of 12:40. According to Table 5.8, this VO_{2max} would place her in the good cardiorespiratory fitness category.

Figure 5.1 Procedure for the 1.5-Mile Run Test.

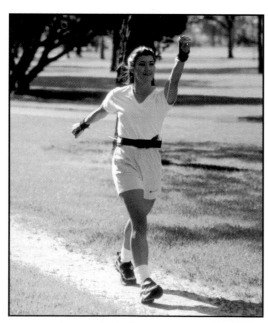

Even moderate physical activity enhances health and longevity.

Table 5.2 Estimated Maximal Oxygen Uptake for the 1.5-Mile Run Test

Time	VO_{2max} (ml/kg/min)	Time	VO_{2max} (ml/kg/min)
6:10	80.0	12:40	39.8
6:20	79.0	12:50	39.2
6:30	77.9	13:00	38.6
6:40	76.7	13:10	38.1
6:50	75.5	13:20	37.8
7:00	74.0	13:30	37.2
7:10	72.6	13:40	36.8
7:20	71.3	13:50	36.3
7:30	69.9	14:00	35.9
7:40	68.3	14:10	35.5
7:50	66.8	14:20	35.1
8:00	65.2	14:30	34.7
8:10	63.9	14:40	34.3
8:20	62.5	14:50	34.0
8:30	61.2	15:00	33.6
8:40	60.2	15:10	33.1
8:50	59.1	15:20	32.7
9:00	58.1	15:30	32.2
9:10	56.9	15:40	31.8
9:20	55.9	15:50	31.4
9:30	54.7	16:00	30.9
9:40	53.5	16:10	30.5
9:50	52.3	16:20	30.2
10:00	51.1	16:30	29.8
10:10	50.4	16:40	29.5
10:20	49.5	16:50	29.1
10:30	48.6	17:00	28.9
10:40	48.0	17:10	28.5
10:50	47.4	17:20	28.3
11:00	46.6	17:30	28.0
11:10	45.8	17:40	27.7
11:20	45.1	17:50	27.4
11:30	44.4	18:00	27.1
11:40	43.7	18:10	26.8
11:50	43.2	18:20	26.6
12:00	42.3	18:30	26.3
12:10	41.7	18:40	26.0
12:20	41.0	18:50	25.7
12:30	40.4	19:00	25.4

Source: Adapted from "A Means of Assessing Maximal Oxygen Intake," by K. H. Cooper, in *Journal of the American Medical Association,* 203(1968), 201-204; *Health and Fitness Through Physical Activity*, by M. L. Pollock, J. H. Wilmore, and S. M. Fox III (New York: John Wiley & Sons, 1978); and *Training for Sport and Activity*, by J. H. Wilmore and D. L. Costill (Dubuque, IA: Wm. C. Brown Publishers, 1988).

1.0-Mile Walk Test

This test can be used by individuals who are unable to run because of low fitness levels or injuries. All that is required is a brisk 1-mile walk that will elicit an exercise heart rate of at least 120 beats per minute at the end of the test.

You will need to know how to take your heart rate by counting your pulse. This can be done on the wrist by placing two fingers over the radial artery (inside the wrist on the side of the thumb) or over the carotid artery in the neck just below the jaw, next to the voice box.

Maximal oxygen uptake is estimated according to a prediction equation that requires the following data: 1.0-mile walk time, exercise heart rate at the end of the walk, age, gender, and body weight in pounds. The procedure for this test and the equation are given in Figure 5.2.

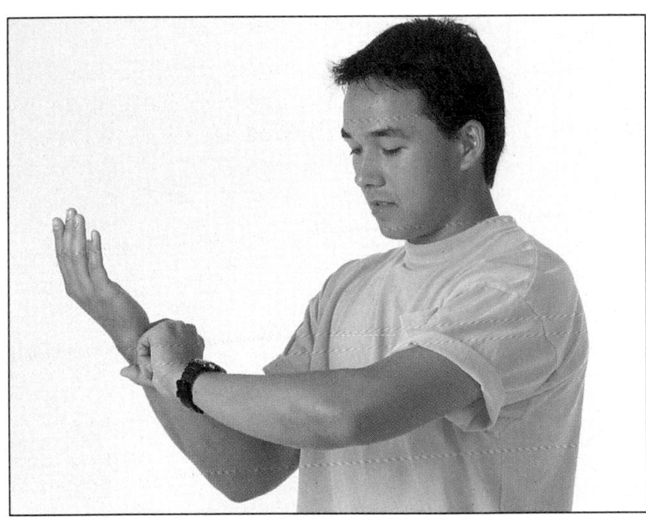

Pulse taken at the radial artery.

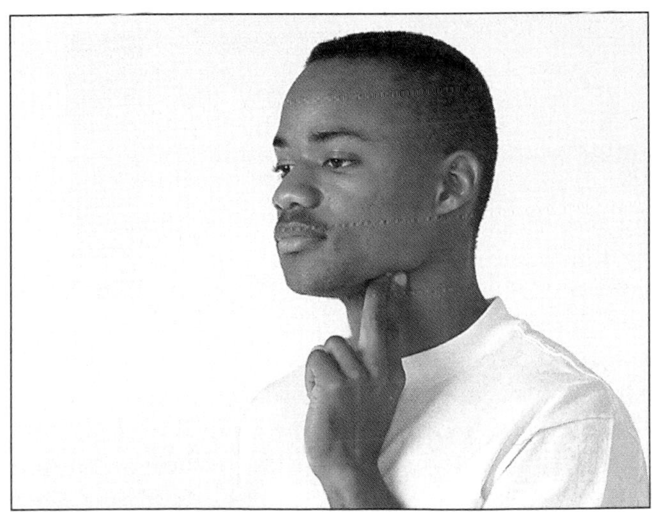

Pulse taken at the carotid artery.

1.0-MILE WALK TEST

1. Select the testing site. Use a 440-yard track (4 laps to a mile) or a premeasured 1.0-mile course.
2. Determine your body weight in pounds prior to the test.
3. Have a stopwatch available to determine total walking time and exercise heart rate.
4. Walk the 1.0-mile course at a brisk pace (the exercise heart rate at the end of the test should be above 120 beats per minute).
5. At the end of the 1.0-mile walk, check your walking time and immediately count your pulse for 10 seconds. Multiply the 10-second pulse count by 6 to obtain the exercise heart rate in beats per minute.
6. Convert the walking time from minutes and seconds to minute units. Because each minute has 60 seconds, divide the seconds by 60 to obtain the fraction of a minute. For instance, a walking time of 12 minutes and 15 seconds would equal $12 + (15 \div 60)$, or 12.25 minutes.
7. To obtain the estimated maximal oxygen uptake (VO_{2max}) in ml/kg/min, plug your values in the following equation:

   $VO_{2max} = 132.853 - (.0769 \times W) - (.3877 \times A) + (6.315 \times G) - (3.2649 \times T) - (.1565 \times HR)$

   Where:

   W = Weight in pounds
   A = Age in years
   G = Gender (use 0 for women and 1 for men)
   T = Total time for the one-mile walk in minutes (see item 6 above)
   HR = Exercise heart rate in beats per minute at the end of the 1.0-mile walk

8. Example: A 19-year-old female who weighs 140 pounds completed the 1.0-mile walk in 14 minutes 39 seconds and with an exercise heart rate of 148 beats per minute. The estimated VO_{2max} would be:

   W = 140 lbs
   A = 19
   G = 0 (female gender = 0)
   T = $14{:}39 = 14 + (39 \div 60) = 14.65$ min
   HR = 148 bpm

   $VO_{2max} = 132.853 - (.0769 \times 140) - (.3877 \times 19) + (6.315 \times 0) - (3.2649 \times 14.65) - (.1565 \times 148)$

   $VO_{2max} = 43.7$ ml/kg/min

Source: "Estimation of VO_{2max} from a One-mile Track Walk, Gender, Age, and Body Weight," by G. Kline et al., *Medicine and Science in Sports and Exercise,* 19:3 (1987), 253–259. © American College of Sports Medicine.

Figure 5.2 Procedure for the 1.0-Mile Walk Test.

5

Step Test

The Step Test requires little time and equipment and can be administered to almost anyone, as a submaximal workload is used to estimate maximal oxygen uptake. Symptomatic and diseased individuals should not take this test. Significantly overweight individuals and those with joint problems in the lower extremities may have difficulty performing the test.

The actual test takes only 3 minutes. A 15-second recovery heart rate is taken between 5 and 20 seconds following the test (see Figure 5.3 and Table 5.3). The equipment required is a bench or gymnasium bleacher 16¼ inches high, a stopwatch, and a metronome.

You also will need to know how to take your heart rate by counting your pulse (explained under the 1.0-Mile Walk Test). By teaching people to take their own heart rate, a large group of people can be tested at once, using gymnasium bleachers.

STEP TEST

1. Conduct the test with a bench or gymnasium bleacher 16¼ inches high.
2. Perform the stepping cycle to a four-step cadence (up-up-down-down). Men should perform 24 complete step-ups per minute, regulated with a metronome set at 96 beats per minute. Women perform 22 step-ups per minute, or 88 beats per minute on the metronome.
3. Allow a brief practice period of 5 to 10 seconds to familiarize yourself with the stepping cadence.
4. Begin the test and perform the step-ups for exactly 3 minutes.
5. Upon completing the 3 minutes, remain standing and take your heart rate for a 15-second interval from 5 to 20 seconds into recovery. Convert recovery heart rate to beats per minute (multiply 15-second heart rate by 4).
6. Maximal oxygen uptake (VO_{2max}) in ml/kg/min is estimated according to the following equations:

   Men:

   $VO_{2max} =$
   $111.33 - (0.42 \times \text{recovery heart rate in bpm})$

   Women:

   $VO_{2max} =$
   $65.81 - (0.1847 \times \text{recovery heart rate in bpm})$
7. Example: The recovery 15-second heart rate for a male following the 3-minute step test is found to be 39 beats. VO_{2max} is estimated as follows:

   15-second heart rate = 39 beats
   Minute heart rate = $39 \times 4 = 156$ bpm
   $VO_{2max} =$
   $111.33 - (0.42 \times 156) = 45.81$ ml/kg/min
8. VO_{2max} also can be obtained according to recovery heart rates in Table 5.3.

From *Exercise Physiology: Energy, Nutrition, and Human Performance,* by W. D. McArdle et al., (Philadelphia: Lea & Febiger, 1991).

Figure 5.3 Procedure for the Step Test.

Table 5.3 Predicted Maximal Oxygen Uptake for the Step Test

15-Sec HR	HR-bpm	VO_{2max} Men (ml/kg/min)	VO_{2max} Women (ml/kg/min)
30	120	60.9	43.6
31	124	59.3	42.9
32	128	57.6	42.2
33	132	55.9	41.4
34	136	54.2	40.7
35	140	52.5	40.0
36	144	50.9	39.2
37	148	49.2	38.5
38	152	47.5	37.7
39	156	45.8	37.0
40	160	44.1	36.3
41	164	42.5	35.5
42	168	40.8	34.8
43	172	39.1	34.0
44	176	37.4	33.3
45	180	35.7	32.6
46	184	34.1	31.8
47	188	32.4	31.1
48	192	30.7	30.3
49	196	29.0	29.6
50	200	27.3	28.9

HR = heart rate
bpm = beats per minute

Astrand-Ryhming Test

Because of its simplicity and practicality, the Astrand-Ryhming has become one of the most popular tests used to estimate maximal oxygen uptake in the laboratory setting. The test is conducted on a bicycle ergometer, and, similar to the Step Test, it requires only submaximal workloads and little time to administer.

The cautions given for the Step Test also apply to the Astrand-Ryhming Test. Nevertheless, because the participant does not have to support his or her own body weight while riding the bicycle, overweight individuals and those with limited joint problems in the lower extremities can take this test.

The bicycle ergometer to be used for this test should allow for the regulation of workloads (see the test procedure in Figure 5.4 and Tables 5.4, 5.5, and 5.6). Besides the bicycle ergometer, a stopwatch and an additional technician to monitor the heart rate are needed to conduct the test.

The heart rate is taken every minute for 6 minutes. At the end of the test, the heart rate should be in the range given for each workload in Tables 5.4, 5.5, and 5.6 (generally between 120 and 170 beats per minute).

When administering the test to older people, good judgment is essential. Low workloads should be used, because if the higher heart rates are reached (around 150 to 170 bpm), these individuals could be working near or at their maximal capacity, making it an unsafe test without adequate medical supervision. When choosing workloads for older people, final exercise heart rates should not exceed 130 to 140 bpm.

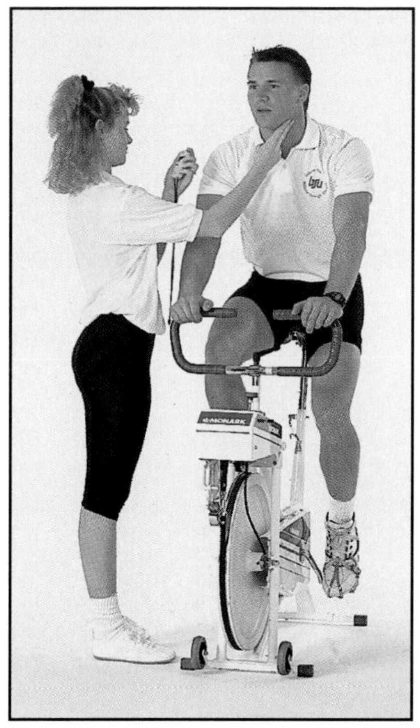

Heart rate monitoring on the carotid artery during the Astrand-Ryhming Test.

ASTRAND-RYHMING TEST

1. Adjust the bike seat so the knees are almost completely extended as the foot goes through the bottom of the pedaling cycle.
2. During the test, keep the speed constant at 50 revolutions per minute. Test duration is 6 minutes.
3. Select the appropriate workload for the bike based on age, weight, health, and estimated fitness level. For unconditioned individuals: women, use 300 kpm (kilopounds per meter) or 450 kpm; men, 300 kpm or 600 kpm. Conditioned adults: women, 450 kpm or 600 kpm; men, 600 kpm or 900 kpm.[a]
4. Ride the bike for 6 minutes and check the heart rate every minute, during the last 10 seconds of each minute. Determine heart rate by recording the time it takes to count 30 pulse beats, and then converting to beats per minute using Table 5.4.
5. Average the final two heart rates (5th and 6th minutes). If these two heart rates are not within five beats per minute of each other, continue the test for another few minutes until this is accomplished. If the heart rate continues to climb significantly after the 6th minute, stop the test and rest for 15 to 20 minutes. You may then retest, preferably at a lower workload. The final average heart rate should also fall between the ranges given for each workload in Table 5.5 (men: 300 kpm = 120 to 140 beats per minute; 600 kpm – 120 to 170 beats per minute).
6. Based on the average heart rate of the final 2 minutes and your workload, look up the maximal oxygen uptake (VO_{2max}) in Table 5.5 (for example: men: 600 kpm and average heart rate = 145, VO_{2max} = 2.4 liters/minute).
7. Correct VO_{2max} using the correction factors found in Table 5.6 (if VO_{2max} = 2.4 and age 35, correction factor = .870. Multiply 2.4 × .870 and final corrected VO_{2max} = 2.09 liters/minute).
8. To obtain VO_{2max} in ml/kg/min, multiply the VO_{2max} by 1,000 (to convert liters to milliliters) and divide by body weight in kilograms (to obtain kilograms, divide your body weight in pounds by 2.2046).
9. Example: Corrected VO_{2max} = 2.09 liters/minute
   Body weight = 132 pounds or 60 kilograms (132 ÷ 2.2046 = 60)
   $$VO_{2max} \text{ in ml/kg/min} = \frac{2.09 \times 1{,}000}{60} = 39.8 \text{ ml/kg/min}$$
   2,090 divided by 60 = 34.8 ml/kg/min

[a] On the Monarch bicycle ergometer, when riding at a speed of 50 revolutions per minute, a load of 1 kp = 300 kpm, 1.5 kp = 450, 2 kp = 600 kpm, and so forth, with increases of 150 kpm to each half kp.

Figure 5.4 Procedure for the Astrand-Ryhming Test.

Table 5.4 Conversion of Time for 30 Pulse Beats to Pulse Rate Per Minute

Sec.	bpm	Sec.	bpm	Sec.	bpm	Sec.	bpm	Sec.	bpm	Sec.	bpm	Sec.	bpm
22.0	82	19.9	90	17.8	101	15.7	115	13.6	132	11.5	157	9.4	191
21.9	82	19.8	91	17.7	102	15.6	115	13.5	133	11.4	158	9.3	194
21.8	83	19.7	91	17.6	102	15.5	116	13.4	134	11.3	159	9.2	196
21.7	83	19.6	92	17.5	103	15.4	117	13.3	135	11.2	161	9.1	198
21.6	83	19.5	92	17.4	103	15.3	118	13.2	136	11.1	162	9.0	200
21.5	84	19.4	93	17.3	104	15.2	118	13.1	137	11.0	164	8.9	202
21.4	84	19.3	93	17.2	105	15.1	119	13.0	138	10.9	165	8.8	205
21.3	85	19.2	94	17.1	105	15.0	120	12.9	140	10.8	167	8.7	207
21.2	85	19.1	94	17.0	106	14.9	121	12.8	141	10.7	168	8.6	209
21.1	85	19.0	95	16.9	107	14.8	122	12.7	142	10.6	170	8.5	212
21.0	86	18.9	95	16.8	107	14.7	122	12.6	143	10.5	171	8.4	214
20.9	86	18.8	96	16.7	108	14.6	123	12.5	144	10.4	173	8.3	217
20.8	87	18.7	96	16.6	108	14.5	124	12.4	145	10.3	175	8.2	220
20.7	87	18.6	97	16.5	109	14.4	125	12.3	146	10.2	176	8.1	222
20.6	87	18.5	97	16.4	110	14.3	126	12.2	148	10.1	178	8.0	225
20.5	88	18.4	98	16.3	110	14.2	127	12.1	149	10.0	180		
20.4	88	18.3	98	16.2	111	14.1	128	12.0	150	9.9	182		
20.3	89	18.2	99	16.1	112	14.0	129	11.9	151	9.8	184		
20.2	89	18.1	99	16.0	113	13.9	129	11.8	153	9.7	186		
20.1	90	18.0	100	15.9	113	13.8	130	11.7	154	9.6	188		
20.0	90	17.9	101	15.8	114	13.7	131	11.6	155	9.5	189		

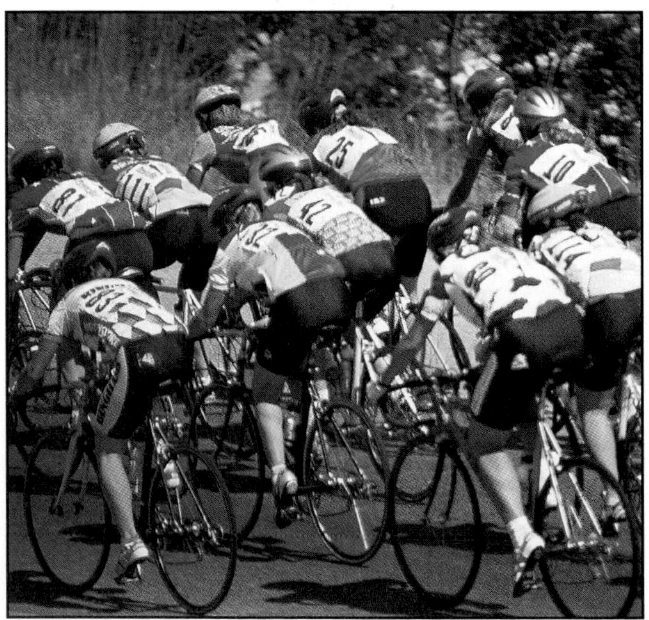

Vigorous exercise is required to achieve the high physical fitness standard.

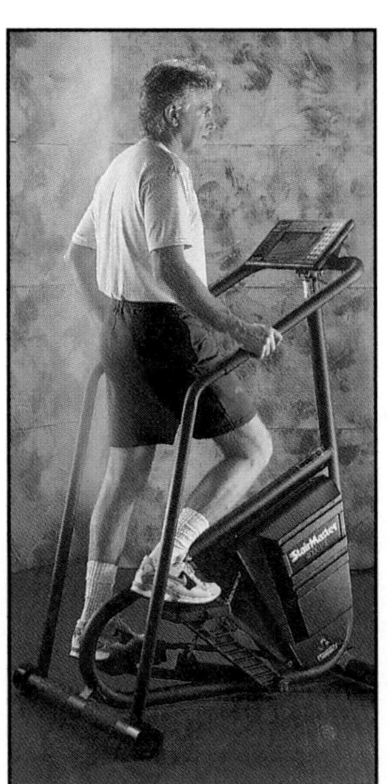

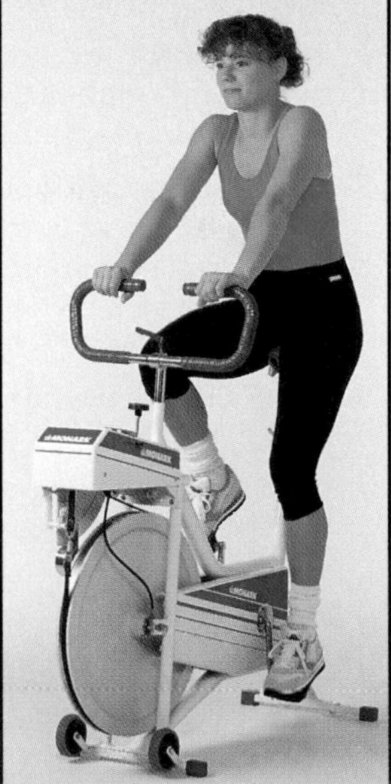

Maximal oxygen uptake can be improved with aerobic exercise.

Table 5.5 Maximal Oxygen Uptake (VO_{2max}) Estimates for the Astrand-Ryhming Test

	MEN l/min					WOMEN l/min				
Heart Rate	**300**	**600**	**900**	**1200**	**1500**	**300**	**450**	**600**	**750**	**900**
120	2.2	3.4	4.8			2.6	3.4	4.1	4.8	
121	2.2	3.4	4.7			2.5	3.3	4.0	4.8	
122	2.2	3.4	4.6			2.5	3.2	3.9	4.7	
123	2.1	3.4	4.6			2.4	3.1	3.9	4.6	
124	2.1	3.3	4.5	6.0		2.4	3.1	3.8	4.5	
125	2.0	3.2	4.4	5.9		2.3	3.0	3.7	4.4	
126	2.0	3.2	4.4	5.8		2.3	3.0	3.6	4.3	
127	2.0	3.1	4.3	5.7		2.2	2.9	3.5	4.2	
128	2.0	3.1	4.2	5.6		2.2	2.8	3.5	4.2	4.8
129	1.9	3.0	4.2	5.6		2.2	2.8	3.4	4.1	4.8
130	1.9	3.0	4.1	5.5		2.1	2.7	3.4	4.0	4.7
131	1.9	2.9	4.0	5.4		2.1	2.7	3.4	4.0	4.6
132	1.8	2.9	4.0	5.3		2.0	2.7	3.3	3.9	4.5
133	1.8	2.8	3.9	5.3		2.0	2.6	3.2	3.8	4.4
134	1.8	2.8	3.9	5.2		2.0	2.6	3.2	3.8	4.4
135	1.7	2.8	3.8	5.1		2.0	2.6	3.1	3.7	4.3
136	1.7	2.7	3.8	5.0		1.9	2.5	3.1	3.6	4.2
137	1.7	2.7	3.7	5.0		1.9	2.5	3.0	3.6	4.2
138	1.6	2.7	3.7	4.9		1.8	2.4	3.0	3.5	4.1
139	1.6	2.6	3.6	4.8		1.8	2.4	2.9	3.5	4.0
140	1.6	2.6	3.6	4.8	6.0	1.8	2.4	2.8	3.4	4.0
141		2.6	3.5	4.7	5.9	1.8	2.3	2.8	3.4	3.9
142		2.5	3.5	4.6	5.8	1.7	2.3	2.8	3.3	3.9
143		2.5	3.4	4.6	5.7	1.7	2.2	2.7	3.3	3.8
144		2.5	3.4	4.5	5.7	1.7	2.2	2.7	3.2	3.8
145		2.4	3.4	4.5	5.6	1.6	2.2	2.7	3.2	3.7
146		2.4	3.3	4.4	5.6	1.6	2.2	2.6	3.2	3.7
147		2.4	3.3	4.4	5.5	1.6	2.1	2.6	3.1	3.6
148		2.4	3.2	4.3	5.4	1.6	2.1	2.6	3.1	3.6
149		2.3	3.2	4.3	5.4		2.1	2.6	3.0	3.5
150		2.3	3.2	4.2	5.3		2.0	2.5	3.0	3.5
151		2.3	3.1	4.2	5.2		2.0	2.5	3.0	3.4
152		2.3	3.1	4.1	5.2		2.0	2.5	2.9	3.4
153		2.2	3.0	4.1	5.1		2.0	2.4	2.9	3.3
154		2.2	3.0	4.0	5.1		2.0	2.4	2.8	3.3
155		2.2	3.0	4.0	5.0		1.9	2.4	2.8	3.2
156		2.2	2.9	4.0	5.0		1.9	2.3	2.8	3.2
157		2.1	2.9	3.9	4.9		1.9	2.3	2.7	3.2
158		2.1	2.9	3.9	4.9		1.8	2.3	2.7	3.1
159		2.1	2.8	3.8	4.8		1.8	2.2	2.7	3.1
160		2.1	2.8	3.8	4.8		1.8	2.2	2.6	3.0
161		2.0	2.8	3.7	4.7		1.8	2.2	2.6	3.0
162		2.0	2.8	3.7	4.6		1.8	2.2	2.6	3.0
163		2.0	2.8	3.7	4.6		1.7	2.2	2.6	2.9
164		2.0	2.7	3.6	4.5		1.7	2.1	2.5	2.9
165		2.0	2.7	3.6	4.5		1.7	2.1	2.5	2.9
166		1.9	2.7	3.6	4.5		1.7	2.1	2.5	2.8
167		1.9	2.6	3.5	4.4		1.6	2.1	2.4	2.8
168		1.9	2.6	3.5	4.4		1.6	2.0	2.4	2.8
169		1.9	2.6	3.5	4.3		1.6	2.0	2.4	2.8
170		1.8	2.6	3.4	4.3		1.6	2.0	2.4	2.7

l/min = liters per minute

From Astrand, I. *Acta Physiologica Scandinavica* 49(1960). Supplementum 169:45-60.

Table 5.6 Age-Based Correction Factors for Maximal Oxygen Uptake (VO_{2max}) for the Astrand-Ryhming Test

Age	Correction Factor	Age	Correction Factor	Age	Correction Factor	Age	Correction Factor
14	1.11	27	.974	40	.830	53	.726
15	1.10	28	.961	41	.820	54	.718
16	1.09	29	.948	42	.810	55	.710
17	1.08	30	.935	43	.800	56	.704
18	1.07	31	.922	44	.790	57	.698
19	1.06	32	.909	45	.780	58	.692
20	1.05	33	.896	46	.774	59	.686
21	1.04	34	.883	47	.768	60	.680
22	1.03	35	.870	48	.762	61	.674
23	1.02	36	.862	49	.756	62	.668
24	1.01	37	.854	50	.750	63	.662
25	1.00	38	.846	51	.742	64	.656
26	.987	39	.838	52	.734	65	.650

Adapted from Astrand, I. *Acta Physiologica Scandinavica* 49(1960). Supplementum 169:45-60.

5

12-Minute Swim Test

Similar to the 1.5-Mile Run test, the 12-Minute Swim Test is considered a maximal exercise test, and the same precautions apply. The objective is to swim as far as possible during the 12-minute test.

A swimming test (Figure 5.5) is practical only for those who are planning to take part in a swimming program. Unlike land-based tests, predicting maximal oxygen uptake through a swimming test is difficult. Differences in skill level, swimming conditioning, and body composition greatly affect the energy requirements (oxygen uptake) of swimming.

A skilled swimmer is able to swim more efficiently and expend much less energy than an unskilled swimmer. Improper breathing patterns cause premature fatigue. Overweight individuals are more buoyant in the water, and the larger surface area (body size) produces greater friction against movement in the water medium.

Lack of conditioning affects swimming test results as well. An unconditioned skilled swimmer who is in good cardiorespiratory shape because of a regular jogging program will not perform as effectively in a swimming test. Swimming conditioning is important for adequate performance on this test.

Because of these limitations, maximal oxygen uptake cannot be estimated for a swimming test and the fitness categories given in Table 5.7 are only estimated ratings. This test should be limited to people who cannot perform any of the other tests and whose primary aerobic exercise will be a swimming program. Unskilled and unconditioned swimmers can expect lower cardiorespiratory fitness ratings than those obtained with a land-based test.

12-MINUTE SWIM TEST

1. Enlist a friend to time the test. The only other requisites are a stopwatch and a swimming pool. Do not attempt to do this test in an unsupervised pool.
2. Warm up by swimming slowly and doing a few stretching exercises before taking the test.
3. Start the test and swim as many laps as possible in 12 minutes. Pace yourself throughout the test, and do not swim to the point of complete exhaustion.
4. After completing the test, cool down by swimming another two or three minutes at a slower pace.
5. Determine the total distance you swam during the test, and look up your fitness category in Table 5.7.

Figure 5.5 Procedure for the 12-Minute Swim Test.

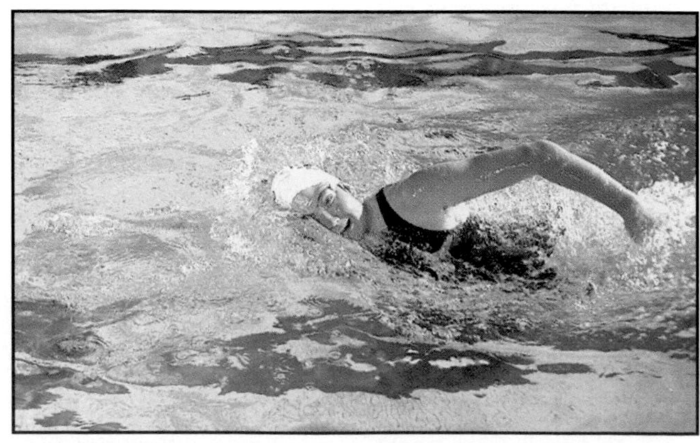

Swimming efficiency requires skill and proper conditioning.

Table 5.7 12-Minute Swim Test Fitness Categories

Distance (yards)	Fitness Category
≥700	Excellent
500–700	Good
400–500	Average
200–400	Fair
≤200	Poor

Adapted from *The Aerobics Program for Total Well-Being*, by K. H. Cooper (New York: Bantam Books, 1982).

University of Houston Non-Exercise Test

The University of Houston Non-Exercise Test (N-Ex) is a method used to estimate maximal oxygen uptake that does not involve any form of exercise testing. As indicated earlier, this protocol can be used as an initial estimate of maximal oxygen uptake and for mass screening purposes. The information for this test is collected through self-reports.

This N-Ex test is especially useful when testing individuals who are taking high blood pressure medication. Hypertensive medication lowers the heart rate. Therefore, tests based on heart rate (walk test, step test, and Astrand-Ryhming) cannot be used with these people. Maximal exercise tests (1.5-Mile Run) also are not to be administered to hypertensive people. The N-Ex equations to predict maximal oxygen uptake have a high degree of accuracy with men on anti-hypertensive medication.

The non-exercise test is based on research findings in exercise physiology indicating that maximal oxygen uptake is related negatively to age and body composition but related positively to exercise habits. Based on these variables, multiple regression equations were developed to estimate maximal oxygen uptake in ml/kg/min. The procedure for the Houston Non-Exercise Test is outlined in Figures 5.6 and 5.7. The test is suitable for men and women alike.

Good cardiorespiratory fitness has been linked to better health and increased longevity.

Interpreting Your Maximal Oxygen Uptake Results

After obtaining your maximal oxygen uptake, you can determine your current level of cardiorespiratory fitness by consulting Table 5.8. Locate the maximal oxygen uptake in your age category, and on the top row you will find your present level of cardiorespiratory fitness. For example, a 19-year-old male with a maximal oxygen uptake of 35 ml/kg/min would be classified in the average cardiorespiratory fitness category. After you initiate your personal cardiorespiratory exercise program (see Chapter 6), you may

5

UNIVERSITY OF HOUSTON NON-EXERCISE TEST

Use the appropriate number (0-7) which best describes your general physical activity rating (PAR) for the previous month:

I. Do not participate regularly in programmed recreation sport or physical activity.

0 Avoid walking or exertion, e.g., always use elevator, drive whenever possible instead of walking.

1 Walk for pleasure, routinely use stairs, occasionally exercise sufficiently to cause heavy breathing or perspiration.

II. Participate regularly in recreation or work requiring modest physical activity, such as golf, horseback riding, calisthenics, gymnastics, table tennis, bowling, weight lifting, yard work.

2 10 to 60 minutes per week.

3 Over one hour per week.

III. Participate regularly in heavy physical exercise such as running or jogging, swimming, cycling, rowing, skipping rope, running in place or engaging in vigorous aerobic activity type exercise such as tennis, basketball or handball.

4 Run less than one mile per week or spend less than 30 minutes per week in comparable physical activity.

5 Run 1 to 5 miles per week or spend 30 to 60 minutes per week in comparable physical activity.

6 Run 5 to 10 miles per week or spend 1 to 3 hours per week in comparable physical activity.

7 Run over 10 miles per week or spend over 3 hours per week in comparable physical activity.

Figure 5.6 Physical activity code for University of Houston Non-Exercise Test.

UNIVERSITY OF HOUSTON NON-EXERCISE TEST*

Multiple regression equations have been developed to estimate maximal oxygen uptake in ml/kg/min according to physical activity rating (PAR), age (A), and percent body fat (%Fat) or body mass index (BMI). The first equation uses percent body fat determined through skinfolds (N-EX %Fat). The procedure to determine percent body fat through skinfolds is outlined in Figure 3.3 in Chapter 3. The second equation uses body mass index (N-Ex BMI). The N-Ex %Fat equation is slightly more accurate than the N-Ex BMI equation. The physical activity rating code provided in Figure 5.6 is used for a global, self-rating of physical activity. The subject uses the code to rate his or her physical activity during the past month. The selected number is a global rating of the subject's exercise habits. This value is used in the equation. The regression equations are as follows:

N-Ex %Fat Model

Men $VO_{2max} = 56.370 - (.289 \times A) - (.552 \times \%Fat) + (1.589 \times PAR)$

Women $VO_{2max} = 50.513 - (.289 \times A) - (.552 \times \%Fat) + (1.589 \times PAR)$

N-Ex BMI Model (BMI = Weight in pounds × 705 ÷ Height in inches ÷ Height in inches

Men $VO_{2max} = 67.350 - (.381 \times A) - (.754 \times BMI) + (1.951 \times PAR)$

Women $VO_{2max} = 56.363 - (.381 \times A) - (.754 \times BMI) + (1.951 \times PAR)$

Examples

The N-Ex %fat model is illustrated with a 40-year-old man with 17% body fat and an activity rating of 6. Estimated Max VO_2 for the man would be:

$$VO_{2max} = 56.37 - (.289 \times 40) - (.552 \times 17) + (1.589 \times 6)$$

$$VO_{2max} = 45.0 \text{ ml/kg/min}$$

The N-Ex BMI for a 30-year-old woman who weighs 130 pounds, with a height of 64 inches, and a physical activity rating of 5 would be:

BMI = Weight in pounds × 705 ÷ Height in inches ÷ Height in inches [or weight in kilograms × (height in meters)^2]

BMI = 130 × 705 ÷ 64 ÷ 64 = 22.38

$$VO_{2max} = 56.363 - (.381 \times 30) - (.754 \times 22.38) + (1.951 \times 5)$$

$$VO_{2max} = 37.8 \text{ ml/kg/min}$$

* University of Houston Non-Exercise Test reproduced with permission from *Exercise Concepts, Calculations, & Computer Applications* by R. M. Ross and A. S. Jackson. Camel, IN: Benchmark Press, Inc.,(1990) pp. 108–110.

Figure 5.7 Procedure for the University of Houston Non-Exercise Test.

Table 5.8 Cardiorespiratory Fitness Classification According to Maximal Oxygen Uptake

Gender	Age	FITNESS CLASSIFICATION (based on VO_{2max} in ml/kg/min)				
		Poor	Fair	Average	Good	Excellent
Men	≤29	≤24.9	25–33.9	34–43.9	44–52.9	≥53
	30–39	≤22.9	23–30.9	31–41.9	42–49.9	≥50
	40–49	≤19.9	20–26.9	27–38.9	39–44.9	≥45
	50–59	≤17.9	18–24.9	25–37.9	38–42.9	≥43
	60–69	≤15.9	16–22.9	23–35.9	36–40.9	≥41
Women	≤29	≤23.9	24–30.9	31–38.9	39–48.9	≥49
	30–39	≤19.9	20–27.9	28–36.9	37–44.9	≥45
	40–49	≤16.9	17–24.9	25–34.9	35–41.9	≥42
	50–59	≤14.9	15–21.9	22–33.9	34–39.9	≥40
	60–69	≤12.9	13–20.9	21–32.9	33–36.9	≥37

High physical fitness standard

Health fitness standard

See Chapter 1, Fitness Standards: Health versus Physical Fitness, page 7.

wish to retest yourself periodically to evaluate your progress.

Heart Rate and Blood Pressure Assessment

You will learn, in Lab 5B how to determine your heart rate and blood pressure. As mentioned previously, heart rate can be obtained by counting your pulse either on the wrist over the radial artery or over the carotid artery in the neck.

You may count your pulse for 30 seconds and multiply by 2 or take it for a full minute. The heart rate usually is at its lowest point (resting heart rate) late in the evening after you have been sitting quietly for about half an hour watching a relaxing TV show or reading in bed, or early in the morning just before you get out of bed.

Unless you have a pathological condition, a lower resting heart rate indicates a stronger heart. To adapt to cardiorespiratory or aerobic exercise, the heart enlarges and the muscle gets stronger. A bigger and stronger heart can pump more blood with fewer strokes.

If in doubt, consult your doctor before initiating, continuing, or increasing your level of physical activity.

Resting heart rate ratings are given in Table 5.9. Although resting heart rate decreases with training, the extent of **bradycardia** depends not only on the amount of training but also on genetic factors. Although most highly trained athletes have a resting heart rate around 40 beats per minute, Jim Ryan, world record holder for the 1-mile run in the 1960s, had a consistent resting heart rate in the 70s even during peak training months during his athletic career. For most individuals, however, the resting heart rate decreases as the level of cardiovascular endurance increases.

Table 5.9 Resting Heart Rate Ratings

Heart Rate (beats/minute)	Rating
≤59	Excellent
60-69	Good
70-79	Average
80-89	Fair
≥90	Poor

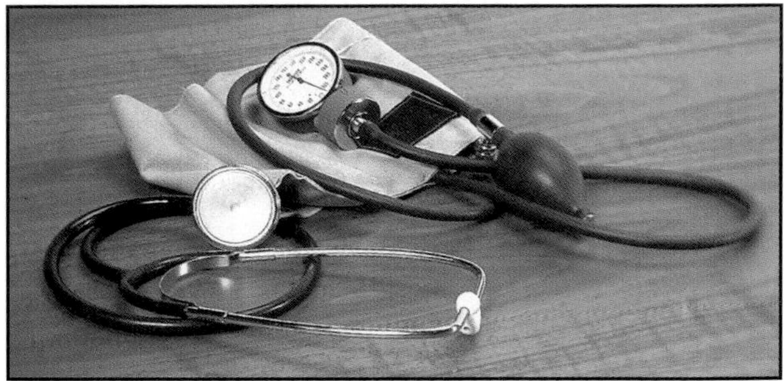

Blood pressure can be measured with an aneroid blood pressure gauge and stethoscope.

Blood pressure is assessed using a **sphygmomanometer** and a stethoscope. A cuff of the appropriate size must be used to get accurate readings. Size is determined by the width of the inflatable bladder, which should be about 40% of the circumference of the midpoint of the arm.

Blood pressure usually is measured while the person is in the sitting position, with the forearm and the manometer at the same level as the heart. At first, the pressure is recorded from each arm, and after that from the arm with the highest reading.

The cuff should be applied approximately an inch above the antecubital space (natural crease of the elbow), with the center of the bladder directly over the medial (inner) surface of the arm. The stethoscope head should be applied firmly, but with little pressure, over the brachial artery in the antecubital space. The arm should be flexed slightly and placed on a flat surface.

The bladder can be inflated while feeling the radial pulse to about 30 to 40 mmHg above the point at which the pulse disappears. The cuff should not be overinflated, as this may cause blood vessel spasm, resulting in higher blood pressure readings. The pressure should be released at a rate of 2 mmHg per second.

As the pressure is released, systolic blood pressure is determined at the point where the initial pulse sound is heard. The diastolic pressure is determined at the point where the sound disappears. The recordings should be expressed as systolic over diastolic pressure — for example, 124/80.

When taking more than one reading, the bladder should be completely deflated, and at least one

Bradycardia Slower heart rate than normal.

Sphygmomanometer An inflatable bladder contained within a cuff and a mercury gravity manometer (or an aneroid manometer) from which the pressure is read.

minute should be allowed before making the next recording. The person measuring the pressure also should note whether the pressure was recorded from the left or the right arm. Resting blood pressure ratings are given in Table 5.10.

In some cases the pulse sounds become less intense (point of muffling sounds) and still can be heard at a lower pressure (50 or 40 mmHg) or even all the way down to zero. In this situation the diastolic pressure is recorded at the point of a clear, definite change in the loudness of the sound (also referred to as fourth phase), and at complete disappearance of the sound (fifth phase) (for example, 120/78/60 or 120/82/0).

When measuring resting heart rate and blood pressure, several readings should be taken by different people or at different times of the day, to establish the real values. A single reading may not be an accurate value because of the various factors that can affect blood pressure.

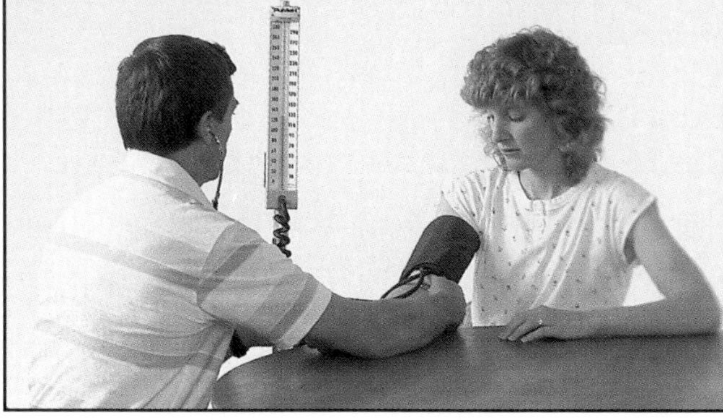

A mercury gravity manometer can be used to assess blood pressure.

Table 5.10 Blood Pressure Ratings

Systolic (in mm/Hg)	Diastolic (in mm/Hg)	Rating
≤120	≤80	Very Low Risk
121-130	81-89	Low Risk
131-140	90-99	Moderate Risk
141-150	100-105	High Risk
≥151	≥106	Very High Risk

Ratings are expressed in terms of risk for cardiovascular disease.

Laboratory Experience

LAB 5A
Cardiorespiratory Endurance Assessment

Lab Preparation
Wear appropriate exercise clothing and jogging or walking shoes as required. Be prepared to take the 1.5-Mile Run Test, 1.0-Mile Walk Test, Step Test, Astrand-Ryhming Test, or 12-Minute Swim Test. Avoid vigorous physical activity 24 hours prior to this lab.

LAB 5B
Heart Rate and Blood Pressure Assessment

Lab Preparation
Wear exercise clothing, including a shirt with short or loose-fitting sleeves to allow the blood pressure cuff to be placed around the upper arm. Do not engage in any form of exercise several hours prior to this lab.

Suggested Readings

American College of Sports Medicine. *Guidelines for Exercise Testing and Prescription.* Philadelphia: Lea & Febiger, 1991.

American College of Sports Medicine. "The Recommended Quantity and Quality of Exercise for Developing and Maintaining Cardiorespiratory and Muscular Fitness in Healthy Adults." *Medicine and Science in Sports and Exercise,* 22 (1990), 265-274.

American Heart Association Committee on Exercise. *Exercise Testing and Training of Apparently Healthy Individuals: A Handbook for Physicians.* New York: AHA, 1972.

Astrand, I. *Acta Physiologica Scandinavica,* 49 (1960), Supplementum 169:45-60.

Astrand, P. O., and K. Rodahl. *Textbook of Work Physiology.* New York: McGraw-Hill, 1986.

Cooper, K. H. "A Means of Assessing Maximal Oxygen Intake." *Journal of the American Medical Association,* 203 (1968), 201-204.

Cooper, K. H. *The Aerobics Program for Total Well-Being.* New York: Mount Evans and Co., 1982.

Fox, E. L., R. W. Bowers, and H. L. Foss. *The Physiological Basis of Physical Education and Athletics.* Philadelphia: Saunders College Publishing, 1988.

Hoeger, W. W. K., and S. A. Hoeger. *Lifetime Fitness & Wellness: A Personalized Program.* Englewood, CO: Morton Publishing, 1995.

Kline, G., et al. "Estimation of VO_{2max} from a One-Mile Track Walk, Gender, Age, and Body Weight." *Medicine and Science in Sports and Exercise* 19:3 (1987), 253-259.

McArdle, W. D., F. I. Katch, and V. L. Katch. *Exercise Physiology: Energy, Nutrition and Human Performance.* Philadelphia: Lea & Febiger, 1991.

Wilmore, J. H., and D. L. Costill. *Training for Sport and Activity.* Dubuque, IA: Wm. C. Brown Publishers, 1988.

Principles of Cardiorespiratory Exercise Prescription

6

LABS

There is no drug in current or prospective use that holds as much promise for sustained health as a lifetime program of physical exercise.[1]

A sound cardiorespiratory endurance program contributes greatly to enhancing and maintaining good health. With the exception of older adults, cardiorespiratory endurance is the single most important component of health-related physical fitness (see Chapter 1). A person needs a certain amount of muscular strength and flexibility to engage in normal daily activities. Nevertheless, a person can get by without a lot of strength and flexibility but cannot do without a good cardiorespiratory system.

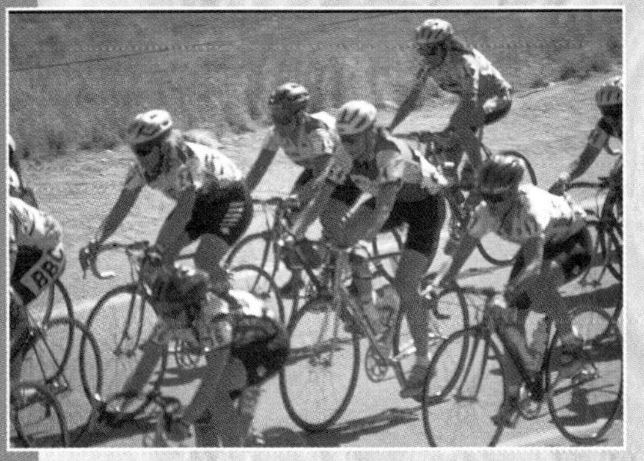

Aerobic exercise is especially important in preventing coronary heart disease. A poorly conditioned heart, which has to pump more often just to keep a person alive, is subject to more wear-and-tear than a well-conditioned heart. In situations that place strenuous demands on the heart, such as doing yard work, lifting heavy objects or weights, or running to catch a bus, the unconditioned heart may not be able to sustain the strain. Regular participation in cardiorespiratory endurance activities also helps a person achieve and maintain recommended body weight, the fourth component of health-related physical fitness.

Objectives

- Determine readiness to start an exercise program.
- Learn the principles that govern cardiorespiratory exercise prescription: intensity, mode, duration, and frequency.
- Clarify misconceptions related to cardiorespiratory endurance training.
- Learn concepts for preventing and treating injuries.
- Learn basic skills to enhance adherence to exercise.
- Learn to predict oxygen uptake and caloric expenditure from exercise heart rate.

Readiness for Exercise

Currently, more than half of the adult population reports little or no regular leisure physical activity.[2] Further, surveys indicate that more than half of the people who start exercising drop out during the first 6 months of the program. Sports psychologists are trying to find out why some people exercise habitually and many do not. All of the benefits of exercise cannot help unless people commit to a lifetime program of physical activity.

Cardiorespiratory endurance is the most important component of health-related physical fitness.

If you are not exercising now, are you willing to give exercise a try? The first step is to decide positively that you will try. Lab 6A will help you make this decision.

Make a list of the advantages and disadvantages of incorporating exercise into your lifestyle. Your list of advantages may include things such as:

1. It will make me feel better.
2. I will lose weight.
3. I will have more energy.
4. It will lower risk for chronic diseases.

Your list of disadvantages might include:

1. I don't want to take the time.
2. I'm too out of shape.
3. There's no good place to exercise.
4. I don't have the willpower to do it.

When the reasons for exercise outweigh the reasons for not exercising, it will become easier to try.

The four basic variables in improving the cardiorespiratory system are intensity, mode, duration, and frequency of exercise.

Lab 6B may answer the question: Am I ready to start an exercise program? You are evaluated in four categories: mastery (self-control), attitude, health, and commitment. The higher you score in any category — mastery, for example — the more important that reason is for you to exercise.

Scores can vary from 4 to 16. A score of 12 and above is a strong indicator that that factor is important to you, whereas 8 and below is low. If you score 12 or more points in each category, your chances of initiating and sticking to an exercise program are good. If you do not score at least 12 points in three categories, your chances of succeeding at exercise may be slim. You need to be better informed about the benefits of exercise, and a retraining process may be helpful. More tips on how you can become committed to exercise are provided later in the chapter.

Guidelines for Cardiorespiratory Exercise Prescription

All too often, individuals who exercise regularly and then take a cardiorespiratory endurance test are surprised to find their maximal oxygen uptake is not as good as they think it is. Although these individuals may be exercising regularly, they most likely are not following the basic principles for cardiorespiratory exercise prescription. Therefore, they do not reap significant improvements in cardiorespiratory endurance.

To develop the cardiorespiratory system, the heart muscle has to be overloaded like any other muscle in the human body. Just as the biceps muscle in the upper arm is developed through strength-training exercises, the heart muscle has to be exercised to increase in size, strength, and efficiency. To better understand how the cardiorespiratory system can be developed, we have to be familiar with four variables: intensity, mode, duration, and frequency of exercise.

Before discussing the cardiorespiratory prescription variables, you should be aware that the American College of Sports Medicine recommends that a medical exam and a diagnostic exercise stress test be administered prior to vigorous exercise by apparently healthy men over age 40 and women over age 50.[3]

The American College of Sports Medicine has defined *vigorous exercise* as an exercise intensity above 60% of maximal oxygen uptake. This intensity is the equivalent of exercise that provides a "substantial challenge" to the participant or one that cannot be maintained for 20 continuous minutes.

Intensity of Exercise

When trying to develop the cardiorespiratory system, **intensity** of exercise is the factor that perhaps is ignored most often. For muscles to develop, they have to be overloaded to a given point. The training stimulus to develop the biceps muscle, for example, can be accomplished with arm curl-up exercises. Likewise, the cardiorespiratory system is stimulated by making the heart pump faster for a specified period of time.

Cardiorespiratory development occurs when working between 50% and 85% of heart rate reserve.[4] Working closer to 85% of heart rate reserve yields quicker results. For this reason, many experts prescribe exercise between 70% and 85% for young people. Exercise intensity can be calculated easily, and training can be monitored by checking your pulse.

Determining Training Intensity

To determine the intensity of exercise or cardiorespiratory training zone:

1. Estimate your **maximal heart rate (MHR)**. The maximal heart rate depends on the person's age and can be estimated according to the formula: MHR = 220 minus age (220 − age)
2. Check your **resting heart rate (RHR)** sometime after you have been at rest for 15 to 20 minutes. You may take your pulse for 30 seconds and multiply by 2, or take it for a full minute.
3. Determine the **heart rate reserve (HRR)**. This is done by subtracting the resting heart rate from the maximal heart rate (HRR = MHR − RHR). HRR indicates the number of beats available to go from a resting condition to an all-out maximal effort.
4. Calculate the training intensities (TI) at 50%, 70%, and 85%. Multiply the heart rate reserve by the respective 50, 70, and 85 percentages, and then add the resting heart rate to these three figures (for example, 85% TI = HRR × .85 + RHR).

   Example: The 50%, 70%, and 85% training intensities for a 20-year-old person with a resting heart rate of 68 bpm is:

   MHR: 220 − 20 = 200 beats per minute (bpm)
   RHR = 68 bpm
   HRR: 200 − 68 = 132 beats
   50% TI = (132 × .50) + 68 = 134 bpm
   70% TI = (132 × .70) + 68 = 160 bpm
   85% TI = (132 × .85) + 68 = 180 bpm
   Cardiorespiratory training zone: 134 to 180 bpm

The cardiorespiratory training zone indicates that whenever you exercise to improve the cardiorespiratory system, you should maintain your heart rate between the 50% and 85% training intensities to obtain adequate development (Figure 6.1). If you have been physically inactive, you should train around the 50% intensity during the first 4 to 6 weeks of the exercise program. After the first few weeks, you should exercise between 70% and 85% training intensity.

Following a few weeks of training, you may have a considerably lower resting heart rate (10 to 20 beats in 8 to 12 weeks). Therefore, you should recompute your target zone periodically. Once you have reached an ideal level of cardiorespiratory endurance, training in the 50% to 85% range will allow you to maintain your fitness level.

> ***Maintain your heart rate between the 50 percent and 85 percent training intensities to obtain adequate cardiorespiratory development.***

During the first few weeks of an exercise program, you should monitor your exercise heart rate regularly to make sure you are training in the proper zone. Wait until you are about 5 minutes into your exercise session before taking your first rate. When you check your heart rate, count your pulse for 10 seconds, and then multiply by 6 to get the per-minute pulse rate. Exercise heart rate will remain at the same level for about 15 seconds following exercise. After 15 seconds, your heart rate will drop rapidly. Do not hesitate to stop during your exercise bout to check your pulse. If the rate is too low, increase the intensity of exercise. If the rate is too high, slow down.

To develop the cardiorespiratory system, you do not have to exercise above the 85% rate. From a fitness standpoint, training above this percentage will not produce extra benefits and actually may be unsafe for some individuals. For unconditioned people and older adults, cardiorespiratory training should be around the 50% rate. This lower rate is recommended to avoid potential problems associated with high-intensity exercise.

Health Fitness Versus Physical Fitness

Training benefits can be obtained by exercising at the 50% training intensity. Training at this lower percentage, however, may place a person in only an

Intensity In cardiorespiratory exercise, how hard a person has to exercise to improve or maintain fitness.

Maximal heart rate (MHR) Highest heart rate for a person, primarily related to age.

Resting heart rate (RHR) Rate after a person has been sitting quietly for 15–20 minutes.

Heart rate reserve (HRR) The difference between the maximal heart rate and the resting heart rate.

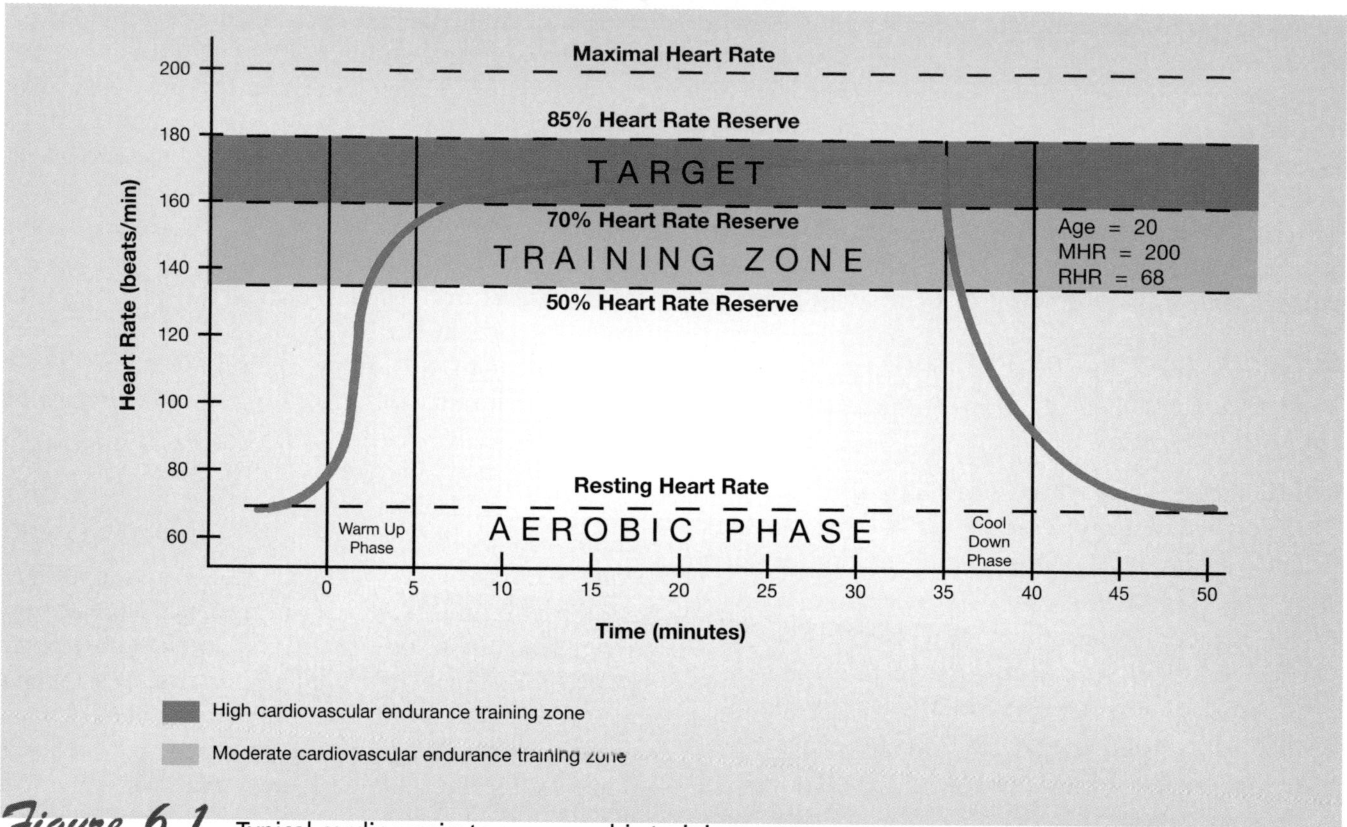

Figure 6.1 Typical cardiorespiratory or aerobic training pattern.

average or a "moderately fit" category (see Table 5.8, page 104). As will be discussed under Specific Exercise Considerations, question 1, exercising at this lower intensity lowers the risk for cardiovascular mortality (health fitness) but does not allow the person to achieve a high cardiorespiratory fitness rating (physical fitness). The latter ratings are obtained by exercising closer to the 85% threshold.

Rate of Perceived Exertion

Because many people do not check their heart rate during exercise, an alternative method of prescribing intensity of exercise has become more popular recently. This method uses a **rate of perceived exertion (RPE)** scale developed by Gunnar Borg. Using the scale in Figure 6.2, a person subjectively rates the perceived exertion or difficulty of exercise when training in the appropriate target zone. The exercise heart rate then is associated with the corresponding RPE value.

For example, if the training intensity requires a heart rate zone between 150 and 170 bpm, the person associates this with training between "hard" and "very hard." Some individuals, however, may perceive less exertion than others when training in the correct zone. Therefore, you have to associate your own inner perception of the task with the phrases given on the scale. You then may proceed to exercise at that rate of perceived exertion.

6	
7	Very, very light
8	
9	Very light
10	
11	Fairly light
12	
13	Somewhat hard
14	
15	Hard
16	
17	Very Hard
18	
19	Very, very hard
20	

From "Perceived Exertion: A Note on History and Methods," by G. Borg, *Medicine and Science in Sports and Exercise,* 5 (1983), 90–93.

Figure 6.2 Rate of Perceived Exertion Scale.

You must be sure to cross-check your target zone with your perceived exertion in the first weeks of your exercise program. To help you develop this association, you should keep a regular record of your activities using the form provided in Figure 6.9 at the end of this chapter. After several weeks of training, you should be able to predict your exercise heart rate just by your own perceived exertion of the exercise intensity.

Whether you monitor the intensity of exercise by checking your pulse or through rate of perceived exertion, you should be aware that changes in normal exercise conditions will affect the training zone. For example, exercising on a hot/humid day or at high altitude increases the heart rate response to a given task requiring adjustments in the intensity of your exercise.

Mode of Exercise

The **mode** of exercise that develops the cardiorespiratory system has to be aerobic in nature. Once you have established your cardiorespiratory training zone, any activity or combination of activities that will get your heart rate up to that training zone and keep it there for as long as you exercise will give you adequate development. Examples of these activities are walking, jogging, aerobics, swimming, water aerobics, cross-country skiing, rope skipping, cycling, racquetball, stair climbing, and stationary running or cycling.

The activity you choose should be based on your personal preferences, what you most enjoy doing, and your physical limitations. Choose low-impact activities, as such greatly decreases the risk for injuries. Most injuries to beginners are related to high-impact activities. General strength conditioning (see Chapter 8) is also recommended prior to initiating an aerobic exercise program for individuals who have been inactive. Strength conditioning will significantly reduce the incidence of injuries.

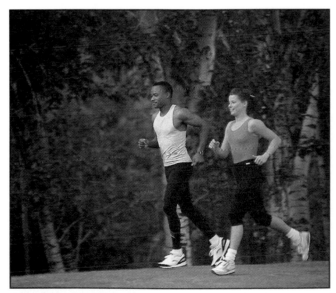

Aerobic exercise promotes cardiorespiratory development and helps decrease the risk for chronic diseases.

The amount of strength or flexibility you develop through various activities differs, but in terms of cardiorespiratory development, the heart doesn't know whether you are walking, swimming, or cycling. All the heart knows is that it has to pump at a certain rate, and as long as that rate is in the desired range, your cardiorespiratory fitness will improve.

From a health fitness point of view, training in the lower end of the cardiorespiratory zone will yield optimal health benefits. The closer the heart rate is to the higher end of the cardiorespiratory training zone, however, the greater will be the improvements in maximal oxygen uptake (high physical fitness).

Aerobic exercise has to involve the major muscle groups of the body, and it has to be rhythmic and continuous. As the amount of muscle mass involved during exercise increases, so does the effectiveness of the activity in providing cardiorespiratory development.

Cross-country skiing is regarded as the prime exercise modality for aerobic development. Several major muscle groups are used during this activity because it requires both upper and lower body work. Research has shown that, of all elite athletes, cross-country skiers have the highest maximal oxygen uptake.

Because of the greater amount of muscle mass involved, more oxygen and energy (calories) are used during cross-country skiing than with most other aerobic activities. A limitation of this activity, of course, is the lack of year-round conditions for skiing, and commercially available cross-country skiing simulating equipment is not readily available to most people.

A new mode of aerobic exercise is *Aero-belt exercise*. The Aero-belt* (Aerobic Endurance Resistance Overloader) consists of a belt with an elastic band that slides freely through the belt and attaches to the wrists. The objective of using the Aero-belt is

*AERO-BELT is a registered trademark of Nurge Fitness Systems, P. O. Box 889, Ketchum, ID 83340 Phone: 1-800-TRY-TO-XL

Rate of perceived exertion (RPE) A perception scale to monitor or interpret the intensity of aerobic exercise.

Mode Form of exercise.

6

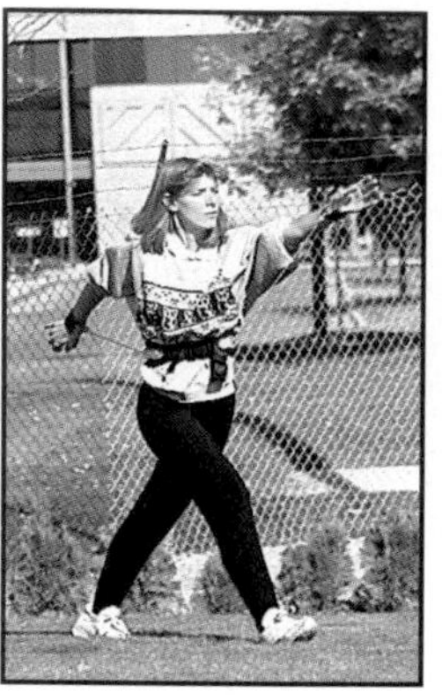

Aero-belt walking

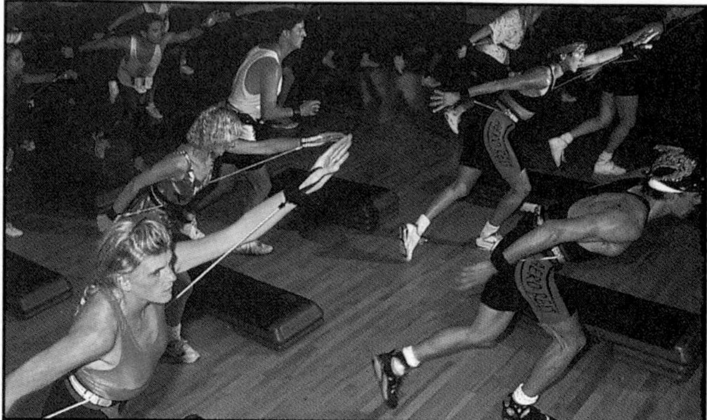

Aero-belt step-aerobics

Aero-belt Exercise: A new exercise modality designed to provide resistance to the arms during lower body physical activity; thereby increasing the person's oxygen consumption, energy expenditure, and upper body strength development during aerobic exercise. (For more information call 1-800-TRY-TO-XL.)

to provide resistance to the arms during lower body physical activity; thereby increasing the person's oxygen consumption, energy expenditure, and upper body strength and endurance development during aerobic exercise. As in cross-country skiing, the Aero-belt provides resistance to the arms while walking, jogging, bounding, stair stepping, riding a stationary bicycle, or doing aerobics.

Using the Aero-belt actually can provide greater upper body conditioning benefits than cross-country skiing. Depending on individual strength and fitness levels, three different tension grades for the elastic cord are available. Medium and high tension are mainly for strength conditioning, and low tension is for developing endurance.

The physiologic responses to Aero-belt walking (4.0 and 4.2 mph), jogging (6.0 mph), and step aerobics were investigated at Boise State University.[5,6,7] Increases in heart rate, oxygen uptake, and caloric expenditure ranged from 32% to 54% from regular walking, jogging, and step-aerobics to walking, jogging, and step-aerobics with an Aero-belt (see Figure 6.3).

Duration of Exercise

The general recommendation is that a person train between 20 and 60 minutes per session. The **duration** is based on how intensely a person trains. If the training is done around 85%, 20 minutes are sufficient. At 50% intensity, the person should train at least 30 minutes. As mentioned under Intensity of Exercise, unconditioned people and older adults should train at lower percentages; therefore, the activity should be carried out over a longer time.

Although most experts recommend 20 to 30 minutes of aerobic exercise per session, research

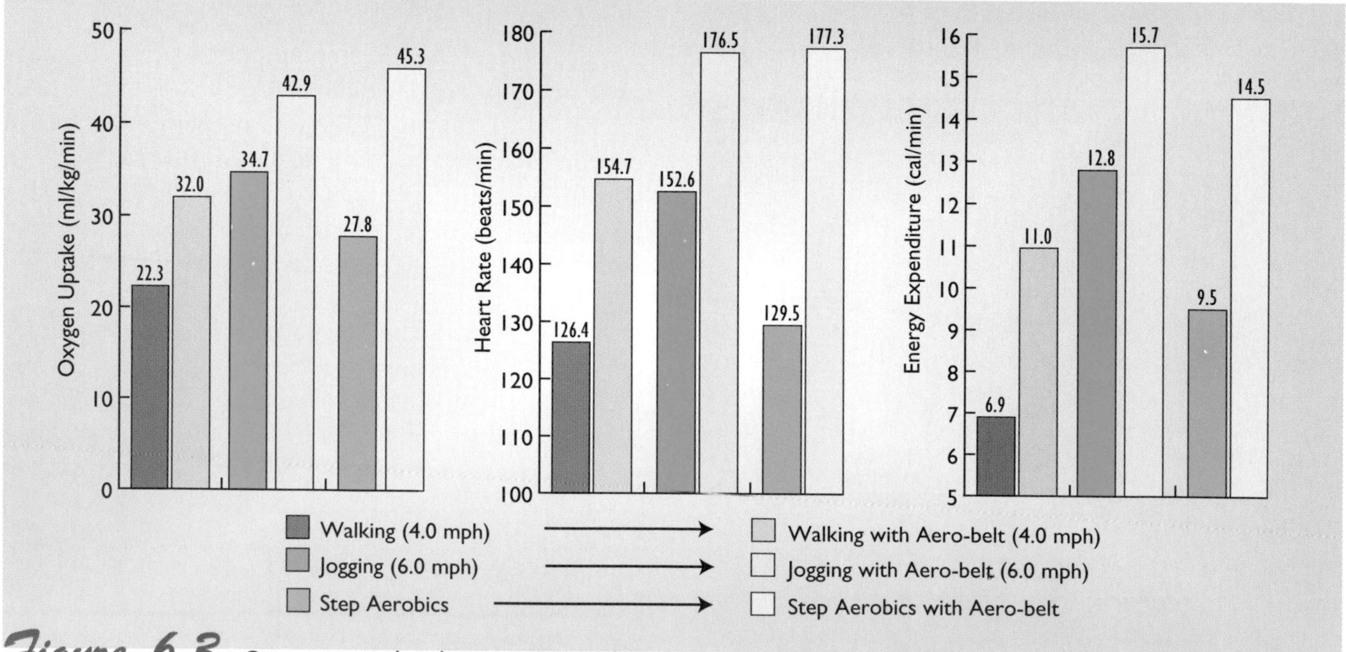

Figure 6.3 Oxygen uptake, heart rate, and energy expenditure responses to walking, jogging, and step aerobics with and without an Aero-belt.

indicates that three 10-minute exercise sessions per day (separated by at least 4 hours), at approximately 70% of maximal heart rate, also produce training benefits.[8]

Although the increases in maximal oxygen uptake with the latter program were not as large (57%) as those found in a group performing a continuous 30-minute bout of exercise per day, the researchers concluded that moderate-intensity exercise training, conducted for 10 minutes, three times per day, benefits the cardiorespiratory system significantly.

Results of this study are meaningful because people often mention lack of time as the reason for not taking part in an exercise program. Many think they have to exercise at least 20 continuous minutes to get any benefits at all. Even though 20 to 30 minutes are ideal, short, intermittent exercise bouts also are beneficial to the cardiorespiratory system.

Exercise sessions always should be preceded by a 5-minute warm-up and followed by a 5-minute cool-down period (see Figure 6.1). The **warm-up** should consist of general calisthenics, stretching exercises, or exercising at a lower intensity level than the actual target zone. The **cool-down** means decreasing the intensity of exercise *gradually*. Abruptly stopping causes blood to pool in the exercised body parts, diminishing the return of blood to the heart. Less blood return can cause dizziness and faintness or even bring on cardiac abnormalities.

Frequency of Exercise

When starting an exercise program, a **frequency** of three to five 20- to 30-minute training sessions per week are recommended to improve maximal oxygen uptake. When training is conducted more than 5 days a week, further improvements are minimal.

For individuals on a weight-loss program, 45- to 60-minute exercise sessions of low to moderate intensity, conducted five to six days per week, are recommended. Longer exercise sessions increase caloric expenditure for faster weight reduction (see Chapter 4, page 80). Three 20- to 30-minute training sessions per week, on nonconsecutive days, will maintain cardiorespiratory fitness as long as the heart rate is in the appropriate target zone. A summary of the cardiorespiratory exercise prescription guidelines according to the American College of Sports Medicine is provided in Figure 6.4.

Although three training sessions per week will maintain cardiorespiratory fitness, the importance of regular physical activity in preventing disease and enhancing quality of life was pointed out clearly in July 1993 at a news briefing held at the National Press Club in Washington, DC. At this briefing the American College of Sports Medicine and the U.S. Centers for Disease Control and Prevention, in conjunction with the President's Council on Physical Fitness and Sports, provided the American public with a set of recommendations on the types of physical activity needed for maintaining and promoting health.[9]

In this summary statement every American is encouraged to accumulate at least 30 minutes of moderate-intensity physical activity almost daily. This daily routine has been promoted as an effective way to improve health. The entire contents of this statement on the benefits of physical activity are given in Figure 6.5.

Ideally, a person should engage in physical activity six to seven times per week. Based on the above discussion, to reap both the high-fitness and health-fitness benefits of exercise, a person needs to exercise a minimum of three times per week in the appropriate target zone for high fitness maintenance and three to four additional times per week in moderate-intensity activities to enjoy the full benefits of health fitness. All exercise/activity sessions should last about 30 minutes.

Activity:	Aerobic (examples: walking, jogging, cycling, swimming, aerobics, racquetball, soccer, stair climbing)
Intensity:	50%–85% heart rate reserve
Duration:	20–60 minutes of continuous aerobic activity
Frequency:	3 to 5 days per week

Source: "The Recommended Quantity and Quality of Exercise for Developing and Maintaining Cardiorespiratory and Muscular Fitness in Healthy Adults by the American College of Sports Medicine," *Medicine and Science in Sports and Exercise*, 22 (1990), 265–274.

Figure 6.4 Cardiorespiratory exercise prescription guidelines.

Duration How long a person exercises.

Warm-up Starting a workout slowly.

Cool-down Tapering off an exercise session slowly.

Frequency How often a person engages in an exercise session.

6

— SUMMARY STATEMENT —
Workshop On
Physical Activity and Public Health

Sponsored By:
U. S. Centers for Disease Control and Prevention
and
American College of Sports Medicine

In Cooperation with the President's Council on Physical Fitness and Sports

Regular physical activity is an important component of a healthy lifestyle — preventing disease and enhancing health and quality of life. A persuasive body of scientific evidence, which has accumulated over the past several decades, indicates that regular, moderate-intensity physical activity confers substantial health benefits. Because of this evidence, the U.S. Public Health Service has identified increased physical activity as a priority in Healthy People 2000, our national health objectives for the year 2000.

A primary benefit of regular physical activity is protection against coronary heart disease. In addition, physical activity appears to provide some protection against several other chronic diseases such as adult-onset diabetes, hypertension, certain cancers, osteoporosis, and depression. Furthermore, on average, physically active people outlive inactive people, even if they start their activity late in life. It is estimated that more than 250,000 deaths per year in the U.S. can be attributed to lack of regular physical activity, a number comparable to the deaths attributed to other chronic disease risk factors such as obesity, high blood pressure, and elevated blood cholesterol.

Despite the recognized value of physical activity, few Americans are regularly active. Only 22% of adults engage in leisure time physical activity at the level recommended for health benefits in Healthy People 2000. Fully 24% of adult Americans are completely sedentary and are badly in need of more physical activity. The remaining 54% are inadequately active and they too would benefit from more physical activity. Participation in regular physical activity appears to have gradually increased during the 1960s, 1970s, and early 1980s, but has plateaued in recent years. Among ethnic minority populations, older persons, and those with lower incomes or levels of education, participation in regular physical activity has remained consistently low.

Why are so few Americans physically active? Perhaps one answer is that previous public health efforts to promote physical activity have overemphasized the importance of high-intensity exercise. The current low rate of participation may be explained, in part, by the perception of many people that they must engage in vigorous, continuous exercise to reap health benefits. Actually the scientific evidence clearly demonstrates that regular, moderate-intensity physical activity provides substantial health benefits. A group of experts brought together by the U.S. Centers for Disease Control and Prevention (CDC) and the American College of Sports Medicine (ACSM) reviewed the pertinent scientific evidence and formulated the following recommendation:

Every American adult should accumulate 30 minutes or more of moderate-intensity physical activity over the course of most days of the week. Incorporating more activity into the daily routine is an effective way to improve health. Activities that can contribute to the 30-minute total include walking up stairs (instead of taking the elevator), gardening, raking leaves, dancing, and walking part or all of the way to or from work. The recommended 30 minutes of physical activity may also come from planned exercise or recreation such as jogging, playing tennis, swimming, and cycling. One specific way to meet the standard is to walk two miles briskly.

Because most adult Americans fail to meet this recommended level of moderate-intensity physical activity, almost all should strive to increase their participation in moderate or vigorous physical activity. Persons who currently do not engage in regular physical activity should begin by incorporating a few minutes of increased activity into their day, building up gradually to 30 minutes of additional physical activity. Those who are irregularly active should strive to adopt a more consistent pattern of activity. Regular participation in physical activities that develop and maintain muscular strength and joint flexibility is also recommended.

This recommendation has been developed to emphasize the important health benefits of moderate physical activity. But recognizing the benefits of physical activity is only part of the solution to this important public health problem. Today's high-tech society entices people to be inactive. Cars, television, and labor-saving devices have profoundly changed the way many people perform their jobs, take care of their homes, and use their leisure time. Furthermore, our surroundings often present significant barriers to participation in physical activity. Walking to the corner store proves difficult if there are no sidewalks; riding a bicycle to work is not an option unless safe bike lanes or paths are available.

Many Americans will not change their lifestyles until the environmental and social barriers to physical activity are reduced or eliminated. Individuals can help to overcome these barriers by modifying their own lifestyles and by encouraging family members and friends to become more active. In addition, local, state, and federal public health agencies; recreation boards; school groups; professional organizations; and fitness and sports organizations should work together to disseminate this critical public health message and to promote national, community, worksite, and school programs that help Americans become more physically active.

The American College of Sports Medicine and the U. S. Centers for Disease Control and Prevention, in cooperation with the President's Council on Physical Fitness and Sports, released this statement July 29, 1993, at the National Press Club in Washington, D.C.

Figure 6.5 Summary Statement: Workshop On Physical Activity and Public Health.

Rating the Fitness Benefits of Aerobic Activities

The fitness contributions of different aerobic activities to the health-related components of fitness vary. Although an accurate assessment of the contributions to each fitness component is difficult to establish, a summary of likely benefits of several activities is provided in Table 6.1. Instead of a single rating or number, ranges are given for some of the categories. The benefits derived are based on the person's effort while participating in the activity.

The nature of the activity often dictates the potential aerobic development. For example, jogging is much more strenuous than walking. The effort during

Table 6.1 Ratings for Aerobic Activities

Activity	Recommended Starting Fitness Level[1]	Injury Risk[2]	Potential Cardiovascular Endurance Development (VO_{2max})[3, 5]	Upper Body Strength Development[3]	Lower Body Strength Development[3]	Upper Body Flexibility Development[3]	Lower Body Flexibility Development[3]	Weight Control[3]	MET Level[4, 5, 6]	Caloric Expenditure (cal/hour)[5,6]
Walking	B	L	1–2	1	2	1	1	3	4–6	300–450
Walking/Water/Chest-Deep	I	L	2–4	2	3	1	1	3	6–10	450–750
Hiking	B	L	2–4	1	3	1	1	3	6–10	450–750
Jogging	I	M	3–5	1	3	1	1	5	6–15	450–1125
Jogging/Deep Water	A	L	3–5	2	2	1	1	5	8–15	600–1125
High Impact Aerobics	A	H	3–4	2	4	3	2	4	6–12	450–900
Low Impact Aerobics	B	L	2–4	2	3	3	2	3	5–10	375–750
Step Aerobics	I	M	2–4	2	3–4	3	2	3–4	5–12	375–900
Moderate Impact Aerobics	I	M	2–4	2	3	3	2	3	6–12	450–900
Swimming (front crawl)	B	L	3–5	4	2	3	1	3	6–12	450–900
Water Aerobics	B	L	2–4	3	3	3	2	3	6–12	450–900
Stationary Cycling	B	L	2 4	1	4	1	1	3	6–10	450–750
Road Cycling	I	M	2–5	1	4	1	1	3	6–12	450–900
Cross Training	I	M	3–5	2–3	3–4	2–3	1–2	3–5	6–15	450–1125
Rope Skipping	I	H	3–5	2	4	1	2	3–5	8–15	600–1125
Cross-Country Skiing	B	M	4–5	4	4	2	2	4–5	10–16	750–1200
Aero-belt Exercise	B	M	4–5	4	4	3	2	4–5	10 16	750–1200
In-Line Skating	I	M	2–4	2	4	2	2	3	6–10	450–750
Rowing	B	L	3–5	4	2	3	1	4	8–14	600–1050
Stair Climbing	B	L	3–5	1	4	1	1	4–5	8–15	600–1125
Racquet Sports	I	M	2–4	3	3	3	2	3	6–10	450–750

[1] B = Beginner, I = Intermediate, A = Advanced

[2] L = Low, M = Moderate, H = High

[3] 1 = Low, 2 = Fair, 3 = Average, 4 = Good, 5 = excellent

[4] One MET represents the rate of energy expenditure at rest (3.5 ml/kg/min). Each additional MET is a multiple of the resting value. For example, 5 METs represents an energy expenditure equivalent to five times the resting value or about 17.5 ml/kg/min.

[5] Varies according to the person's effort (exercise intensity) during exercise.

[6] Varies according to body weight.

exercise also has an impact on the amount of physiological development. The training benefits of just going through the motions of a low-impact aerobics routine, as compared to accentuating all motions, are of a different magnitude.

Table 6.1 indicates a starting fitness level for each aerobic activity. Attempting to participate in high-intensity activities without proper conditioning often leads to injuries and discouragement. Beginners should start with low-intensity activities that carry a minimum risk for injuries.

In some cases, such as in high-impact aerobics and rope skipping, the risk for injuries remains high even if the participants have adequate conditioning. These activities should be supplemental only and are not recommended as the sole mode of exercise. Most exercise-related injuries occur as a result of high impact activities and not a high exercise intensity.

Physicians who work with cardiac patients frequently use **METs** as an alternative method of prescribing exercise intensity. One MET represents the rate of energy expenditure at rest or the equivalent of an oxygen uptake of 3.5 ml/kg/min. The MET range for the various activities is included in Table 6.1. A 10-MET activity requires a tenfold increase in the resting energy requirement, or approximately 35 ml/kg/min. MET levels for a given activity vary according to the effort expended. The harder a person exercises, the higher is the MET level.

The effectiveness of various aerobic activities in weight management also is provided in Table 6.1. As a general rule, the greater the muscle mass involved in exercise, the better are the results. Rhythmic and continuous activities that involve large amounts of muscle mass are most effective in burning calories.

Higher intensity activities increase caloric expenditure as well. Exercising longer, however, compensates for lower intensities. If carried out long enough (45 to 60 minutes five to six times per week), even walking can be an excellent exercise mode for weight loss. Additional information on a comprehensive weight management program is given in Chapter 4.

Specific Exercise Considerations

In addition to many of the exercise-related issues discussed to this point, many other concerns require clarification or are somewhat controversial. Let's examine some of these issues.

1. *Does aerobic exercise make a person immune to heart and blood vessel disease?* Although aerobically fit individuals as a whole have a lower incidence of cardiovascular disease, a regular aerobic exercise program by itself does not offer an absolute guarantee against cardiovascular disease. Overall risk factor management is the best way to minimize the risk for cardiovascular disease (see Chapter 12). Many factors including a genetic predisposition, can increase the person's risk. Experts believe, however, that a regular aerobic exercise program not only will delay the onset of cardiovascular problems but also that the chances of surviving a heart attack are much better for those who exercise regularly.

   Even moderate increases in aerobic fitness lower the incidences of premature cardiovascular deaths significantly. Data from the Aerobics Research Institute in Dallas, Texas (see Figure 1.6, page 5) indicate that the decrease in cardiovascular mortality is greatest between the unfit (group 1) and the moderately fit (2 and 3) groups. A further decrease in cardiovascular mortality is observed between the moderately fit and the highly fit groups (4 and 5), but the difference is not as much as that between the unfit and moderately fit groups.

2. *How much aerobic exercise is required to decrease the risk for cardiovascular disease?* Although research has not yet indicated the exact amount of aerobic exercise required to lower the risk for cardiovascular disease, some general recommendations have been set forth. In their study, "Cause-Specific Death Rates per 10,000 Man-Years of Observation Among 16,936 Harvard Alumni, 1962 to 1968, by Physical Activity Index" Dr. Ralph Paffenbarger and co-researchers showed that 2,000 calories expended per week as a result of physical activity yielded the lowest risk for cardiovascular disease among this group of almost 17,000 Harvard alumni (see Figure 1.5, page 5). Two thousand calories per week represents about 300 calories per daily exercise session.

3. *Do people get a "physical high" during aerobic exercise?* During vigorous exercise, **endorphines** are released from the pituitary gland in the brain. They can create feelings of euphoria and natural well-being.

   Higher levels of endorphines often are seen as a result of aerobic endurance activities and may remain elevated for as long as 30 to 60 minutes following exercise. Many experts believe these higher levels explain the physical high some people get during and after prolonged exercise.

Endorphine levels also have been shown to be elevated during pregnancy and delivery. Endorphines act as pain killers, these higher levels could explain why a woman has more tolerance for the pain and discomfort of natural childbirth and her pleasant feelings shortly after the baby's birth. Several reports have indicated that well-conditioned women have shorter and easier labor. These women possibly attain higher endorphine levels during delivery, making childbirth less traumatic than it is for untrained women.

4. *Is exercise safe during pregnancy?* Women should not forsake exercise during pregnancy. If anything, they should exercise to strengthen the body and prepare for delivery. Moderate exercise during pregnancy helps to prevent excessive weight gain and speed up recovery following birth.

   Pregnant women in American Indian tribes continue to do all of their difficult work chores up to the very day of delivery, and a few hours after the baby's birth they resume their normal activities. Several women athletes have competed in sports during the early stages of pregnancy. Nevertheless, the woman and her personal physician should make the final decision regarding her exercise program.

   Stretching exercises are to be performed gently because hormonal changes during pregnancy increase the laxity of muscles and connective tissue. These changes facilitate delivery, but they also make women more susceptible to injuries during exercise.

   Among the American College of Obstetricians and Gynecologists recommendations for exercise during pregnancy with no additional risk factors are:[10]

   - Continue to exercise at a mild-to-moderate pace throughout the pregnancy, but decrease exercise intensity by about 25% from the pre-pregnancy program.
   - Exercise regularly a minimum of three times a week instead of doing occasional bouts of exercise.
   - Pay attention to the body's signals of discomfort and distress. Stop exercise when tired. Never exercise to exhaustion. Stop if unusual symptoms arise. These include pain of any kind, cramping, nausea, bleeding or leaking amniotic fluid, faintness, dizziness, palpitations, numbness in any part of the body, or decreased fetal activity.
   - After the first trimester, avoid exercises that require you to lie on your back. This position can block blood flow to the uterus and the baby.
   - Do non-weight-bearing activities such as cycling, swimming, or water aerobics, which minimize the risk of injury and may allow you to continue exercise throughout the pregnancy.
   - Avoid activities that could lead to a loss of balance or cause even mild trauma to the abdomen.
   - Get proper nourishment. Pregnancy requires approximately 300 extra calories per day.
   - During the first 3 months in particular, avoid exercise in the heat. Wear clothing that allows for proper heat dissipation, and drink plenty of water.

5. *Does exercise help relieve* ***dysmenorrhea****?* Exercise has not been shown to either cure or aggravate painful menstruation, but it has been shown to relieve menstrual cramps because it improves circulation to the uterus. Less severe menstrual cramps also could be related to higher increased levels of endorphines produced during prolonged physical activity, which may counteract pain. Particularly, stretching exercises of the muscles in the pelvic region seem to reduce and prevent painful menstruation that is not the result of disease.[11]

6. *Does participation in exercise hinder menstruation?* In some instances, highly trained athletes may develop amenorrhea (cessation of menstruation) during training and competition. This condition is seen most often in extremely lean women who also engage in sports that require strenuous physical effort over a sustained time, but it is by no means irreversible. At present, we

6

MET Represents the rate of resting energy expenditure at rest; one MET is the equivalent of 3.5 ml/kg/min.

Endorphines Morphine-like substances released from the pituitary gland in the brain during prolonged aerobic exercise. They are thought to induce feelings of euphoria and natural well-being.

Dysmenorrhea Painful menstruation.

do not know whether the condition is caused by physical or emotional stress related to high-intensity training, excessively low body fat, or other factors.

Although, on the average, women have a lower physical capacity during menstruation, medical surveys at the Olympic games have shown that women have broken Olympic and world records at all stages of the menstrual cycle. Menstruation should not keep a woman from participating in athletics, and it will not necessarily have a negative impact on performance.

7. *Does exercise offset the detrimental effects of cigarette smoking?* Physical exercise often motivates toward smoking cessation but does not offset any ill effects of smoking. If anything, smoking greatly decreases the ability of the blood to transport oxygen to working muscles.

Oxygen is carried in the circulatory system by hemoglobin, the iron-containing pigment of the red blood cells. Carbon monoxide, a by-product of cigarette smoke, has 210 to 250 times greater affinity for hemoglobin over oxygen. Consequently, carbon monoxide combines much faster with hemoglobin, decreasing the oxygen-carrying capacity of the blood.

Chronic smoking also increases airway resistance, requiring the respiratory muscles to work much harder and consume more oxygen just to ventilate a given amount of air. If a person quits smoking, exercise does help increase the functional capacity of the pulmonary system.

A regular exercise program does seem to be a powerful incentive to quit smoking. A random survey of 1,250 runners conducted at the 6.2-mile Peachtree Road Race in Atlanta provided impressive results. The results indicated that 81% and 75% of the men and women who smoked cigarettes when they started running had quit before the race date.

8. *What type of clothing should I wear when I exercise?* The type of clothing you wear during exercise is important. In general, clothing should fit comfortably and allow free movement of the various body parts. Select clothing according to air temperature, humidity, and exercise intensity. Avoid nylon and rubberized materials and tight clothes that interfere with the cooling mechanism of the human body or obstruct normal blood flow. Fabrics made from polypropylene, Capilene, Thermax, and synthetics are best.

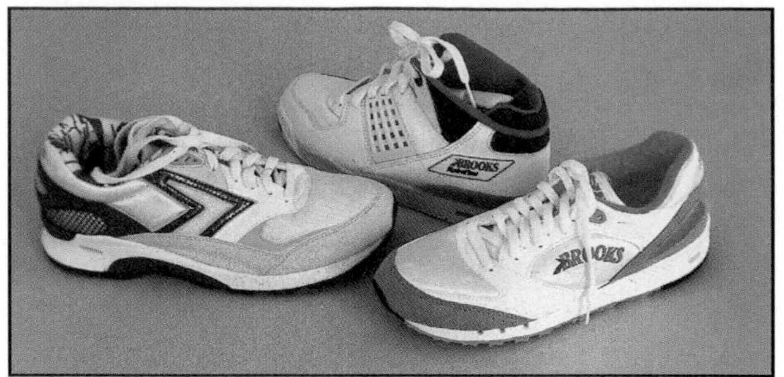

Activity-specific shoes are recommended to prevent lower-extremity injuries.

These types of fabrics draw moisture away from the skin, enhancing evaporation and cooling of the body. Exercise intensity is also important because the harder you exercise, the more heat the body produces.

When exercising in the heat, avoid the hottest time of the day, between 11:00 a.m. and 5:00 p.m. Surfaces such as asphalt, concrete, and artificial turfs absorb heat, which then radiates to the body. Therefore, these surfaces are not recommended. (Also see the discussion on exercise in hot and humid conditions in this chapter).

Only a minimal amount of clothing is necessary during exercise in the heat, to allow for maximal evaporation. Clothing should be lightweight, light-colored, loose-fitting, airy, and absorbent. Examples of commercially available products that can be used during exercise in the heat include Asci's Perma Plus, Cool-max, and Nike's Dri-F.I.T. Double-layer acrylic socks are more absorbent than cotton and help to prevent blistering and chafing of the feet. A straw-type hat can be worn to protect the eyes and head from the sun. Clothing for exercise in the cold is discussed later in this chapter.

A good pair of shoes is vital to prevent injuries to lower-limbs. Shoes manufactured specifically for your choice of activity are a must. (See Figure 6.6). When selecting proper footwear, body type, tendency toward pronation (rotating foot outward) or supination (rotating foot inward), and exercise surfaces must be considered. Shoes should have good stability, motion control, and comfortable fit. Purchase shoes in the middle of the day when feet have expanded and might be one-half size larger. For increased breatheability, choose shoes with nylon or mesh uppers. Generally, salespeople at

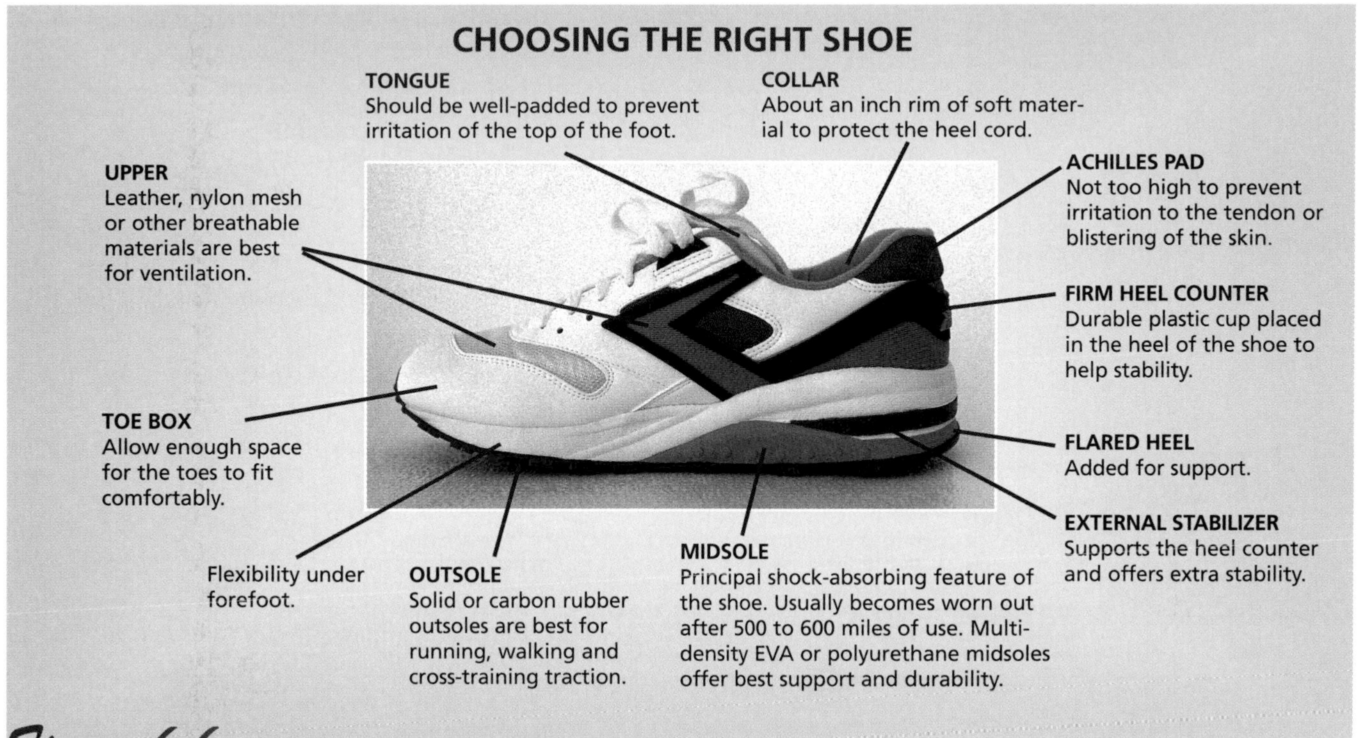
CHOOSING THE RIGHT SHOE
TONGUE
Should be well-padded to prevent irritation of the top of the foot.
COLLAR
About an inch rim of soft material to protect the heel cord.
UPPER
Leather, nylon mesh or other breathable materials are best for ventilation.
ACHILLES PAD
Not too high to prevent irritation to the tendon or blistering of the skin.
FIRM HEEL COUNTER
Durable plastic cup placed in the heel of the shoe to help stability.
TOE BOX
Allow enough space for the toes to fit comfortably.
FLARED HEEL
Added for support.
EXTERNAL STABILIZER
Supports the heel counter and offers extra stability.
Flexibility under forefoot.
OUTSOLE
Solid or carbon rubber outsoles are best for running, walking and cross-training traction.
MIDSOLE
Principal shock-absorbing feature of the shoe. Usually becomes worn out after 500 to 600 miles of use. Multi-density EVA or polyurethane midsoles offer best support and durability.

Figure 6.6 What to look for in a good pair of jogging shoes.

reputable athletic shoe stores are knowledgeable and can help select a good shoe that fits your needs. Examine your shoes after 500 miles or 6 months, and obtain a new pair if they are worn out. Old shoes frequently are responsible for lower-limb injuries.

9. *How long should a person wait after a meal before exercising strenuously?* The length of time to wait before exercising after a meal depends on the amount of food eaten. On the average, after a regular meal, you should wait about 2 hours before participating in strenuous physical activity. A walk or some other light physical activity is fine following a meal, though. If anything, it helps burn extra calories and may help the body metabolize fats more efficiently.

10. *What time of the day is best for exercise?* You can do intense exercise almost any time of the day, with the exception of about 2 hours following a heavy meal, or the noon and early afternoon hours on hot and humid days. Moderate exercise seems to be beneficial shortly after a meal, because exercise enhances the **thermogenic response.** A walk after a meal burns more calories than a walk several hours after a meal.

    Many people enjoy exercising early in the morning because it gives them a boost to start the day. People who exercise in the morning also seem to stick with it more than others. Some prefer the lunch hour for weight-control reasons. By exercising at noon, they do not eat as big a lunch, which helps keep daily caloric intake down. Highly stressed people seem to like the evening hours because of the relaxing effects of exercise.

11. *Why is exercising in hot and humid conditions unsafe?* When a person exercises, only 30% to 40% of the energy the body produces is used for mechanical work or movement. The rest of the energy (60% to 70%) is converted into heat. If this heat cannot be dissipated properly because the weather either is too hot or the relative humidity is too high, body temperature increases and, in extreme cases, can result in death.

    The specific heat of body tissue (the heat required to raise the temperature of the body by 1°C) is .38 calories per pound of body weight per 1°C (.38 cal/lb/°C). This indicates that if no body heat is dissipated, a 150-pound person needs to burn only 57 calories (150 × .38) to increase total body temperature by 1°C. If this

Thermogenic response The amount of energy required to digest food.

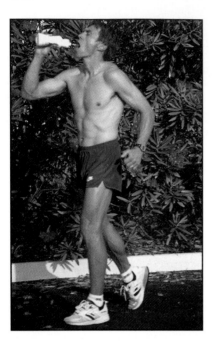

Fluid and carbohydrate replacement are essential during exercise of prolonged duration.

person were to conduct an exercise session requiring 300 calories (about 3 miles running) without any heat dissipation, the inner body temperature would increase by 5.3°C, which is the equivalent of going from 98.6°F to 108.1°F.

This example illustrates clearly the need for caution when exercising in hot or humid weather. If the relative humidity is too high, body heat cannot be lost through evaporation because the atmosphere already is saturated with water vapor. In one instance, a football casualty occurred at a temperature of only 64°F but at a relative humidity of 100%. People must be cautious when air temperature is above 90°F and the relative humidity is above 60%.

The American College of Sports Medicine recommends that individuals should not engage in strenuous physical activity when the readings of a wet-bulb globe thermometer exceed 82.4°F. With this type of thermometer, the wet bulb is cooled by evaporation, and on dry days it shows a lower temperature than the regular (dry) thermometer. On humid days the cooling effect is less because of less evaporation; hence, the difference between the wet and dry readings is not as great.

The American Running and Fitness Association offers the following descriptions and first-aid measures for three signs of trouble when exercising in the heat:

- **Heat cramps.** Symptoms include spasms and muscle twitching in the legs, arms, and abdomen. To relieve heat cramps, stop exercising, get out of the heat, massage the painful area, slowly stretch, and drink plenty of fluids.
- **Heat exhaustion.** Symptoms include fainting, dizziness, profuse sweating, cold, clammy skin, weakness, headache, and a rapid, weak pulse. If you experience any of these symptoms, stop and find a cool place to rest. Drink plenty of cool fluids. Loosen or remove clothing, and rub your body with a cool, wet towel. Stay out of the heat for the rest of the day, and possibly for the next 2 or 3 days.
- **Heat stroke.** Symptoms include serious disorientation, warm, dry skin, no sweating, rapid, full pulse, vomiting, diarrhea, unconsciousness, and high body temperature. As the temperature climbs, unexplained anxiety sets in. When the body temperature reaches 104°F to 105°F, the individual may get goose bumps, feel a cold sensation in the trunk of the body, nausea, throbbing in the temples, and numbness in the extremities. After this stage, most people become incoherent. When body temperature reaches 105°F to 106°F, disorientation, loss of fine-motor control, and muscular weakness set in. If the temperature exceeds 106°F, serious neurologic injury and death may be imminent.

  Heat stroke requires immediate emergency medical attention. Someone should request help (call 911) and get the person out of the sun. While you're waiting for the person to be taken to the hospital's emergency room, spray the person with cool water and rub the body with cool towels. Fan the person and give him or her plenty of cold liquids.

12. *What should a person do to replace fluids lost during prolonged aerobic exercise?* The main objective of fluid replacement during prolonged aerobic exercise is to maintain the blood volume so circulation and sweating can continue at normal levels. Adequate water replacement is the most important factor in preventing heat disorders. Drinking about 6 to 8 ounces of cool water every 15 to 20 minutes during exercise seems to be ideal to prevent **dehydration.** Cold fluids seem to be absorbed more rapidly from the stomach.

Other relevant points are the following.

- Commercial fluid-replacement solutions (such as Exceed and Gatorade) contain about 6% to 8% glucose, which seems to be optimal for fluid absorption and performance. Sugar does not become available to the muscles until about 30 minutes after drinking a glucose solution.
- Drinks high in fructose or with a glucose concentration above 8% will slow down water absorption when exercising in the heat.
- Most soft drinks (cola, non-cola) contain between 10% and 12% glucose, an amount that is too high for proper rehydration during exercise in the heat (also see carbohydrate loading in Chapter 2, page 48).
- Commercially prepared sports drinks are recommended when exercise will be strenuous and carried out for more than an hour. For exercise lasting less than an hour, water is just as effective in replacing fluid loss. The sports drinks you select should be based on your personal preference. Try different drinks at 6% to 8% glucose concentration to see which drink you tolerate best and suits your tastes as well.

13. *What precautions must a person take when exercising in the cold?* When exercising in the cold, the two factors to consider are frostbite and **hypothermia.** In contrast to hot and humid conditions, exercising in the cold usually does not threaten one's health because clothing for heat conservation can be selected, and exercise itself increases the production of body heat.

    Most people actually overdress for exercise in the cold. Because exercise increases body temperature, a moderate workout on a cold day makes a person feel that the temperature is 20°–30° warmer than it actually is. Overdressing for exercise can make the clothes damp from excessive perspiration. The risk for hypothermia increases when a person is wet or not moving around sufficiently to increase body heat. Initial warning signs of hypothermia include shivering, loss of coordination, and difficulty speaking. With a continued drop in body temperature, shivering stops, the muscles weaken and stiffen, and the person has feelings of elation or intoxication and eventually loses consciousness. To prevent hypothermia, use common sense, dress properly, and be aware of environmental conditions.

    The popular belief that exercising in cold temperatures (32°F and lower) freezes the lungs is false because the air is warmed properly in the air passages before it reaches the lungs. Cold is not what poses a threat. Rather, wind velocity is what affects the chill factor greatly.

    For example, exercising at a temperature of 25°F with adequate clothing is not too cold, but if the wind is blowing at 25 miles per hour, the chill factor lowers the actual temperature to −5°F. This effect is even worse if a person is wet and exhausted. When the weather is windy, exercise (jog, cycle) against the wind on the way out and with the wind when you return.

    Even though the lungs are under no risk when exercising in the cold, the face, head, hands, and feet should be protected, as they are subject to frostbite. Watch for signs of frostbite: numbness and discoloration. In cold temperatures, about 30% of the body's heat is lost through the head's surface area if it is unprotected. A wool or synthetic cap, hood, or hat will help to hold in body heat. Mittens are better than gloves because they keep the fingers together, so the surface area from which to lose heat is less. Inner linings of synthetic material to wick (draw) moisture away from the skin are recommended.

    Wearing several layers of lightweight clothing is preferable to wearing one single, thick layer because warm air is trapped between layers of clothes, enabling greater heat conservation. As body temperature increases, you can remove layers as necessary. For lengthy or long-distance workouts (cross-country skiing or long runs), take a small backpack to carry the clothing that is removed. You also can carry extra warm and dry clothes in case you stop exercising away from shelter. If you remain outdoors following exercise, added clothing and continuous body movement are essential.

    The first layer of clothes should wick moisture away from the skin. Polypropylene,

6

Heat cramps Muscle spasms caused by heat-induced changes in electrolyte balance in muscle cells.

Heat exhaustion Heat-related fatigue.

Heat stroke Heat-related emergency.

Dehydration Loss of body water below normal volume.

Hypothermia A breakdown in the body's ability to generate heat with a drop in temperature below 95°F.

Capilene, and Thermax are recommended materials. Next, a layer of wool, dacron, or polyester fleece insulates well even when wet. Lycra tights or sweatpants help protect the legs. The outer layer should be waterproof, wind-resistant, and breatheable. A synthetic material such as Gortex is best so moisture still can escape from the body. A ski mask or face mask helps protect the face. In extremely cold conditions, exposed skin, such as the nose, cheeks, or around the eyes, can be insulated with petroleum jelly.

Managing Exercise-Related Injuries

To enjoy and maintain physical fitness, preventing injury during a conditioning program is essential. Exercise-related injuries, nonetheless, are common in individuals who participate in exercise programs. Surveys indicate that more than half of all new participants suffer injuries during the first 6 months of the conditioning program.

The four most common causes of injuries are: (a) high-impact activities, (b) rapid conditioning programs — doing too much too quick, (c) improper shoes or training surfaces, and (d) anatomical predisposition (body propensity). High-impact activities and a significant increase in quantity, intensity, and duration of activities are by far the most common causes of injuries. The body requires time to adapt to more intense activities. Most of these injuries can be prevented through a more gradual and correct conditioning (low-impact) program.

Proper shoes for specific activities are essential. Shoes should be replaced when they show a lot of wear and tear. Softer training surfaces, such as grass and dirt, produce less trauma than asphalt and concrete.

Few people have perfect body alignment, so injuries may occur eventually. These types of injuries often are associated with overtraining. In case of injury, proper treatment can avert a lengthy recovery process. A summary of common exercise-related injuries and how to manage them follows.

Acute Sports Injuries

The best treatment always has been prevention itself. If an activity causes unusual discomfort or chronic irritation, you need to treat the cause by decreasing the intensity, switching activities, substituting equipment, or upgrading clothing, such as proper-fitting shoes.

In cases of acute injury, the standard treatment is rest, cold application, compression or splinting (or both), and elevation of the affected body part. This commonly is referred to as RICE: R = rest, I = ice application, C = compression, and E = elevation. Cold should be applied three to five times a day for 15 to 20 minutes at a time during the first 24 to 36 hours, by submerging the injured area in cold water, using an ice bag, or applying ice massage to the affected part. An elastic bandage or wrap can be used for compression. Elevating the body part decreases blood flow to it.

The purpose of these treatment modalities is to minimize swelling in the area, which hastens recovery time. After the first 36 to 48 hours, heat can be used if the injury shows no further swelling or inflammation. If you have doubts regarding the nature or seriousness of the injury (such as suspected fracture), you should seek a medical evaluation.

Obvious deformities (such as in fractures, dislocations, or partial dislocations) call for splinting, cold application with an ice bag, and medical attention. Never try to reset any of these conditions by yourself, as muscles, ligaments, and nerves could be damaged further. Treatment of these injuries always should be in the hands of specialized medical personnel. A quick reference guide for the signs or symptoms and treatment of exercise-related problems is provided in Table 6.2.

Muscle Soreness and Stiffness

Individuals who begin an exercise program or participate after a long layoff from exercise often develop muscle soreness and stiffness. The acute soreness that sets in the first few hours after exercise is thought to be related to a lack of blood (oxygen) flow and general fatigue of the exercised muscles.

Delayed muscle soreness that appears several hours after exercise (usually about 12 hours later) and lasts 2 to 4 days may be related to actual tiny tears in muscle tissue, muscle spasms that increase fluid retention stimulating the pain nerve endings, and overstretching or tearing of connective tissue in and around muscles and joints.

Mild stretching before and adequately stretching after exercise helps to prevent soreness and stiffness. Gradually progressing into an exercise program is important, too. A person should not attempt to do

Table 6.2 Reference Guide for Exercise-Related Problems

Injury	Signs/Symptoms	Treatment*
Bruise (contusion)	Pain, swelling, discoloration	Cold application, compression, rest
Dislocations Fractures	Pain, swelling, deformity	Splinting, cold application, seek medical attention
Heat cramps	Cramps, spasms and muscle twitching in the legs, arms, and abdomen	Stop activity, get out of the heat, stretch, massage the painful area, drink plenty of fluids
Heat exhaustion	Fainting, profuse sweating, cold/clammy skin, weak/rapid pulse, weakness, headache	Stop activity, rest in a cool place, loosen clothing, rub body with cool/wet towel, drink plenty of fluids, stay out of heat for 2–3 days
Heat stroke	Hot/dry skin, no sweating, serious disorientation, rapid/full pulse, vomiting, diarrhea, unconsciousness, high body temperature	**Seek immediate medical attention**, request help and get out of the sun, bathe in cold water/spray with cold water/rub body with cold towels, drink plenty of cold fluids
Joint sprains	Pain, tenderness, swelling, loss of use, discoloration	Cold application, compression, elevation, rest, heat after 36 to 48 hours (if no further swelling)
Muscle cramps	Pain, spasm	Stretch muscle(s), use mild exercises for involved area
Muscle soreness and stiffness	Tenderness, pain	Mild stretching, low-intensity exercise, warm bath
Muscle strains	Pain, tenderness, swelling, loss of use	Cold application, compression, elevation, rest, heat after 36 to 48 hours (if no further swelling)
Shin splints	Pain, tenderness	Cold application prior to and following any physical activity, rest, heat (if no activity is carried out)
Side stitch	Pain on the side of the abdomen below the rib cage	Decrease level of physical activity or stop altogether, gradually increase level of fitness
Tendonitis	Pain, tenderness, loss of use	Rest, cold application, heat after 48 hours

* Cold should be applied three to four times a day for 15 minutes. Heat can be applied three times a day for 15 to 20 minutes.

too much too quickly. To relieve pain, mild stretching, low-intensity exercise to stimulate blood flow, and a warm bath might help.

Exercise Intolerance

When starting an exercise program, participants should stay within the safe limits. The best method to determine whether you are exercising too strenuously — exercise intolerance — is to check your heart rate and make sure it does not exceed the limits of your target zone. Exercising above this target zone may not be safe for unconditioned or high-risk individuals. You do not need to exercise beyond your target zone to gain the desired cardiorespiratory benefits.

Several physical signs will tell you when you are exceeding your functional limitations. Signs of intolerance include rapid or irregular heart rate, difficult breathing, nausea, vomiting, lightheadedness,

6

headache, dizziness, pale skin, flushness, extreme weakness, lack of energy, shakiness, sore muscles, cramps, and tightness in the chest. Learn to listen to your body. If you notice any of these symptoms, seek medical attention before continuing your exercise program.

Recovery heart rate is another indicator of overexertion. To a certain extent, recovery heart rate is related to fitness level. The higher your cardiovascular fitness level, the faster your heart rate will decrease following exercise. As a rule of thumb, heart rate should be below 120 beats per minute 5 minutes into recovery. If your heart rate is above 120, you most likely have overexerted yourself or possibly could have some other cardiac abnormality. If you lower the intensity or duration of exercise, or both, and you still have a fast heart rate 5 minutes into recovery, you should consult your physician.

Side Stitch

Side stitch happens primarily in the early stages of exercise participation. The exact cause is unknown. Some experts suggest that it could relate to a lack of blood flow to the respiratory muscles during strenuous physical exertion. Side stitch occurs primarily in unconditioned beginners and in trained individuals when they exercise at higher intensities than usual. As one's physical condition improves, this condition tends to disappear unless training is intensified. Some people, however, encounter side stitch during downhill running. If side stitch is a problem for you, slow down, and if it persists, stop altogether. Lying down on your back and gently bringing both knees to the chest and holding that position for 30 to 60 seconds also helps.

Some people also get side stitch if they eat or drink juice shortly before exercise. Drinking only water an hour to two prior to exercise sometimes prevents side stitch. Other individuals have problems with commercially available carbohydrate solutions during high-intensity exercise. Unless carbohydrate replacement is crucial to complete an event (marathon, triathlon), drink cool water for fluid replacement, or try a different carbohydrate solution. Fluid and carbohydrate replacement during prolonged exercise or exercise in the heat is discussed elsewhere in this chapter.

Shin Splints

The **shin splint**, one of the most common injuries to the lower limbs, usually results from one or more of the following: (a) lack of proper and gradual conditioning, (b) doing physical activities on hard surfaces (wooden floors, hard tracks, cement, and asphalt), (c) fallen arches in the feet, (d) chronic overuse, (e) muscle fatigue, (f) faulty posture, (g) improper shoes, and (h) participating in weight-bearing activities when excessively overweight.

To manage shin splints:

1. Remove or reduce the cause (exercise on softer surfaces, wear better shoes or arch supports, or completely stop exercise until the shin splints heal).
2. Do stretching exercises before and after physical activity.
3. Use ice massage for 10 to 20 minutes before and after physical exercise.
4. Apply active heat (whirlpool and hot baths) for 15 minutes, two to three times a day.
5. Use supportive taping during physical activity (the proper taping technique can be learned readily from a qualified athletic trainer).

Muscle Cramps

Muscle cramps are caused by the body's depletion of essential electrolytes or a breakdown in the coordination between opposing muscle groups. If you have a muscle cramp, you should attempt first to stretch the muscles involved. For example, in the case of the calf muscle, pull your toes up toward the knees. After stretching the muscles, rub them down gently, and, finally, do some mild exercises requiring the use of those muscles.

In pregnant and lactating women, muscle cramps often are related to a lack of calcium. If women get cramps during these times, calcium supplements usually relieve the problem. Tight clothing also can cause cramps, by decreasing blood flow to active muscle tissue.

Leisure-Time Physical Activity

Although individuals have notable differences, the average person in developed countries has about 3.5 hours of "free" or leisure time daily. Unfortunately, in our current automated society, most of this time is spent in sedentary living. People would be better off doing some physical activities, based on personal interests. Motivational factors include health, aesthetics, weight control, competition and challenge, fun, social interaction, mental arousal, relaxation, and stress management.

Frequently, **leisure-time physical activity** does not include exercise performed during a regular exercise program. It consists of activities such as walking, hiking, gardening, yard work, occupational work and chores, and moderate sports such as tennis, table tennis, badminton, golf, or croquet.

Every small increase in daily physical activity contributes to better health and wellness. Small increases in physical activity have a large impact in decreasing early risk for disease and premature death. Therefore, a new, concerted effort must be made to spend leisure-time in activities that will promote the expenditure of energy, provide a break from daily tasks, and contribute to health-related fitness.

Getting Started and Adhering to a Lifetime Exercise Program

Having learned the basic principles of cardiorespiratory exercise prescription, you can proceed to Lab 6C and fill out your own prescription. This exercise prescription calls for a gradual increase in intensity, duration, and frequency.

If you have not been exercising regularly, you could go ahead and attempt to train five or six times a week for 30 minutes at a time. You may find this discouraging, however, and may drop out before getting too far because you probably will develop some muscle soreness and stiffness and possibly incur minor injuries.

Muscle soreness and stiffness and the risk for injuries can be lessened or eliminated by increasing the intensity, duration, and frequency of exercise progressively as outlined in Lab 6C. Or, if using the computer software available with this book, you can obtain a printout of your personalized cardiorespiratory exercise prescription (see Figure 6.7). You also can create and regularly update a computer file to keep a record of your activity program (see Figure 6.8). This file is based on the EXLOG computer program.

Once you have determined your exercise prescription, the difficult part begins: starting and sticking to a lifetime exercise program. Although you may be motivated after reading the benefits to be gained from physical activity, lifelong dedication and perseverance are necessary to reap and maintain good fitness.

The first few weeks are probably the most difficult, but where there's a will, there's a way. Once you begin to see positive changes, it won't be as hard. Soon you will develop a habit for exercise that will be deeply satisfying and will bring about a sense of self-accomplishment. The following suggestions have been used successfully to help change behavior and adhere to a lifetime exercise program.

Tips to Start and Adhere to an Exercise Program

1. *Select aerobic activities you enjoy.* If you pick an activity you don't enjoy, you will be less likely to keep exercising. Don't be afraid to try out a new activity, even if that means learning new skills.
2. *Combine different activities.* You can train by doing two or three different activities the same week. This **cross-training** may deter the monotony of repeating the same activity every day. Try lifetime sports. Many endurance sports such as racquetball, basketball, soccer, badminton, roller skating, cross-country skiing, and surfing (paddling the board) provide a nice break from regular workouts.
3. *Set aside a regular time for exercise.* If you don't plan ahead, it is a lot easier to skip. Holding your exercise hour "sacred" helps you adhere to the program.
4. *Use the proper clothing and equipment for exercise.* A poor pair of shoes, for example, can make you more prone to injury, discouraging you from the beginning.
5. *Find a friend or group of friends to exercise with.* Social interaction will make exercise more fulfilling. Besides, it's harder to skip if someone else is waiting for you.
6. *Set goals, and share them with others.* Quitting is tougher when someone else knows what you are trying to accomplish. When you reach a

6

Side stitch A sharp pain in the side of the abdomen.

Shin splints Injury to the lower leg characterized by pain and irritation in the shin region or front of the leg.

Leisure-time physical activity Any activity undertaken during an individual's discretionary time that helps to increase resting energy or caloric expenditure.

Cross-training Combining two or more activities to achieve a similar training effect.

PERSONALIZED CARDIORESPIRATORY EXERCISE PRESCRIPTION
Fitness and Wellness Series - Ver 3.96

Jane K. Johnston Age: 18 Date: 04-11-1996
Maximal heart rate: 202 bpm Resting heart rate: 74 bpm
Present cardiorespiratory fitness level: Fair

The following is your personal program for cardiorespiratory fitness development and maintenance. If you have been exercising regularly and you are in the average or good category, you may start at week five. If you are in the excellent category, you can start at week nine.

Week	Time (min.)	Frequency (per week)	Training Intensity (beats per minute)	Pulse (10 sec. count)
1	15	3	About 138	23 beats
2	15	4	About 138	23 beats
3	20	4	About 138	23 beats
4	20	5	About 138	23 beats
5	20	4	138 to 164	23 to 27
6	20	5	138 to 164	23 to 27
7	30	4	138 to 164	23 to 27
8	30	5	138 to 164	23 to 27
9	30	4	164 to 183	27 to 31
10	30	5	164 to 183	27 to 31
11	30--40	5	164 to 183	27 to 31
12	30--40	5-6	164 to 183	27 to 31

You may participate in any combination of activities which are aerobic and continuous in nature, such as walking, jogging, swimming, cross country skiing, rope skipping, cycling, aerobic dancing, racquetball, stair climbing, stationary running or cycling, etc. As long as the heart rate reaches the desired rate, and it stays at that level for the period of time indicated, the cardiorespiratory system will improve.

Following the twelve week program, in order to maintain your fitness level, you should exercise between 164 and 183 bpm for about 30 minutes, a minimum of three times per week on nonconsecutive days.

When you exercise, allow about 5 minutes for a gradual warm-up period and another 5 for gradual cool-down. Also, when you check your exercise heart rate, only count your pulse for 10 seconds (start counting with 0) and then refer to the above 10 sec. pulse count. You may also multiply by 6 to obtain your rate in beats per minute.

Good cardiorespiratory fitness will greatly contribute toward the enhancement and maintenance of good health. It is especially important in the prevention of cardiovascular disease. We encourage you to be persistent in your exercise program and to participate regularly.

Figure 6.7 Sample computerized exercise prescription.

FITNESS & WELLNESS SERIES
by Werner W.K. Hoeger and Sharon A. Hoeger
Morton Publishing Company - Englewood, Colorado
Ver 3.96

MONTHLY EXERCISE LOG

Jim R. Johnson

Month of October 1996

Date	Body Weight	Type of Exercise	Exercise Heart Rate	Duration of Exercise	Distance (miles)	Calories Burned
1	179.5	Walking (4.5 mph)	120	30 min.	2.0	242
		Running (11 min/mile)	156	34 min.	3.0	427
3	179.0	Running (11 min/mile)	156	33 min.	3.0	413
5	179.0	Tennis/Moderate	126	60 min.		483
		Running (11 min/mile)	162	38 min.	3.5	476
7	178.5	Running (8.5 min/mile)	180	12 min.	1.5	193
9	178.0	Water Aerobics/Vigorous	156	45 min.		561
11	177.5	Running (8.5 min/mile)	174	28 min.	3.0	447
12	177.0	Racquetball	144	60 min.		690
		Swimming (25 yds/min)	138	25 min.	0.5	177
14	176.0	Running (8.5 min/mile)	174	29 min.	3.0	459
16	176.0	Aero-belt Step-Aerobics	144	45 min.		832
		Calisthenics	102	15 min.		87
18	175.5	Running (8.5 min/mile)	174	26 min.	3.0	411
19	175.0	Soccer	136	60 min.		620
		Golf	102	90 min.		473
21	175.0	Running (7 min/mile)	172	18 min.	2.5	321
23	174.5	Step-Aerobics	144	60 min.		733
24	175.0	Bowling	102	90 min.		473
25	174.5	Basketball/Moderate	150	60 min.		482
		Dance/Moderate	102	120 min.		628
26	174.0	Running (7 min/mile)	168	30 min.	4.0	532
		Skiing/Downhill	114	60 min.		626
28	174.0	Running (7 min/mile)	168	30 min.	4.0	532
		Strength Training	138	60 min.		522
30	173.5	Stationary Cycling/Vig.	156	60 min.		729

MONTHLY SUMMARY

Average body weight:	176.2 lbs.
Average exercise heart rate:	145 bpm
Total number of days exercised:	18 days
Average exercise time/day:	68 min.
Total number of calories burned:	12,570
Average number of calories per day exercised:	698
Total number of miles jogged:	30.5
Total number of miles swum:	0.5
Total number of miles walked:	2.0

Figure 6.8 Sample monthly exercise record using the EXLOG (Exercise Log) computer program.

6

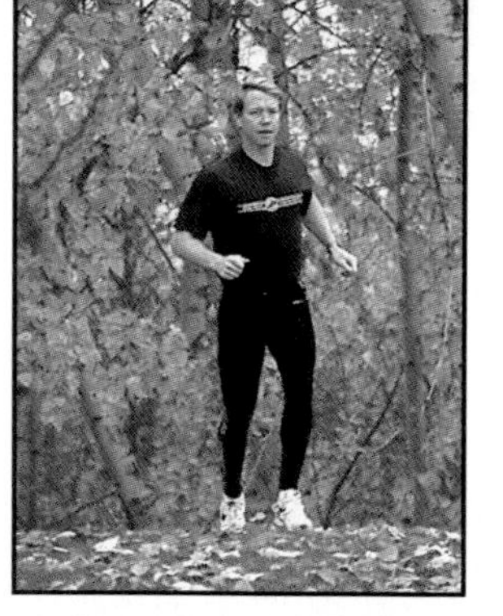

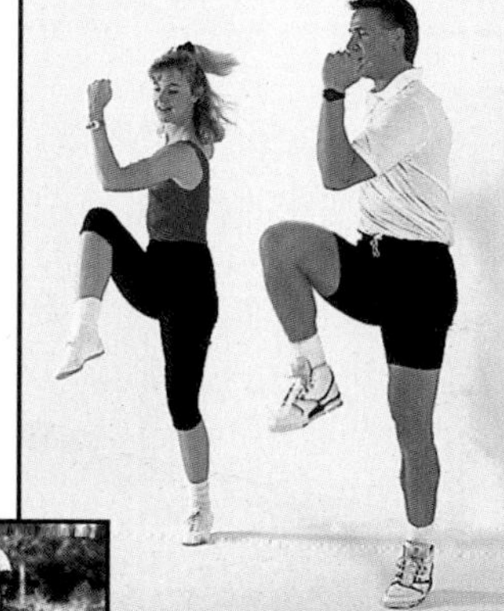

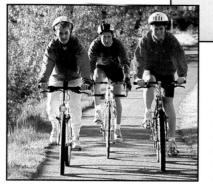

Cross-training enhances fitness, decreases the rate of injuries, and eliminates the monotony of single-activity programs.

targeted goal, reward yourself with a new pair of shoes or a jogging suit.

7. *Don't become a chronic exerciser.* Learn to listen to your body. Overexercising can lead to chronic fatigue and injuries. Exercise should be enjoyable, and in the process you should *stop and smell the roses.*
8. *Exercise in different places and facilities.* This will add variety to your workouts.
9. *Keep a regular record of your activities.* Keeping a record allows you to monitor your progress and compare it against previous months and years (see Figure 6.9).
10. *Conduct periodic assessments.* Improving to a higher fitness category is a reward in itself.
11. *If a health problem arises, see a physician.* When in doubt, it's better to be safe than sorry.

Predicting Oxygen Uptake and Caloric Expenditure

As pointed out in Chapter 5, oxygen uptake can be expressed in liters per minute (l/min) or milliliters per kilogram per minute (ml/kg/min). The latter is used to classify individuals into the various cardiorespiratory fitness categories (see Table 5.8, page 104).

Oxygen uptake expressed in l/min is valuable in determining the caloric expenditure of physical activity. The human body burns about 5 calories for each liter of oxygen consumed. During aerobic exercise the average person trains between 50% and 70% of maximal oxygen uptake.

A person with a maximal oxygen uptake of 3.5 l/min who trains at 60% of maximum uses 2.1 (3.5 × .60) liters of oxygen per minute of physical activity. This indicates that 10.5 calories are burned each minute of exercise (2.1 × 5). If the activity is carried out for 30 minutes, 315 calories (10.5 × 30) have been burned.

Applying the principle of 5 calories burned per liter of oxygen consumed, you can determine with reasonable accuracy your own caloric output for walking and jogging. Table 6.3 contains the oxygen requirement (uptake) for walking speeds between 50 and 100 meters per minute and for jogging speeds in excess of 80 meters per minute.

There is a transition period from walking to jogging for speeds in the range of 80 to 134 meters per minute. Consequently, the person must be truly jogging at these lower speeds to use the estimated oxygen uptakes for jogging in Table 6.3. Because these uptakes are expressed in ml/kg/min, you will need to convert this figure to l/min to predict caloric output. This is done by multiplying the oxygen uptake in ml/kg/min by your body weight in kilograms (kg) and then dividing by 1000.

For example, let's estimate the caloric cost for an individual who weighs 145.5 pounds and runs 3 miles in 21 minutes. Each mile is about 1600 meters, or four laps around a 400-meter (440-yard) track. Three miles then would be 4,800 meters (1600 × 3). Therefore, 3 miles (4800 meters) at a speed of 21 minutes represents a pace of 228.6 meters per minute (4800 ÷ 21).

Table 6.3 indicates an oxygen requirement (uptake) of 49.5 ml/kg/min for a speed of 228.6 meters per minute. A weight of 145.5 pounds equals 66 kilograms (145.5 ÷ 2.2046). The oxygen uptake in l/min now can be calculated by multiplying the value

Table 6.3 Oxygen Requirement Estimates for Selected Walking and Jogging Speeds*

WALKING		JOGGING			
Speed (m/min)	VO_2 (ml/kg/min)	Speed (m/min)	VO_2 (ml/kg/min)	Speed (m/min)	VO_2 (ml/kg/min)
50	8.5	80	19.5	210	45.5
52	8.7	85	20.5	215	46.5
54	8.9	90	21.5	220	47.5
56	9.1	95	22.5	225	48.5
58	9.3	100	23.5	230	49.5
60	9.5	105	24.5	235	50.5
62	9.7	110	25.5	240	51.5
64	9.9	115	26.5	245	52.5
66	10.1	120	27.5	250	53.5
68	10.3	125	28.5	255	54.5
70	10.5	130	29.5	260	55.5
72	10.7	135	30.5	265	56.5
74	10.9	140	31.5	270	57.5
76	11.1	145	32.5	275	58.5
78	11.3	150	33.5	280	59.5
80	11.5	155	34.5		
82	11.7	160	35.5		
84	11.9	165	36.5		
86	12.1	170	37.5		
88	12.3	175	38.5		
90	12.5	180	39.5		
92	12.7	185	40.5		
94	12.9	190	41.5		
96	13.1	195	42.5		
98	13.3	200	43.5		
100	13.5	205	44.5		

m/min = meters per minute
ml/kg/min = milliliters per kilogram per minute

*Table developed using the metabolic calculations contained in *Guidelines for Exercise Testing and Exercise Prescription,* by the American College of Sports Medicine (Philadelphia: Lea & Febiger, 1995).

in ml/kg/min by body weight in kg and dividing by 1000. In our example, it is 49.5 by 66 and divided by 1,000, which equals 3.3 l/min. This oxygen uptake in 21 minutes represents a total of 347 calories ($3.3 \times 5 \times 21$).

In Lab 6D (page 327) you have an opportunity to determine your own oxygen uptake and caloric expenditure for walking and jogging. Using your oxygen uptake information in conjunction with exercise heart rates allows you to estimate your caloric expenditure for almost any activity, as long as the heart rate ranges from 110 to 180 beats per minute. To make an accurate estimate, you have to be skilled in assessing exercise heart rate. Also, as your level of fitness improves, you will need to reassess your exercise heart rate because it will drop (at the same workload) with improved physical condition.

A Lifetime Commitment to Fitness

The benefits of fitness can be maintained only through a regular lifetime program. Exercise is not like putting money in the bank. It does not help much to exercise 4 or 5 hours on Saturday and not do anything else the rest of the week. If anything, exercising only once a week is unsafe for unconditioned adults.

Even the greatest athletes on earth, if they were to stop exercising, would be, after just a few years, at a risk for disease similar to someone who never has done any physical activity. Staying with a physical fitness program long enough brings about positive physiological and psychological changes, and once you are there, you will not want to have it any other way.

6

The time involved in losing the benefits of exercise varies among the different components of physical fitness and also depends on the person's condition before the interruption. In regard to cardiorespiratory endurance, it has been estimated that 4 weeks of aerobic training are completely reversed in two consecutive weeks of physical inactivity. On the other hand, if you have been exercising regularly for months or years, two weeks of inactivity will not hurt you as much as it will someone who has exercised only a few weeks.

As a rule of thumb, after 48 to 72 hours of aerobic inactivity, the cardiorespiratory system starts to lose some of its capacity. Flexibility can be maintained with two or three stretching sessions per week. Strength is easily retained with just one maximal training session per week.

To maintain fitness, you should keep up a regular exercise program, even during vacations. If you have to interrupt your program for reasons beyond your control, you should not attempt to resume training at the same level you left off but, rather, build up gradually again.

Laboratory Experience

LAB 6A
Advantages and Disadvantages of Adding Exercise to Your Lifestyle

Lab Preparation
None required.

LAB 6B
Exercise Readiness Questionnaire

Lab Preparation
None required.

LAB 6C
Cardiorespiratory Exercise Prescription

Lab Preparation
None required.

LAB 6D
Exercise Heart Rate and Caloric Cost of Physical Activity

Lab Preparation
Wear exercise clothing, including jogging shoes. Do not engage in vigorous physical activity before the lab. Bring your own stopwatch or a watch with a second hand. Prior to this lab, read the information in this chapter on predicting caloric expenditure from exercise heart rate.

Notes

1. W. M. Bortz II, "Disuse and Aging," *Journal of the American Medical Association*, 248 (1982), 1203–1208.
2. National Institutes of Health, *Consensus Development Conference Statement: Physical Activity and Cardiovascular Health*, December 18–20, 1995.
3. American College of Sports Medicine, *Guidelines for Exercise Testing and Prescription* (Baltimore: Williams & Wilkins, 1995).
4. American College of Sports Medicine, "The Recommended Quantity and Quality of Exercise for Developing and Maintaining Cardiorespiratory and Muscular Fitness in Healthy Adults," *Medicine and Science in Sports and Exercise*, 22 (1990), 265–274.
5. W. W. K. Hoeger, M. L. Chupurdia, W. J. Nurge, and D. E. Van Zee, "Physiologic Responses to Step Aerobics and Aero-Belt Step Aerobics," *Medicine and Science in Sports and Exercise*, 26 (1994), S43, 246.
6. D. R. Hopkins, W. W. K. Hoeger, D. E. Van Zee, and W. J. Nurge, "Physiologic Responses to Aero-belt Walking," *Medicine and Science in Sports and Exercise*, 26 (1994), 243:245.
7. W. J. Nurge, D. E. Van Zee, and W. W. K. Hoeger. "Physiologic Responses to Aero-belt Walking and Jogging," *Medicine and Science in Sports and Exercise*, 26 (1994), 243:247.
8. R. F. DeBusk, U. Stenestrand, M. Sheehan, and W. L. Haskell. "Training Effects of Long Versus Short Bouts of Exercise in Healthy Subjects," American Journal of Cardiology, 65 (1990), 1010-1013.
9. U. S. Centers for Disease Control and Prevention and American College of Sports Medicine, "Summary Statement: Workshop on Physical Activity and Public Health," *Sports Medicine Bulletin*, 28 (1993), 7.
10. American College of Obstetricians and Gynecologists, *Guidelines for Exercise During Pregnancy*, 1994.
11. University of California at Berkeley, *The Wellness Guide to Lifelong Fitness* (New York: Random House, 1993), p. 198.

Suggested Readings

Arnheim, D. D., and W. Prentice. *Modern Principles of Athletic Training*. St. Louis: Mosby Year Book, 1993.

Borg, G. "Perceived Exertion: A Note on History and Methods." *Medicine and Science in Sports and Exercise*, 5 (1993), 90–93.

Coleman, E. *Eating for Endurance*. Palo Alto, CA: Bull Publishing, 1992.

Cooper, K. H. *The Aerobics Program for Total Well-Being*. New York: Mount Evans and Co., 1982.

Fox, E. L., R. W. Bowers, and M. L. Fossand. *The Physiological Basis for Exercise and Sport*. Philadelphia: Saunders College Publishing, 1993.

Heyward, V. H. *Advanced Fitness Assessment & Exercise Prescription*. Champaign, IL: Human Kinetic, 1991.

Karvonen, M. J., E. Kentala, and O. Mustala. "The Effects of Training on the Heart Rate, a Longitudinal Study." *Annales Medicinae Experimetalis et Biologiae Fenniae*, 35 (1957), 307-315.

McArdle, W. D., F. I. Katch, and V. L. Katch. *Essentials of Exercise Physiology*. Philadelphia: Lea & Febiger, 1994.

Metcalf, J. A. "Exercising During Pregnancy." *Certified News*, 5:2 (1995), 10–11.

Pfeiffer, R. P, and B. C. Mangus. *Concepts of Athletic Training*. Boston: Jones and Bartlett Publishers, 1995.

Teitz, C. C. "Overuse Injuries," in *Scientific Foundations of Sports Medicine* (C. C. Teitz Editor), pp. 299–328). Philadelphia: B. C. Decker, 1989.

Wilmore, J. H., and D. L. Costill. *Physiology of Sport and Exercise*. Champaign, IL: Human Kinetics, 1994.

Month ____________________

Date	Body Weight	Exercise Heart Rate	Type of Exercise	Distance In Miles	Time Hrs/Min	RPE*
1						
2						
3						
4						
5						
6						
7						
8						
9						
10						
11						
12						
13						
14						
15						
16						
17						
18						
19						
20						
21						
22						
23						
24						
25						
26						
27						
28						
29						
30						
31						
			Total			

*Rate of perceived exertion.

Month ____________________

Date	Body Weight	Exercise Heart Rate	Type of Exercise	Distance In Miles	Time Hrs/Min	RPE*
1						
2						
3						
4						
5						
6						
7						
8						
9						
10						
11						
12						
13						
14						
15						
16						
17						
18						
19						
20						
21						
22						
23						
24						
25						
26						
27						
28						
29						
30						
31						
			Total			

*Rate of perceived exertion.

Figure 6.9 Cardiorespiratory exercise record form.

6

Month ____________

Date	Body Weight	Exercise Heart Rate	Type of Exercise	Distance In Miles	Time Hrs/Min	RPE*
1						
2						
3						
4						
5						
6						
7						
8						
9						
10						
11						
12						
13						
14						
15						
16						
17						
18						
19						
20						
21						
22						
23						
24						
25						
26						
27						
28						
29						
30						
31						
			Total			

*Rate of perceived exertion.

Month ____________

Date	Body Weight	Exercise Heart Rate	Type of Exercise	Distance In Miles	Time Hrs/Min	RPE*
1						
2						
3						
4						
5						
6						
7						
8						
9						
10						
11						
12						
13						
14						
15						
16						
17						
18						
19						
20						
21						
22						
23						
24						
25						
26						
27						
28						
29						
30						
31						
			Total			

*Rate of perceived exertion.

Figure 6.9 Continued.

Principles of Strength and Endurance Assessment

7

LABS

Evidence of the benefits of strength training in enhancing health and well-being is well-documented. Nevertheless, some people are still under the impression that strength is necessary only for highly trained athletes and other individuals who hold jobs that require heavy muscular work.

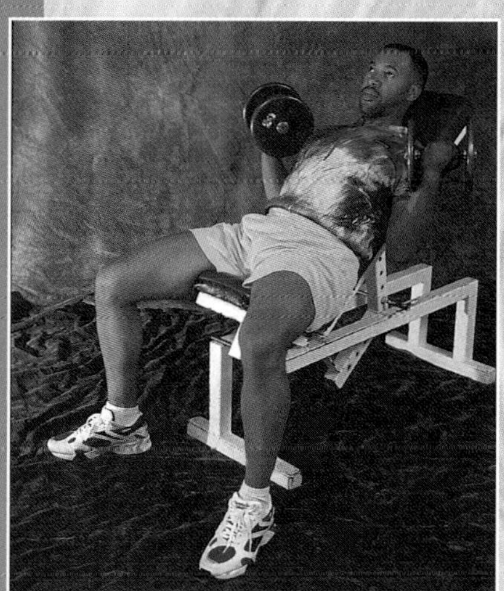

As a basic component of fitness and wellness, ***muscular strength*** *is crucial for optimal performance in daily activities such as sitting, walking, running, lifting and carrying objects, doing housework, and even enjoying recreational activities. Strength also is of great value in improving posture, personal appearance and self-image, in developing sports skills, and in meeting certain emergencies in life in which strength is necessary to cope effectively. From a health standpoint, strength helps to maintain muscle tissue and a higher resting metabolism, lessens the risk for occupational and exercise-related injuries, helps to prevent and eliminate chronic low back pain, and is a key factor in childbearing.*

Muscular strength also seems to be the most important health-related component of physical fitness in the older-adult population. While proper cardiovascular endurance helps maintain a healthy heart, good strength levels will do more toward independent living than any other fitness component. More than anything else, older

Objectives

- Understand the importance of adequate strength levels in maintaining good health and well-being.
- Clarify misconceptions about women who engage in strength-training programs.
- Define muscular strength and muscular endurance.
- Be able to assess muscular strength and endurance through two different strength testing protocols.
- Learn to interpret strength testing results according to health fitness and physical fitness standards.

adults want to enjoy good health and function independently. Many of them, however, are, confined to nursing homes because they lack sufficient strength to move about. They cannot walk very far, and many have to be helped in and out of beds, chairs, and tubs.

A strength-training program can have a tremendous impact in enhancing quality of life. Research has shown leg strength improvements as high as 200% in previously inactive adults over the age of 90.[1] As strength improves, so does the ability to move about, the capacity for independent living, and enjoyment of life during the "golden years."

Relationship Between Strength and Metabolism

Perhaps one of the most significant benefits of maintaining a good strength level is its relationship to human **metabolism.** A primary outcome of a strength-training program is an increase in muscle mass or size known as muscle **hypertrophy.**

Muscle tissue uses energy even at rest. In contrast, fatty tissue uses very little energy and may be considered metabolically inert from the point of view of caloric use. As muscle size increases, so does **resting metabolism.** Even small increases in muscle mass may affect resting metabolism. Each additional pound of muscle tissue increases resting metabolic rate by an estimated 35 calories per day.[2] All other factors being equal, if two individuals both weigh 150 pounds but have different amounts of muscle mass — let's say 5 pounds — the one with more muscle mass will have a higher resting metabolic rate, allowing this person to ingest more calories to maintain the muscle tissue.

Aging and Metabolic Rate

Loss of lean tissue also is thought to be the main reason for the decrease in metabolism as people grow older. Contrary to some beliefs, metabolism does not have to slow down significantly with aging. It is not so much that metabolism slows down. It's that we slow down.

Lean body mass decreases with sedentary living, which in turn slows down the resting metabolic rate. If people continue eating at the same rate, body fat increases. The average decrease in resting metabolism from age 26 to age 60 is about 360 calories per day.[3] Hence, participating in a strength-training program is important in preventing and reducing excess body fat.

Gender Differences

One of the most common misconceptions about physical fitness is related to women and strength training. Because of the increase in muscle mass commonly seen in men, some women think a strength-training program will be counterproductive because they, too, will develop large musculature.

Even though the quality of muscle in men and women is the same, endocrinological differences do not allow women to achieve the same amount of muscle hypertrophy as men. Men also have more muscle fibers, and because of the male sex-specific hormones, each individual fiber has more potential for hypertrophy.

The idea that strength training allows women to develop muscle hypertrophy to the same extent as men do is as false as the notion that playing basketball will turn women into giants. Masculinity and femininity are established by genetic inheritance, not by the amount of physical activity.

Variations in the extent of masculinity and femininity are determined by individual differences in hormonal secretions of androgen, testosterone, estrogen, and progesterone. Women with a bigger-than-average build often are inclined to participate in sports because of their natural physical advantage. As a result, many women have associated participation in sports and strength training with large muscle size.

As the number of women who participate in sports has increased steadily during the last few years, the myth that strength training in women leads to large increases in muscle size has abated somewhat. For example, per pound of body weight, women gymnasts are considered to be among the strongest athletes in the world. These athletes engage regularly in serious strength training programs. Yet, female gymnasts have some of the most well-toned and graceful figures of all women.

In recent years, improved body appearance has become the rule rather than the exception for women who participate in strength-training programs. Some of the most attractive women movie stars also train with weights to further improve their personal image. Many beauty pageant participants engage in some sort of strength-training program as they prepare for the pageant. A survey at a state beauty pageant revealed that 86% of the participants (38 of 44 contestants) exercised with weights![4]

At the same time, you may ask, "If weight training does not masculinize women, why do so many

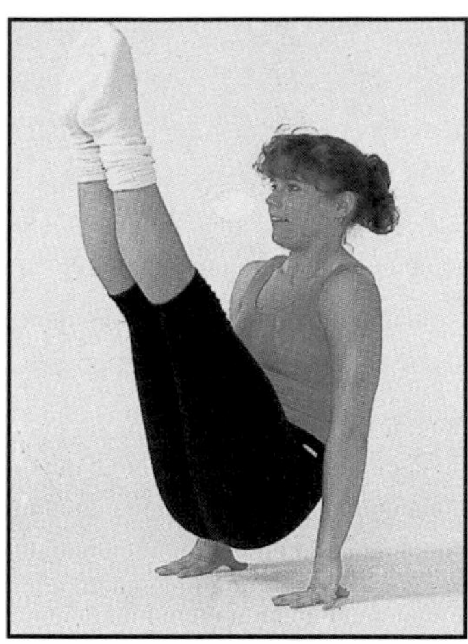

Female gymnast performs a strength skill in the floor exercise event.

women body builders develop such heavy musculature?" In the sport of body building, the athletes follow intense training routines consisting of two or more hours of constant weight lifting with short rest intervals between sets. Many times, body building training routines call for back-to-back exercises using the same muscle groups. The objective of this type of training is to "pump" extra blood into the muscles, which makes the muscles appear much bigger than they really are in a resting condition. Based on the intensity and the length of the training session, the muscles can remain filled with blood, appearing measurably larger for several hours after completing the training session. Therefore, in real life, these women are not as muscular as they seem when they are "pumped up" for a contest.

Improved body appearance has become the rule rather than the exception for women who participate in strength-training programs.

In the sport of body building, a big point of controversy is the use of **anabolic steroids** and human growth hormones, even among women participants. These hormones produce detrimental and undesirable side effects in women (hypertension, fluid retention, decreased breast size, deepening of the voice, facial whiskers, and body hair growth) which some women deem tolerable. Anabolic steroid use in general, except for medical reasons and when monitored carefully by a physician, can lead to serious health consequences.

Use of anabolic steroid by women body builders is widespread. According to several sports medicine physicians and women body builders, about 80% of women body builders have used steroids. Furthermore, according to several women's track-and-field coaches, as many as 95% of women athletes in this sport around the world had used anabolic steroids to remain competitive at the international level.

Women who take steroids will build heavy musculature, and, if the steroids are taken long enough, they will produce masculinizing effects. As a result,

Selected detrimental effects of anabolic steroid use

- Liver tumors
- Hepatitis
- Hypertension
- Reduction of high density lipoprotein (HDL) cholesterol
- Elevation of low density lipoprotein (LDL) cholesterol
- Hyperinsulinism
- Impaired pituitary function
- Impaired thyroid function
- Mood swings
- Aggressive behavior
- Increased irritability
- Acne
- Fluid retention
- Decreased libido
- HIV infection (via injectable steroids)
- Prostate problems (men)
- Testicular atrophy (men)
- Reduced sperm count (men)
- Clitoral enlargement (women)
- Decreased breast size (women)
- Increased body and facial hair (nonreversible in women)
- Deepening of the voice (nonreversible in women)

Muscular strength The ability of a muscle to exert maximum force against resistance (for example, 1 repetition maximum or 1 RM on the bench press exercise).

Metabolism All energy and material transformations that occur within living cells necessary to sustain life.

Hypertrophy An increase in the size of the cell (for example, muscle hypertrophy).

Resting metabolism The amount of energy (expressed in milliliters of oxygen per minute or total calories per day) an individual requires during resting conditions to sustain proper body function.

Anabolic steroids Synthetic versions of the male sex hormone testosterone, which promotes muscle development and hypertrophy.

the International Federation of Body Building instituted a mandatory steroid-testing program for women participating in the Miss Olympia contest. When drugs are not used to promote development, improved body image is the rule rather than the exception among women who participate in body building, strength training, or sports in general.

Body Composition Changes

Another benefit of strength training, accentuated even more when combined with aerobic exercise, is a decrease in adipose or fatty tissue around muscle fibers themselves. The decrease in fatty tissue often is greater than the amount of muscle hypertrophy (see Figure 7.1). Therefore, losing inches but not body weight is common.

Because muscle tissue is more dense than fatty tissue, and despite the fact that inches are lost during a combined strength-training and aerobic program, people, especially women, often become discouraged because they cannot see the results readily on the scale. They can offset this discouragement by determining their body composition regularly to monitor changes in percent body fat rather than simply measure changes in total body weight.

7

Assessment of Muscular Strength and Endurance

Although muscular strength and endurance are interrelated, they do differ.

Muscular endurance (also referred to as localized muscular endurance) depends to a large extent on muscular strength. Weak muscles cannot repeat an action several times or sustain it for a long time. Keeping these principles in mind, strength tests and training programs have been designed to measure and develop absolute muscular strength or muscular endurance, or a combination of the two.

Muscular strength usually is measured by **one repetition maximum (1 RM)**. This assessment yields a good measure of absolute strength, but it does require a considerable amount of time, as the 1 RM is determined through trial and error. For example, strength of the chest muscles frequently is measured through the bench press exercise. If the individual has not trained with weights, he or she may try 100 pounds and lift this resistance quite easily. After adding 50 pounds, the person fails to lift the resistance. The resistance then is decreased by 10 or 20 pounds. Finally, after several trials the 1 RM is established.

A true 1 RM might be difficult to obtain the first time an individual is tested because fatigue becomes a factor. By the time the 1 RM is established, the person already has made several maximal or near-maximal attempts.

Muscular endurance commonly is established by the number of repetitions an individual can perform against a submaximal resistance or by the length of time a given contraction can be sustained. For example: How many push-ups can an individual do? Or how many times can he or she lift 50 pounds? Or how long can a person hold the chin above a bar while holding on to the bar?

In strength testing, several body sites should be tested. Because different body parts have different strength levels, no single strength test provides a good assessment of overall body strength. As a minimum, a strength profile should include the upper body, the lower body, and the abdominal muscles.

If time is a factor and only one test item can be done, the Hand Grip Test, described in Figure 7.2, is used commonly to assess strength. Even this test, though, provides only a weak correlation with overall body strength. Lab 7A provides the opportunity

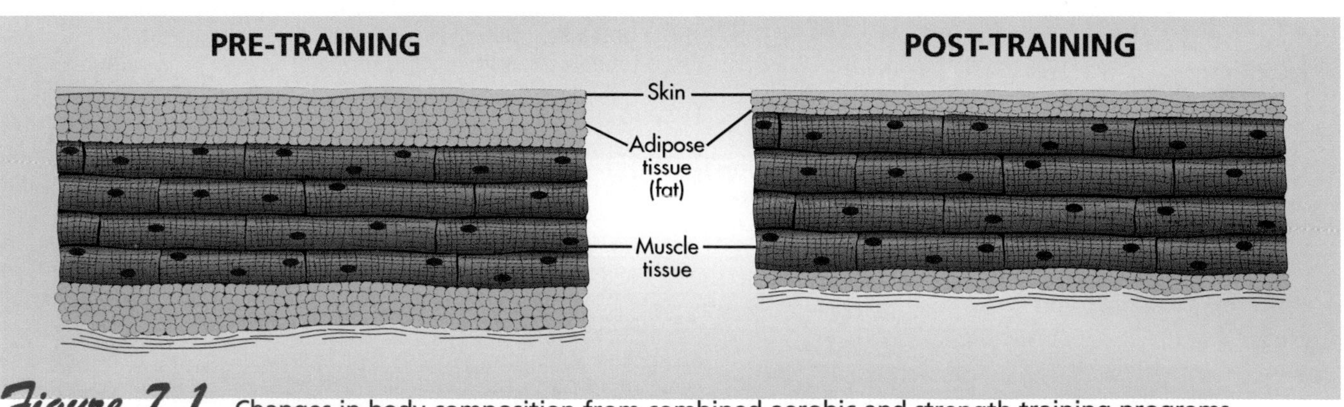

Figure 7.1 Changes in body composition from combined aerobic and strength training programs.

to assess your own level of muscular strength or endurance, through three tests. You may take one or more of these tests according to your time and the facilities available.

Muscular strength and endurance are both highly specific. A high degree of strength or endurance in one body part does not necessarily indicate this is the case in other parts. Accordingly, exercises for the strength tests in Lab 7A were selected to obtain a profile including the upper body, lower body, and mid-body regions.

Before taking the strength test, you should become familiar with the procedures for the respective tests (Figures 7.2, 7.3, and 7.4). For safety reasons, always take a friend or group of friends with you whenever you train with weights or conduct any type of strength assessment. Also, these are different tests, so to make valid comparisons, the same test should be used for pre- and post-assessments. The following are your options.

Hand Grip Test

As indicated, when time is a factor, the Hand Grip Test (Figure 7.2) can be used to provide a rough estimate of strength. (Mode of Training, Chapter 8, page 144, provides further information on isometric training). Unlike the other two tests in this chapter, this is a static contraction (isometric) test. If the proper grip is used, no finger or body movement should occur during the test.

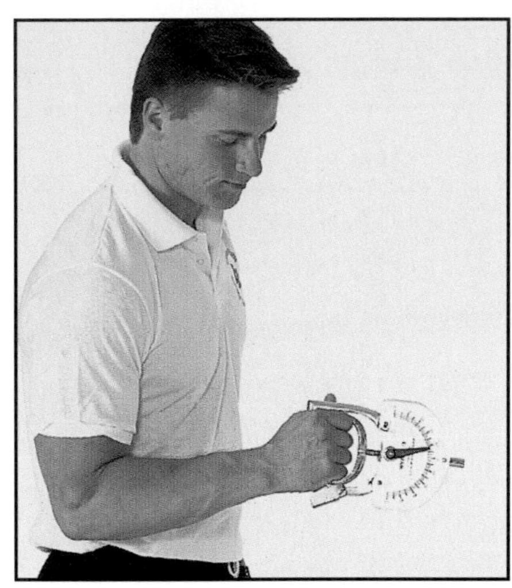

The hand grip tests strength.

Changes in strength may be more difficult to evaluate with this test. Most strength-training programs are dynamic in nature (body segments are moved through a range of motion), and this test provides an isometric assessment. Further, grip-strength exercises seldom are used in strength training, and

Muscular endurance The ability of a muscle to exert submaximal force repeatedly over time.

One repetition maximum (1 RM) The maximum amount of resistance an individual is able to lift in a single effort.

7

HAND GRIP STRENGTH TEST

1. Adjust the width of the dynamometer* so the middle bones of your fingers rest on the distant end of the dynamometer grip.

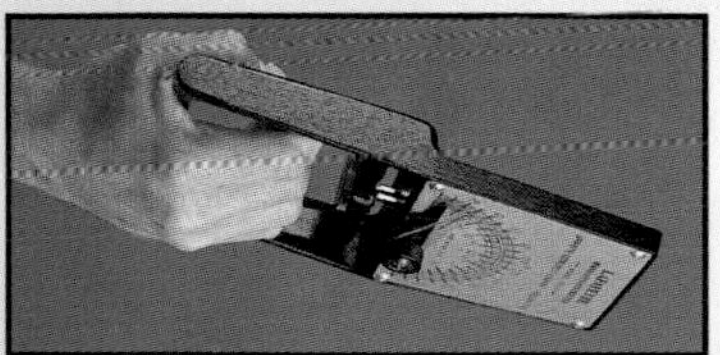

2. Use your dominant hand for this test. Place your elbow at a 90° angle and about 2" away from the body.
3. Now grip as hard as you can for a few seconds. Do not move any other body part as you perform the test (do not flex or extend the elbow, do not move the elbow away or toward the body, and do not lean forward or backward during the test).
4. Record the dynamometer reading in pounds (if reading is in kilograms, multiply by 2.2046).
5. Three trials are allowed for this test. Use the highest reading for your final test score. Look up your percentile rank for this test in Table 7.1.
6. Based on your percentile rank, obtain the hand grip strength fitness category according to the following guidelines:

Percentile Rank	Fitness Classification
≥81	Excellent
61–80	Good
41–60	Average
21–40	Fair
≤20	Poor

* A Lafayette model 78010 dynamometer is recommended for this test (Lafayette Instruments Co., Sagamore and North 9th Street, Lafayette, IN 47903).

Figure 7.2 Procedure for the Hand Grip Strength Test.

Table 7.1 Grip Strength Scoring Table

Percentile Rank	MEN	WOMEN
99	153	101
95	145	94
90	141	91
80	139	86
70	132	80
60	124	78
50	122	74
40	114	71
30	110	66
20	100	64
10	91	60
5	76	58

High physical fitness standard
Health fitness standard

increases in strength are specific to the body parts exercised. This test, however, provides a rough estimate of strength and also can be used to supplement the other strength tests discussed in this chapter.

Muscular Strength and Endurance Test

On this test you will lift a submaximal resistance as many times as possible on five different strength-training exercises, and you also will perform an abdominal crunch test. All of these exercises are illustrated at the end of Chapter 8. The resistance for each lift is determined according to selected percentages of body weight (see Figure 7.3).

A strength/endurance rating is determined according to the maximum number of repetitions you are able to do on each exercise. A 16-station, fixed-resistance, Universal Gym apparatus is necessary to administer all but the abdominal crunch exercise on

7

MUSCULAR STRENGTH AND ENDURANCE TEST

A 16-station, fixed resistance, Universal Gym apparatus is required to perform this test, along with a partner.

1. Familiarize yourself with the six lifts used for this test: lat pull-down, leg extension, bench press, abdominal crunch, leg curl, and arm curl. For the leg curl exercise, the knees should be flexed to 90°. A description and illustration of the abdominal crunch exercise is provided in Figure 7.4. For the lat pull-down exercise, use a sitting position and have your partner hold you down by the waist or shoulders. On the leg extension lift, maintain the trunk in an upright position.
2. Determine your body weight in pounds.
3. Determine the amount of resistance to be used on each lift. To obtain this number, multiply your body weight by the percent given below for each lift.

Lift	Percent of Body Weight	
	Men	Women
Lat Pull-Down	.70	.45
Leg Extension	.65	.50
Bench Press	.75	.45
Abdominal Crunch	NA*	NA*
Leg Curl	.32	.25
Arm Curl	.35	.18

*NA = not applicable — *see* Figure 7.4

4. Perform the maximum continuous number of repetitions possible.
5. Based on the number of repetitions performed, look up the percentile rank for each lift in the far left column of Table 7.2.
6. Obtain an overall strength fitness category by determining an average percentile score for all six lifts. Determine your overall muscular endurance fitness category according to the following ratings:

Average Percentile Score	Fitness Classification
≥81	Excellent
61–80	Good
41–60	Average
21–40	Fair
≤20	Poor

Figure 7.3 Procedure for the Muscular Strength and Endurance Test.

this test (see Chapter 8, Mode of Training, for an explanation of fixed-resistance equipment).

For individuals who do only a few repetitions, the test will primarily measure absolute strength. For those who are able to do a lot of repetitions, the test will be an indicator of muscular endurance. A percentile rank for each exercise is given in Table 7.2 according to the number of repetitions performed. An overall muscular strength/endurance rating can be determined by taking an average of the percentile ranks obtained for each exercise.

If no fixed-resistance Universal Gym equipment is available, you still can perform the test using different equipment. In that case, though, the percentile rankings and strength fitness categories may not be accurate because a certain resistance (for example, 50 pounds) is seldom the same on two different weight machines. The industry has no standard calibration procedure for strength equipment. Consequently, if you lift a certain weight on one machine, you may or may not be able to lift the same amount on a different piece of equipment.

Even though the percentile ranks may not be valid when using different equipment, test results still can be used to evaluate changes in fitness. For example, you may be able to do seven repetitions on the equipment available to you (whereas you might have done 10 on Universal Gym fixed resistance), but if you can perform 14 repetitions after 12 weeks of training, that's a measure of improvement. When performing this test on different equipment, you should disregard the percentile ranks and use the test results to assess *changes* in fitness only.

Muscular Endurance Test

The exercises given in Figure 7.4 were selected to assess the endurance of the upper body, lower body, and mid-body muscle groups. The advantage of this test is that it does not require strength-training equipment. For this test you will need a stopwatch, a metronome, a bench or gymnasium bleacher 16¼" high, a cardboard strip 3½" wide by 30" long, and a partner. As with the Muscular Strength and Endurance Test, a percentile rank is given for each exercise according to the number of repetitions performed (see Table 7.3). An overall endurance rating can be obtained through the average percentile rank for the three exercises.

7

Table 7.2 Muscular Strength and Endurance Scoring Table

	MEN						WOMEN					
Percentile Rank	Lat Pull-Down	Leg Extension	Bench Press	Abdominal Crunch	Leg Curl	Arm Curl	Lat Pull-Down	Leg Extension	Bench Press	Abdominal Crunch	Leg Curl	Arm Curl
99	30	25	26	100	24	25	30	25	27	100	20	25
95	25	20	21	100	20	21	25	20	21	100	17	21
90	19	19	19	100	19	19	21	18	20	69	12	20
80	16	15	16	66	15	15	16	13	16	49	10	16
70	13	14	13	45	13	12	13	11	13	37	9	14
60	11	13	11	38	11	10	11	10	11	34	7	12
50	10	12	10	33	10	9	10	9	10	31	6	10
40	9	10	7	29	8	8	9	8	5	27	5	8
30	7	9	5	26	6	7	7	7	3	24	4	7
20	6	7	3	22	4	5	6	5	1	21	3	6
10	4	5	1	18	3	3	3	3	0	15	1	3
5	3	3	0	16	1	2	2	1	0	0	0	2

High physical fitness standard
Health fitness standard

MUSCULAR ENDURANCE TEST

Three exercises are conducted on this test: bench-jumps, modified dips (men) or modified push-ups (women), and abdominal crunches. All exercises should be conducted with the aid of a partner. The correct procedure for performing each exercise is as follows:

Bench-jump. Using a bench or gymnasium bleacher 16¼" high, attempt to jump up and down the bench as many times as possible in 1-minute. If you cannot jump the full minute, you may step up and down. A repetition is counted each time both feet return to the floor.

Modified dip. Men only: Using a bench or gymnasium bleacher, place the hands on the bench with the fingers pointing forward. Have a partner hold your feet in front of you. Bend the hips at approximately 90° (you also may use three sturdy chairs, put your hands on two chairs placed by the sides of your body, and place your feet on the third chair in front of you). Lower your body by flexing the elbows until you reach a 90° angle at this joint, then return to the starting position. Perform the repetitions to a two-step cadence (down-up) regulated with a metronome set at 56 beats per minute. Perform as many continuous repetitions as possible. Do not count any more repetitions if you fail to follow the metronome cadence.

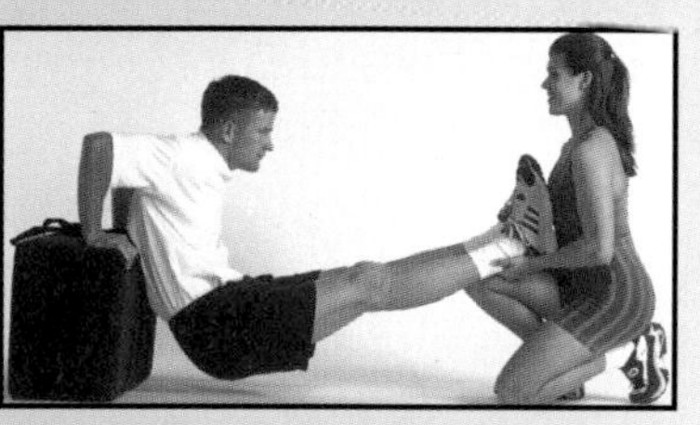

Modified push-up. Women only: Lie down on the floor (face down), bend the knees (feet up in the air), and place the hands on the floor by the shoulders with the fingers pointing forward. The lower body will be supported at the knees (as opposed to the feet) throughout the test. The chest must touch the floor on each repetition. As with the modified-dip exercise (above), perform the repetitions to a two-step cadence (up-down) regulated with a metronome set at 56 beats per minute. Perform as many continuous repetitions as possible. Do not count any more repetitions if you fail to follow the metronome cadence.

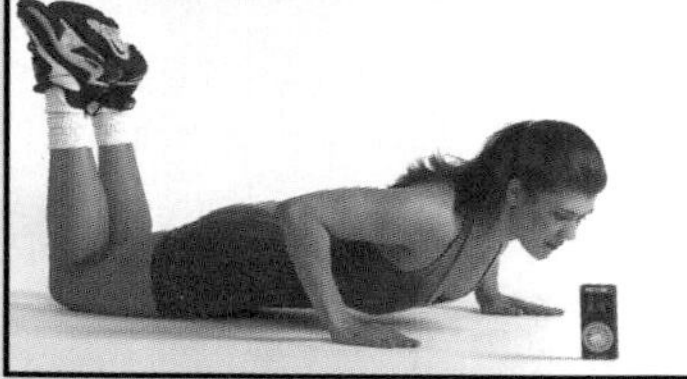

Abdominal crunch. Tape a 3½" × 30" strip of cardboard onto the floor. Lie down on the floor in a supine position (face up) with the knees bent at approximately 100° and the legs slightly apart. The feet should be on the floor, and you must hold them in place yourself throughout the test. Straighten out your arms, and place them on the floor alongside the trunk with the palms down and the fingers fully extended. The fingertips of both hands should barely touch the closest edge of the cardboard. Bring the head off the floor until the chin is 1" to 2" away from your chest. Keep the head in this position during the entire test (do not move the head by flexing or extending the neck). You now are ready to begin the test.

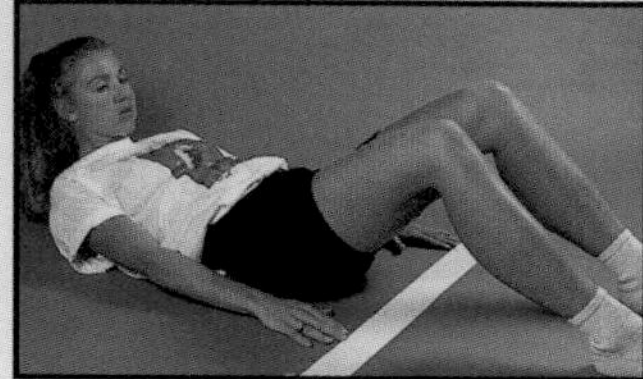

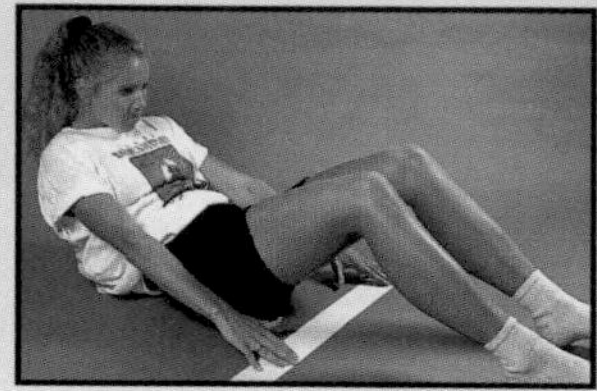

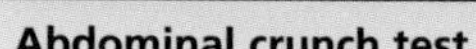

Abdominal crunch test

Perform the repetitions to a two-step cadence (up-down) regulated with a metronome set at 60 beats per minute. As you curl up, slide the fingers over the cardboard until the fingertips reach the far end (3½") of the board, then return to the starting position.

Allow a brief practice period of 5 to 10 seconds to familiarize yourself with the cadence. Initiate the up movement with the first beat and the down movement with the next beat. Accomplish one repetition every two beats of the metronome. Count as many repetitions as you are able to perform following the proper cadence. You may not count a repetition if the fingertips fail to reach the distant end of the cardboard.

Terminate the test if: (a) you fail to maintain the appropriate cadence, (b) the heels come off the floor, (c) the chin is not kept close to the chest, (d) you accomplish 100 repetitions, or (e) you no longer can perform the test. Have your partner check the angle at the knees throughout the test to make sure the 100° angle is maintained as closely as possible.

For this test you also may use a Crunch-Ster Curl-Up Tester, available from Novel Products.* An illustration of the test performed with this equipment is provided below.

According to the results, look up your percentile rank for each exercise in the far left column of Table 7.3.

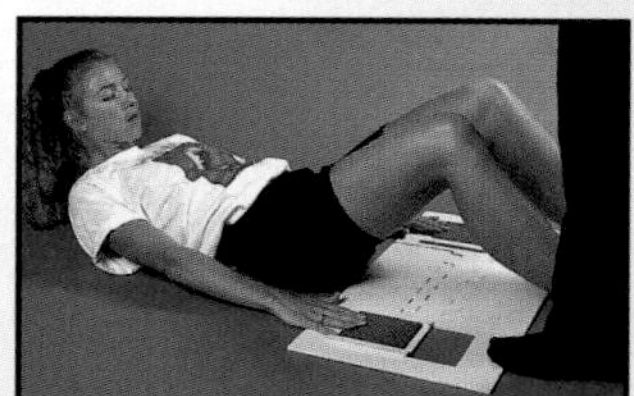

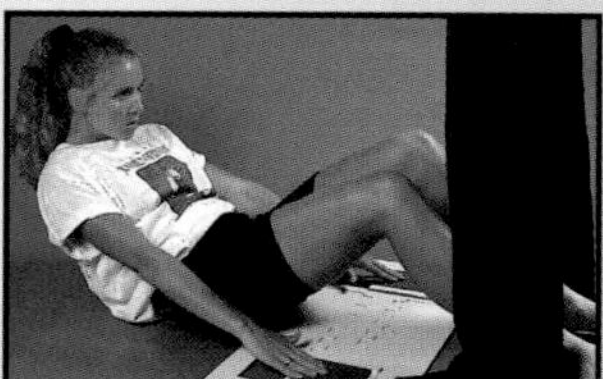

Abdominal crunch test performed with a Crunch-Ster Curl-up Tester

Total the percentile scores obtained for each exercise, and divide by 3 to obtain an average score. Determine your overall muscular endurance fitness category according to the following ratings:

Average Percentile Score	Fitness Classification
>81	Excellent
61-80	Good
41-60	Average
21-40	Fair
<20	Poor

*Novel Products, Inc. Figure Finder Collection. P. O. Box 408, Rockton, IL 61072-0408. 1-800-323-5143, FAX 815-624-4866.

Figure 7.4 Procedure for the Muscular Endurance Test.

Table 7.3 Muscular Endurance Scoring Table

Percentile Rank	MEN Bench Jumps	MEN Modified Dips	MEN Abdominal Crunches	WOMEN Bench Jumps	WOMEN Modified Push-ups	WOMEN Abdominal Crunches
99	66	54	100	58	95	100
95	63	50	100	54	70	100
90	62	38	100	52	50	69
80	58	32	66	48	41	49
70	57	30	45	44	38	37
60	56	27	38	42	33	34
50	54	26	33	39	30	31
40	51	23	29	38	28	27
30	48	20	26	36	25	24
20	47	17	22	32	21	21
10	40	11	18	28	18	15
5	34	7	16	26	15	0

High physical fitness standard
Health fitness standard

7

Laboratory Experience

LAB 7A
Muscular Strength and Endurance Assessment

Lab Preparation
Wear exercise clothing and be prepared to take the Muscular Strength and Endurance Test, the Muscular Endurance Test, or the Hand Grip Test. Avoid strenuous strength training 48 hours before doing this lab.

Notes

1. "Exercise, Nutrition and Aging," by W. J. Evans, in *Journal of Nutrition*, 122 (1992), 796–801.
2. W. W. Campbell, M. C. Crim, V. R. Young, and W. J. Evans, "Increased Energy Requirements and Changes in Body Composition with Resistance Training in Older Adults," *American Journal of Clinical Nutrition*, 60 (1994), 167–175.
3. P. E. Allsen, *Strength Training* (Dubuque, IA: Kendall/Hunt Publishing Company, 1996).
4. J. L. Hesson, *Weight Training for Life* (Englewood, CO: Morton Publishing, 1995).

Suggested Readings

Caltin, D., et al. "Assessing the Threat of Anabolic Steroids." *Physician and Sportsmedicine,* 21 (1993), 37–44.

Fox, E. L., R. W. Bowers, and M. L. Fossand. *The Physiological Basis for Exercise and Sport.* Philadelphia: Saunders College Publishing, 1993.

Getchell, B. *Physical Fitness: A Way of Life.* New York: Macmillan, 1992.

Hesson, J. L. *Weight Training for Life.* Englewood, CO: Morton Publishing, 1995.

Heyward, V. H. *Advanced Fitness Assessment & Exercise Prescription.* Champaign, IL: Human Kinetic Press, 1991.

Hoeger, W. W. K., and S. A. Hoeger. *Lifetime Physical Fitness and Wellness: A Personalized Program.* Englewood, CO: Morton Publishing, 1995.

Hoeger, W. W. K., D. R. Hopkins, S. L. Barette, & D. F. Hale. "Relationship Between Repetitions and Selected Percentages of One Repetition Maximum: A Comparison Between Untrained and Trained Males and Females." *Journal of Applied Sport Science Research,* 4:2 (1990), 47–51.

McArdle, W. D., F. I. Katch, and V. L. Katch. *Exercise Physiology: Energy, Nutrition and Human Performance.* Philadelphia: Lea and Febiger, 1997.

Silvester, L. J. *Weight Training for Strength and Fitness.* Boston: Jones and Bartlett Publishers, 1992.

Wilmore, J. H., and D. L. Costill. *Physiology of Sport and Exercise.* Champaign, IL: Human Kinetics, 1994.

Principles of Strength Training

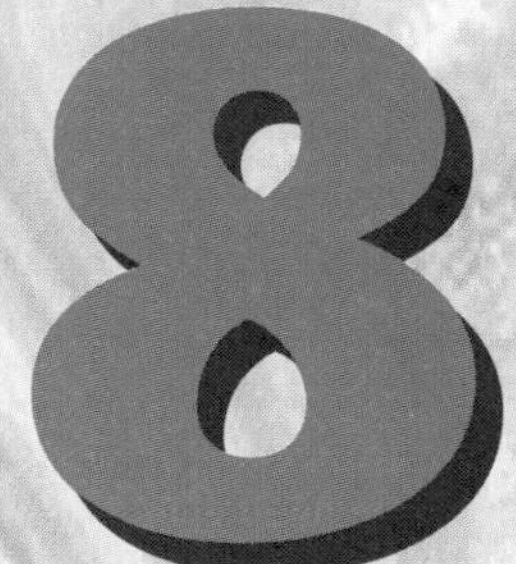

*The capacity of muscle cells to exert force increases and decreases according to the demands placed upon the muscular system. If muscle cells are overloaded beyond their normal use, such as in strength-training programs, the cells increase in size (**hypertrophy**) and strength. If the demands placed on the muscle cells decrease, such as in sedentary living or required rest because of illness or injury, the cells **atrophy** and lose strength. A good level of muscular strength is important to develop and maintain fitness, health, and total well-being.*

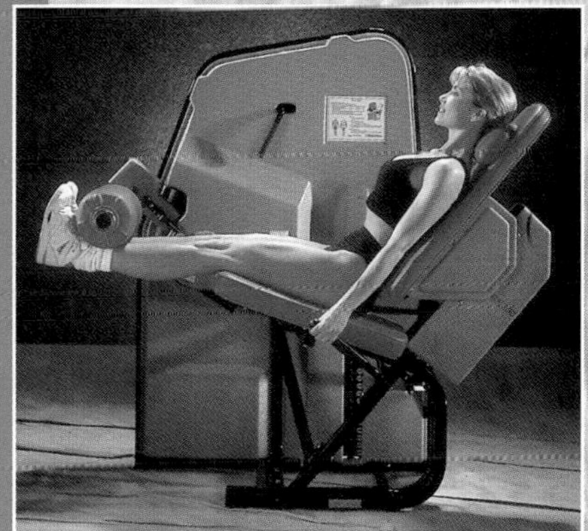

Factors That Affect Strength

LABS

Several physiological factors are related to muscle contraction and subsequent strength gains: neural stimulation, type of muscle fiber, the overload principle, and specificity of training. Basic knowledge of these concepts is important in understanding the principles involved in strength training.

Neural Stimulation

*Within the neuromuscular system, single **motor neurons** branch and attach to multiple muscle fibers. The combination of a motor neuron and the fibers it innervates is called a* motor unit. *The number of fibers a motor neuron can innervate varies from just a few in muscles that require precise control (eye muscles, for example) to as many as 1,000 or more in large muscles that do not perform refined or precise movements.*

Objectives

- Identify the factors that affect strength.
- Name the different types of muscle fibers.
- Understand the overload principle for strength development.
- Recognize the variables that govern development of muscular strength and muscular endurance (mode, resistance, sets, frequency).
- Become acquainted with three distinct strength-training programs.

Stimulation of a motor neuron causes the muscle fibers to contract maximally or not at all. Variations in the number of fibers innervated and the frequency of their stimulation determine the strength of the muscle contraction. As the number of fibers innervated and frequency of stimulation increases, so does the strength of the muscular contraction.

Types of Fiber

Two basic types of muscle fibers determine muscle response: (a) slow-twitch or red fibers, and (b) fast-twitch or white fibers. **Slow-twitch fibers** have a greater capacity for aerobic work. **Fast-twitch fibers** have a greater capacity for anaerobic work and produce more overall force. The latter are important for quick and powerful movements commonly used in strength-training activities.

The proportion of slow- and fast-twitch fibers is determined genetically, and consequently varies from one person to another. Nevertheless, training increases the functional capacity of both types of fiber, and more specifically, strength training increases their ability to exert force.

During muscular contraction slow-twitch fibers always are recruited first. As the force and speed of muscle contraction increase, the relative importance of the fast-twitch fibers also increases. To activate the fast-twitch fibers, an activity must be intense and powerful.

Overload Principle

Strength gains are achieved in two ways:

1. Through increased ability of individual muscle fibers to generate a stronger contraction.
2. By recruiting a greater proportion of the total available fibers for each contraction.

These two factors combine in the **overload principle**. Just like all other organs and systems of the human body, to increase in physical capacity, muscles have to be taxed beyond their accustomed loads. Because of this principle, strength training also is called *progressive resistance training*.

Specificity of Training

The principle of **specificity of training** states that, for a muscle to increase in strength or endurance, the training program must be specific to obtain the desired effects. In like manner, to increase static (isometric) strength versus dynamic strength, an individual must use static against dynamic training to achieve the desired results.

Variables Involved in Strength Training

Because muscular strength and endurance are important in developing and maintaining overall fitness and well-being, the principles necessary to develop a strength-training program have to be followed, as in the prescription of cardiorespiratory exercise. These principles are: mode, resistance, sets, and frequency of training.

Mode of Training

Muscular strength seems to be the most important health-related component of physical fitness in the older-adult population.

Two basic types of training methods are used to improve strength: static (**isometric**) and **dynamic.** Isometric training does not require much equipment. Its popularity of several years ago has waned. Because strength gains with isometric training are specific to the angle of muscle contraction, this type of training is beneficial in a sport such as gymnastics, which requires regular static contractions during routines.

Dynamic training programs can be conducted without weights or with **free weights**, fixed-resistance

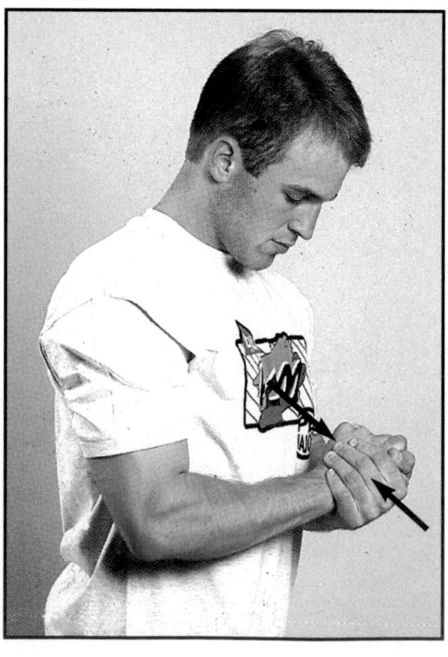

Isometric training.

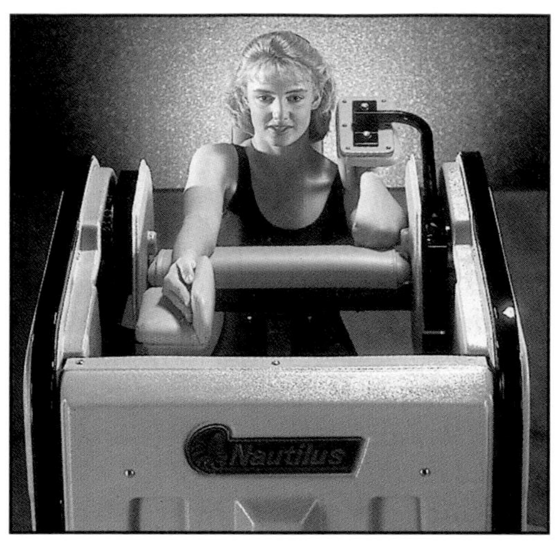

Dynamic strength training.

machines, variable-resistance machines, and isokinetic equipment. When performing dynamic exercises without weights (for example, pull-ups, push-ups), with free weights, or with **fixed-resistance** machines, a constant resistance is moved through a joint's full **range of motion.** The greatest resistance that can be lifted equals the maximum weight that can be moved at the weakest angle of the joint. This is because of changes in muscle length and angle of pull as the joint moves through its range of motion.

As strength training became more popular, new strength-training machines were developed. This technology brought about isokinetic and **variable-resistance** training programs with the intent of overloading the muscle group maximally through the entire range of motion. In **isokinetic** training, in comparison, the speed of the muscle contraction is kept constant. The mode of training an individual selects depends mainly on the type of equipment available and the specific objective the training program is attempting to accomplish.

Dynamic training is the most popular mode for strength training. The primary advantage is that strength is gained through the full range of motion. Most daily activities are dynamic in nature. We are constantly lifting, pushing, and pulling objects, and strength is needed through a complete range of motion. Another advantage is that improvements are measured easily by the amount lifted.

The benefits of isokinetic and variable-resistance training are similar to the other dynamic training methods. Theoretically, strength gains should be better because maximum resistance is applied at all angles. Research, however, has shown that this type of training is not more effective than other modes of dynamic training. A possible advantage, though, is that specific speeds used in various sport skills can be duplicated more closely with isokinetic strength training, which may enhance performance (specificity of training). A disadvantage is that the equipment is not readily available to many people, and, in the case of athletes, it does not resemble the specific actions they encounter in their sports. Most sports involve ballistic contractions that can be duplicated more easily with constant resistance.

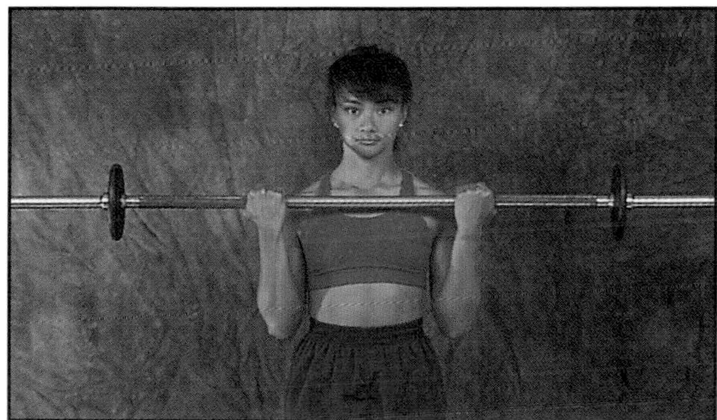
Strength-training with free weights.

Hypertrophy Increase in cell size.

Atrophy Decrease in the size of a cell.

Motor neurons Nerves traveling from the central nervous system to the muscle.

Slow-twitch fibers Muscle fibers with greater aerobic potential and slow speed of contraction.

Fast-twitch fibers Muscle fibers with greater anaerobic potential and fast speed of contraction.

Overload principle Training concept stating that the demands placed on a system (cardiorespiratory, muscular) must be increased systematically and progressively over a period of time to cause physiologic adaptation (development or improvement).

Specificity of training A principle stating that training must be done with the specific muscle the person is attempting to improve.

Isometric Strength training method referring to a muscle contraction that produces little or no movement, such as pushing or pulling against an immovable object.

Dynamic strength training Strength training method referring to a muscle contraction with movement.

Free weights Barbells and dumbbells.

Fixed resistance Type of exercise in which a constant resistance is moved through a joint's full range of motion.

Range of motion Range of movement of a given joint.

Variable resistance Training using special machines equipped with mechanical devices that provide differing amounts of resistance through the range of motion.

Isokinetic Strength-training method in which the speed of the muscle contraction is kept constant because the equipment (machine) provides an accommodating resistance to match the user's force (maximal) through the range of motion.

Perhaps the only exercise that calls for more than 12 repetitions is the abdominal group of exercises. The abdominal muscles are considered primarily antigravity or postural muscles. Hence, a little more endurance may be required. When doing abdominal work, most people perform about 20 repetitions.

If time is a concern in completing a strength-training exercise program, the American College of Sports Medicine[1] recommends as a minimum: (a) one set of 8 to 12 repetitions performed to near fatigue, and (b) 8 to 10 exercises involving the major muscle groups of the body, conducted twice a week. The recommendation is based on research showing that this training generates 70% to 80% of the improvements reported in other programs using three sets of about 10 RM.

Laboratory Experience

LAB 8A
Sample Strength-Training Program

Lab Preparation
Wear exercise clothing and prepare to participate in a sample strength-training exercise session.

8

Note

1. "The Recommended Quantity and Quality of Exercise for Developing and Maintaining Cardiorespiratory and Muscular Fitness in Healthy Adults," *Medicine and Science in Sports and Exercise*, 22 (1990), 265–274.

Suggested Readings

Allsen, P. E. *Strength Training.* Dubuque, IA: Kendall/Hunt Publishing Company, 1996.

Fox, E. L., R. W. Bowers, and M. L. Fossand. *The Physiological Basis for Exercise and Sport.* Philadelphia: Saunders College Publishing, 1993.

Getchell, B. *Physical Fitness: A Way of Life.* New York: Macmillan, 1992.

Hesson, J. L. *Weight Training for Life.* Englewood, CO: Morton Publishing, 1995.

Heyward, V. H. *Advanced Fitness Assessment & Exercise Prescription.* Champaign, IL: Human Kinetic Press, 1991.

Hoeger, W. W. K., and S. A. Hoeger. *Lifetime Physical Fitness and Wellness: A Personalized Program.* Englewood, CO: Morton Publishing, 1995.

McArdle, W. D., F. I. Katch, and V. L. Katch. *Exercise Physiology: Energy, Nutrition and Human Performance.* Philadelphia: Lea and Febiger, 1997.

Munnings, F. "Strength Training: Not Only for the Young." *Physician and Sportsmedicine,* 21 (1993) 133–140.

Silvester, L. J. *Weight Training for Strength and Fitness.* Boston,: Jones and Bartlett Publishers, 1992.

Wilmore, J. H., and D. L. Costill. *Physiology of Sport and Exercise.* Champaign, IL: Human Kinetic Press, 1994.

Name________________________________

Date										
Exercise	St/Reps/Res*	St/Reps/Res*	St/Reps/Res*	St/Reps/Res*	St/Reps/Res*	St/Reps/Res*	St/Reps/Res*	St/Reps/Res*	St/Reps/Res*	St/Reps/Res*

*St/Reps/Res = Sets, Repetitions, Resistance (e.g., 1/6/125 = 1 set of 6 repetitions with 125 pounds)

Figure 8.3 Strength-training record form.

Name____________________

Date										
Exercise	St/Reps/Res*	St/Reps/Res*	St/Reps/Res*	St/Reps/Res*	St/Reps/Res*	St/Reps/Res*	St/Reps/Res*	St/Reps/Res*	St/Reps/Res*	St/Reps/Res*

*St/Reps/Res = Sets, Repetitions, and Resistance (e.g., 1/6/125 = 1 set of 6 repetitions with 125 pounds)

Figure 8.3 Strength-training record form.

Strength-Training Exercise without Weights

1

Step-Up

Action Step up and down using a box or chair approximately 12 to 15 inches high (a). Conduct one set using the same leg each time you go up, and then conduct a second set using the other leg. You also could alternate legs on each step-up cycle. You may increase the resistance by holding an object in your arms (b). Hold the object close to the body to avoid increased strain in the lower back.

Muscles Developed Gluteal muscles, quadriceps, gastrocnemius, and soleus

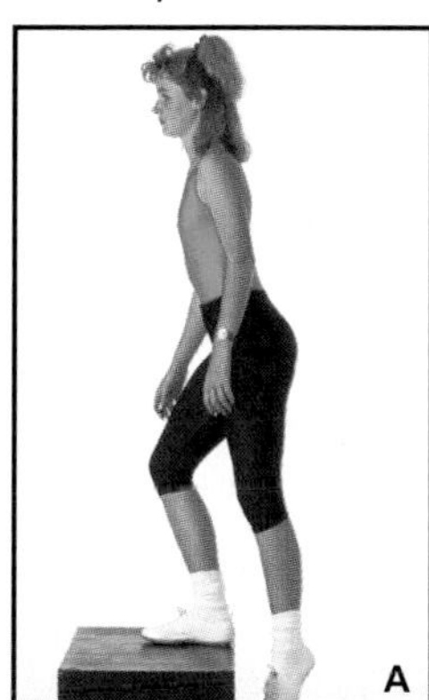

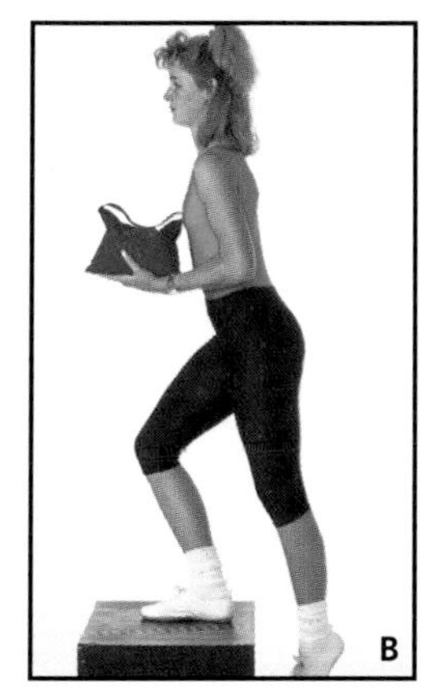

2

High-Jumper

Action Start with the knees bent at approximately 150° (a) and jump as high as you can, raising both arms simultaneously (b).

Muscles Developed Gluteal muscles, quadriceps, gastrocnemius, and soleus

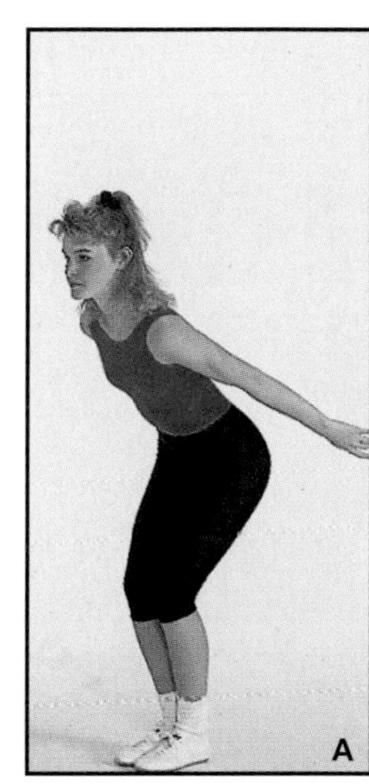

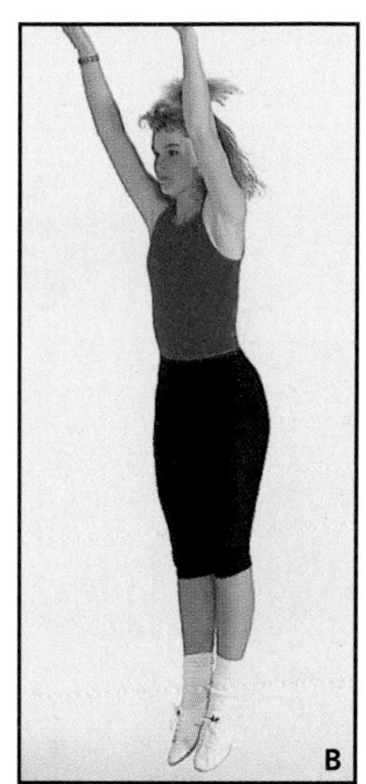

3

Push-Up

Action Maintaining your body as straight as possible (a), flex the elbows, lowering the body until you almost touch the floor (b), then raise yourself back up to the starting position. If you are unable to perform the push-up as indicated, decrease the resistance by supporting the lower body with the knees rather than the feet (c) or using an incline plane and supporting your hands at a higher point than the floor (d). If you wish to increase the resistance, have someone else add resistance to your shoulders as you are coming back up (e).

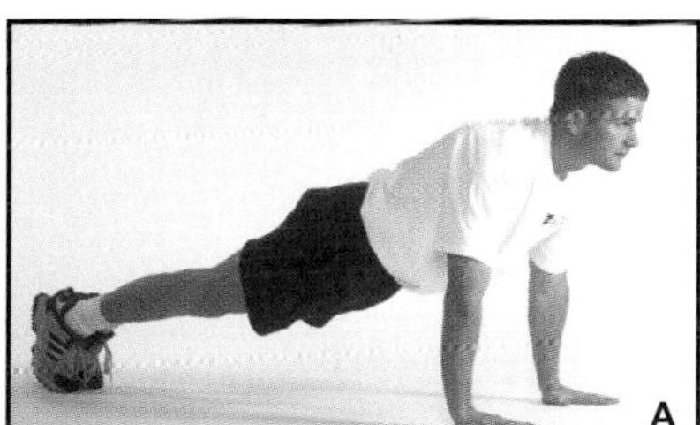

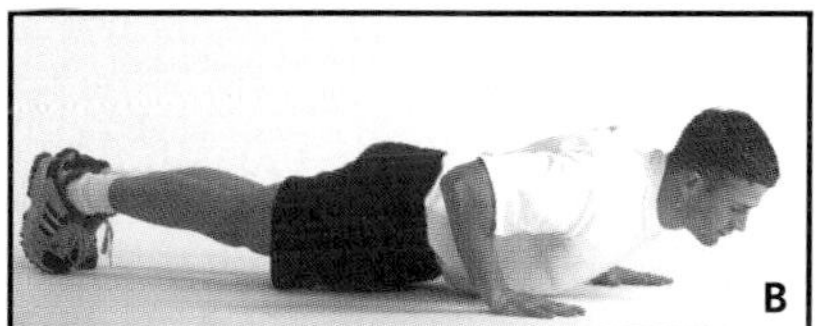

Muscles Developed Triceps, deltoid, pectoralis major, erector spinae, and abdominals

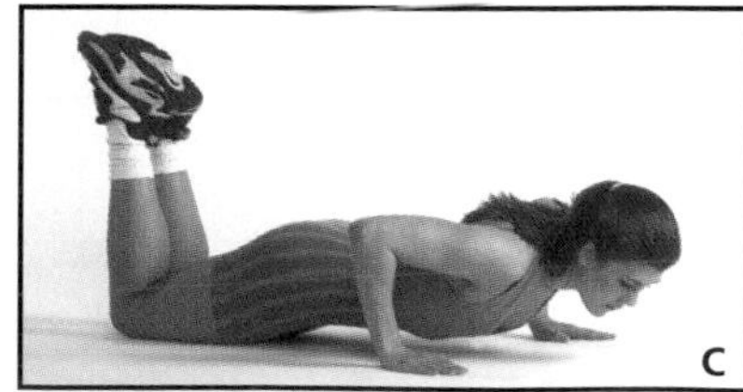

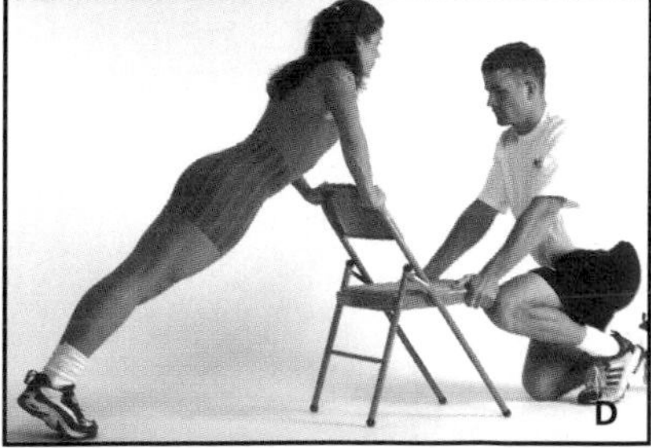

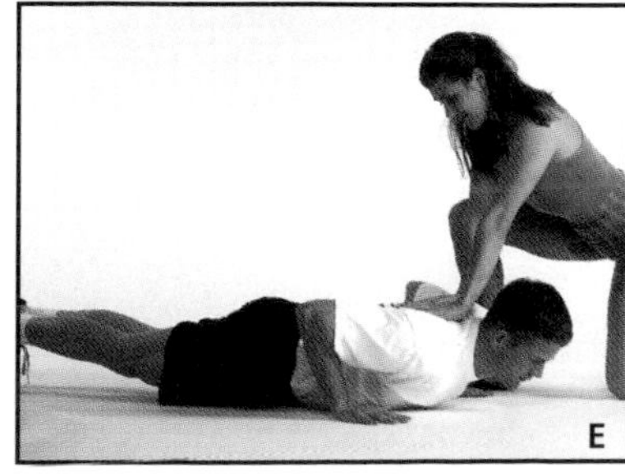

4

Abdominal Crunch and Abdominal Curl-Up

Action Start with your head and shoulders off the floor, arms crossed on your chest, and knees slightly bent (a). The greater the flexion of the knee, the more difficult the curl-up. Now curl up to about 30° (**abdominal crunch** — illustration b) or curl up all the way (**abdominal curl-up** — illustration c), then return to the starting position without letting the head or shoulders touch the floor or allowing the hips to come off the floor. If you allow the hips to raise off the floor and the head and shoulders to touch the floor, you most likely will "swing up" on the next crunch or curl-up, which minimizes the work of the abdominal muscles. If you cannot curl up with the arms on the chest, place the hands by the side of the hips or even help yourself up by holding on to your thighs (illustrations d and e). Do not perform the sit-up exercise with your legs completely extended, as this will strain the lower back. For additional resistance during the abdominal crunch, have a partner add slight resistance to your shoulders as you "crunch up."

Muscles Developed Abdominal muscles and hip flexors

NOTE: The abdominal curl-up exercise should be used only by individuals of at least average fitness without a history of lower back problems. New participants and those with a history of lower back problems should use the abdominal crunch exercise in its place.

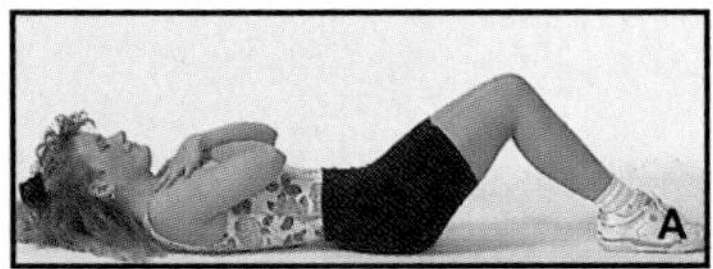
A

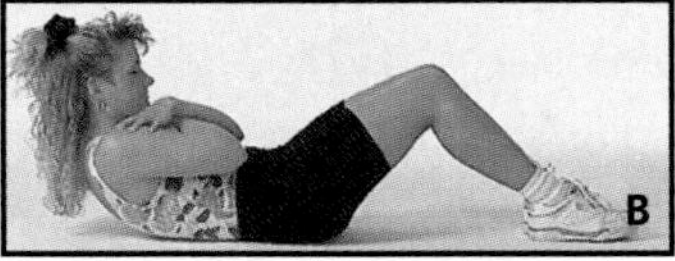
B

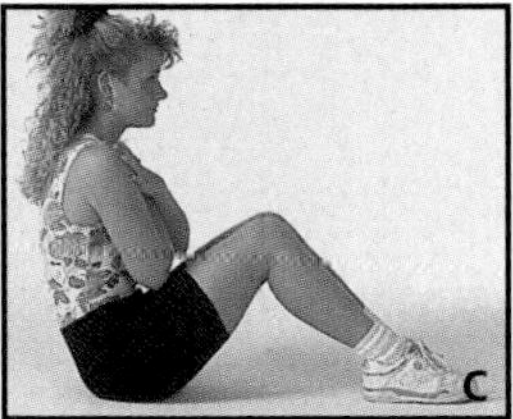
C

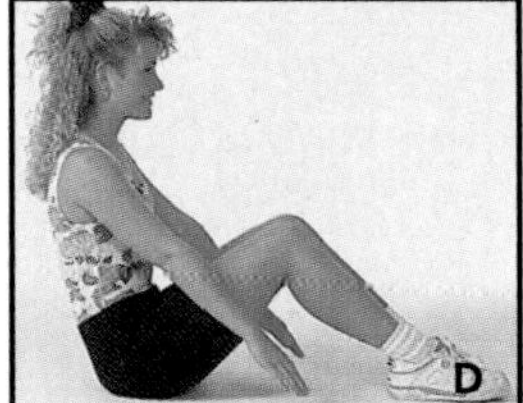
D

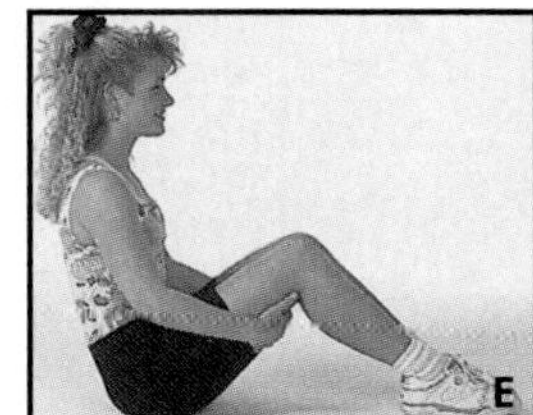
E

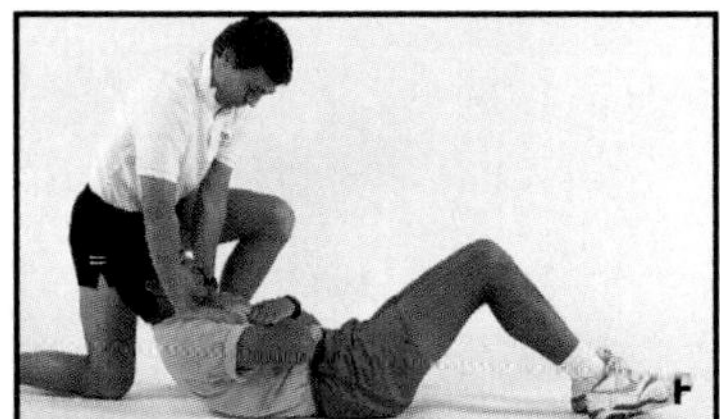
F

8

5

Leg Curl

Action Lie on the floor face down. Cross the right ankle over the left heel (a). Apply resistance with your right foot while you bring the left foot up to 90° at the knee joint (b). Apply enough resistance so the left foot can only be brought up slowly. Repeat the exercise, crossing the left ankle over the right heel.

Muscles Developed Hamstrings (and quadriceps)

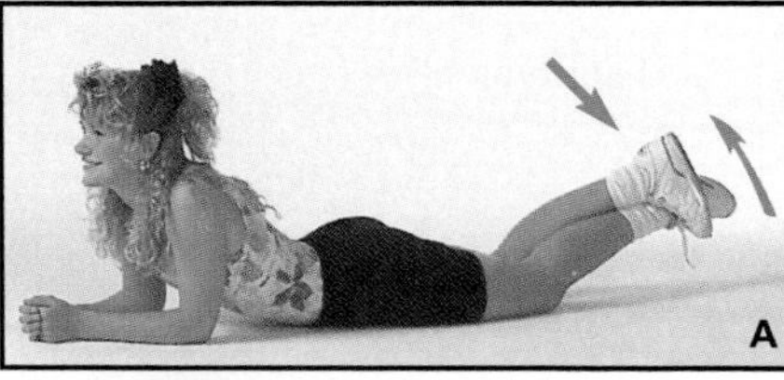
A

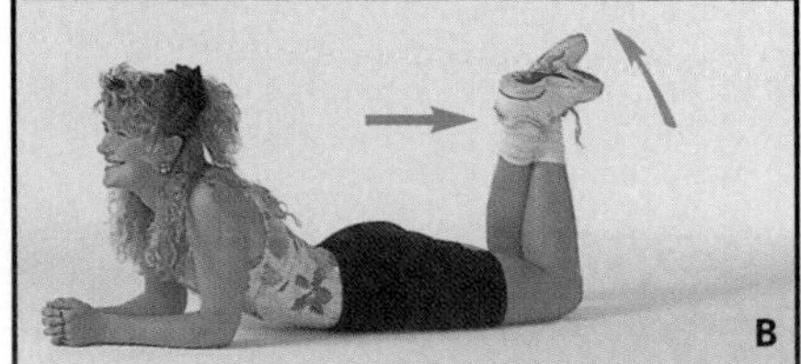
B

6

Modified Dip

Action Place your hands and feet on opposite chairs with knees slightly bent (make sure that the chairs are well stabilized). Dip down at least to a 90° angle at the elbow joint, then return to the initial position. To increase the resistance, have someone else hold you down by the shoulders on the way up (see illustration c). You may also perform this exercise using a gymnasium bleacher or box and with the help of a partner, as illustrated in photo d.

Muscles Developed Triceps, deltoid, and pectoralis major

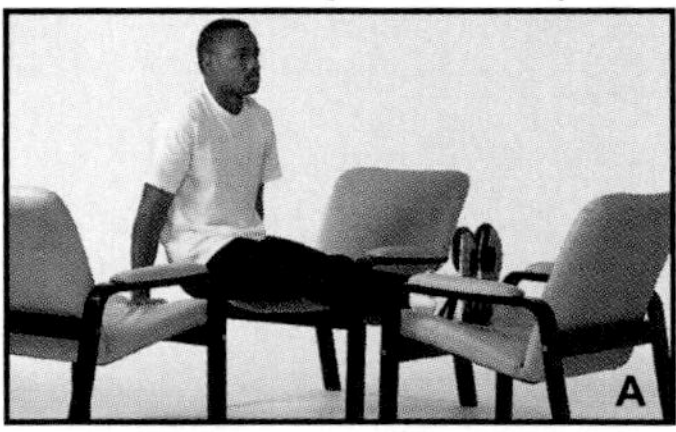
A

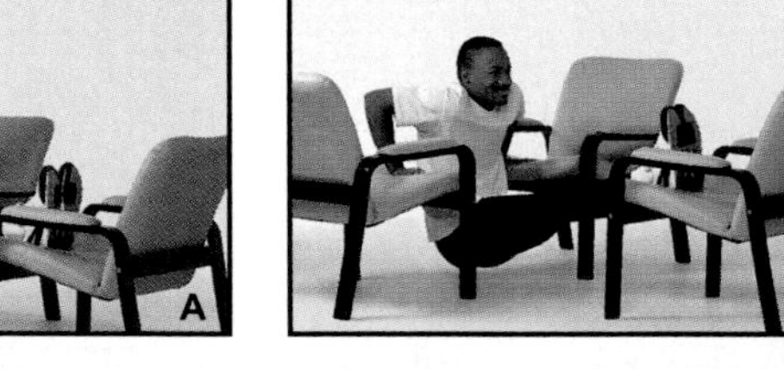
B

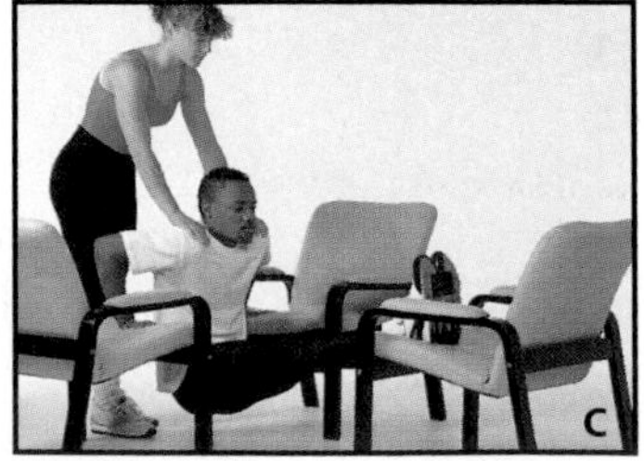
C

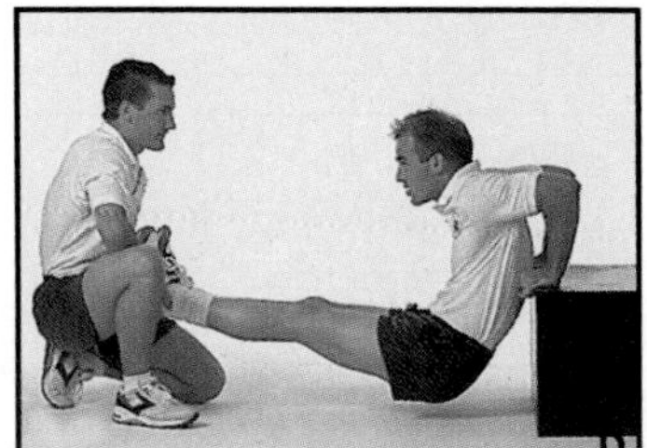
D

7

Pull-Up

Action Suspend yourself from a bar with a pronated (thumbs in) grip (a). Pull your body up until your chin is above the bar (b), then lower the body slowly to the starting position. If you are unable to perform the pull-up as described, either have a partner hold your feet to push off and facilitate the movement upward (illustrations c and d) or use a lower bar and support your feet on the floor (e).

Muscles Developed Biceps, brachioradialis, brachialis, trapezius, and latissimus dorsi

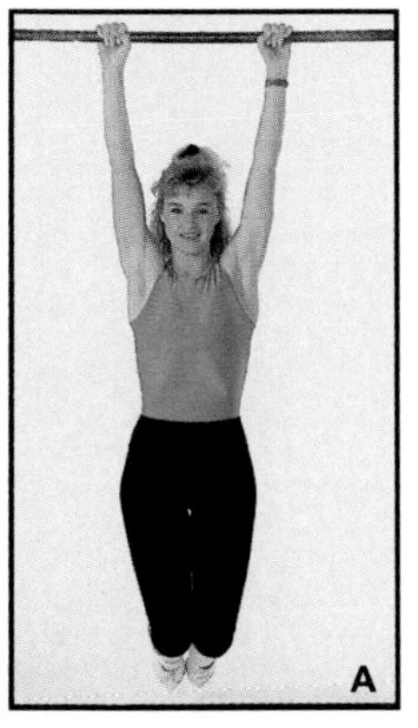
A

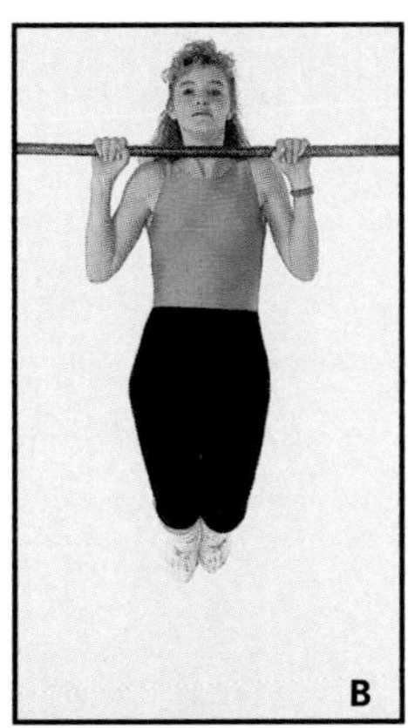
B

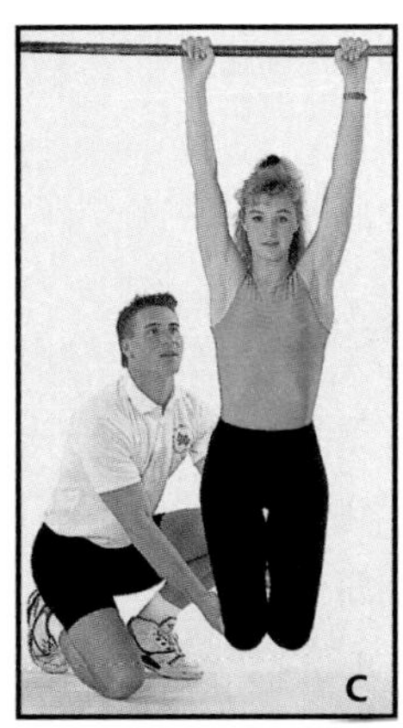
C

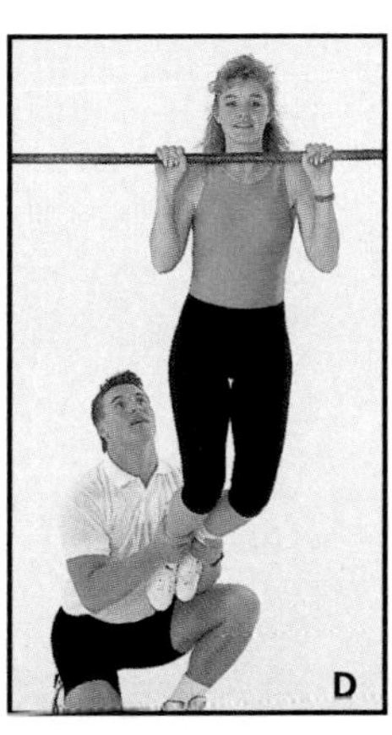
D

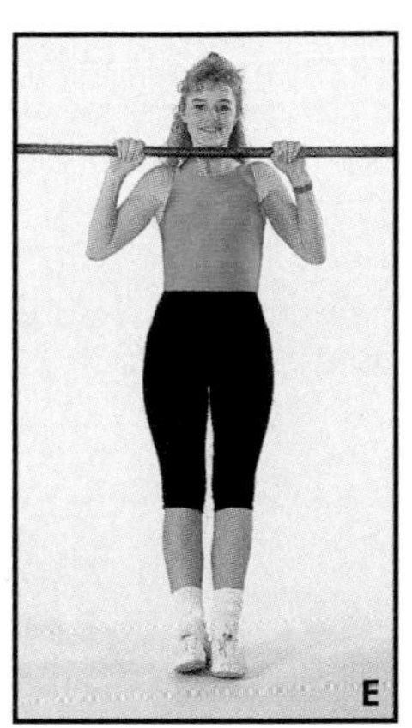
E

8

Arm Curl

Action Using a palms-up grip, start with the arm completely extended, and with the aid of a sandbag or bucket filled (as needed) with sand or rocks (a), curl up as far as possible, then return to the initial position (b). Repeat the exercise with the other arm.

Muscles Developed Biceps, brachioradialis, and brachialis

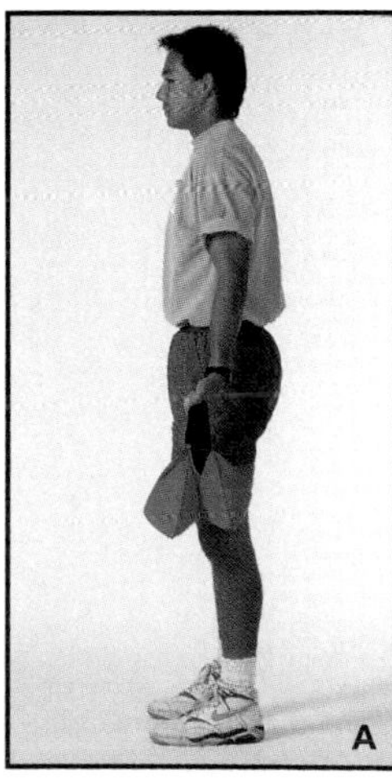
A

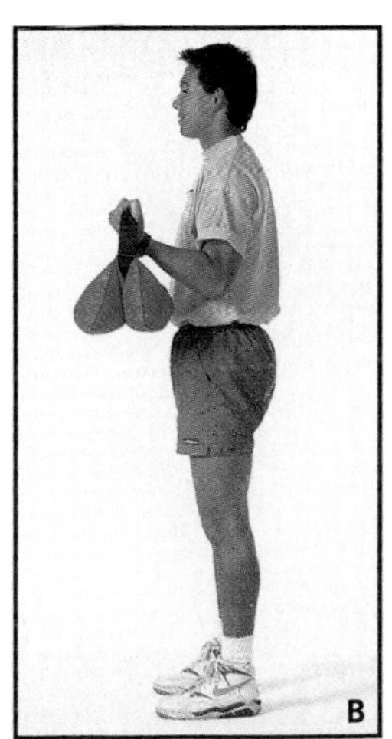
B

9

Heel Raise

Action From a standing position with feet flat on the floor (a), raise and lower your body weight by moving at the ankle joint only (b). For added resistance, have someone else hold your shoulders down as you perform the exercise.

Muscles Developed Gastrocnemius and soleus

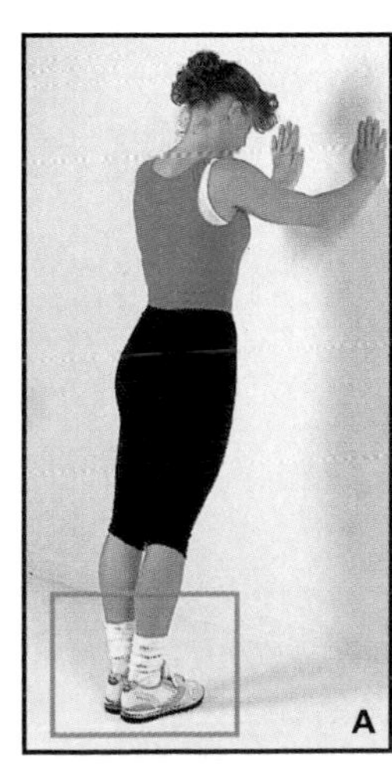
A

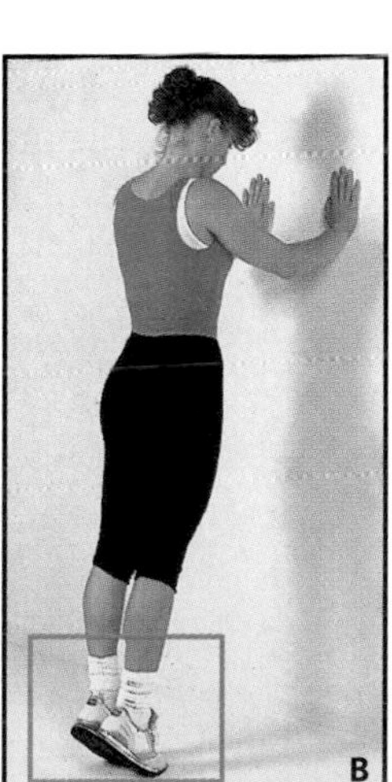
B

10

Leg Abduction and Adduction

Action Both participants sit on the floor. The person on the left places the feet on the inside of the other person's feet. Simultaneously, the person on the left presses the legs laterally (to the outside — abduction), while the person on the right presses the legs medially (adduction). Hold the contraction for 5 to 10 seconds. Repeat the exercise at all three angles, and then reverse the pressing sequence. The person on the left places the feet on the outside and presses inward, while the person on the right presses outward.

Muscles Developed Hip abductors (rectus femoris, sartori, gluteus medius and minimus), and adductors (pectineus, gracilis, adductor magnus, adductor longus, and adductor brevis)

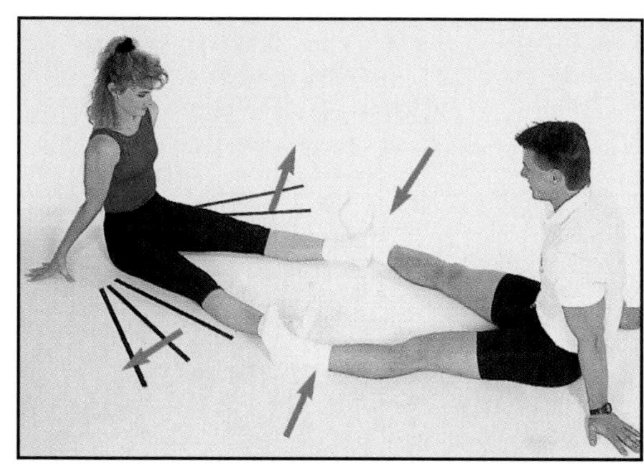

11

Reverse Crunch

Action Lie on your back with arms crossed on your chest and knees and hips flexed at 90° (a). Now attempt to raise the pelvis off the floor by lifting vertically from the knees and lower legs (b). This is a challenging exercise that may be difficult for beginners to perform.

Muscles Developed Abdominals

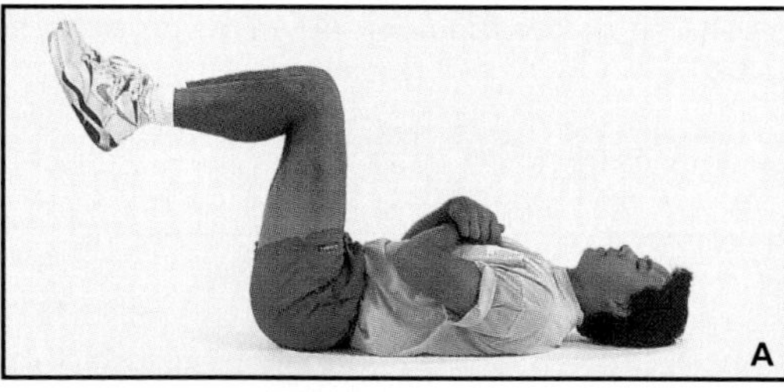
A

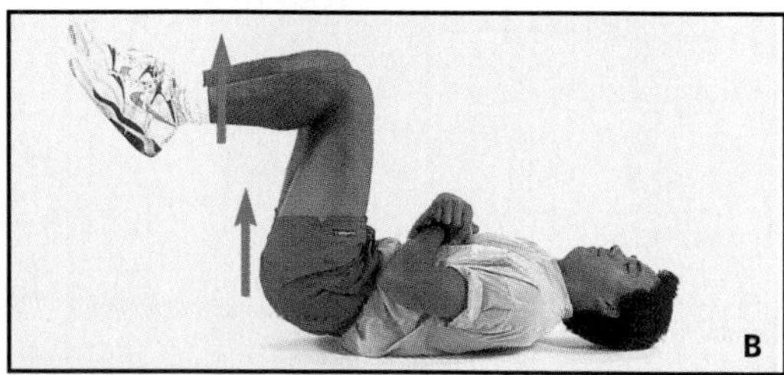
B

12

Pelvic Tilt

Action Lie flat on the floor with the knees bent at about a 90° angle (a). Tilt the pelvis by tightening the abdominal muscles, flattening your back against the floor, and raising the lower gluteal area ever so slightly off the floor (b). Hold the final position for several seconds. The exercise can also be performed against a wall (c).

Areas Stretched Low-back muscles and ligaments

Areas Strengthened Abdominal and gluteal muscles

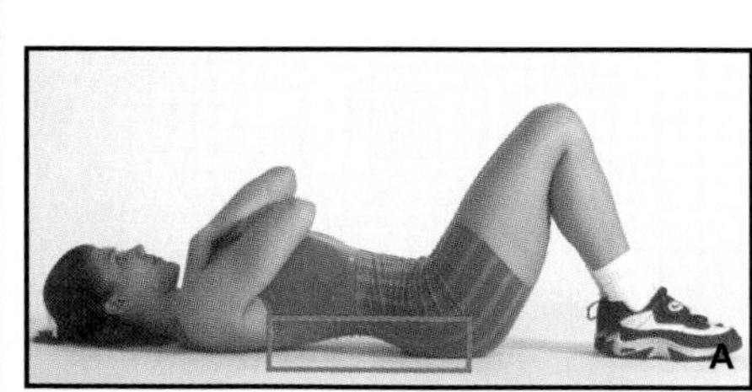
A

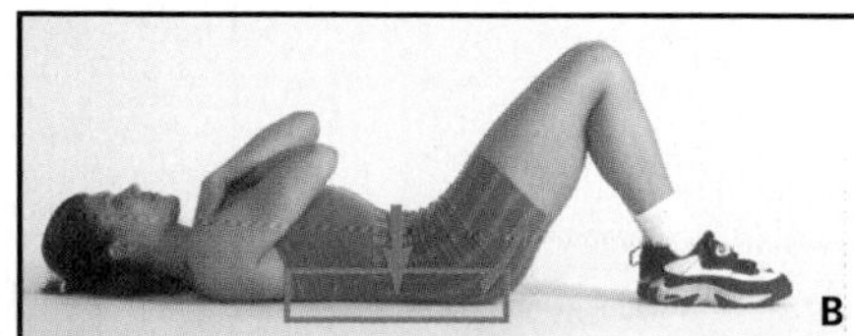
B

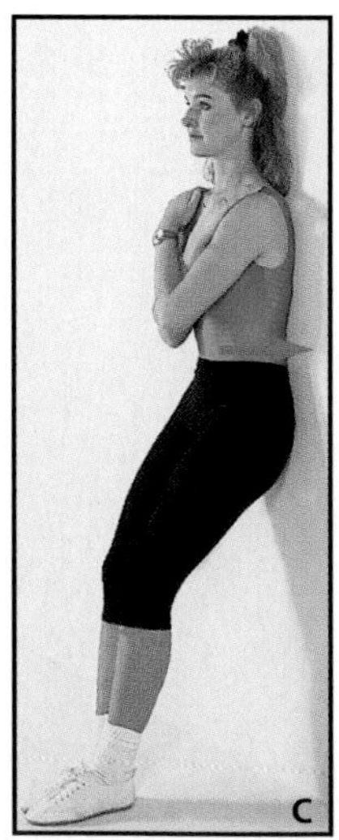
C

8

Strength-Training Exercises with Weights

13

Bench Press

Action Lie down on the bench with the head by the weight stack, the bench press bar above the chest, and the knees bent so the feet rest on the far end of the bench (a). Grasp the bar handles and press upward until the arms are completely extended (b), then return to the original position. Do not arch the back during this exercise.

Muscles Developed Pectoralis major, triceps, and deltoid

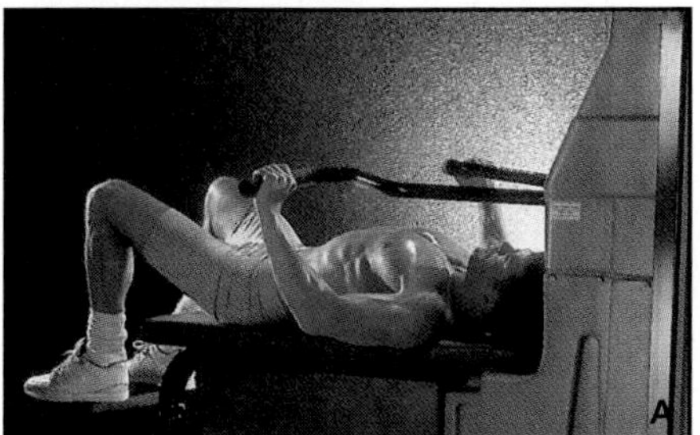
A

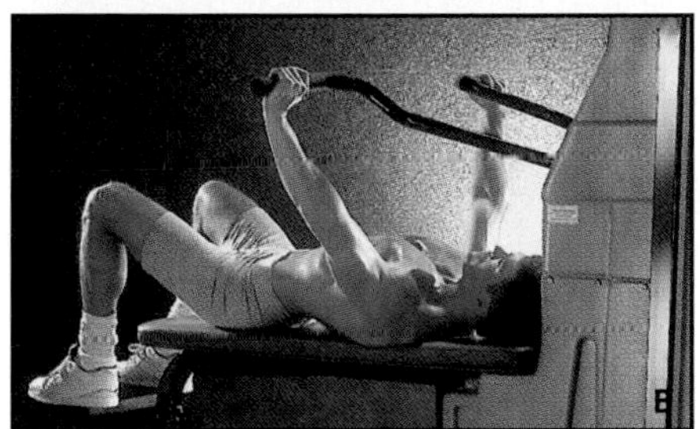
B

14

Leg Press

Action From a sitting position with the knees flexed at about 90° and both feet on the footrest (a), extend the legs fully (b), then return slowly to the starting position.

Muscles Developed Quadriceps and gluteal muscles

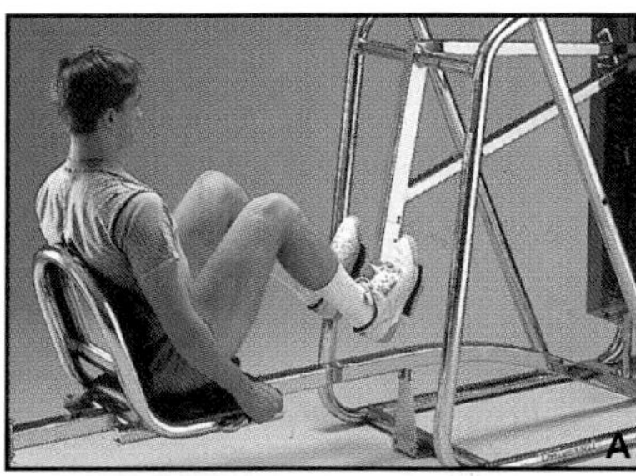
A

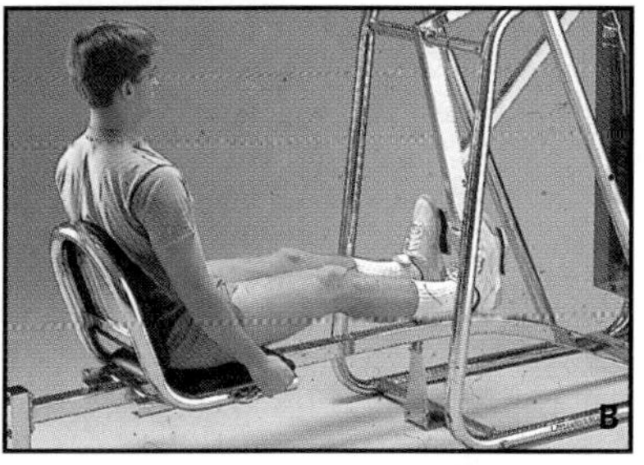
B

8

15

Abdominal Crunch

Action Sit in an upright position. Grasp the handles over your shoulders and crunch forward. Return slowly to the original position.

Muscles Developed Abdominals

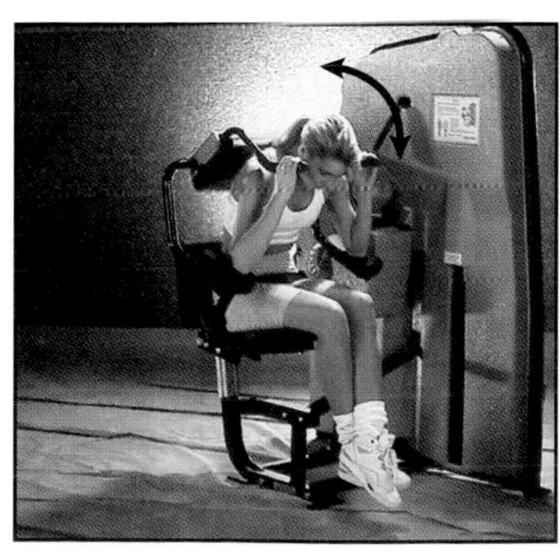

16

Rowing Torso

Action Sit in the machine with your arms in front of you, elbows bent and resting against the padded bars (a). Press back as far as possible, drawing the shoulder blades together (b). Return to the original position.

Muscles Developed Posterior deltoid, rhomboids, and trapezius

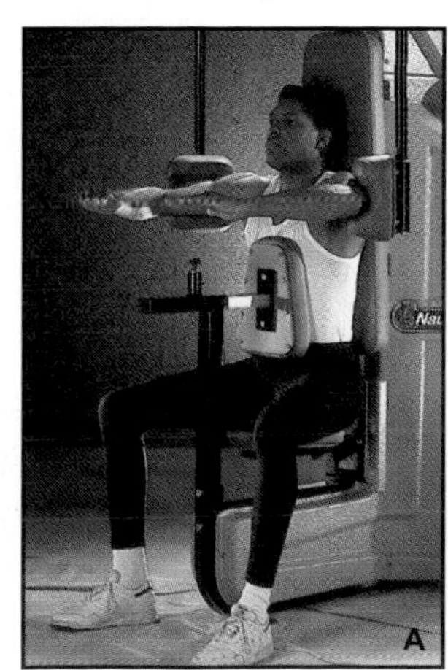
A

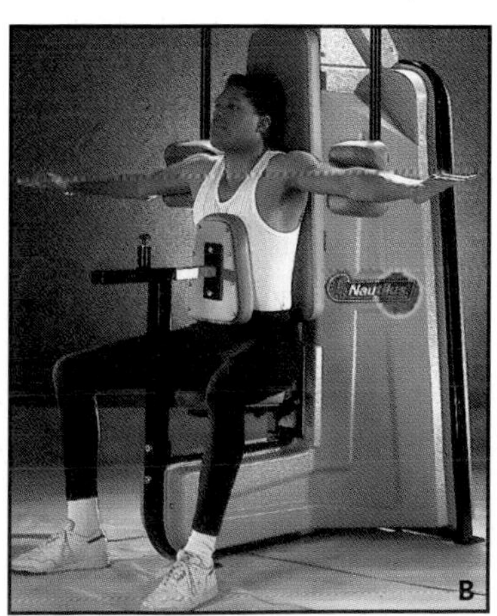

B

17

Arm Curl

Action Using a supinated or palms-up grip, start with the arms almost completely extended (a). Curl up as far as possible (b), then return to the starting position.

Muscles Developed Biceps, brachioradialis, and brachialis

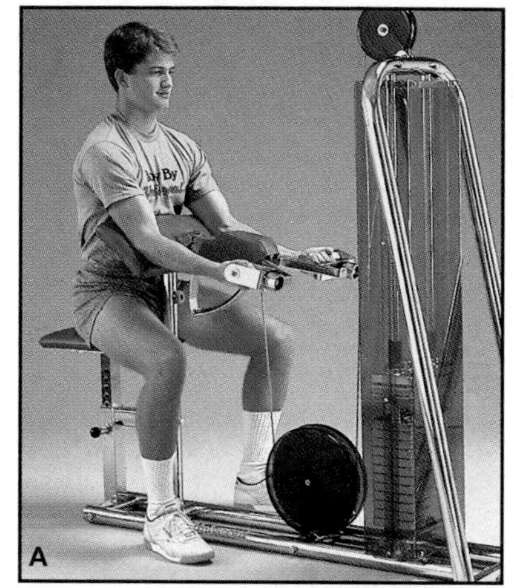
A

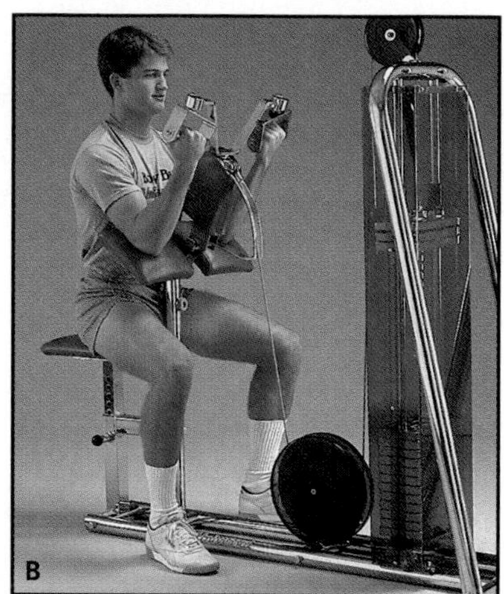
B

18

Leg Curl

Action Lie with the face down on the bench, legs straight, and place the back of the feet under the padded bar (a). Curl up to at least 90° (b), and return to the original position.

Muscles Developed Hamstrings

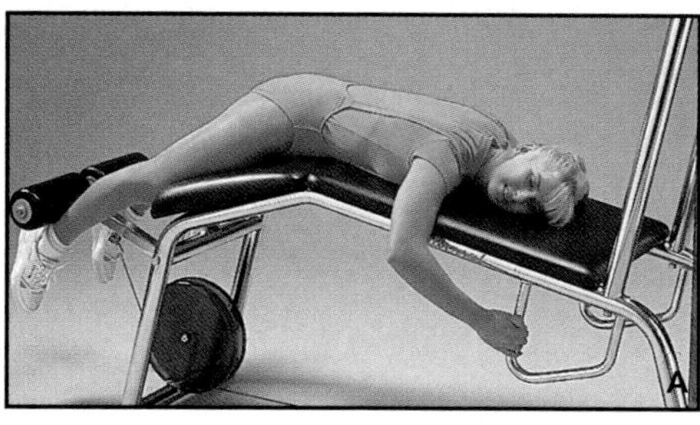
A

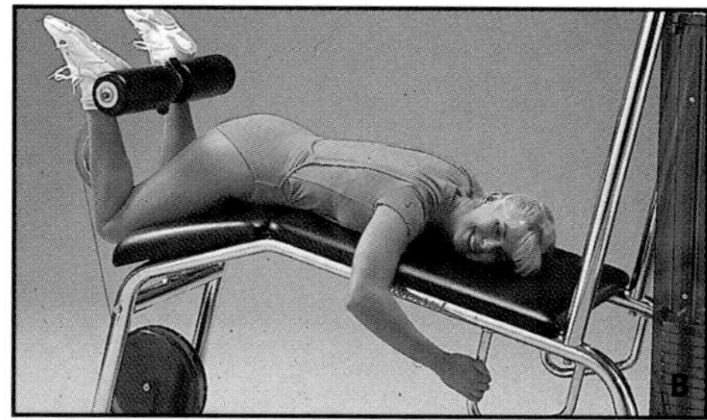
B

19

Seated Back

Action Sit in the machine with your trunk flexed and the upper back against the shoulder pad. Place the feet under the padded bar and hold on with your hands to the bars on the sides (a). Start the exercise by pressing backward, simultaneously extending the trunk and hip joints (b). Slowly return to the original position.

Muscles Developed Erector spinae and gluteus maximus

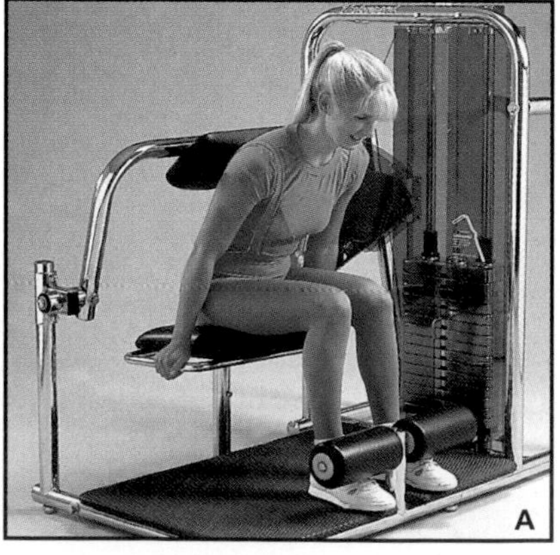
A

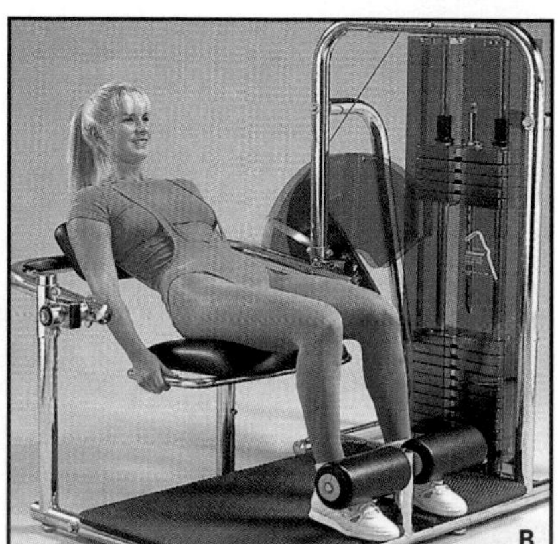
B

20

Heel Raise

Action Start with your feet either flat on the floor or the front of the feet on an elevated block (a), then raise and lower yourself by moving at the ankle joint only (b). If additional resistance is needed, you can use a squat strength-training machine.

Muscles Developed Quadriceps

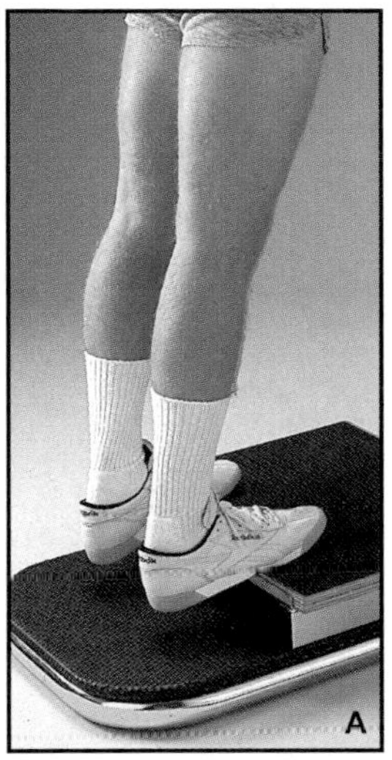
A

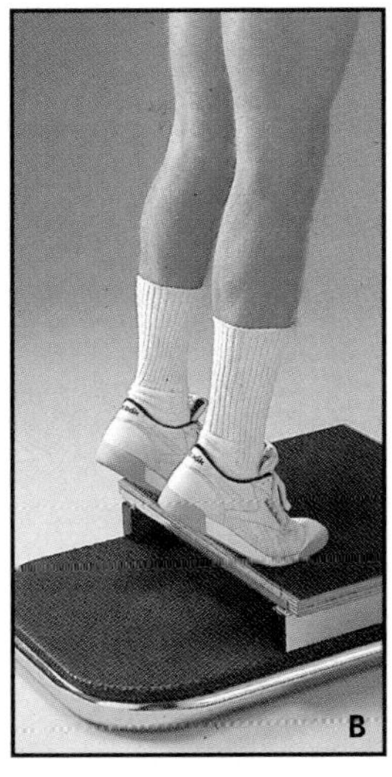
B

21

Lat Pull-Down

Action Starting from a sitting position, hold the exercise bar with a wide grip (a). Pull the bar down until it touches the base of the neck (b), then return to the starting position. (If heavy resistance is used, stabilization of the body may be required either by using equipment as shown or by having someone else hold you down by the waist or shoulders.

Muscles Developed Latissimus dorsi, pectoralis major, and biceps

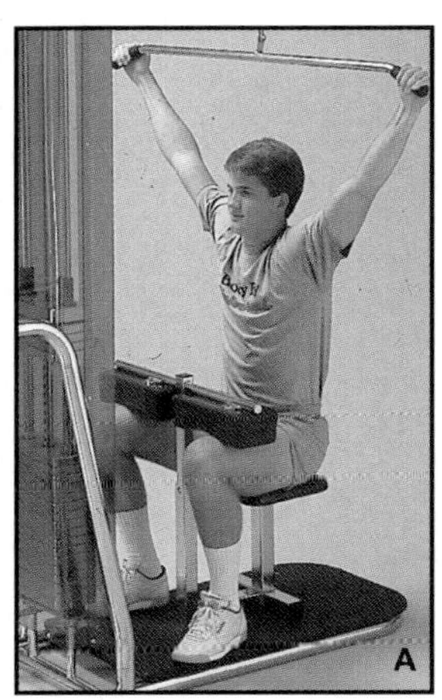
A

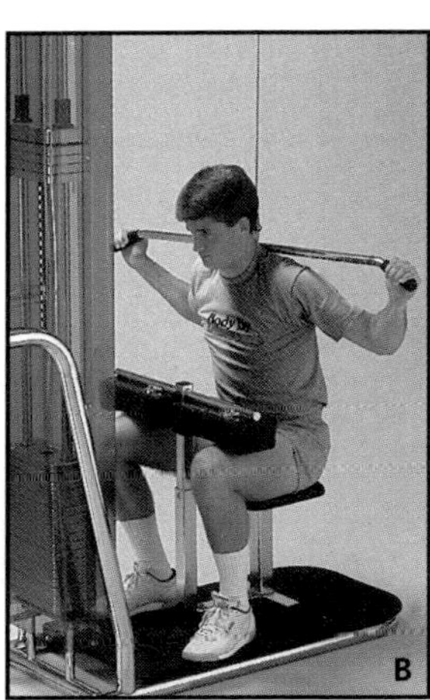
B

8

22

Rotary Torso

Action Sit upright into the machine and place the elbows behind the padded bars (a). Rotate the torso as far as possible to one side (b) and then return slowly to the starting position. Repeat the exercise to the opposite side.

Muscles Developed Internal and external obliques (abdominal muscles).

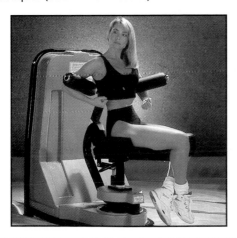

23

Triceps Extension

Action Sit in an upright position, arms up, elbows bent, and place the little finger side of the hands and wrists against the pads, palms of the hands facing each other (a). Fully extend one arm at a time (b), and then return to the original position. Repeat with the other arm.

Muscles Developed Triceps

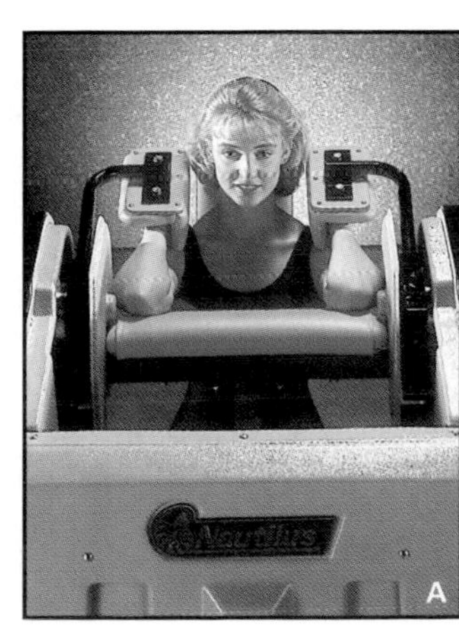

A

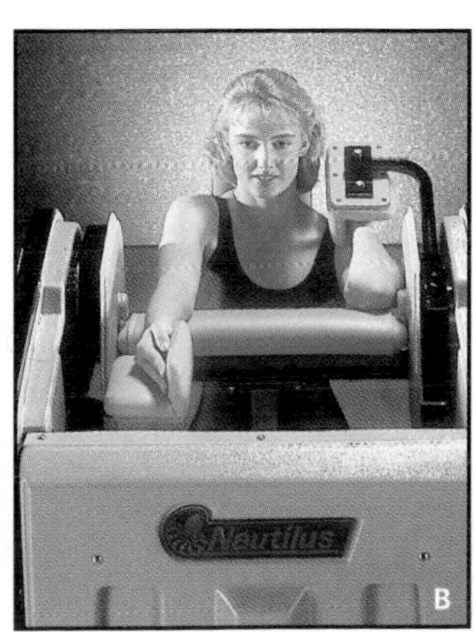

B

24

Leg Extension

Action Sit in an upright position with the feet under the padded bar and grasp the handles at the sides (a). Extend the legs until they are completely straight (b), then return to the starting position.

Muscles Developed Quadriceps

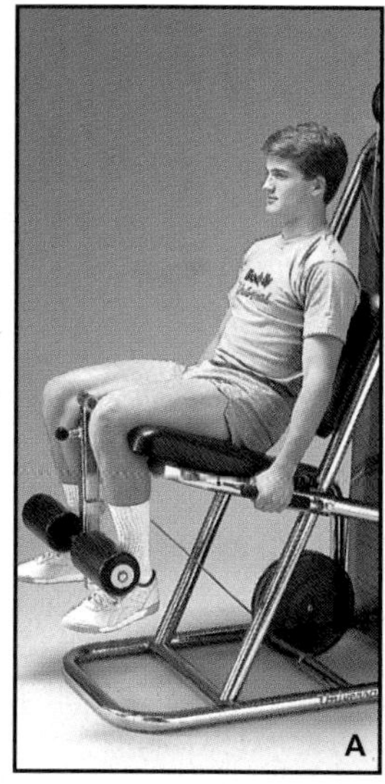

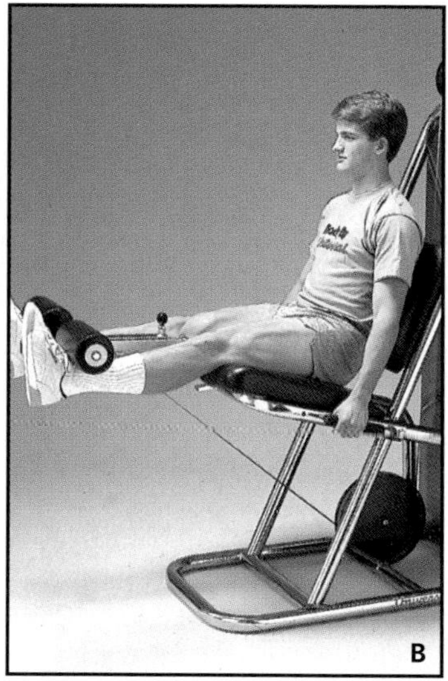

25

Shoulder Press

Action Sit in an upright position and grasp the bar wider than shoulder width (a). Press the bar all the way up until the arms are fully extended (b), then return to the initial position.

Muscles Developed Triceps, deltoid, and pectoralis major

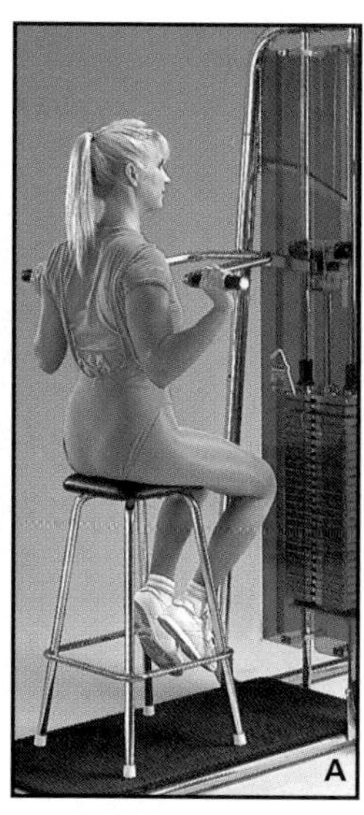

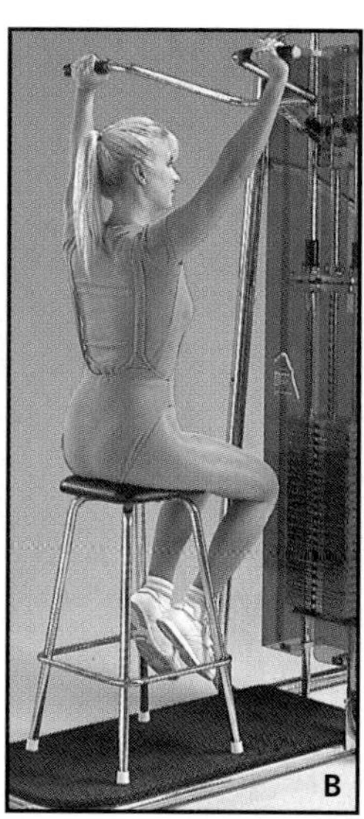

26

Chest Press

Action Start with the arms up to the side, hands resting against the handle bars, and elbows bent at 90° (a). Press the movement arms forward as far as possible, leading with the elbows (b). Slowly return to the starting position.

Muscles Developed Pectoralis major and deltoid

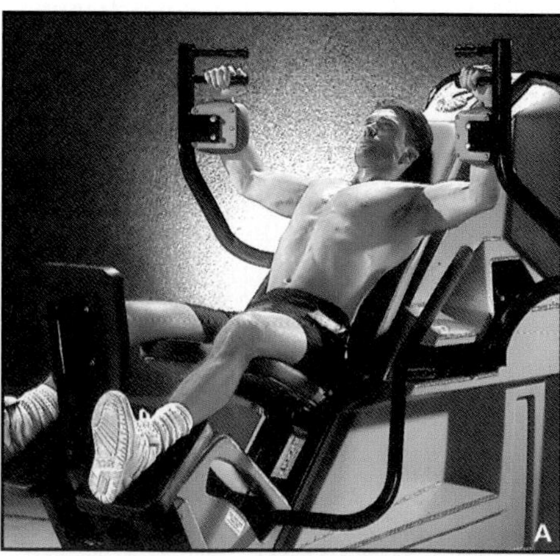

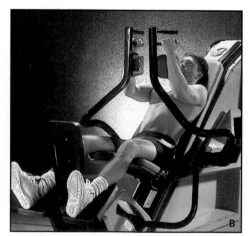

27

Squat

Action Sit in an upright position with the feet under the padded bar and grasp the handles at the sides (a). Extend the legs until they are completely straight (b), then return to the starting position.

Muscles Developed Quadriceps

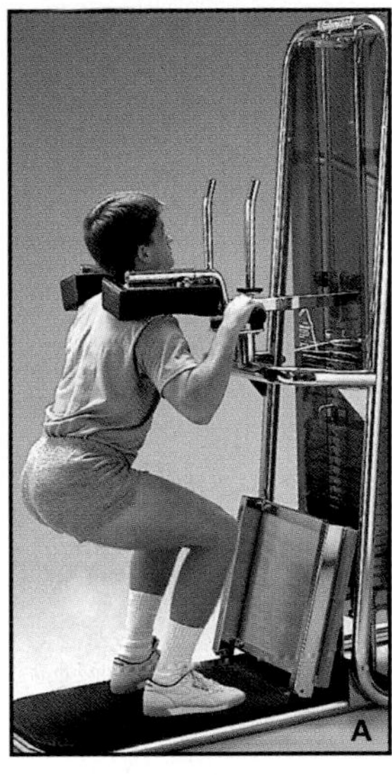
A

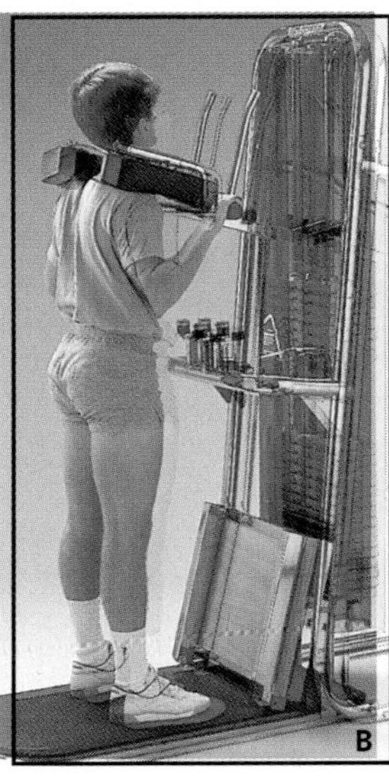
B

28

Upright Rowing

Action Start with the arms extended and grip the handles with the palms down (a). Pull all the way up to the chin (b), then return to the starting position.

Muscles Developed Biceps, brachioradialis, brachialis, deltoid, and trapezius

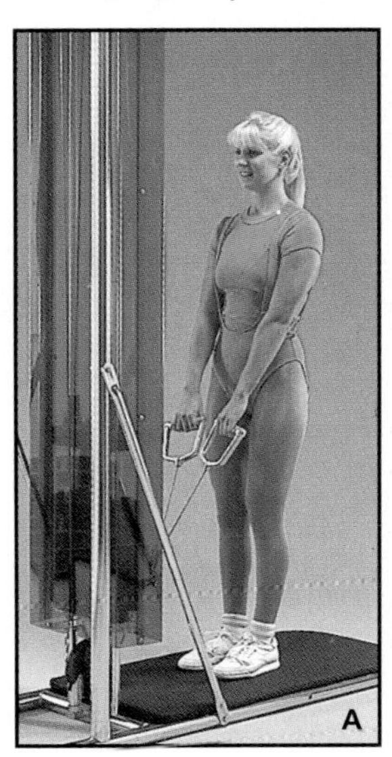
A

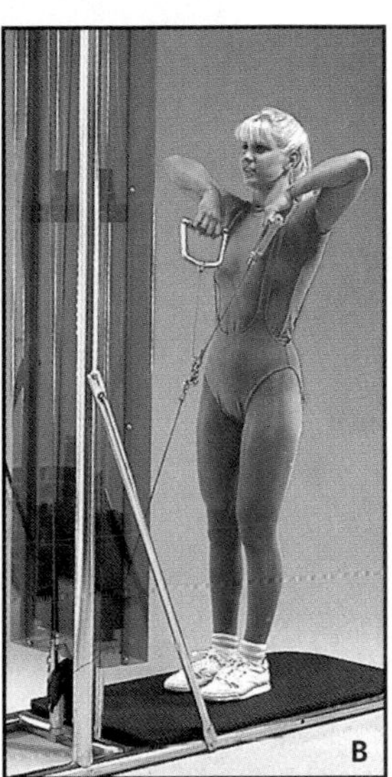
B

29

Seated Leg Curl

Action Sit in the unit and place the strap over the upper thighs. With legs extended, place the back of the feet over the padded rollers (a). Flex the knees until you reach a 90° to 100° angle (b). Slowly return to the starting position.

Muscles Developed Hamstrings

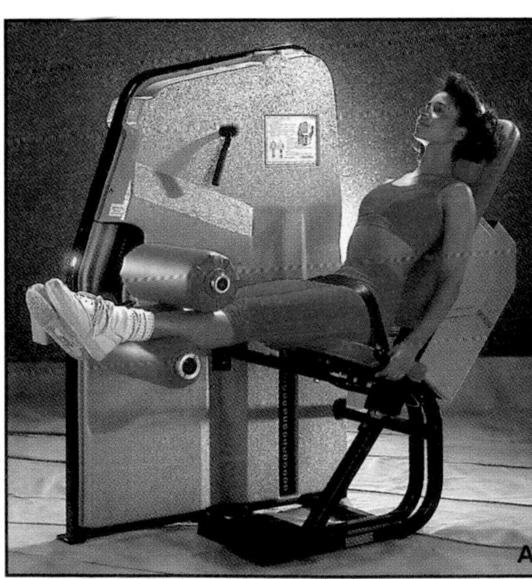
A

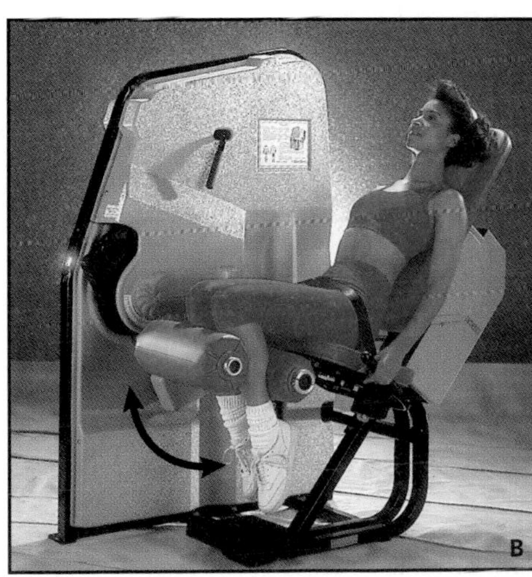
B

30

Bent-arm Pullover

Action Sit back into the chair and grasp the bar behind your head (a). Pull the bar over your head all the way down to your abdomen (b), and slowly return to the original position.

Muscles Developed Latissimus dorsi, pectoral muscles, deltoid, and serratus anterior

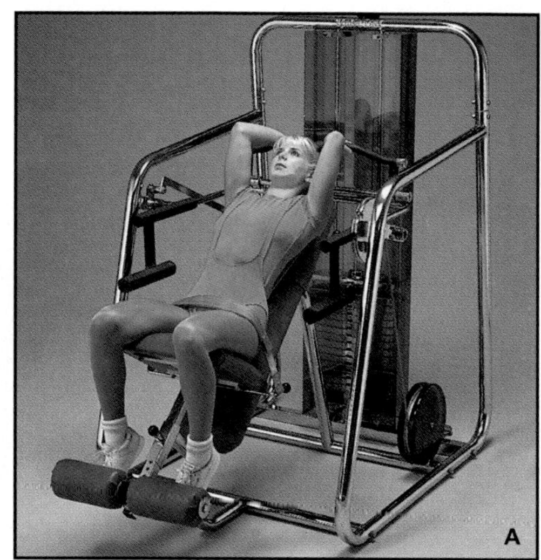
A

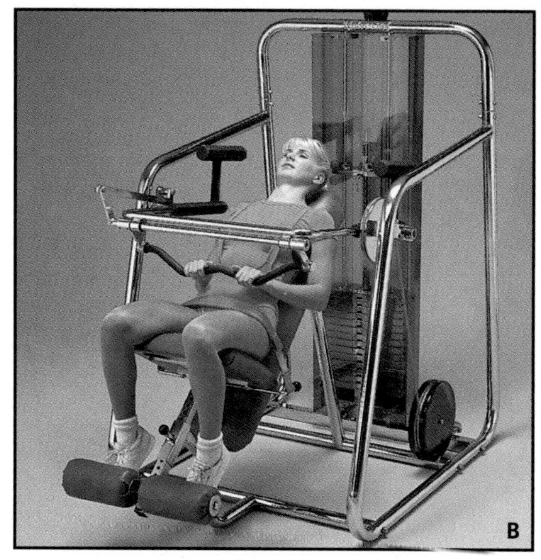
B

31

Triceps Extension

Action Using a palms-down grip, grasp the bar slightly closer than shoulder width, and start with the elbows almost completely bent (a). Extend the arms fully (b), then return to starting position.

Muscles Developed Triceps

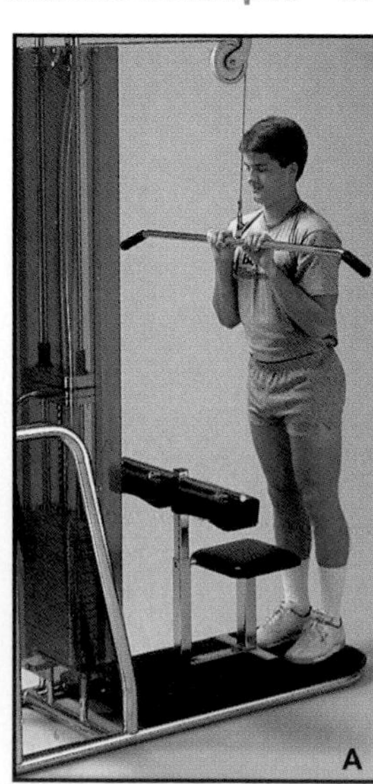
A

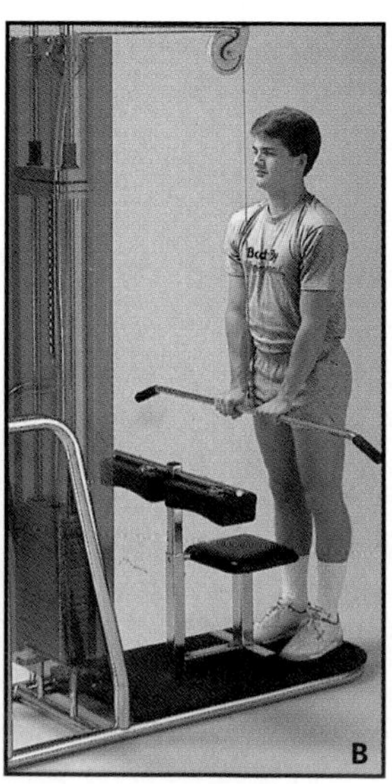
B

32

Dip

Action Start with the elbows flexed (a), then extend the arms fully and return slowly to the initial position.

Muscles Developed Triceps, deltoid, and pectoralis major

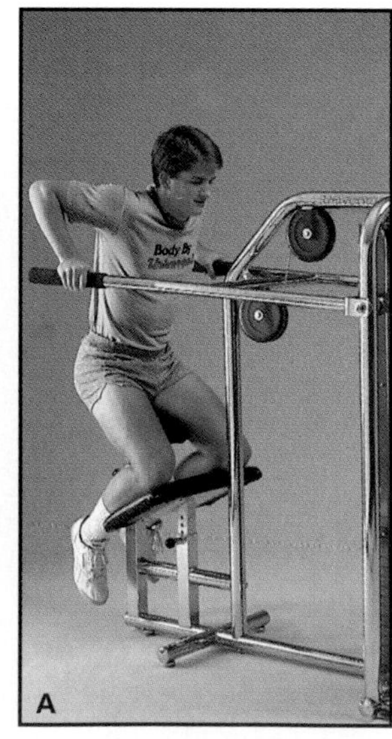
A

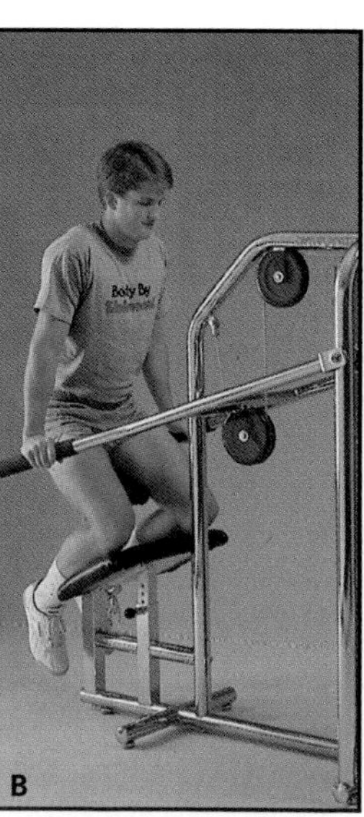
B

Muscular Flexibility Assessment

9

Health-care professionals and practitioners generally have underestimated and overlooked the contribution of good muscular ***flexibility*** *to overall fitness and preventive health care. In daily life, we often have to make rapid or strenuous movements that we are not accustomed to making, which may cause injury. Improper body mechanics often are the result of poor flexibility. Sports medicine specialists believe that many muscular/skeletal problems and injuries, especially in adults, may be related to a lack of flexibility.*

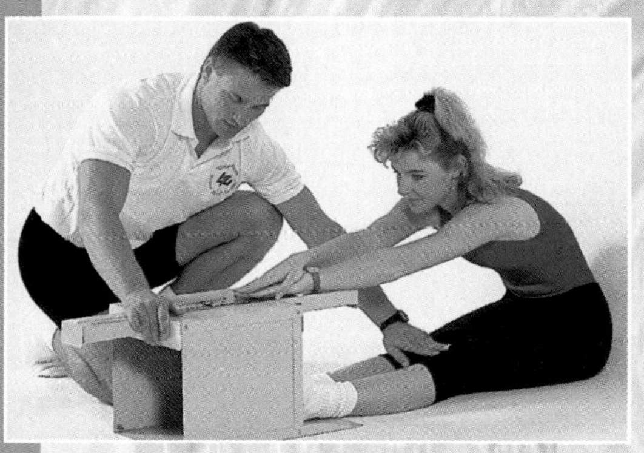

Approximately 80% of all low-back problems in the United States stem from improper alignment of the vertebral column and pelvic girdle, a direct result of inflexible and weak muscles. This backache syndrome costs American industry billions of dollars each year in lost productivity, health services, and worker's compensation.[1]

LABS

Improving and maintaining good range of motion in the joints is important to enhance the quality of life. Participating in a regular flexibility program will:

- *help maintain good joint mobility*
- *increase resistance to muscle injury and soreness*
- *prevent low-back and other spinal column problems*

Objectives

- Understand the importance of muscular flexibility to adequate fitness and preventive health care.
- Identify the factors that affect muscular flexibility.
- Introduce a battery of muscular flexibility tests to assess overall body flexibility (Modified Sit-and-Reach Test, Body Rotation Test, Shoulder Rotation Test).
- Learn to interpret flexibility test results according to health fitness and physical fitness standards.
- Learn to evaluate body posture.

- improve and maintain good postural alignment
- promote proper and graceful body movement
- improve personal appearance and self-image
- help to develop and maintain motor skills throughout life.

In addition, flexibility exercises have been prescribed successfully to treat dysmenorrhea[2] (painful menstruation) and general neuromuscular tension (stress).

Further, **stretching** exercises, in conjunction with calisthenics, are helpful in warm-up routines to prepare the human body for more vigorous aerobic or strength training exercises, as well as cool-down routines following exercise to help the person return to a normal resting state. Fatigued muscles tend to contract to a shorter than average resting length. Stretching exercises help fatigued muscles reestablish their normal resting length.

Similar to muscular strength, good range of motion is critical in older life. Because of a lack of flexibility, some older adults are unable to perform simple daily tasks such as bending forward or turning. Many older adults do not turn their head or rotate their trunk to look over their shoulder but, rather, step around 90° to 180° to see behind them.

Physical activity and exercise also can be hampered severely by lack of good range of motion. Because of the pain involved with activity, older people who have tight hip flexors (muscles) cannot jog or walk very far. A vicious circle ensues, because the condition usually worsens with further inactivity. A simple stretching program can alleviate or prevent this problem and help people return to an exercise program.

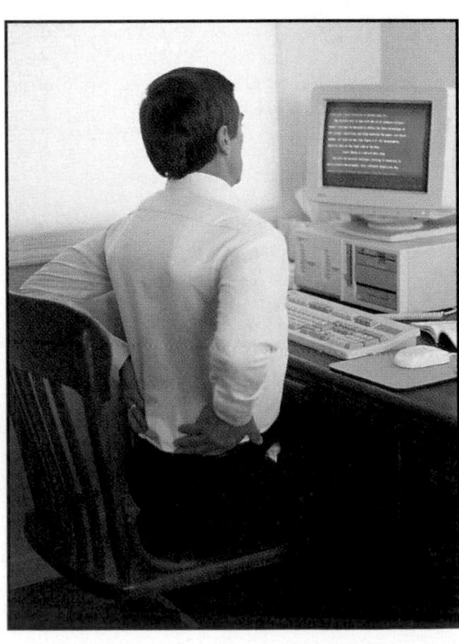

Lack of physical conditioning frequently leads to chronic back pain.

Factors Affecting Flexibility

Total range of motion around a joint is highly specific and varies from one joint to another (hip, trunk, shoulder), as well as from one individual to the next. Muscular flexibility relates primarily to genetic factors and to physical activity. Beyond that, factors such as joint structure, ligaments, tendons, muscles, skin, tissue injury, adipose tissue (fat), body temperature, age, and sex influence range of motion about a joint. Because of the specificity of flexibility, to indicate what constitutes an ideal level of flexibility is difficult. Nevertheless, flexibility is important to health and independent living.

Plastic elongation is permanent lengthening of soft tissue. Elastic elongation is temporary lengthening of soft tissue.

The range of motion about a given joint depends mostly on the structure of that joint. Greater range of motion, however, can be attained through plastic and elastic elongation. Plastic elongation is permanent lengthening of soft tissue. Even though joint capsules, ligaments, and tendons are basically nonelastic, they can undergo plastic elongation. This permanent lengthening, accompanied by increases in range of motion, is best attained through slow-sustained stretching exercises.

Elastic elongation refers to temporary lengthening of soft tissue. Muscle tissue has elastic properties and responds to stretching exercises by undergoing elastic or temporary lengthening. Elastic elongation increases the extensibility of the muscles.

Changes in muscle temperature can increase or decrease flexibility by as much as 20%. Properly warmed-up individuals have more flexibility than non-warmed-up people. Cool temperatures have the opposite effect, impeding joint range of motion. Because of the effects of temperature on muscular flexibility, many people prefer to do their stretching exercises after the aerobic phase of their workout. Aerobic activities raise body temperature, facilitating plastic elongation.

Another factor that influences flexibility is the amount of adipose (fat) tissue in and around joints and muscle tissue. A lot of adipose tissue not only increases resistance to movement, but the added bulk also hampers joint mobility because of the contact between body surfaces.

On the average, women are more flexible than men, and they seem to retain this advantage throughout life. Aging does decrease the extensibility of soft tissue, though, resulting in less flexibility in both sexes as they get older.

The two most significant contributors to lower flexibility levels are sedentary living and lack of exercise. With less physical activity, muscles lose their elasticity and tendons and ligaments tighten and shorten. Inactivity also tends to be accompanied by an increase in adipose tissue, which further decreases joint range of motion. Finally, injury to muscle tissue, and tight skin from excessive scar tissue, has a negative effect on joint range of motion.

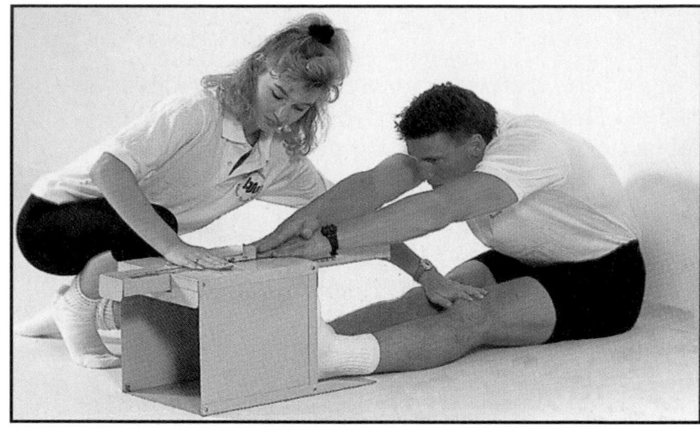

Modified Sit-and-Reach Test.

Assessment of Flexibility

Most of the flexibility tests developed over the years are specific to certain sports and are not practical for the general population. Their application in health and fitness programs is limited. For example, the Front-to-Rear Splits Test and the Bridge-Up Test may have applications in sports such as gymnastics and several track-and-field events, but they do not represent the actions of most people in daily life.

Because of the lack of practical flexibility tests, most health/fitness centers have relied strictly on the Sit-and-Reach Test as an indicator of overall flexibility. This test measures flexibility of the hamstring muscles (back of the thigh) and, to a lesser extent, the lower-back muscles.

Because flexibility is joint-specific and a lot of flexibility in one joint does not necessarily indicate the same is true in other joints, two additional tests — indicators of everyday movements such as reaching, bending, and turning — are included to determine your flexibility profile. These tests are the Total Body Rotation Test and the Shoulder Rotation Test.

The procedure for the Sit-and-Reach Test, as modified from the traditional test, is given in Figure 9.1. Unlike the traditional Sit-and-Reach Test, arm and leg lengths are taken into consideration to determine the score. In the original Sit-and-Reach Test, the 15-inch mark of the yardstick on top of the box always is set at the edge of the box where the feet are placed. This procedure does not differentiate between individuals with long arms and/or short legs or those with short arms and/or long legs, or both.[3,4,5] All other factors being equal, an individual with longer arms or shorter legs, or both, receives a better rating because of the structural advantage.

The procedures and norms for the battery of flexibility tests are given in Figures 9.1 through 9.3 and Tables 9.1 through 9.3. Note that the flexibility test results in these three tables are provided both in inches and centimeters (cm). Be sure to use the proper column to read your percentile score based on your test results (either in inches or cm.) For the flexibility profile, instead of a choice of tests, you should take all three. You will be able to assess your flexibility profile in Lab 9A.

9

Flexibility The ability of a joint to move freely through its full range of motion.

Stretching Moving the joints beyond the accustomed range of motion.

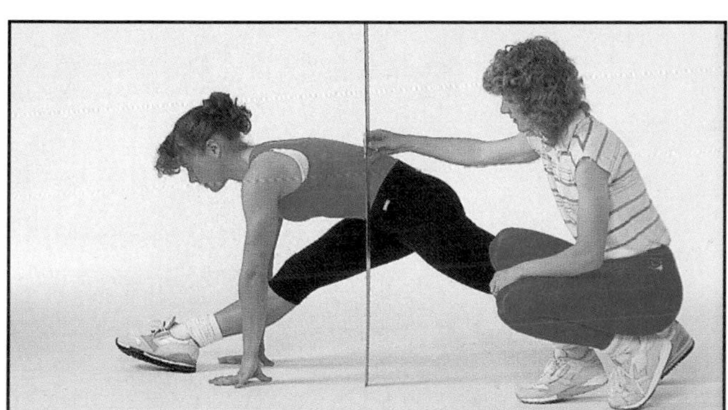

Front-to-Rear Splits Test

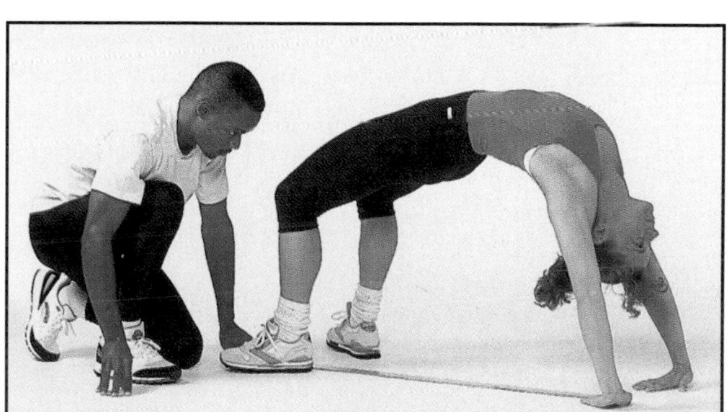

Bridge-Up Test

MODIFIED SIT-AND-REACH TEST

To perform this test, you will need the Acuflex I* Sit-and-Reach Flexibility Tester, or you may simply place a yardstick on top of a box approximately 12" high.

1. Warm up properly before the first trial.
2. Remove your shoes for the test. Sit on the floor with the hips, back, and head against a wall, the legs fully extended, and the bottom of the feet against the Acuflex I or sit-and-reach box.
3. Place the hands one on top of the other, and reach forward as far as possible without letting the head and back come off the wall (the shoulders may be rounded as much as possible, but neither the head nor the back should come off the wall at this time). The technician then can slide the reach indicator on the Acuflex I (or yardstick) along the top of the box until the end of the indicator touches the participant's fingers. The indicator then must be held firmly in place throughout the rest of the test.
4. Now your head and back can come off the wall. Gradually reach forward three times, the third time stretching forward as far as possible on the indicator (or yardstick) and holding the final position for at least 2 seconds. Be sure that during the test you keep the backs of the knees flat against the floor.

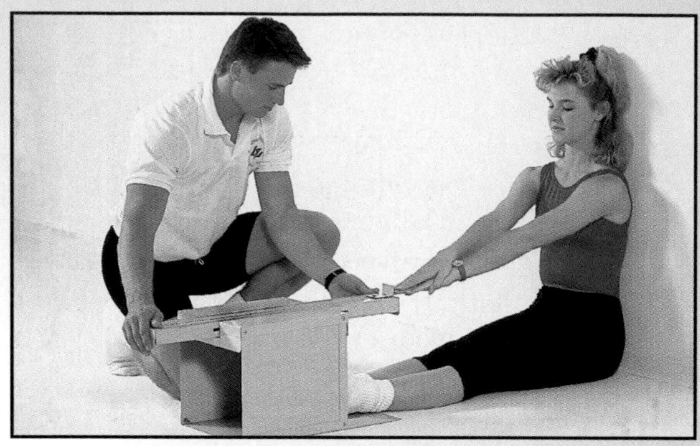

Determining the starting position for the Modified Sit-and-Reach Test.

5. Record the final number of inches reached to the nearest one-half inch.

You are allowed two trials, and an average of the two scores is used as the final test score. The respective percentile ranks and fitness categories for this test are given in Tables 9.1 and 9.4.

*The Acuflex I Flexibility Tester for the Modified Sit-and-Reach Test can be obtained from Figure Finder Collection, Novel Products, P. O. Box 408, Rockton, IL 61072-0480. Phone: 800-323-5143, FAX 815-624-4866.

Figure 9.1 Procedure for the Modified Sit-and-Reach Test.

Table 9.1 Percentile Ranks for the Modified Sit-and-Reach Test

Men

Percentile Rank	≤18 in.	≤18 cm	19–35 in.	19–35 cm	36–49 in.	36–49 cm	≥50 in.	≥50 cm
99	20.8	52.8	20.1	51.1	18.9	48.0	16.2	41.1
95	19.6	49.8	18.9	48.0	18.2	46.2	15.8	40.1
90	18.2	46.2	17.2	43.7	16.1	40.9	15.0	38.1
80	17.8	45.2	17.0	43.2	14.6	37.1	13.3	33.8
70	16.0	40.6	15.8	40.1	13.9	35.3	12.3	31.2
60 (shaded)	15.2	38.6	15.0	38.1	13.4	34.0	11.5	29.2
50	14.5	36.8	14.4	36.6	12.6	32.0	10.2	25.9
40	14.0	35.6	13.5	34.3	11.6	29.5	9.7	24.6
30	13.4	34.0	13.0	33.0	10.8	27.4	9.3	23.6
20	11.8	30.0	11.6	29.5	9.9	25.1	8.8	22.4
10	9.5	24.1	9.2	23.4	8.3	21.1	7.8	19.8
05	8.4	21.3	7.9	20.1	7.0	17.8	7.2	18.3
01	7.2	18.3	7.0	17.8	5.1	13.0	4.0	10.2

Women

Percentile Rank	≤18 in.	≤18 cm	19–35 in.	19–35 cm	36–49 in.	36–49 cm	≥50 in.	≥50 cm
99	22.6	57.4	21.0	53.3	19.8	50.3	17.2	43.7
95	19.5	49.5	19.3	49.0	19.2	48.8	15.7	39.9
90	18.7	47.5	17.9	45.5	17.4	44.2	15.0	38.1
80	17.8	45.2	16.7	42.4	16.2	41.1	14.2	36.1
70	16.5	41.9	16.2	41.1	15.2	38.6	13.6	34.5
60 (shaded)	16.0	40.6	15.8	40.1	14.5	36.8	12.3	31.2
50	15.2	38.6	14.8	37.6	13.5	34.3	11.1	28.2
40	14.5	36.8	14.5	36.8	12.8	32.5	10.1	25.7
30	13.7	34.8	13.7	34.8	12.2	31.0	9.2	23.4
20	12.6	32.0	12.6	32.0	11.0	27.9	8.3	21.1
10	11.4	29.0	10.1	25.7	9.7	24.6	7.5	19.0
05	9.4	23.9	8.1	20.6	8.5	21.6	3.7	9.4
01	6.5	16.5	2.6	6.6	2.0	5.1	1.5	3.8

High physical fitness standard

Health fitness standard (shaded)

TOTAL BODY ROTATION TEST

An Acuflex II* Total Body Rotation Flexibility Tester or a measuring scale with a sliding panel is needed to administer this test. The Acuflex II or scale is placed on the wall at shoulder height and should be adjustable to accommodate individual differences in height. If you need to build your own scale, use two measuring tapes and glue them above and below the sliding panel centered at the 15" mark. Each tape should be at least 30" long. If no sliding panel is available, simply tape the measuring tapes onto a wall. A line also must be drawn on the floor and centered with the 15" mark.

1. Warm up properly before beginning this test.
2. Stand sideways, an arm's length away from the wall, with the feet straight ahead, slightly separated, and the toes right up to the corresponding line drawn on the floor. Hold out the arm opposite to the wall horizontally from the body, making a fist with the hand. The Acuflex II, measuring scale, or tapes should be shoulder height at this time.
3. Rotate the trunk, the extended arm going backward (always maintaining a horizontal plane) and making contact with the panel, gradually sliding it forward as far as possible. If no panel is available, slide the fist alongside the tapes as far as possible. Hold the final position at least 2 seconds. Position the hand with the little finger side forward during the entire sliding movement. **Proper hand position is crucial. Many people attempt to open the hand, or push with extended fingers, or slide the panel with the knuckles — none of which is acceptable.** During the test the knees can be bent slightly, but **the feet cannot be moved, always pointing straight forward.** The body must be kept as straight (vertical) as possible.
4. Conduct the test on either the right or the left side of the body. Perform two trials on the selected side. Record the farthest point reached, measured to the nearest half inch and held for at least 2 seconds. Use the average of the two trials as the final test score. Referring to Tables 9.2 and 9.4, determine the percentile rank and flexibility fitness classification for this test.

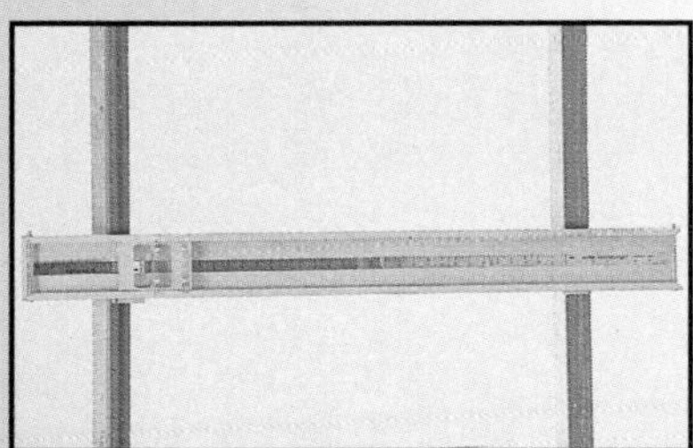

Acuflex II measuring device for the Total Body Rotation Test.

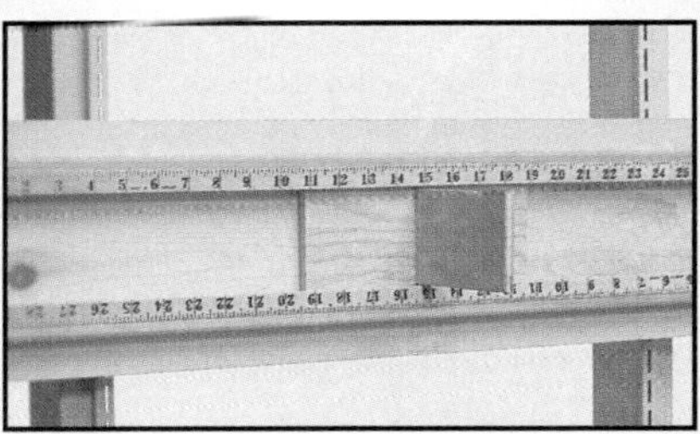

Homemade measuring device for the Total Body Rotation Test.

* The Acuflex II Flexibility Tester for the Total Body Rotation Test can be obtained from Figure Finder Collection, Novel Products, P.O. Box 408, Rockton, IL 61072-0408. Phone: 800-323-5143, FAX 815-624-4866.

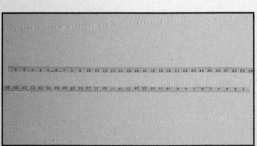

Measuring tapes for the Total Body Rotation Test.

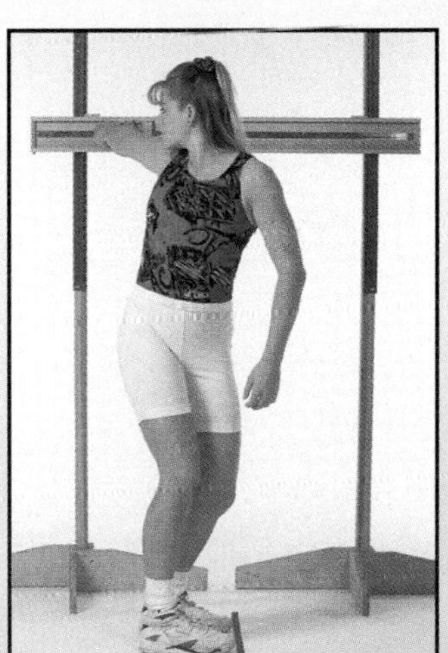
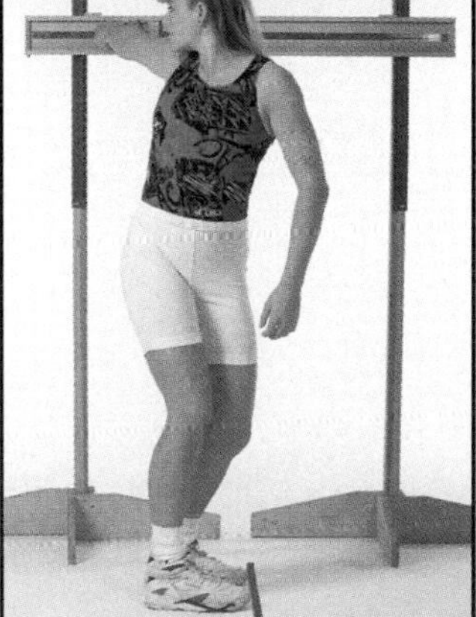

Total Body Rotation Test.

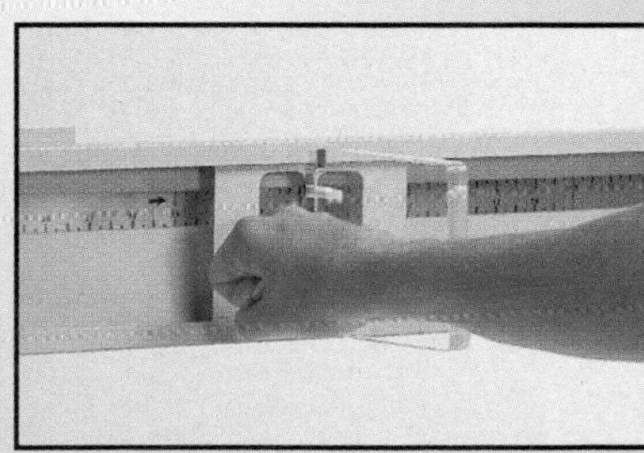

Proper hand position for the Total Body Rotation Test.

Figure 9.2 Procedure for the Total Body Rotation Test.

Table 9.2 Percentile Ranks for the Total Body Rotation Test

	Percentile Rank	Left Rotation								Right Rotation							
		≤18		19–35		36–49		≥50		≤18		19–35		36–49		≥50	
		in.	cm	in.	cm	in.	cm	in.	cm	in.	cm	in.	cm	in.	cm	in.	cm
Men	99	29.1	73.9	28.0	71.1	26.6	67.6	21.0	53.3	28.2	71.6	27.8	70.6	25.2	64.0	22.2	56.4
	95	26.6	67.6	24.8	63.0	24.5	62.2	20.0	50.8	25.5	64.8	25.6	65.0	23.8	60.5	20.7	52.6
	90	25.0	63.5	23.6	59.9	23.0	58.4	17.7	45.0	24.3	61.7	24.1	61.2	22.5	57.1	19.3	49.0
	80	22.0	55.9	22.0	55.9	21.2	53.8	15.5	39.4	22.7	57.7	22.3	56.6	21.0	53.3	16.3	41.4
	70	20.9	53.1	20.3	51.6	20.4	51.8	14.7	37.3	21.3	54.1	20.7	52.6	18.7	47.5	15.7	39.9
	60	19.9	50.5	19.3	49.0	18.7	47.5	13.9	35.3	19.8	50.3	19.0	48.3	17.3	43.9	14.7	37.3
	50	18.6	47.2	18.0	45.7	16.7	42.4	12.7	32.3	19.0	48.3	17.2	43.7	16.3	41.4	12.3	31.2
	40	17.0	43.2	16.8	42.7	15.3	38.9	11.7	29.7	17.3	43.9	16.3	41.4	14.7	37.3	11.5	29.2
	30	14.9	37.8	15.0	38.1	14.8	37.6	10.3	26.2	15.1	38.4	15.0	38.1	13.3	33.8	10.7	27.2
	20	13.8	35.1	13.3	33.8	13.7	34.8	9.5	24.1	12.9	32.8	13.3	33.8	11.2	28.4	8.7	22.1
	10	10.8	27.4	10.5	26.7	10.8	27.4	4.3	10.9	10.8	27.4	11.3	28.7	8.0	20.3	2.7	6.9
	05	8.5	21.6	8.9	22.6	8.8	22.4	0.3	0.8	8.1	20.6	8.3	21.1	5.5	14.0	0.3	0.8
	01	3.4	8.6	1.7	4.3	5.1	13.0	0.0	0.0	6.6	16.8	2.9	7.4	2.0	5.1	0.0	0.0
Women	99	29.3	74.4	28.6	72.6	27.1	68.8	23.0	58.4	29.6	75.2	29.4	74.7	27.1	68.8	21.7	55.1
	95	26.8	68.1	24.8	63.0	25.3	64.3	21.4	54.4	27.6	70.1	25.3	64.3	25.9	65.8	19.7	50.0
	90	25.5	64.8	23.0	58.4	23.4	59.4	20.5	52.1	25.8	65.5	23.0	58.4	21.3	54.1	19.0	48.3
	80	23.8	60.5	21.5	54.6	20.2	51.3	19.1	48.5	23.7	60.2	20.8	52.8	19.6	49.8	17.9	45.5
	70	21.8	55.4	20.5	52.1	18.6	47.2	17.3	43.9	22.0	55.9	19.3	49.0	17.3	43.9	16.8	42.7
	60	20.5	52.1	19.3	49.0	17.7	45.0	16.0	40.6	20.8	52.8	18.0	45.7	16.5	41.9	15.6	39.6
	50	19.5	49.5	18.0	45.7	16.4	41.7	14.8	37.6	19.5	49.5	17.3	43.9	14.6	37.1	14.0	35.6
	40	18.5	47.0	17.2	43.7	14.8	37.6	13.7	34.8	18.3	46.5	16.0	40.6	13.1	33.3	12.8	32.5
	30	17.1	43.4	15.7	39.9	13.6	34.5	10.0	25.4	16.3	41.4	15.2	38.6	11.7	29.7	8.5	21.6
	20	16.0	40.6	15.2	38.6	11.6	29.5	6.3	16.0	14.5	36.8	14.0	35.6	9.8	24.9	3.9	9.9
	10	12.8	32.5	13.6	34.5	8.5	21.6	3.0	7.6	12.4	31.5	11.1	28.2	6.1	15.5	2.2	5.6
	05	11.1	28.2	7.3	18.5	6.8	17.3	0.7	1.8	10.2	25.9	8.8	22.4	4.0	10.2	1.1	2.8
	01	8.9	22.6	5.3	13.5	4.3	10.9	0.0	0.0	8.9	22.6	3.2	8.1	2.8	7.1	0.0	0.0

9

High physical fitness standard

Health fitness standard

SHOULDER ROTATION TEST

This test can be done using the Acuflex III* Flexibility Tester, which consists of a shoulder caliper and a measuring device for shoulder rotation. If unavailable, you can construct your own device quite easily. The caliper can be built with three regular yardsticks. Nail and glue two of the yardsticks at one end at a 90° angle, and use the third one as the sliding end of the caliper. Construct the rotation device by placing a 60" measuring tape on an aluminum or wood stick, starting at about 6" or 7" from the end of the stick.

1. Warm up before the test.
2. Using the shoulder caliper, measure the biacromial width to the nearest fourth inch (use the top scale on the Acuflex III). Measure biacromial width between the lateral edges of the acromion processes of the shoulders.

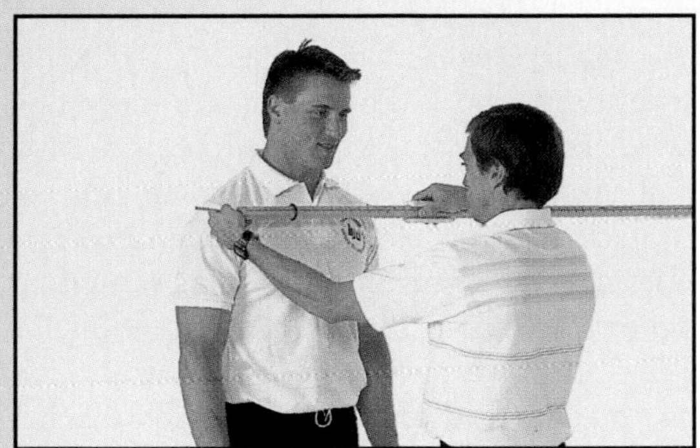

Measuring biacromial width.

3. Place the Acuflex III or homemade device behind the back and use a reverse grip (thumbs out) to hold on to the device. Place the right hand next to the zero point of the scale or tape (lower scale on the Acuflex III) and hold it firmly in place throughout the test. Place the left hand on the other end of the measuring device, as wide as needed.
4. Standing straight up and extending both arms to full length, with elbows locked, slowly bring the measuring device over the head until it reaches forehead level. For subsequent trials, depending on the resistance encountered when rotating the shoulders, move the left grip in ½" to 1" at a time, and repeat the task until you no longer can rotate the shoulders without undue strain or start bending the elbows to do so. Always keep the righthand grip against the zero point of the scale. Measure the last successful trial to the nearest half inch. Take this measurement right at the inner edge of the left hand on the side of the little finger.
6. Determine the final score for this test by subtracting the biacromial width from the best score (shortest distance) between both hands on the rotation test. For example, if the best score is 35" and the biacromial width is 15", the final score is 20" (35 – 15 = 20). Using Tables 9.3 and 9.4, determine the percentile rank and flexibility fitness classification for this test.

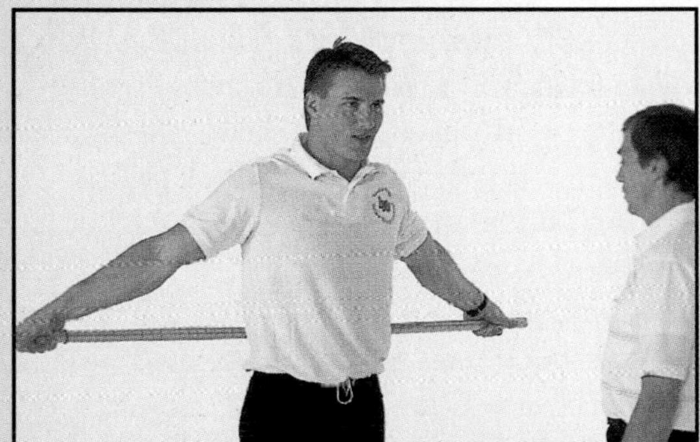

Starting position for the Shoulder Rotation Test (note the reverse grip used for this test).

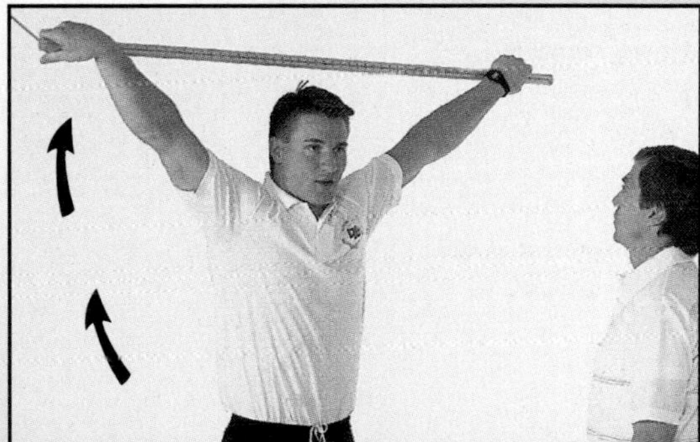

Shoulder Rotation Test.

*The Acuflex III Flexibility Tester for the Shoulder Rotation Test can be obtained from Figure Finder Collection, Novel Products, Inc., P. O. Box 408, Rockton, IL 61072-0408. Phone: (800) 323-5143, FAX 815-624-4866.

Figure 9.3 Procedure for the Shoulder Rotation Test.

Table 9.3 Percentile Ranks for the Shoulder Rotation Test

	Age Category								
	Percentile Rank	≤18 in.	cm	19–35 in.	cm	36–49 in.	cm	≥50	cm
	99	2.2	5.6	−1.0	−2.5	18.1	46.0	21.5	54.6
	95	15.2	38.6	10.4	26.4	20.4	51.8	27.0	68.6
	90	18.5	47.0	15.5	39.4	20.8	52.8	27.9	70.9
	80	20.7	52.6	18.4	46.7	23.3	59.2	28.5	72.4
	70	23.0	58.4	20.5	52.1	24.7	62.7	29.4	74.7
	60	24.2	61.5	22.9	58.2	26.6	67.6	29.9	75.9
Men	50	25.4	64.5	24.4	62.0	28.0	71.1	30.5	77.5
	40	26.3	66.8	25.7	65.3	30.0	76.2	31.0	78.7
	30	28.2	71.6	27.3	69.3	31.9	81.0	31.7	80.5
	20	30.0	76.2	30.1	76.5	33.3	84.6	33.1	84.1
	10	33.5	85.1	31.8	80.8	36.1	91.7	37.2	94.5
	05	34.7	88.1	33.5	85.1	37.8	96.0	38.7	98.3
	01	40.8	103.6	42.6	108.2	43.0	109.2	44.1	112.0
	99	2.6	6.6	−2.4	−6.1	11.5	29.2	13.1	33.3
	95	8.0	20.3	6.2	15.7	15.4	39.1	16.5	41.9
	90	10.7	27.2	9.7	24.6	16.8	42.7	20.9	53.1
	80	14.5	36.8	14.5	36.8	19.2	48.8	22.5	57.1
	70	16.1	40.9	17.2	43.7	21.5	54.6	24.3	61.7
	60	19.2	48.8	18.7	47.5	23.1	58.7	25.1	63.8
Women	50	21.0	53.3	20.0	50.8	23.5	59.7	26.2	66.5
	40	22.2	56.4	21.4	54.4	24.4	62.0	28.1	71.4
	30	23.2	58.9	24.0	61.0	25.9	65.8	29.9	75.9
	20	25.0	63.5	25.9	65.8	29.8	75.7	31.5	80.0
	10	27.2	69.1	29.1	73.9	31.1	79.0	33.1	84.1
	05	28.0	71.1	31.3	79.5	33.4	84.8	34.1	86.6
	01	32.5	82.5	37.1	94.2	34.9	88.6	35.4	89.9

High physical fitness standard
Health fitness standard

Table 9.4 Flexibility Fitness Categories

Percentile Rank	Fitness Category
≥81	Excellent
61–80	Good
41–60	Average
21–40	Fair
≤20	Poor

Interpreting Flexibility Test Results

After obtaining your scores and fitness ratings for each test, you can determine the fitness category for each flexibility test using the guidelines given in Table 9.4. The overall flexibility fitness classification is obtained by computing an average percentile rank from all three tests and using the same guidelines given in Table 9.4.

Evaluating Body Posture

Posture tests are used to detect deviations from normal body alignment and prescribe corrective exercises or procedures to improve alignment. These analyses preferably are conducted early in life, because certain postural deviations are more complex to correct in older people. If deviations are allowed to go uncorrected, they usually become more serious as the person grows older. Consequently, corrective exercises or other medical procedures should be used to stop or slow down postural degeneration.

Faulty posture and weak and inelastic muscles are the leading causes for chronic low-back problems in the United States. An estimated 75 million Americans have low-back problems each year. About 80% of low-back pain is caused by a combination of poor flexibility and improper postural alignment in the lower back and a weak abdominal wall.

A battery of tests to evaluate these areas becomes crucial in preventing and rehabilitating low-back pain. The results of these tests can be used to prescribe corrective exercises.

Adequate body mechanics also aid in reducing chronic low-back pain. Proper body mechanics means using correct positions in all the activities of daily life, including sleeping, sitting, standing, walking, driving, working, and exercising. Because of the high incidence of low-back pain, a series of corrective and preventive exercises, along with illustrations of proper body mechanics, are given in Chapter 10.

Most people are unaware of how faulty their posture is until they see themselves in a photograph. This can be quite a shock to many people and often is enough to motivate them to change.

Besides engaging in the recommended exercises to elicit changes in postural alignment, people need to be continually aware of the corrections they are trying to make. As their posture improves, people

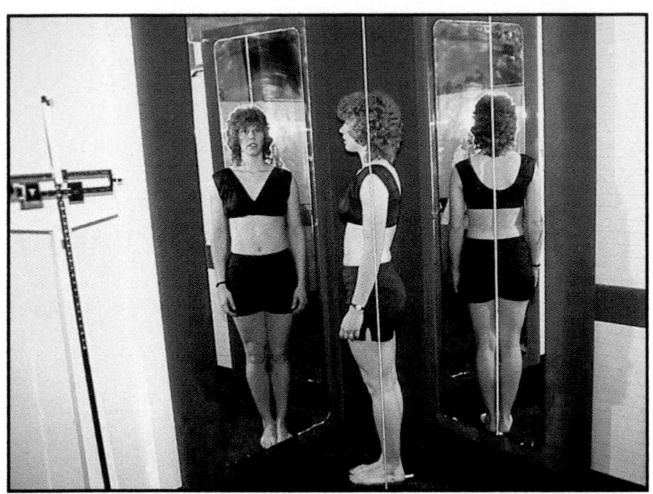

Photographic technique used for posture evaluation.

frequently become motivated to change other aspects, such as improving muscular strength and flexibility and decreasing body fat.

Proper body alignment has been difficult to evaluate because most experts still don't know exactly what constitutes good posture. To objectively analyze a person's posture, an observer either must be adequately trained or must have some guidelines to identify abnormalities and assign ratings according to the amount of deviation from "normal" posture.

A posture rating chart, such as given in Lab 9B, provides simple guidelines for evaluating posture. Assuming the drawings in the left column as proper alignment and the drawings in the right column as extreme deviations from normal, an observer is able to rate each body segment on a scale from 1 to 5.

Faulty posture and weak and inelastic muscles are the leading causes of chronic low-back problems in the United States.

Postural analysis can be done with more precision with the aid of a plumb line, two mirrors, and a Polaroid camera. The mirrors are placed at an 80° to 85° angle, and the plumb line is centered in front of the mirrors. Another line is drawn down the center of the mirror on the right. The person should stand with the left side to the plumb line. The plumb line is used as a reference to divide the body into front and back halves (try to center the line with the hip joint and the shoulder). The line on the back mirror should divide the body into right and left sides. A picture then is taken that can be compared to the rating chart given in Lab 9B.

The photographic procedure allows for a better comparison of the different body segment alignments and a more objective analysis. If no mirrors and camera are available, the participant should stand with his or her side to the line, and then repeat with the back to the line, while the evaluator does the assessment.

A final posture score is determined according to the sum of the ratings obtained for each body segment. Table 9.5 contains the various categories as determined by the final posture score.

Table 9.5 Posture Evaluation Standards

Total Points	Classification
≥45	Excellent
40-44	Good
30-39	Average
20-29	Fair
≤19	Poor

Source: *The Complete Guide for the Development and Implementation of Health Promotion Programs,* by W. W. K. Hoeger (Englewood, CO: Morton Publishing, 1987). Reproduced by permission.

Laboratory Experience

LAB 9A
Muscular Flexibility Assessment

Lab Preparation
Wear loose exercise clothing.

LAB 9B
Posture Evaluation

Lab Preparation
For the posture analysis, men should wear shorts only, and women should wear shorts and a tank top. Prior to the lab, study the posture analysis form given in Lab 9B and review the section on Posture Evaluation in this chapter.

Notes

1. S. A. Plowman, "Physical Fitness and Healthy Low Back Function," *President's Council on Physical Fitness and Sports: Physical Activity and Fitness Research Digest*, Series 1:3 (1993), 3.
2. University of California at Berkeley, *The Wellness Guide to Lifelong Fitness* (New York: Random House, 1993), p. 198.
3. W. W. K. Hoeger and D. R. Hopkins, "A Comparison Between The Sit and Reach and the Modified Sit and Reach in the Measurement of Flexibility in Women," *Research Quarterly for Exercise and Sport*, 63?:191–195.
4. W. W. K. Hoeger, D. R. Hopkins, S. Button, and T. A. Palmer, "Comparing the Sit and Reach with the Modified Sit and Reach in Measuring Flexibility in Adolescents," *Pediatric Exercise Science*, 2 (1990), 156–162.
5. D. R., Hopkins and W. W. K. Hoeger, "A Comparison of the Sit and Reach and the Modified Sit and Reach in the Measurement of Flexibility for Males," *Journal of Applied Sports Science Research*, 6 (1992), 7–10.

Suggested Readings

Billing, H., and E. Loewendahl. *Mobilization of the Human Body*. Palo Alto, CA: Stanford University Press, 1949.

Chapman, E. A., H. A. deVries, and R. Swezey. "Joint Stiffness: Effects of Exercise on Young and Old Men." *Journal of Gerontology*, 27 (1972), 218–221.

Dickerson, R. V. "The Specificity of Flexibility." *Research Quarterly*, 33 (1962), 222–229.

Fleishman, E. A. *Examiners Manual for Basic Fitness Tests*. Englewood Cliffs, NJ: Prentice-Hall, 1964.

Hoeger, W. W. K., S. Button, D. R. Hopkins, and T. A. Palmer. "Relationship Among Four Selected Flexibility Tests for High School-Age Students." *Northwest Journal for Health, Physical Education, Recreation and Dance*, 1:2 (1989), 6–10.

Hoeger, W. W. K., and D. R. Hopkins. "Assessing Muscular Flexibility." *Fitness Management*, 6:2 (1990), 34–36, 42.

Hoeger, W. W. K., and D. R. Hopkins. "A Comparison Between The Sit and Reach and The Modified Sit and Reach in the Measurement of Flexibility in Women." *Research Quarterly for Exercise and Sport*, 63 (1992), 191–195.

Hoeger, W. W. K, D. R. Hopkins, S. Button, and T. A. Palmer. "Comparing the Sit and Reach with the Modified Sit and Reach in Measuring Flexibility in Adolescents." *Pediatric Exercise Science*, 2 (1990), 156–162.

Hopkins, D. R., and W. W. K. Hoeger. "A Comparison of the Sit and Reach and the Modified Sit and Reach in the Measurement of Flexibility for Males." *Journal of Applied Sports Science Research*, 6 (1992), 7–10.

Holt, L. E., T. M. Travis, and T. Okita. "Comparative Study of Three Stretching Techniques." *Perceptual and Motor Skills*, 31 (1970), 611–616.

Johnson, B. L., and J. K. Nelson. *Practical Measurements for Evaluation in Physical Education*. Minneapolis: Burgess Publishing, 1979.

Sapega, A. A., T. C. Quedenfeld, R. A. Moyer, and R. A. Butler. "Biophysical Factors in Range-of-Motion Exercise." *Physician and Sportsmedicine*, 9 (1981), 57–65.

Wright, V., and R. J. Johns. "Physical Factors Concerned with Stiffness of Normal and Diseased Joints." *Bulletin of Johns Hopkins Hospital*, 106 (1960), 215–231.

9

Principles of Muscular Flexibility Prescription

10

Developing and maintaining good range of motion (flexibility) around the joints is important to enhance health and quality of life. Even though hereditary factors play a crucial role in body flexibility, joint mobility can be increased and maintained through a regular flexibility exercise program. Because range of motion is highly specific to each body part (ankle, trunk, shoulder), a comprehensive stretching program should include all body parts and follow the basic guidelines for flexibility development.

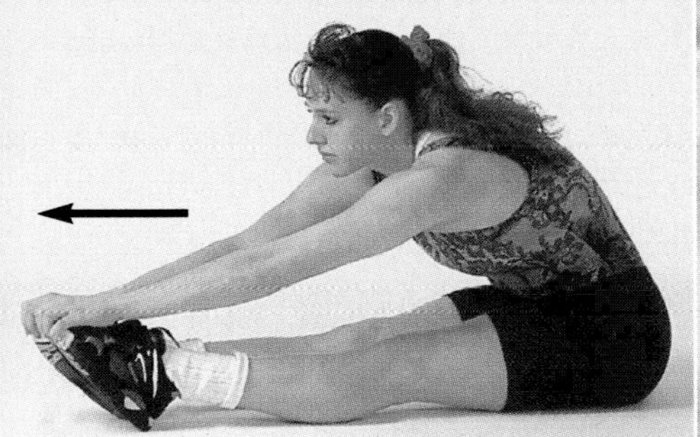

Guidelines for Flexibility Development

The overload and specificity of training principles discussed in conjunction with strength development in Chapter 8 apply as well to the development of muscular flexibility. To increase the total range of motion of a joint, the specific muscles surrounding that joint have to be stretched progressively beyond their accustomed length. The principles of mode, intensity, repetitions, and frequency of exercise also can be applied to flexibility programs.

LABS

Objectives

- Define ballistic stretching, slow-sustained stretching, and proprioceptive neuromuscular facilitation stretching.
- Understand the factors that contribute to the development of muscular flexibility.
- Learn a complete set of exercises for an overall body flexibility-development program.
- Be introduced to a program for preventing and rehabilitating of low back pain.

Mode of Training

Three modes of stretching exercises can increase flexibility:

1. Ballistic stretching.
2. Slow-sustained stretching.
3. Proprioceptive neuromuscular facilitation stretching.

Although research has indicated that all three types of stretching are effective in improving flexibility, each technique has certain advantages.

Ballistic *or* **dynamic stretching** provides the necessary force to lengthen the muscles. This type of stretching helps to develop flexibility, but the ballistic actions may cause muscle soreness and injury from small tears to the soft tissue.

Precautions must be taken not to overstretch ligaments, because they undergo plastic or permanent elongation. If the stretching force cannot be controlled, as in fast, jerky movements, ligaments easily can be overstretched. This, in turn, leads to excessively loose joints, increasing the risk for injuries, including joint dislocation and **subluxation**. Most authorities, therefore, do not recommend ballistic exercises for developing flexibility.

A **slow-sustained stretch** causes the muscles to relax and thereby achieve greater length. This type of stretch causes little pain and has a low risk for injury. Slow-sustained stretching exercises are the most frequently used and recommended for flexibility development programs.

10

Proprioceptive neuromuscular facilitation (PNF) stretching has become more popular in the last few years. This technique, based on a "contract and relax" method, usually requires the assistance of another person, although external resistance could come from the floor, a wall, or other body parts. The procedure is as follows:

1. The person assisting with the exercise provides initial force by pushing slowly in the direction of the desired stretch. This first stretch does not cover the entire range of motion.
2. The person being stretched then applies force in the opposite direction of the stretch, against the assistant, who tries to hold the initial degree of stretch as close as possible. An isometric contraction is being performed at that angle.
3. After 4 or 5 seconds of isometric contraction, the muscle being stretched is relaxed completely. The assistant then increases the degree of stretch slowly to a greater angle.

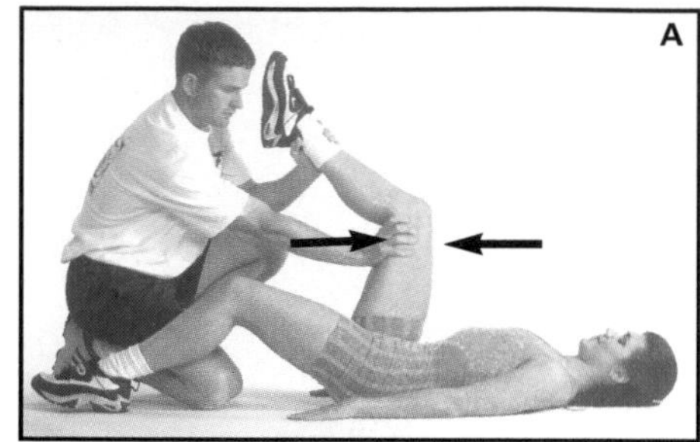

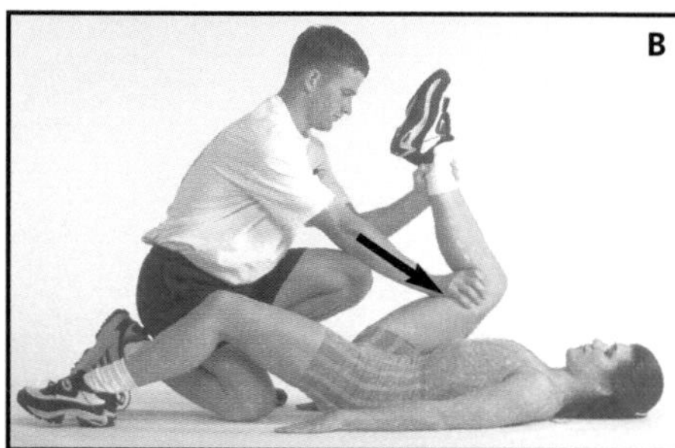

Proprioceptive neuromuscular facilitation stretching technique (a) isometric phase (b) stretching phase.

4. The isometric contraction is repeated for another 4 or 5 seconds, following which the muscle is relaxed again. The assistant then can increase the degree of stretch slowly one more time. Steps 1 to 4 are repeated two to five times, until the exerciser feels mild discomfort. On the last trial the final stretched position should be held for several seconds.

Theoretically, with the PNF technique, the isometric contraction helps relax the muscle being stretched, which results in greater muscle length. Some fitness leaders believe PNF is more effective than slow-sustained stretching. Another benefit of PNF is an increase in strength of the muscle(s) being stretched. Recent research showed an approximate 17% and 35% increase in absolute strength and muscular endurance, respectively, in the hamstring muscle group through 12 weeks of PNF stretching.[1] The results were consistent in both men and women. These increases are attributed to the isometric contractions performed during PNF. The disadvantages are more pain with PNF, a second person, preferably, has to assist, and more time is necessary to conduct each session.

Intensity of Exercise

The **intensity** should be only *to a point of mild discomfort.* Pain does not have to be a part of the stretching routine. Excessive pain is an indication that the load is too great and may lead to injury.

All stretching should be done to slightly below the pain threshold. As participants reach this point, they should try to relax the muscle being stretched as much as possible. After completing the stretch, the body part is brought back gradually to the starting point.

Repetitions

The time required for an exercise session for flexibility development is based on the number of repetitions performed and the length of time each repetition (final stretched position) is held. The general recommendation is that each exercise be done four or five times, holding the final position each time for about 10 to 30 seconds.

As flexibility increases, a person can gradually increase the time each repetition is held, to a maximum of 1 minute. Individuals who are susceptible to flexibility injuries should limit each stretch to 20 seconds.

Frequency of Exercise

Flexibility exercises should be conducted at least three times per week in the early stages of the program. After a minimum of 6 to 8 weeks, flexibility levels can be maintained with only two sessions per week, using about three repetitions of 10 to 15 seconds each.The flexibility development guidelines are summarized in Figure 10.1.

- **Mode**
  Static stretching or proprioceptive neuromuscular facilitation (PNF) to include every major joint of the body
- **Intensity**
  Stretch to the point of mild discomfort
- **Repetitions**
  Repeat each exercise three to five times and hold the final stretched position for 10 to 30 seconds
- **Frequency**
  At least three days per week

Source: ACSM's Guidelines for Exercise Testing and Prescription. Baltimore: Williams & Wilkins, 1995.

Figure 10.1 Guidelines for flexibility development.

When to Stretch?

Many people do not differentiate a warm-up from stretching. Warming up means starting a workout slowly with walking, slow jogging, or light calisthenics. Stretching implies movement of joints through their range of motion.

Before performing flexibility exercises, the muscles should be warmed up properly. Failing to warm up increases the risk for muscle pulls and tears. Surveys have shown that individuals who stretch before workouts without an adequate warm-up actually have a higher rate of injuries than those who do not stretch at all.

A good time to do flexibility exercises is after aerobic workouts. Higher body temperature in itself helps to increase joint range of motion. Muscles also are fatigued following exercise. A fatigued muscle tends to shorten, which can lead to soreness and spasms. Stretching exercises help fatigued muscles reestablish their normal resting length and prevent unnecessary pain.

Flexibility Exercises

To improve body flexibility, each major muscle group should be subjected to at least one stretching exercise. A complete set of exercises for developing muscular flexibility is presented at the end of this chapter.

You may not be able to hold a final stretched position with some of these exercises, such as lateral head tilts and arm circles, but you should still perform the exercise through the joint's full range of motion. Depending on the number and length of the repetitions, a complete workout will last between 15 and 30 minutes.

Preventing and Rehabilitating Low-Back Pain

Few people make it through life without having low-back pain at some point. An estimated 75 million Americans currently suffer from chronic low back pain each year. About 80% of the time, backache

Ballistic or dynamic stretching Exercises done with jerky, rapid, and bouncy movements.

Subluxation Partial dislocation of a joint.

Slow-sustained stretching A technique in which muscles are lengthened gradually through a joint's complete range of motion and the final position is held for a few seconds.

Proprioceptive neuromuscular facilitation (PNF) Stretching technique where muscles are progressively stretched out with intermittent isometric contractions.

Intensity Degree of stretch when doing flexibility exercises.

10

HOW TO PUT YOUR BACK TO BED

For proper bed posture, a firm mattress is essential. Bedboards, sold commercially, or devised at home, may be used with soft mattresses. Bedboards, preferably, should be made of 3/4 inch plywood. Faulty sleeping positions intensify swayback and result not only in backache but in numbness, tingling, and pain in arms and legs.

Incorrect:
Lying flat on back makes swayback worse.

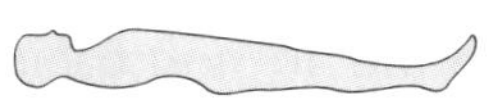

Use of high pillow strains neck, arms, shoulders.

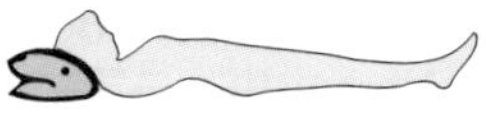

Sleeping face down exaggerates swayback, strains neck and shoulders.

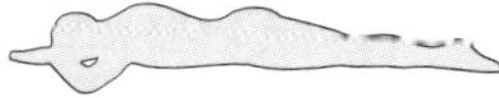

Bending one hip and knee does not relieve swayback.

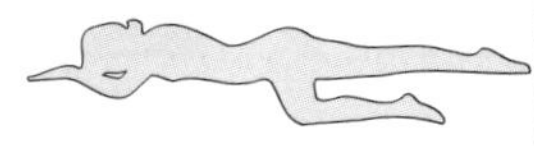

Correct:
Lying on side with knees bent effectively flattens the back. Flat pillow may be used to support neck, especially when shoulders are broad.

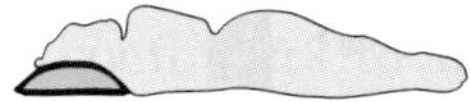

Sleeping on back is restful and correct when knees are properly supported.

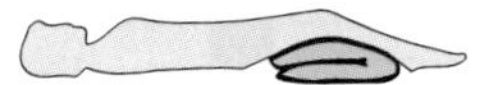

Raise the foot of the mattress eight inches to discourage sleeping on the abdomen.

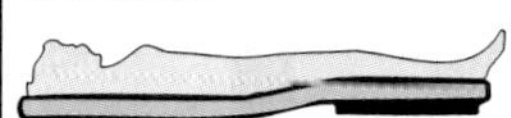

Proper arrangement of pillows for resting or reading in bed.

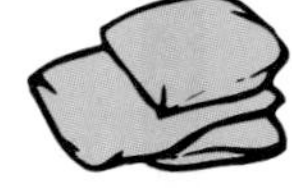

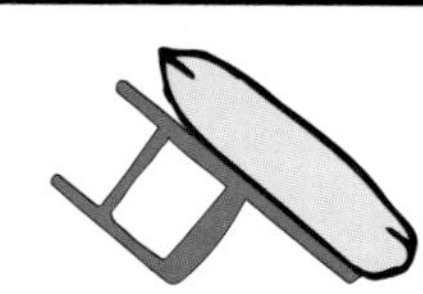

A straight-back chair used behind a pillow makes a serviceable backrest.

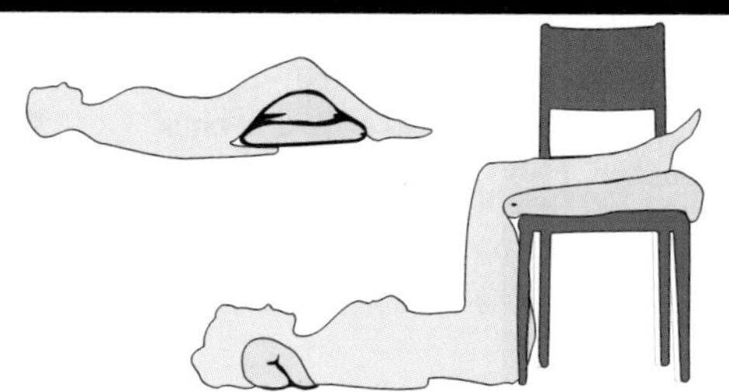

WHEN DOING NOTHING, DO IT RIGHT

Rest is the first rule for the tired, painful back. The following positions relieve pain by taking all pressure and weight off the back and legs.

Note pillows under knees to relieve strain on spine.

For complete relief and relaxing effect, these positions should be maintained from 5 to 25 minutes.

EXERCISE — WITHOUT GETTING OUT OF BED Exercises to be performed while lying in bed are aimed not so much at strengthening muscles as at teaching correct positioning. But muscles used correctly become stronger and in time are able to support the body with the least amount of effort.

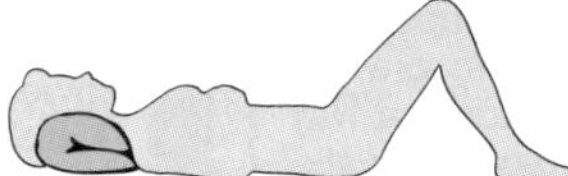

Do all exercises in this position. Legs should not be straightened.

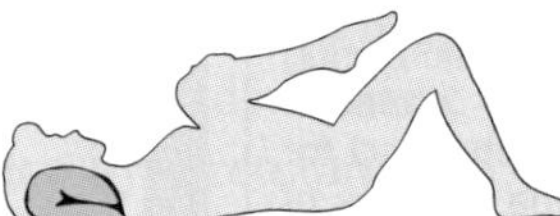

Bring knee up to chest. Lower slowly but do not straighten leg. Relax. Repeat with each leg 10 times.

EXERCISE — WITHOUT ATTRACTING ATTENTION Use these inconspicuous exercises whenever you have a spare moment during the day, both to relax tension and improve the tone of important muscle groups.

1. Rotate shoulders, forward and backward.
2. Turn head slowly side to side.
3. Watch an imaginary plane take off, just below the right shoulder. Stretch neck, follow it slowly as it moves up, around and down, disappearing below the other shoulder. Repeat, starting on left side.
4. Slowly, slowly, touch left ear to left shoulder, right ear to right shoulder. Raise both shoulders to touch ears, drop them as far down as possible.
5. At any pause in the day — waiting for an elevator to arrive, for a specific traffic light to change — pull in abdominal muscles, tighten, hold it for the count of eight without breathing. Relax slowly. Increase the count gradually after the first week, practice breathing normally with the abdomen flat and contracted. Do this sitting, standing, and walking.

Bring both knees slowly up to chest. Tighten muscles of abdomen, press back flat against bed. Hold knees to chest 20 seconds, then lower slowly. Relax. Repeat 5 times. This exercise gently stretches the shortened muscles of the lower back, while strengthening abdominal muscles. Clasp knees, bring them up to chest, at the same time coming to a sitting position. Rock back and forth.

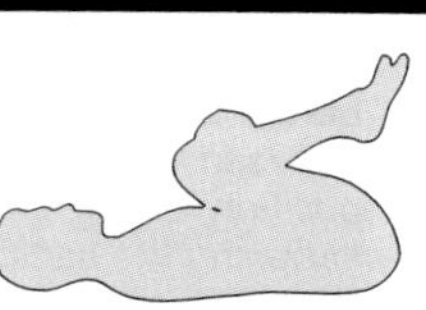

RULES TO LIVE BY - FROM NOW ON

1. Never bend from the waist only; bend the hips and knees.
2. Never lift a heavy object higher than your waist.
3. Always turn and face the object you wish to lift.
4. Avoid carrying unbalanced loads; hold heavy objects close to your body.
5. Never carry anything heavier than you can manage with ease.
6. Never lift or move heavy furniture. Wait for someone to do it who knows the principles of leverage.
7. Avoid sudden movements, sudden "overloading" of muscles. Learn to move deliberately, swinging the legs from the hips.
8. Learn to keep the head in line with the spine, when standing, sitting, lying in bed.
9. Put soft chairs and deep couches on your "don't sit" list. During prolonged sitting, cross your legs to rest your back.
10. Your doctor is the only one who can determine when low back pain is due to faulty posture. He is the best judge of when you may do general exercises for physical fitness. when you do, omit any exercise which arches or overstrains the lower back: backward bends, or forward bends, touching the toes with the knees straight.
11. Wear shoes with moderate heels, all about the same height. Avoid changing from high to low heels.
12. Put a footrail under the desk, and a footrest under the crib.
13. Diaper the baby sitting next to him or her on the bed.
14. Don't stoop and stretch to hand the wash; raise the clothesbasket and lower the washline.
15. Beg or buy a rocking chair. Rocking rests the back by changing the muscle groups used.
16. Train yourself vigorously to use your abdominal muscles to flatten your lower abdomen. In time, this muscle contraction will become habitual, making you the envied possessor of a youthful body-profile!
17. Don't strain to open windows or doors.
18. For good posture, concentrate on strengthening "nature's corset" — the abdominal and buttock muscles. The pelvic roll exercise is especially recommended to correct the postural relation between the pelvis and the spine.

Figure 10.3 Continued.

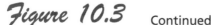

Flexibility Exercises

1

Lateral Head Tilt

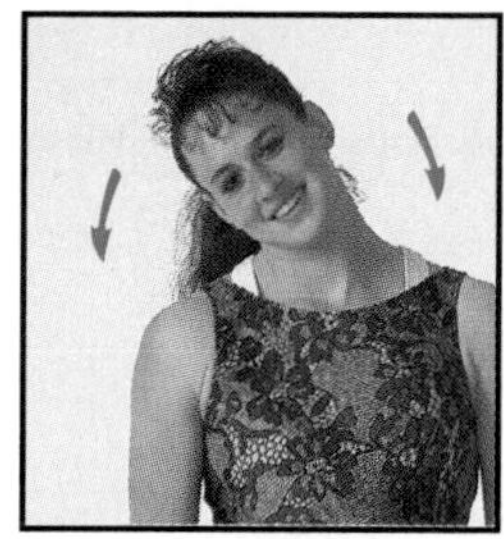

Action Slowly and gently tilt the head laterally. Repeat several times to each side.

Areas Stretched Neck flexors and extensors and ligaments of the cervical spine.

2

Arm Circles

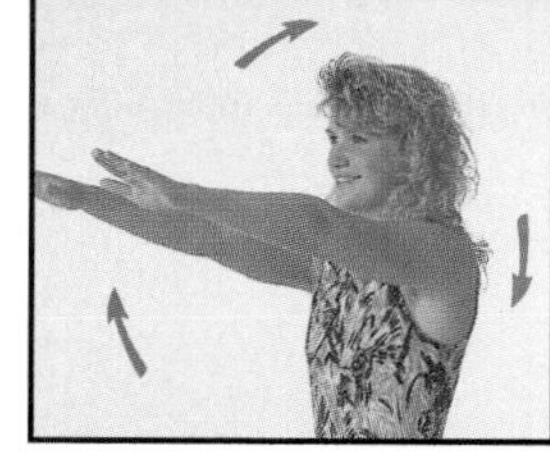

Action Gently circle your arms all the way around. Conduct the exercise in both directions.

Areas Stretched Shoulder muscles and ligaments.

3

Side Stretch

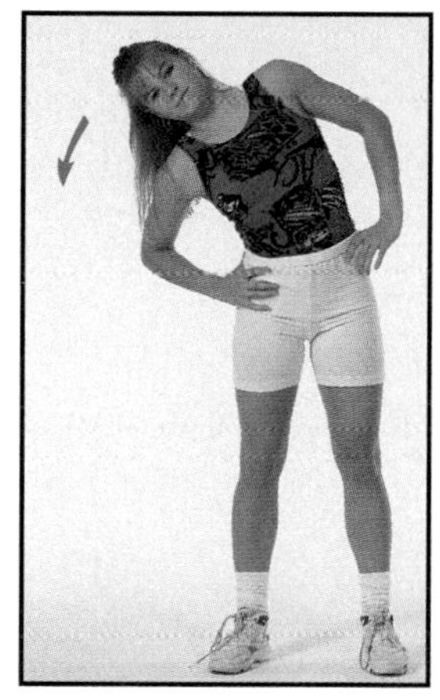

Action Stand straight up, feet separated to shoulder width, and place your hands on your waist. Now move the upper body to one side and hold the final stretch for a few seconds. Repeat on the other side.

Areas Stretched Muscles and ligaments in the pelvic region.

4

Body Rotation

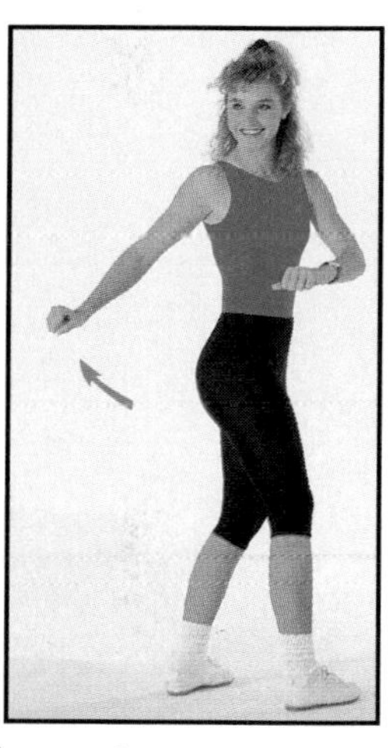

Action Place your arms slightly away from your body ,and rotate the trunk as far as possible, holding the final position for several seconds. Conduct the exercise for both the right and left sides of the body. You also can perform this exercise by standing about 2 feet away from the wall (back toward the wall) and then rotating the trunk, placing the hands against the wall.

Areas Stretched Hip, abdominal, chest, back, neck, and shoulder muscles; hip and spinal ligaments.

5

Chest Stretch

Action Kneel down behind a chair and place both hands on the back of the chair. Gradually push your chest downward and hold for a few seconds.

Areas Stretched Chest (pectoral) muscles and shoulder ligaments.

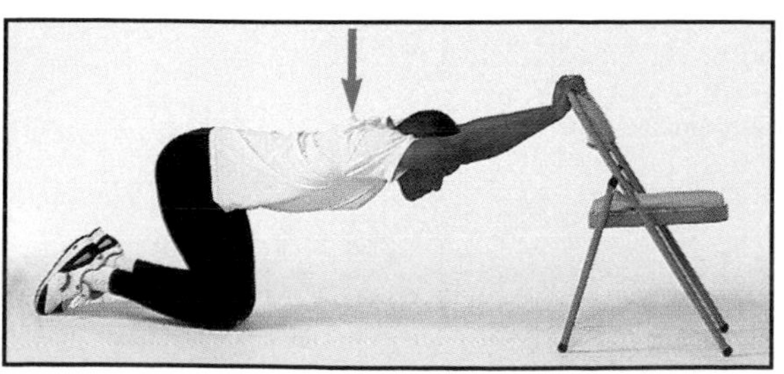

6

Shoulder Hyperextension Stretch

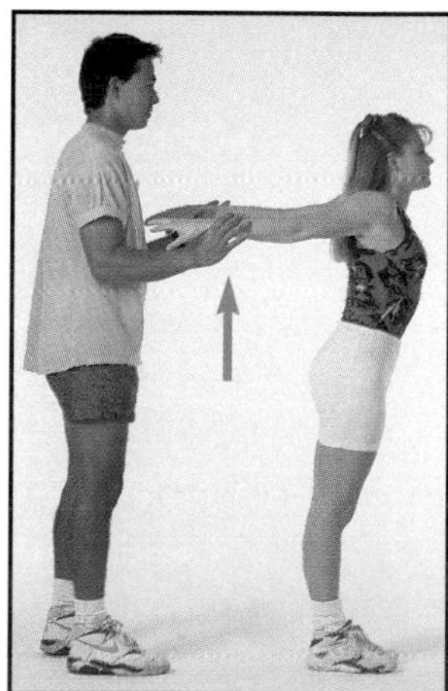

Action Have a partner grasp your arms from behind by the wrists and slowly push them upward. Hold the final position for a few seconds.

Areas Stretched Deltoid and pectoral muscles, and ligaments of the shoulder joint.

7

Shoulder Rotation Stretch

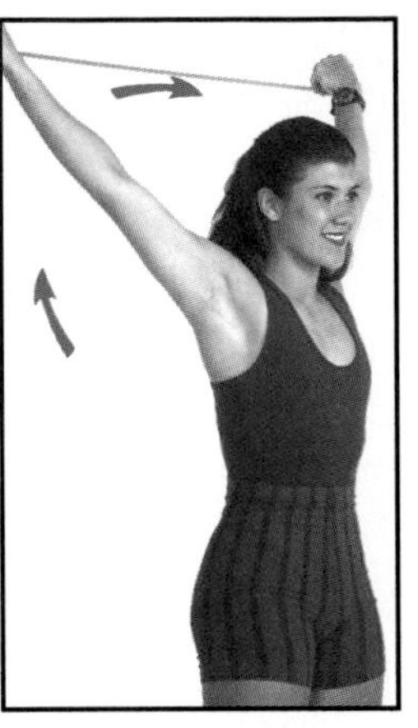

Action With the aid of surgical tubing or an aluminum or wood stick, place the tubing or stick behind your back and grasp the two ends using a reverse (thumbs-out) grip. Slowly bring the tubing or stick over your head, keeping the elbows straight. Repeat several times (bring the hands closer together for additional stretch).

Areas Stretched Deltoid, latissimus dorsi, and pectoral muscles; shoulder ligaments.

8

Quad Stretch

Action Lie on your side and move one foot back by flexing the knee. Grasp the front of the ankle and pull the ankle toward the gluteal region. Hold for several seconds. Repeat with the other leg.

Areas Stretched Quadriceps muscle, and knee and ankle ligaments.

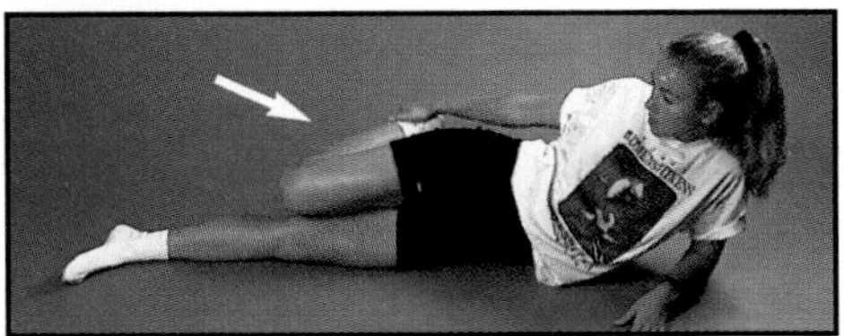

9

Heel Cord Stretch

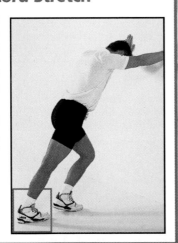

Action Stand against the wall or at the edge of a step, and stretch the heel downward, alternating legs. Hold the stretched position for a few seconds.

Areas Stretched Heel cord (Achilles tendon), gastrocnemius and soleus muscles.

10

Adductor Stretch

Action Stand with your feet about twice shoulder width and place your hands slightly above the knee. Flex one knee and slowly go down as far as possible, holding the final position for a few seconds. Repeat with the other leg.

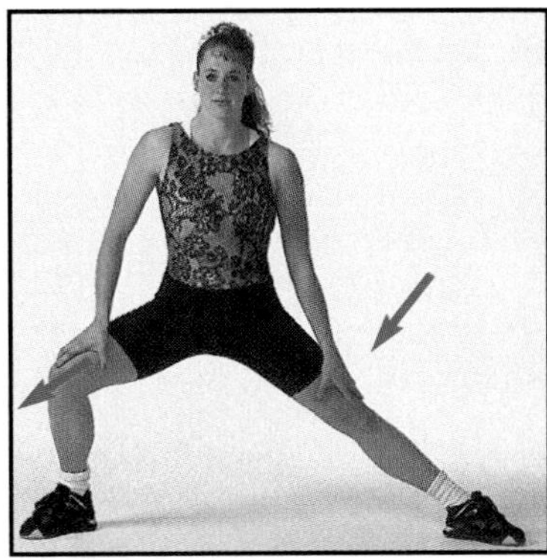

Areas Stretched Hip adductor muscles.

11

Sitting Adductor Stretch

Action Sit on the floor and bring your feet in close to you, allowing the soles of the feet to touch each other. Now place your forearms (or elbows) on the inner part of the thigh and push the legs downward, holding the final stretch for several seconds.

Areas Stretched Hip adductor muscles.

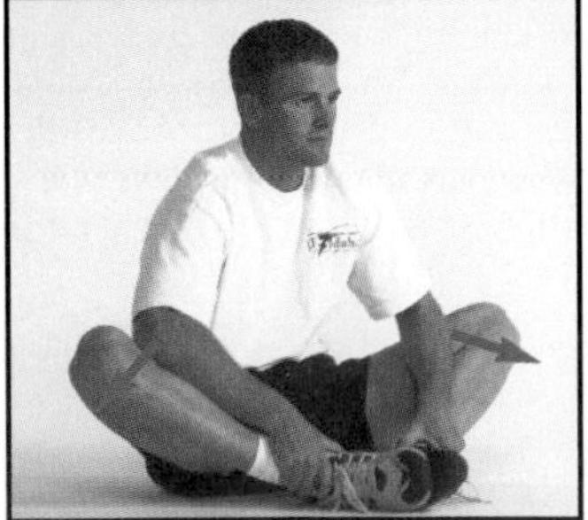

12

Sit-and-Reach Stretch

Action Sit on the floor with legs together and gradually reach forward as far as possible. Hold the final position for a few seconds. This exercise also may be performed with the legs separated, reaching to each side as well as to the middle.

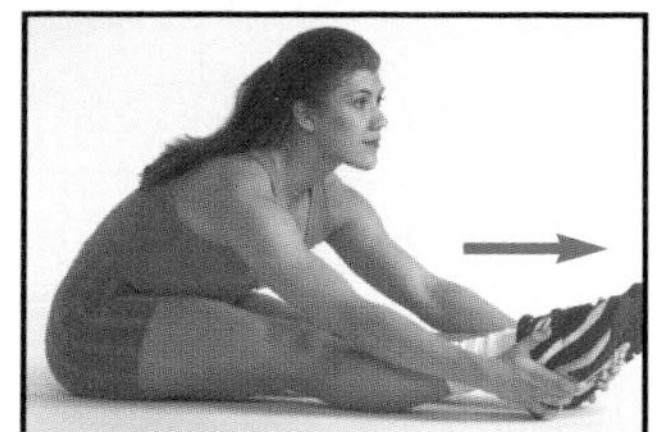

Areas Stretched Hamstrings and lower back muscles, and lumbar spine ligaments.

13

Triceps Stretch

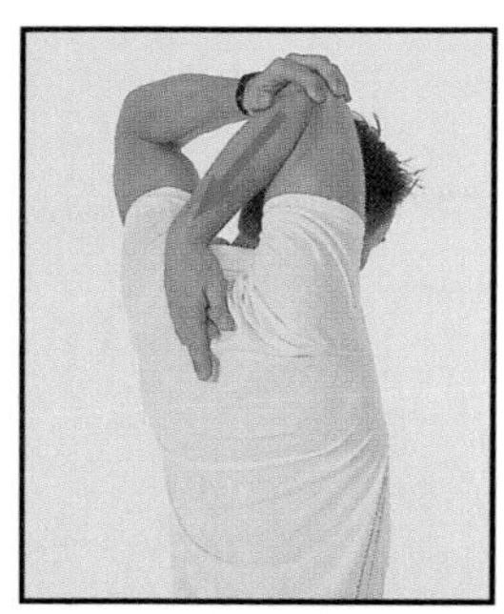

Action Place the right hand behind your neck. Grasp the right arm above the elbow with the left hand. Gently pull the elbow backward. Repeat the exercise with the opposite arm.

Areas Stretched Back of upper arm (triceps muscle) and shoulder joint.

Exercises for the Prevention and Rehabilitation of Low-Back Pain

14

Single-Knee to Chest Stretch

Action Lie down flat on the floor. Bend one leg at approximately 100° and gradually pull the opposite leg toward your chest. Hold the final stretch for a few seconds. Switch legs and repeat the exercise.

Areas Stretched Lower back and hamstring muscles, and lumbar spine ligaments.

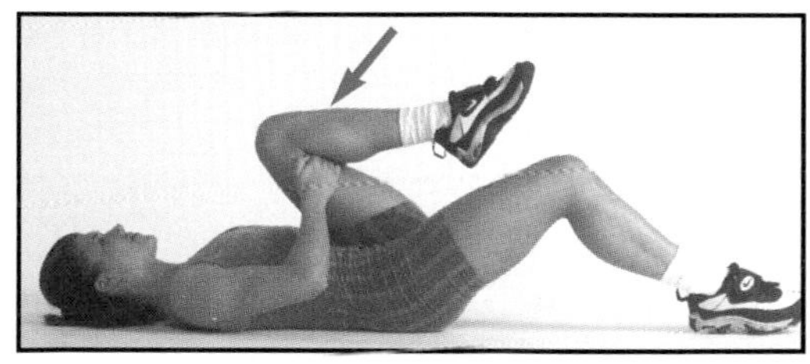

15

Double-Knee to Chest Stretch

Action Lie flat on the floor and then curl up slowly into a fetal position. Hold for a few seconds.

Areas Stretched Upper and lower back and hamstring muscles; spinal ligaments.

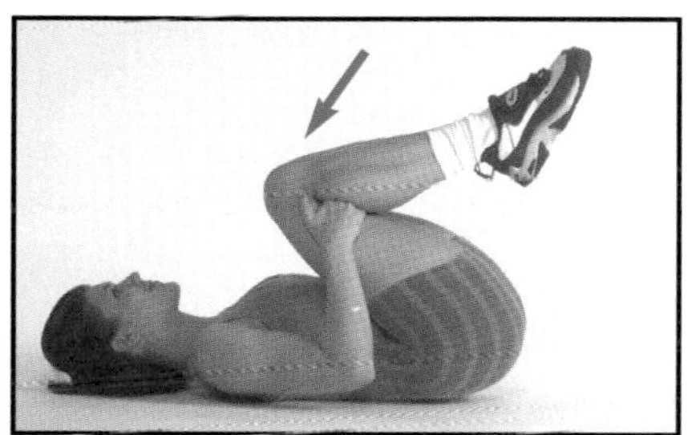

16

Upper and Lower Back Stretch

Action Sit on the floor and bring your feet in close to you, allowing the soles of the feet to touch each other. Holding on to your feet, bring your head and upper chest gently toward your feet.

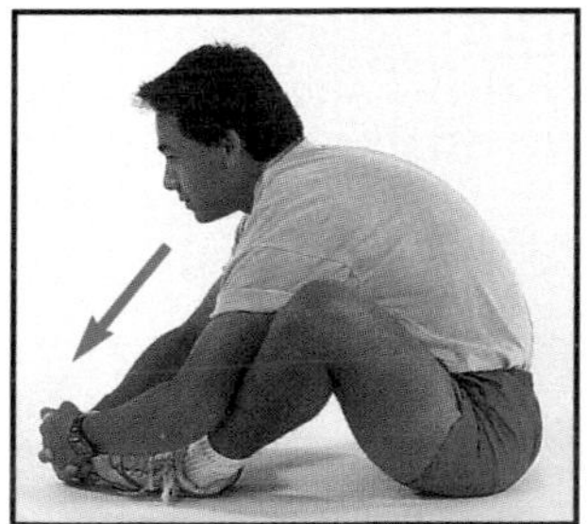

Areas Stretched Upper and lower back muscles and ligaments

17

Sit-and-Reach Stretch

(see Exercise 12 above)

10

18

Gluteal Stretch

Action Sit on the floor, bend your right leg and place your right ankle slightly above the left knee. Grasp the left thigh with both hands and gently pull the leg toward your chest. Repeat the exercise with the opposite leg.

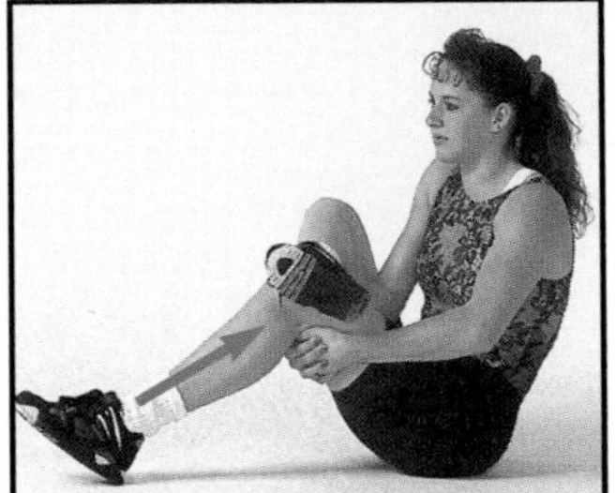

Areas Stretched Buttock area (gluteal muscles).

19

Back Extension Stretch

Action Lie face down on the floor with the elbows by the chest, forearms on the floor, and the hands beneath the chin. Gently raise the trunk by extending the elbows until you reach an approximate 90° angle at the elbow joint. Be sure the forearms remain in contact with the floor at all times. DO NOT extend the back beyond this point. Hyperextension of the lower back may lead to or aggravate an existing back problem. Hold the stretched position for about 10 seconds.

Areas Stretched Abdominal region.

Additional Benefits Restore lower back curvature.

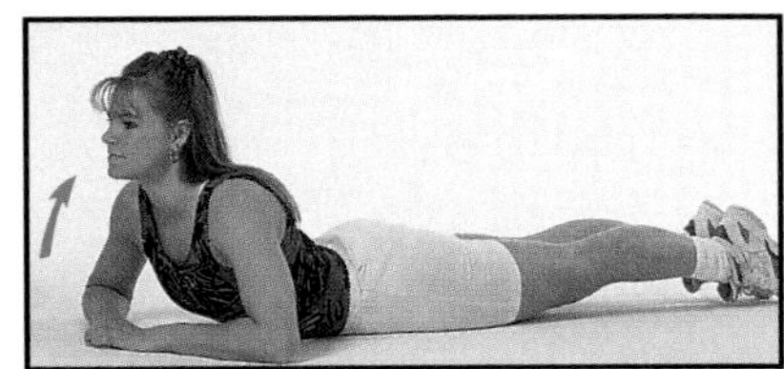

20

Trunk Rotation and Lower Back Stretch

Action Sit on the floor and bend the right leg, placing the right foot on the outside of the left knee. Place the left elbow on the right knee and push against it. At the same time, try to rotate the trunk to the right (clockwise). Hold the final position for a few seconds. Repeat the exercise with the other side.

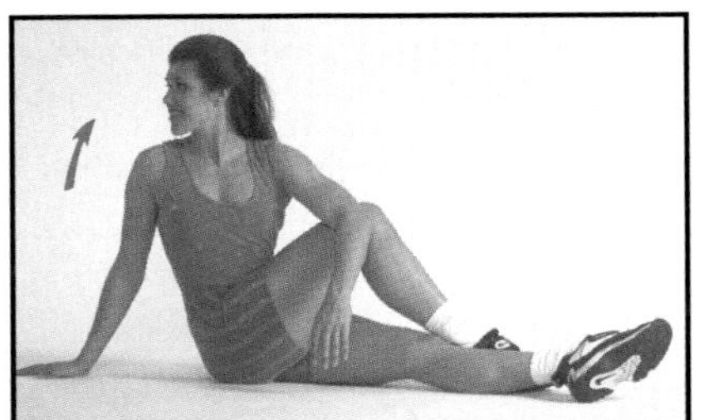

Areas Stretched Lateral side of the hip and thigh; trunk and lower back.

21

Pelvic Tilt

(see Exercise 12 in Chapter 8, page 156)

Note:

This is perhaps the most important exercise for the care of the lower back. It should be included as a part of the your daily exercise routine and should be performed several times throughout the day when pain in the lower back is present as a result of muscle imbalance.

10

22

Cat Stretch

Action Kneel on the floor and place your hands in front of you (on the floor) about shoulder width apart. Relax your trunk and lower back (a). Now arch the spine and pull in your abdomen as far as you can and hold this position for a few seconds (b). Repeat the exercise 4–5 times.

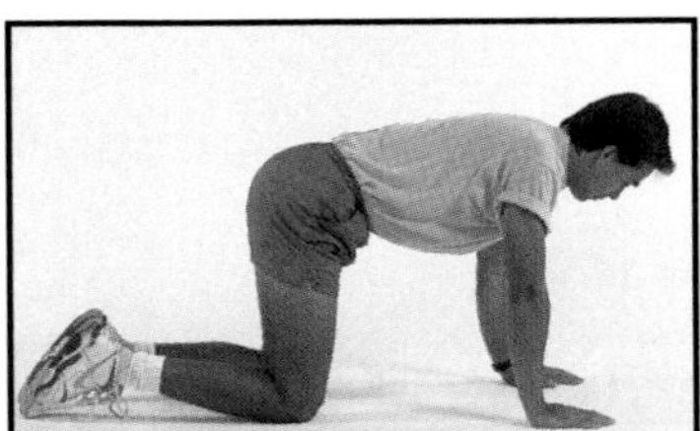

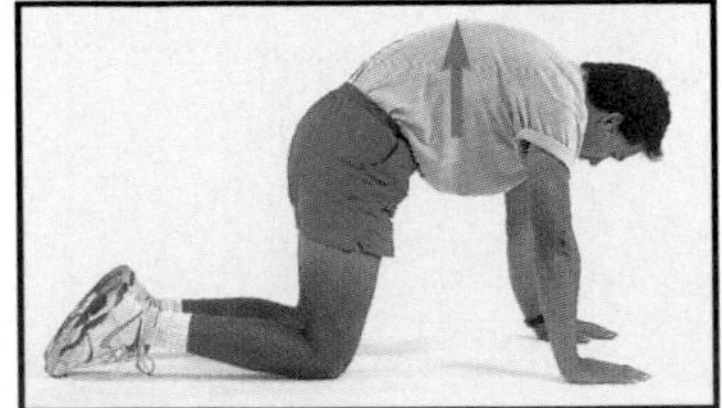

Areas Stretched Low back muscles and ligaments.

Areas Strengthened Abdominal and gluteal muscles.

23

Abdominal Crunch or Abdominal Curl-Up

(see Exercise 4 in Chapter 8, page 154)

It is important that you do not stabilize your feet when performing either of these exercises, because doing so decreases the work of the abdominal muscles. Also, remember not to "swing up" but, rather, to curl up as you perform these exercises.

Skill-Related Components of Physical Fitness

11

Skill-related fitness is important for successful motor performance in athletic events and in lifetime sports and activities such as basketball, racquetball, golf, hiking, soccer, and water skiing. Good **skill-related fitness** also enhances overall quality of life by helping people cope more effectively in emergency situations.

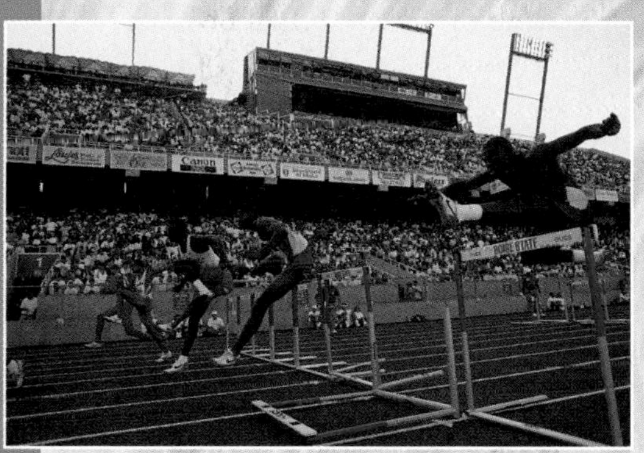

Outstanding gymnasts, for example, must achieve good skill-related fitness in all components. A significant amount of agility is necessary to perform a double back somersault with a full twist — a skill during which the athlete must simultaneously rotate around one axis and twist around a different one. Static balance is essential for maintaining a handstand or a scale. Dynamic balance is needed to perform many of the gymnastics routines (such as balance beam, parallel bars, and pommel horse). Coordination is important to successfully integrate various skills requiring varying degrees of difficulty into one routine. Power and speed are needed to propel the body into the air, such as when tumbling or vaulting. Reaction time is necessary in determining when to end rotation upon a visual clue, such as spotting the floor on a dismount.

LABS

As with the health-related fitness components, the principle of specificity of training applies to skill-related components. In the case of agility, balance, coordination,

Objectives

- Learn the benefits of good skill-related fitness.
- Identify and define the six components of skill-related fitness.
- Become familiar with performance tests to assess skill-related fitness.

and reaction time, development of these components is highly task-specific. To develop a certain task or skill, the individual must practice that same task many times. There seems to be very little crossover learning effect.

For instance, properly practicing of a handstand (balance) will lead eventually to successfully performing the skill, but complete mastery of this skill does not ensure that the person will have immediate success when attempting to perform other static-balance positions in gymnastics. Power and speed may be improved with a specific strength-training program or frequent repetition of the specific task to be improved, or both.

The rate of learning in skill-related fitness varies from person to person, mainly because these components seem to be determined to a large extent by genetics. Individuals with good skill-related fitness tend to do better and learn faster when performing a wide variety of skills. Nevertheless, few individuals enjoy complete success in all skill-related components. Furthermore, though skill-related fitness can be enhanced with practice, improvements in reaction time and speed are limited and seem to be related primarily to genetic endowment.

To develop a given component, the training program must be specific to the type of development the individual is trying to achieve.

Although we do not know how much skill-related fitness is desirable, everyone should attempt to develop and maintain a better-than-average level. As pointed out earlier, this type of fitness is crucial for athletes, and it also enables one to lead a better and happier life. Improving skill-related fitness not only affords an individual more enjoyment and success in lifetime sports (for example, tennis, racquetball, basketball), but it also can help a person cope more effectively in emergency situations. Some of the benefits are as follows:

1. Good reaction time, balance, coordination, and agility can help you avoid a fall or break a fall and thereby minimize injury.
2. The ability to generate maximum force in a short time (power) may be crucial to ameliorate injury or even preserve life in a situation in which you may be called upon to lift a heavy object that has fallen on another person or even on yourself.
3. In our society, where the average lifespan continues to expand, maintaining speed can be especially important for elderly people. Many of these individuals and, for that matter, many unfit/overweight young people no longer have the speed they need to cross an intersection safely before the light changes for oncoming traffic.

Regular participation in a health-related fitness program can heighten performance of skill-related components, and vice versa. For example, significantly overweight people do not have good agility or speed. Because participating in aerobic and strength-training programs helps take off body fat, an overweight individual who loses weight through such an exercise program can improve agility and speed. A sound flexibility program decreases resistance to motion about body joints, which may increase agility, balance, and overall coordination. Improvements in strength definitely help develop power. On the other hand, people who have good skill-related fitness usually participate in lifetime sports and games, which in turn helps develop health-related fitness.

Performance Tests for Skill-Related Fitness

Several performance tests have been developed over the years to assess the various components of skill-related fitness. Results of the performance tests, expressed in percentile ranks, are given in Table 11.1 (men) and Table 11.2 (women), at the end of the chapter. Fitness categories for skill-fitness components are established according to percentile rankings only. The categories are similar to those given for muscular strength and endurance and for flexibility (see Table 11.3).

Agility

Agility is defined as *the ability to quickly and efficiently change body position and direction.* Agility is important in sports such as basketball, soccer, and racquetball, in which the participant must change direction rapidly and also maintain proper body control.

AGILITY TEST

SEMO Agility Test[1]

Objective

To measure general body agility

Procedure

The free-throw area of a basketball court or any other smooth area 12 by 19 feet with adequate

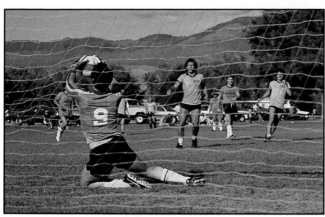

Successful soccer players demonstrate high levels of skill-fitness.

running space around it can be used for this test. Four plastic cones or similar objects are placed on each corner of the free-throw lane, as shown in Figure 11.1.

Start on the outside of the free-throw lane at point A, with your back to the free-throw line. When given the "go" command, sidestep from A to B (do not make crossover steps), backpedal from B to D, sprint forward from D to A, again backpedal from A to C, sprint forward from C to B, and sidestep from B to the finish line at A.

During the test, always go around (outside) each corner cone. A stopwatch is to be started at the "go" command and stopped when crossing the finish line. Use the best of two trials, preceded by a practice trial, as the final test score. Record the time to the nearest tenth of a second.

Figure 11.1 Graphic description of the SEMO test for agility.

Balance

The ability to maintain the body in proper equilibrium, **balance** is vital in activities such as gymnastics, diving, ice skating, skiing, and even football and wrestling, in which the athlete attempts to upset the opponent's equilibrium.

BALANCE TEST

1-Foot Stand Test (preferred foot, without shoes)

Objective

To measure static balance

Procedure

A flat, smooth floor, not carpeted, is used for this test. Remove your shoes and socks, and stand on your preferred foot, placing the other foot on the inside of the supporting knee and the hands on the sides of the hips. When the "go" command is given, raise your heel off the floor and balance yourself as long as possible without moving the ball of the foot from its initial position.

The test is terminated when any of the following conditions occur:

1. The supporting foot moves (shuffles).

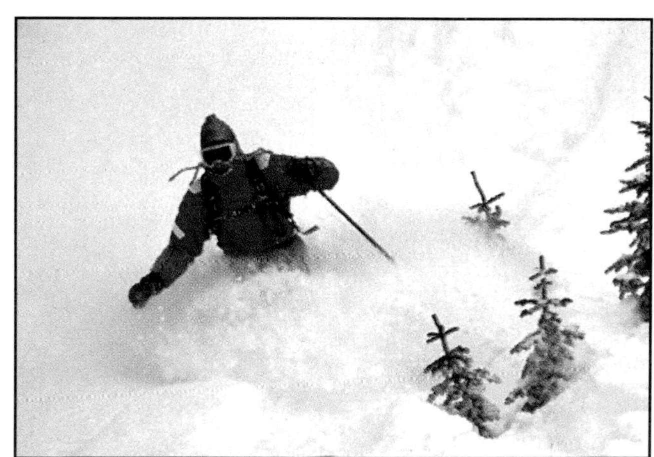

Nordic skiing requires good balance, a skill-related component of fitness.

Skill-related fitness Fitness components important for success in skillful activities and athletic events; encompasses agility, balance, coordination, power, reaction time, and speed.

Agility Ability to change body position and direction quickly and efficiently.

Balance Ability to maintain the body in proper equilibrium.

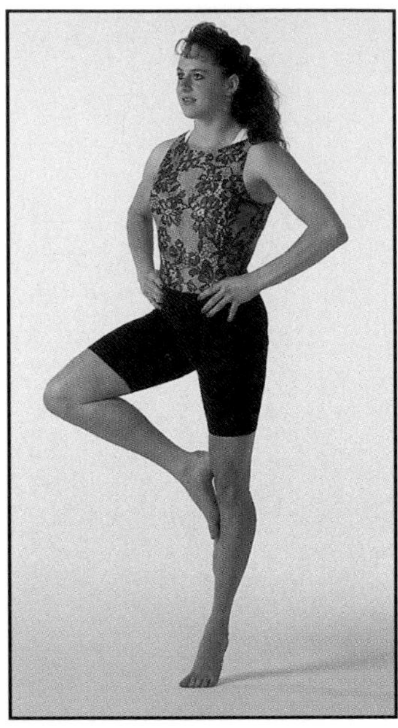

1-Foot Stand Test for balance.

2. The raised heel touches the floor.
3. The hands are moved from the hip.
4. A minute has elapsed.

The test is scored by recording the number of seconds balance is maintained on the selected foot, starting with the "go" command. The best of two trials, preceded by a practice trial, is used as the final performance score. Record the time to the nearest tenth of a second.

Coordination

Coordination can be defined as *the integration of the nervous and the muscular systems to produce correct, graceful, and harmonious body movements.* This component is important in a wide variety of motor activities such as golf, baseball, karate, soccer, and racquetball, in which hand-eye or foot-eye movements, or both, must be integrated.

11

COORDINATION TEST

Soda Pop Test

Objective

To assess overall motor/muscular control and movement time.

Procedure

Administrator: Homemade equipment is necessary to perform this test. Draw a straight line lengthwise through the center of a piece of cardboard approximately 32" long by 5" wide. Draw six marks exactly 5" away from each other on this line (draw the first mark about 2½" from the edge of the cardboard). Using a compass, draw six circles 3¼" in diameter (a radius of 1 centimeter larger than a can of soda pop), which must be centered on the six marks along the line.

For purpose of this test, each circle is assigned a number starting with 1 for the first circle on the right of the testee, all the way to 6 for the last circle on the left. The cardboard, three unopened (full) cans of soda pop, a table, a chair, and a stopwatch are needed to perform the test.

Place the cardboard on a table and have the person sit in front of it with the center of the cardboard bisecting the body. Use the preferred hand for this test. If this is the right hand, place the three cans of soda pop on the cardboard in the following manner: can 1 centered in circle 1 (farthest to the right), can 2 in circle 3, and can 3 in circle 5.

Participant: To start the test, place the right hand, with the thumb up, on can 1 and the elbow joint at about 100°–120°. When the tester gives the signal and the stopwatch is started, proceed to turn the cans of soda pop upside down, placing can 1 inside circle 2, followed by can 2 inside circle 4, and then can 3 inside circle 6. Immediately return all three cans, starting with can 1, then can 2, and can 3, turning them right side up to their original placement. On this "return trip," grasp the cans with the hand in a thumb-down position.

The entire procedure is done twice, without stopping, and is counted as one trial. Two "trips" down and up are required to complete one trial. The watch is stopped when the last can of soda pop is returned to its original position, following the second trip back. The preferred hand (in this case, the right hand) is

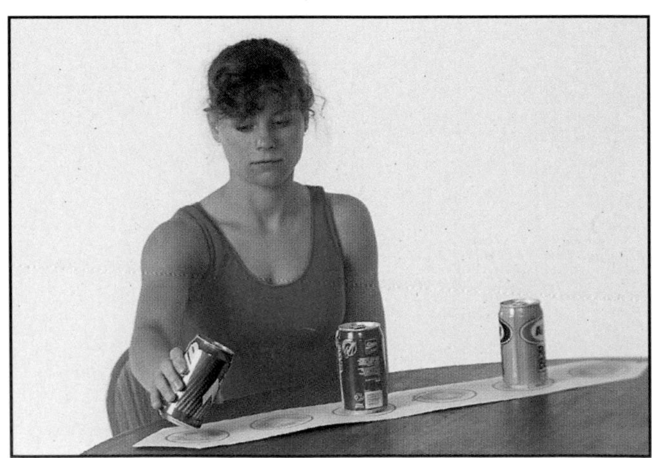

"Soda Pop" Test for coordination.

used throughout the entire task, and the object of the test is to perform the task as fast as possible, making sure the cans always are placed within each circle. If the person misses a circle at any time during the test (a can placed on a line or outside a circle), the trial must be repeated from the start. A graphic illustration of this test is provided in Figure 11.2.

If the participant chooses to use the left hand, the same procedure is followed, except the cans are placed starting from the left, with can 1 in circle 6, can 2 in circle 4, and can 3 in circle 2. The procedure is initiated by turning can 1 upside down onto circle 5, can 2 onto circle 3, and so on.

Two practice trials are allowed prior to initiating the test. Two test trials then are administered, and the best time, recorded to the nearest tenth of a second, is used as the test score. If the person has a mistrial (misses a circle), the test is repeated until two successful trials are accomplished.

Power

Power is defined as *the ability to produce maximum force in the shortest time.* The two components of **power** are speed and force (strength). An effective combination of these two components allows a person to produce explosive movements such as in jumping, putting the shot, and spiking/throwing/hitting a ball.

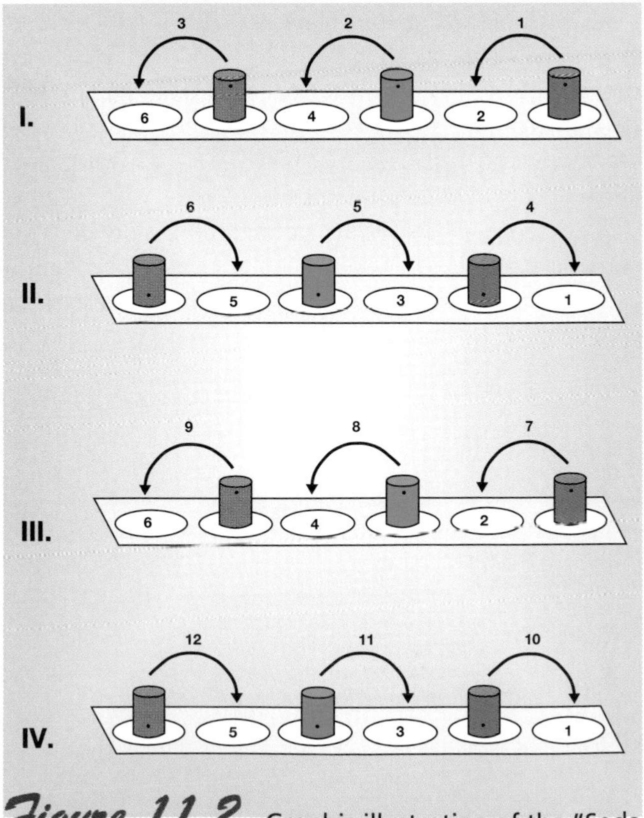

POWER TEST

Standing Long Jump Test[2]

Objective

To measure leg power

Procedure

Administrator: Draw a takeoff line on the floor, and place a 10-foot-long tape measure perpendicular to this line. Have the participant stand with feet several inches apart, centered with the tape measure and toes just behind the takeoff line (see Figure 11.3).

Participant: Prior to the jump, swing your arms backward and bend your knees. Perform the jump by extending your knees and swinging your arms forward at the same time.

The distance is recorded from the takeoff line to the heel or other body part that touches the floor nearest the takeoff line. Three trials are allowed, and the best trial, measured to the nearest inch, becomes the final test score.

Figure 11.2 Graphic illustration of the "Soda Pop" Test.

Reaction Time

Reaction time can be defined as *the time required to initiate a response to a given stimulus.* Good **reaction time** is important for starts in track and swimming, to react quickly when playing tennis at the net, or in sports such as ping pong, boxing, and karate.

REACTION TIME TEST

Yardstick Test (preferred hand)

Objective

To measure hand reaction time in response to a visual stimulus

Procedure

Administrator: For this test you will need a regular yardstick with a shaded "concentration zone" marked on the first 2" of the stick. Administer the test with

Coordination Integration of the nervous and the muscular systems to produce correct, graceful, and harmonious body movements.

Power The ability to produce maximum force in the shortest time.

Reaction time The time required to initiate a response to a given stimulus.

11

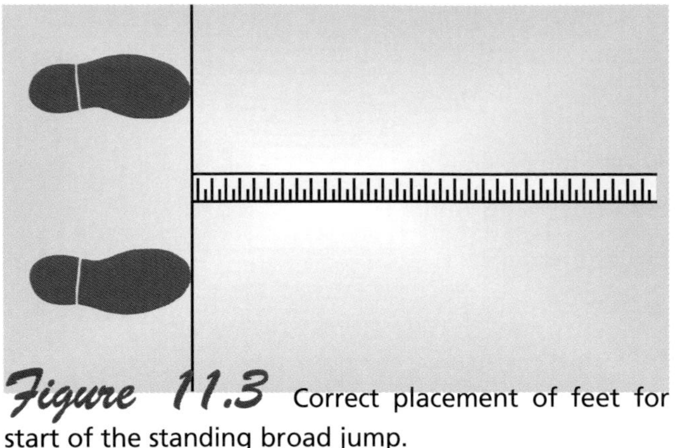

Figure 11.3 Correct placement of feet for start of the standing broad jump.

the participant sitting in a chair adjacent to a table and the preferred forearm and hand resting on the table.

Participant: Hold the tips of the thumb and fingers in a "ready-to-pinch" position, about 1" apart and 3" beyond the edge of the table, with the upper edges of the thumb and index finger parallel to the floor. With the person administering the test holding the yardstick near the end and the zero point of the stick even with the upper edge of your thumb and index finger (the administrator may steady the middle of the stick with the other hand), look at the "concentration zone" and react by catching the stick when it is dropped. Do not look at the administrator's hand or move it up or down while trying to catch the stick.

Twelve trials comprise the test, each preceded by the preparatory command "ready." The administrator makes a random 1– to 3–second count between the "ready" command and each drop of the stick. Each trial is scored to the nearest half inch, read just above the upper edge of the thumb. Three practice trials are given before the actual test to be sure the person understands the procedure. The three lowest and the three highest scores are discarded, and the average of the middle six is used as the final test score. The testing area should be as free from distractions as possible.

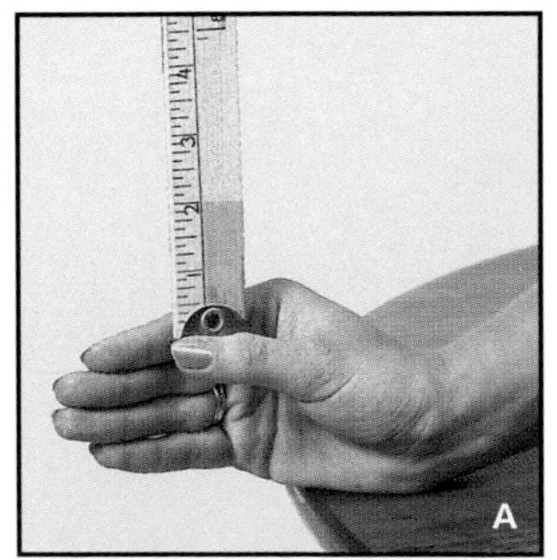

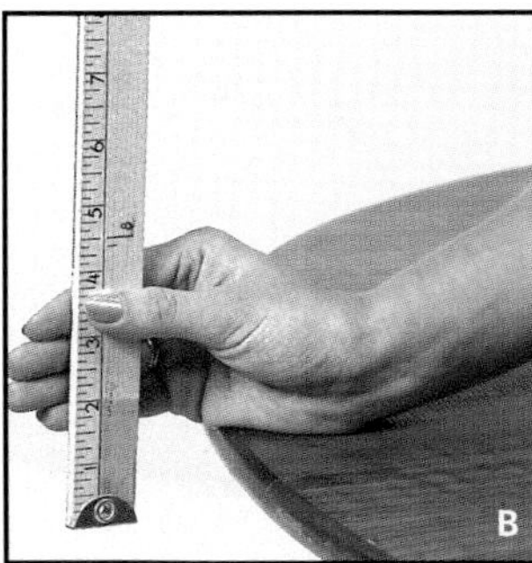

"Yardstick" Test for reaction time.

11

Speed

Speed is *the ability to rapidly propel the body or a part of the body from one point to another.* Sprints in track, stealing a base in baseball, soccer, and basketball are examples of activities that require good **speed** for success.

SPEED TEST

50-Yard Dash[3]

Objective

To measure speed

Procedure

Two participants are preferable. Take your positions behind the starting line. The starter raises one arm and says "Are you ready?" followed by the command "go" while simultaneously swinging an arm downward as a signal for the timer (or timers) who stands at the finish line to start the stopwatch (or stopwatches).

The score is the time that elapses between the starting signal and the moment the participant crosses the finish line, recorded to the nearest tenth of a second.

Speed The ability to propel the body or a part of the body rapidly from one point to another.

Table 11.1 Percentile Ranks and Fitness Classification for Skill-Related Fitness Components — Men

	Agility*	Balance*	Coordination*	Power**	Reaction Time*	Speed**
99	9.5	59.8	5.8	9'10"	3.5	5.4
95	10.3	46.9	7.5	8'5"	4.2	5.9
90	10.6	41.1	7.7	8'2"	4.5	6.0
80	11.1	24.9	8.5	7'10"	4.9	6.3
70	11.5	15.4	8.9	7'7"	5.3	6.4
60	11.7	12.0	9.3	7'5"	5.5	6.5
50	11.9	9.2	9.6	7'2"	5.8	6.6
40	12.1	7.3	9.9	7'0"	6.1	6.8
30	12.4	5.8	10.2	6'8"	6.5	7.0
20	12.9	4.3	10.7	6'4"	6.7	7.1
10	13.7	3.1	11.3	5'10"	7.2	7.5
5	14.0	2.6	11.8	5'3"	7.4	7.9

* Norms developed at Boise State University, Department of Physical Education. Research conducted by Werner W. K. Hoeger, Sherman G. Button, and Troy A. Palmer.
** From *AAHPERD Youth Fitness: Test Manual.* 1976. Reproduced with permission.

Table 11.2 Percentile Ranks and Fitness Classification for Skill-Related Fitness Components — Women

	Agility*	Balance*	Coordination*	Power**	Reaction Time*	Speed**
99	11.1	59.9	7.5	7'6"	3.3	6.4
95	12.0	39.1	8.0	6'9"	4.5	6.8
90	12.2	25.8	8.2	6'6"	4.7	7.0
80	12.5	16.7	8.6	6'2"	5.1	7.3
70	12.9	11.9	9.0	5'11"	5.3	7.5
60	13.2	9.8	9.2	5'9"	5.9	7.6
50	13.4	7.6	9.5	5'5"	6.1	7.9
40	13.9	6.2	9.6	5'3"	6.4	8.0
30	14.2	5.0	9.9	5'0"	6.7	8.2
20	14.8	4.2	10.3	4'9"	7.2	8.5
10	15.5	2.9	10.7	4'4"	7.8	9.0
5	16.2	1.8	11.2	4'1"	8.4	9.5

* Norms developed at Boise State University, Department of Physical Education. Research conducted by Werner W. K. Hoeger, Sherman G. Button, and Troy A. Palmer.
** From *AAHPERD Youth Fitness: Test Manual.* 1976. Reproduced with permission.

Table 11.3 Skill-Fitness Categories

Percentile Rank	Fitness Category
≥81	Excellent
61-80	Good
41-60	Average
21-40	Fair
≤20	Poor

Laboratory Experience

LAB 11A
Assessment of Skill-Related Components of Fitness

Lab Preparation
Bring exercise clothing, including running shoes. Do not exercise strenuously several hours prior to this lab.

11

Notes

1. Kirby, R. F., "A Simple Test of Agility," *Coach and Athlete* (June 1971), 30–31.
2. American Association of Health, Physical Education, Recreation and Dance (AAHPERD), *Youth Fitness: Test Manual* (Reston, VA: AAHPERD, 1976.)
3. AAHPERD.

Suggested Readings

American Association of Health, Physical Education, Recreation and Dance (AAHPERD), *Youth Fitness: Test Manual*. Reston, VA: AAHPERD, 1976.

Kirby, R. F. "A Simple Test of Agility." *Coach and Athlete* (June 1971), 30–31.

A Healthy Lifestyle Approach

12

Most people recognize that participating in fitness programs improves their quality of life. In recent years, however, we came to realize that improving physical fitness alone was not always sufficient to lower the risk for disease and ensure better health.

For example, individuals who run 3 miles (about 5 km) a day, lift weights regularly, participate in stretching exercises, and watch their body weight easily can be classified as having good or excellent fitness. If these same people, however, have high blood pressure, smoke, are under constant stress, consume alcohol excessively, and eat too many fatty foods, they are at risk for cardiovascular disease and may not be aware of these **risk factors.**

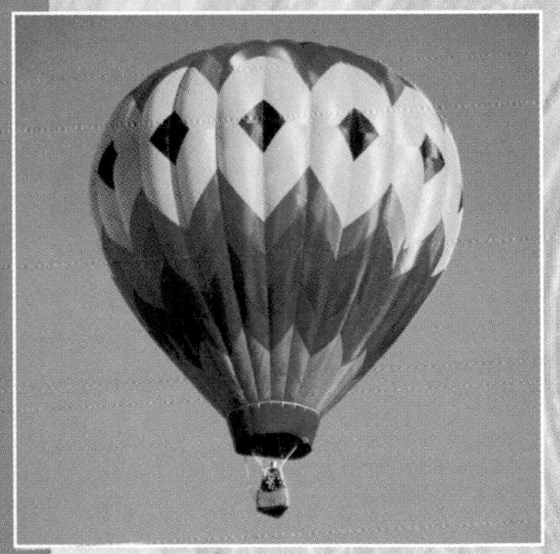

One of the best examples that good fitness does not always provide a risk-free guarantee of a healthy and productive life was the tragic death in 1984 of Jim Fixx, author of the best selling book The Complete Book of Running. At the time of his death by heart attack, Fixx was 52 years old. He been running between 60 and 80 miles a week and had believed that people at his high level of fitness could not die from heart disease.

At age 36, Jim Fixx smoked two packs of cigarettes per day, weighed about 215 pounds, did not participate in regular physical activity, and had a family

LABS

Objectives

- Learn the importance of implementing a healthy lifestyle program.
- Understand the major factors for coronary heart disease.
- Become acquainted with cancer-prevention guidelines.
- Learn how to cope with stress.
- Recognize the relationship between spirituality and wellness.
- Learn the health consequences of chemical abuse and irresponsible sex.

history of heart disease. His father, having had a first heart attack at age 35, later died at age 43.

Perhaps in an effort to lessen his risk for heart disease, Fixx began to raise his level of fitness. He started to jog, lost 50 pounds, and quit cigarette smoking. On several occasions, though, Fixx declined to have an exercise electrocardiogram (ECG) test, which most likely would have revealed his cardiovascular problem. His unfortunate death is a tragic example that exercise programs by themselves will not make high-risk people immune to heart disease, though they may delay the onset of a serious or fatal problem.

Good health, therefore, no longer is viewed as simply the absence of illness. The notion of good health has evolved notably in the last few years and continues to change as scientists learn more about lifestyle factors that bring on illness and affect wellness. Once the idea took hold that fitness by itself would not always decrease the risk for disease and ensure better health, a new wellness concept developed in the 1980s.

The term **wellness** is an all-inclusive umbrella covering a variety of activities aimed at helping individuals recognize components of lifestyle that are detrimental to their health. Wellness living requires implementing positive programs to change behavior to improve health and quality of life, prolong life, and achieve total well-being.

To enjoy a wellness lifestyle, a person needs to practice behaviors that will lead to positive outcomes in the five dimensions of wellness: physical, emotional, intellectual, social, and spiritual (see Figure 12.1). These dimensions are interrelated; one dimension frequently affects the others. For example, a person who is "emotionally down" often has no desire to exercise, study, socialize with friends, or attend church.

In looking at the five dimensions of wellness, high level wellness clearly goes beyond the absence of disease and optimal fitness. Wellness incorporates factors such as adequate fitness, proper nutrition, stress management, disease prevention, spirituality, smoking cessation, personal safety, substance abuse control, regular physical examinations, health education, and environmental support (see Figure 12.2).

For a wellness way of life, not only must individuals be physically fit and manifest no signs of disease, but they also must have no risk factors for disease (such as hypertension, hyperlipidemia, cigarette smoking, negative stress, faulty nutrition, careless sex). Even though an individual tested in a fitness center may demonstrate adequate or even excellent fitness, indulging in unhealthy lifestyle behaviors still will increase the risk for chronic diseases and decrease the person's well-being.

Consequently, our biggest challenge at the end of this century is to learn how to take control of our personal health habits by engaging in positive lifestyle activities. To help you achieve this goal, researchers have pointed out 10 simple lifestyle habits that can increase health and longevity significantly:

1. Participate in a lifetime exercise program.
2. Do not smoke cigarettes.

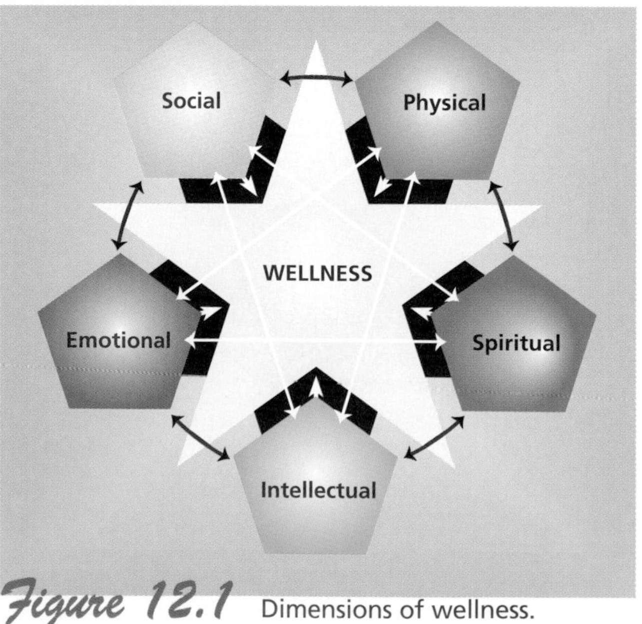

Figure 12.1 Dimensions of wellness.

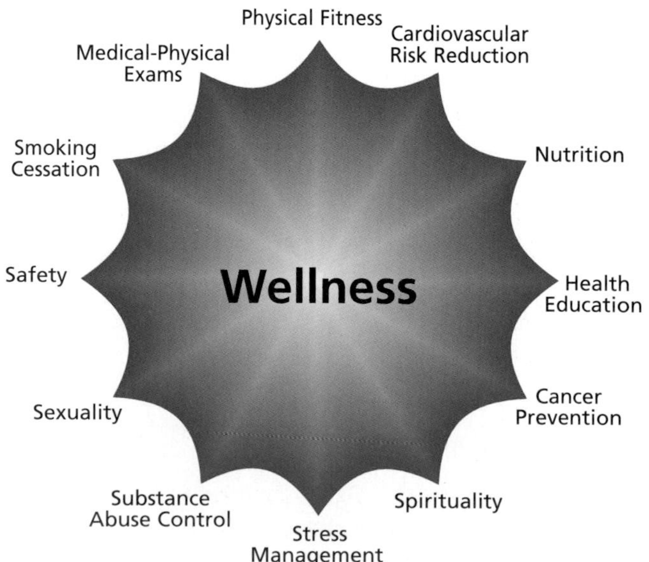

Figure 12.2 Wellness components.

12

3. Eat a balanced diet.
4. Maintain recommended body weight.
5. Sleep 7 to 8 hours each night.
6. Decrease stress levels.
7. Drink alcohol moderately or not at all.
8. Surround yourself with healthy relationships.
9. Be informed about the environment and avoid environmental risk factors.
10. Take personal safety measures.

Major Health Problems in the United States

Of all deaths in the United States, 66% are caused by cardiovascular disease and cancer.[1] Close to 80% of these deaths could be prevented by a healthy lifestyle program. The third and fourth leading causes of death, chronic and obstructive pulmonary disease and accidents, also are preventable, primarily by abstaining from tobacco and other drugs, wearing seat belts, and using common sense.

In looking at the underlying causes of death in the United States, estimates[2] indicate that 9 of the 10 causes are related to lifestyle and lack of common sense (see Figure 12.3). The "big four" — tobacco use, poor diet, inactivity, and alcohol abuse — are responsible for more than 800,000 annual deaths.

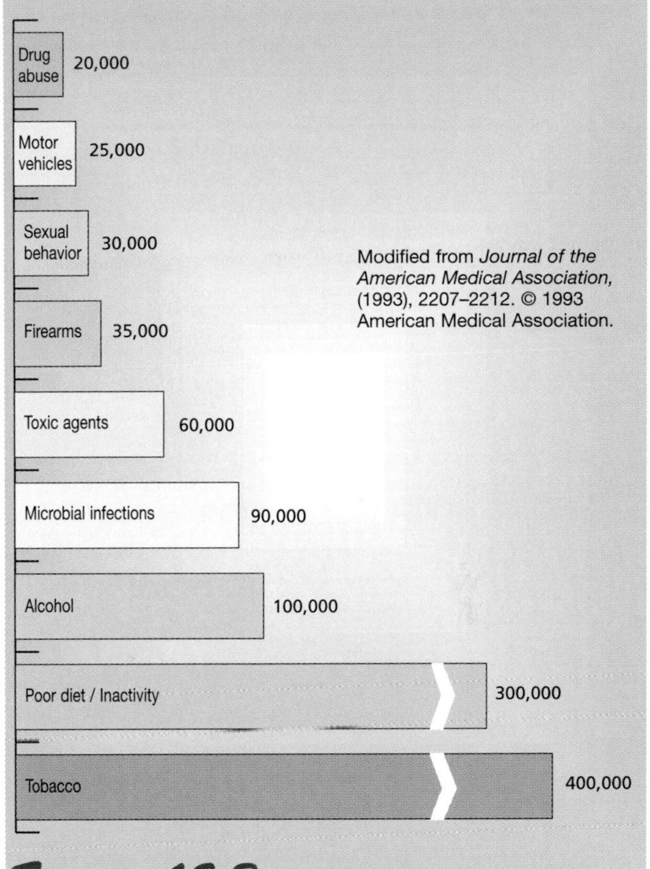

Figure 12.3 Underlying causes of death in the United States.

Cardiovascular Diseases

The most prevalent degenerative conditions in the United States are **cardiovascular diseases.** One in six men and one in eight women age 45 and older have had a heart attack or stroke.[3] Based on 1992 vital statistics, 42% of all deaths in the United States were attributable to heart and blood vessel disease.[4] Some examples of cardiovascular diseases are coronary heart disease, peripheral vascular disease, congenital heart disease, rheumatic heart disease, atherosclerosis, strokes, high blood pressure, and congestive heart failure. Table 12.1 provides the estimated prevalence and annual number of deaths caused by the major types of cardiovascular disease.

According to the American Heart Association, the estimated cost of heart and blood vessel disease in the United States exceeded $135 billion in 1994. More than 1.5 million people have heart attacks each year, and over half a million of them die as a result. About half the time the first symptom of coronary heart disease is the heart attack itself. In one of every five cardiovascular deaths, sudden death is the initial symptom. About half of those who die are men in their most productive years of life — between ages 40 and 65.

Although heart and blood vessel disease is still the number-one health problem in the United States, the incidence has declined by 36% in the last two decades (see Figure 12.4). The main reason for this dramatic decrease is health education. More people now are aware of the risk factors for cardiovascular disease and are changing their lifestyle to lower their potential risk for this disease.

The heart and the coronary arteries are illustrated in Figure 12.5 The major form of cardiovascular

Risk factors Lifestyle and genetic variables that may lead to disease.

Wellness The constant and deliberate effort to stay healthy and achieve the highest potential for well-being.

Cardiovascular diseases Diseases that affect the heart and the blood vessels.

12

Table 12.1 Estimated Prevalence and Yearly Number of Deaths from Cardiovascular Disease in United States, 1992

	Prevalence	Deaths
Major forms of cardiovascular diseases*	58,920,000	925,079
Coronary heart disease	11,200,000**	
Heart attack	1,500,000	480,170
Stroke	3,080,000	143,640
High blood pressure	50,000,000	35,830
Rheumatic heart disease	1,350,000	5,960

*Includes people with one or more forms of cardiovascular disease.
**Number of deaths included under heart attack.

Source: American Heart Association, *Heart and Stroke Facts: 1995* (Statistical Supplement) (Dallas: AHA, 1994).

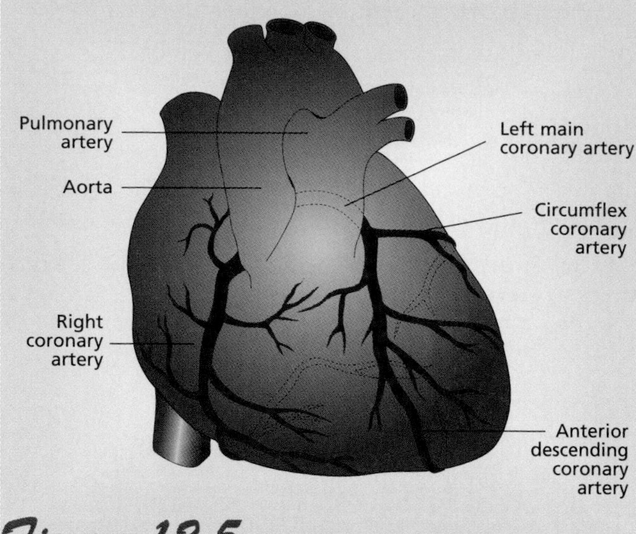

Figure 12.5 The heart and its blood vessels.

disease is **coronary heart disease (CHD)**. Heart attack, angina pectoris, and sudden cardiac death are all included under CHD. Narrowing of the coronary arteries diminishes the blood supply to the heart muscle, which can precipitate a heart attack. CHD is the single leading cause of death in the United States, accounting for approximately a third of all deaths and more than half of all cardiovascular deaths.

The leading contributors to the development of CHD are:

- Physical inactivity
- Low HDL-cholesterol
- High LDL-cholesterol
- Smoking
- High **blood pressure**
- Abnormal electrocardiograms (ECG)
- Personal and family history of cardiovascular disease
- Diabetes
- Excessive body fat
- Elevated triglycerides
- Tension and stress
- Gender
- Age

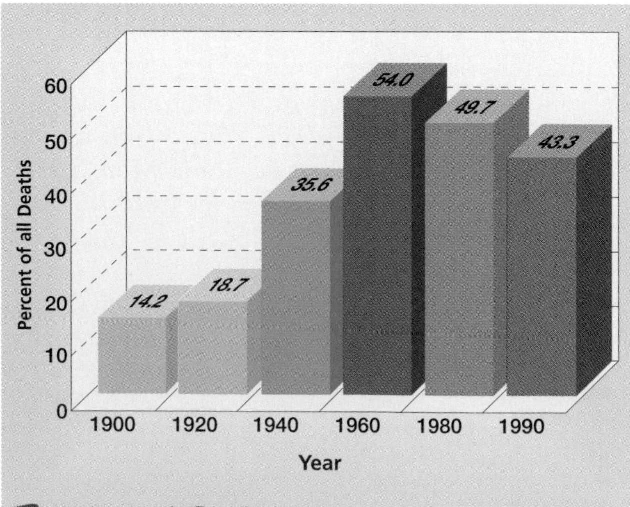

Figure 12.4 Incidence of cardiovascular disease in the United States for selected years.

An important concept in CHD risk management is that, with the exception of age, gender, family history of heart disease, and certain electrocardiographic abnormalities, all other risk factors are preventable and reversible. Individuals can control them by modifying their lifestyle. Approximately 90% of CHD is preventable if people practice healthy lifestyle habits.[5] To aid in implementing a lifetime risk reduction program, the risk factors described next should be considered.

Physical Inactivity

Improving cardiorespiratory endurance through aerobic exercise has perhaps the greatest impact in reducing the overall risk for cardiovascular disease. In this day and age of "mechanized societies," we cannot afford *not* to exercise. Research data on the benefits of aerobic exercise in reducing cardiovascular disease are too impressive to be ignored.

The guidelines for implementing an aerobic exercise program are discussed thoroughly in Chapter 6. These guidelines are ideal for developing proper cardiorespiratory fitness, enhancing health, and extending the lifespan. Even moderate amounts of aerobic exercise, however, can reduce cardiovascular risk considerably. As shown in Figure 12.6, work conducted at the Aerobics Research Institute in Dallas, Texas, showed a much higher incidence of cardiovascular deaths in unfit people (group 1 in Figure 12.6), as compared to moderately fit people (groups 2 and 3).[6]

A regular aerobic exercise program helps to control most of the major risk factors that lead to heart and blood vessel disease. Aerobic exercise will:

- — increase cardiorespiratory endurance.
- — decrease and control blood pressure.
- — reduce body fat.
- — lower blood lipids (cholesterol and triglycerides).
- — improve HDL-cholesterol (see later discussion).
- — help control or decrease the risk for diabetes.
- — increase and maintain good heart function, sometimes improving certain ECG abnormalities.
- — motivate toward smoking cessation.
- — alleviate tension and stress.
- — counteract a personal history of heart disease.

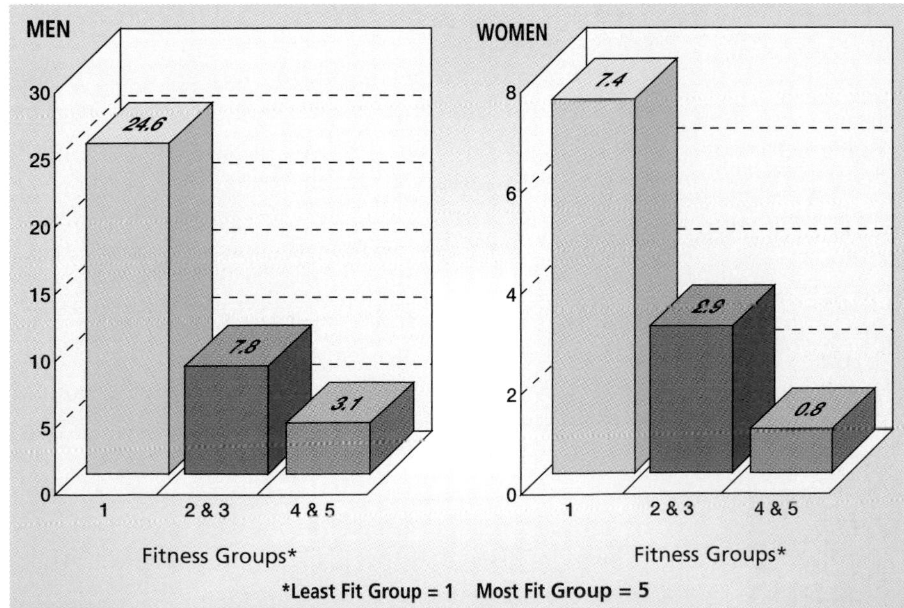

Note: Age-adjusted death rates per 10,000 person-years of follow-up, 1978–1985

From "Physical Fitness and All-Cause Mortality: A Prospective Study of Healthy Man and Woman," by S. N. Blair, H. W. Kohl, III, R. S. Paffenbarger, Jr., D. B. Clark, D. H. Cooper, and L. W. Gibbons, *Journal of the American Medical Association,* 262 (1985), 2395–2401.

Figure 12.6 Relationship between fitness levels and cardiovascular mortality.

The significance of physical inactivity in contributing to cardiovascular risk was shown clearly in 1992 when the American Heart Association added physical inactivity as one of the four major risk factors for cardiovascular disease. The other three are smoking, a poor cholesterol profile, and high blood pressure.

High Blood Pressure

Blood pressure should be checked regularly, regardless of whether it is or is not elevated. The pressure is measured in milliliters of mercury (mm Hg) and usually expressed in two numbers, **systolic pressure** and **diastolic pressure.** Ideal blood pressure is 120/80 or below. The American Heart Association considers all blood pressures over 140/90 as **hypertension.** Regular aerobic exercise, weight control, a low-salt/low-fat diet, smoking cessation, and stress management are the keys to blood pressure control. If needed, medications are used to lower high blood pressure.

Body Composition

As discussed in Chapter 3, body composition is the ratio of lean body weight to fat weight. If too much fat is present, the person is considered obese. Obesity long has been recognized as a

12

Coronary heart disease (CHD) Narrowing of the arteries that supply the heart muscle with oxygen as a result of fatty deposits in artery walls.

Blood pressure The force of the blood exerted against artery walls.

Systolic pressure Blood pressure exerted during the forceful contraction of the heart.

Diastolic pressure Blood pressure during the heart's relaxation phase, when no blood is being ejected.

Hypertension High blood pressure.

risk factor for coronary heart disease. Maintaining recommended body weight (fat percent) is essential in any cardiovascular risk reduction program. Guidelines for a comprehensive weight management program are given in Chapter 4.

Blood Lipids

Because **cholesterol** and triglycerides cannot float around freely in the water-based medium of the blood, they are packaged and transported in the blood by **lipoproteins.**

If you never have had a blood lipid test, it is highly recommended. The blood test should include total cholesterol, **high-density lipoprotein** cholesterol (HDL-cholesterol), **low-density lipoprotein** cholesterol (LDL-cholesterol), and triglycerides. A significant elevation in blood lipids has been linked clearly to heart and blood vessel disease.

A poor blood lipid profile is thought to be the most important predisposing factor in the development of CHD, accounting for almost half of all cases. The general recommendation by the National Cholesterol Education Program (NCEP) is to keep total cholesterol levels below 200 mg/dl (see Table 12.2). Cholesterol levels between 200 and 239 mg/dl are borderline high, and levels of 240 mg/dl and above indicate high risk for disease. Approximately 52%, or 94.6 million American adults, have total cholesterol values of 200 mg/dl or higher and 20% have values at or above 240 mg/dl.[7]

Many preventive medicine practitioners recommend a lower total cholesterol level, ranging between 160 and 180 mg/dl. For children the level always should be below 170 mg/dl. In the Framingham Heart Study, a 40-year ongoing project in the community of Framingham, Massachusetts, not a single individual with a total cholesterol level of 150 mg/dl or lower has had a heart attack.[8]

Perhaps even more significant is the way cholesterol is carried in the bloodstream. Cholesterol is transported primarily by high-density and low-density lipoproteins (HDL and LDL). HDLs act as scavengers, removing cholesterol from the body and preventing **atherosclerosis.** The more HDL-cholesterol, the better. HDL-cholesterol, the "good cholesterol," offers some protection against heart disease.

A poor blood lipid profile is thought to be the most important predisposing factor in the development of CHD.

Evidence suggests that low levels of HDL-cholesterol could be the best predictor of CHD and may be more significant than the total cholesterol value. Substantial research supports the evidence that a low level of HDL-cholesterol has the strongest relationship to CHD at all levels of total cholesterol, including levels below 200 mg/dl. The recommended HDL-cholesterol values to minimize the risk for CHD are 45 mg/dl or higher. A level below 35 mg/dl is viewed as a positive or high risk for CHD. An HDL level above 60 mg/dl is viewed as a negative risk factor, one that decreases the risk of coronary disease.

LDL, on the other hand, releases cholesterol into the bloodstream, enhancing plaque formation. The NCEP guidelines state that an LDL-cholesterol value below 130 mg/dl is desirable, between 130 and 159 mg/dl is borderline-high, and 160 mg/dl and above is high risk for cardiovascular disease.

12

Table 12.2 Standards for Blood Lipids

Total Cholesterol	≤200 mg/dl	Desirable
	201–239 mg/dl	Borderline High
	≥240 mg/dl	High Risk
LDL-Cholesterol	≤130 mg/dl	Desirable
	131–159 mg/dl	Borderline High
	≥160 mg/dl	High Risk
HDL-Cholesterol	≥45 mg/dl	Desirable
	36–44 mg/dl	Borderline High
	≤35 mg/dl	High Risk
Triglycerides	≤125 mg/dl	Desirable
	126–499 mg/dl	Borderline High
	≥500 mg/dl	High Risk

Source: National Cholesterol Education Program

cholesterol profile and decreases the risk for CHD. Habitual aerobic exercise (intensity level above 6 METs), excessive weight loss, and quitting smoking have all been shown to raise HDL-cholesterol. Getting enough beta-carotene, substituting monounsaturated oils for saturated fat in the diet (not to exceed 30% of all calories consumed during the day), and engaging in drug therapy also promote higher HDL-cholesterol levels.

If LDL-cholesterol is higher than ideal, it can be lowered by losing body fat, taking medication, and manipulating the diet. A diet low in fat, saturated fat, and cholesterol and high in fiber is recommended to decrease LDL-cholesterol. The NCEP recommends replacing saturated fat with monounsaturated fat

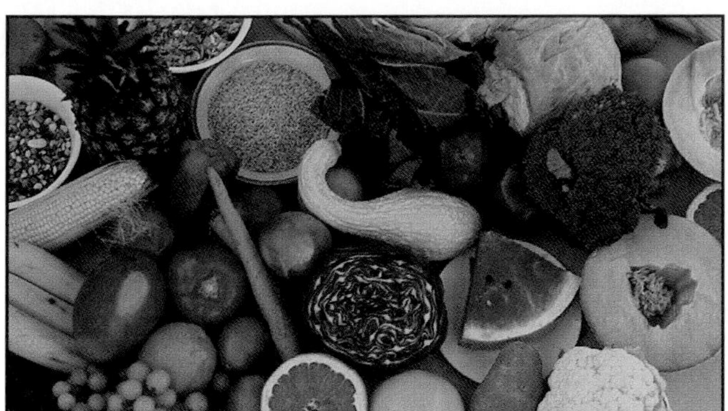

Low-fat foods are necessary to control blood lipids.

(for example, olive, canola, peanut, and sesame oils), because the latter does not cause a reduction in HDL-cholesterol and actually may lower LDL-cholesterol.

Many experts believe that, to have a significant effect in lowering LDL-cholesterol, total fat consumption must be significantly lower than the current 30% of total daily caloric intake guideline. When trying to lower LDL-cholesterol, saturated fat consumption should be much lower than the 10% of total daily caloric intake guideline for "healthy" people. Average cholesterol consumption should be well below 300 mg per day.

Saturated fats are found mostly in meats and dairy products but seldom in foods of plant origin. Poultry and fish contain less saturated fat than beef but should be eaten in moderation (about 3 to 6 ounces per day). Unsaturated fats are mainly of plant origin and cannot be converted to cholesterol.

The antioxidant effect of Vitamins C and E and beta-carotene also can reduce the risk for CHD.[9] Research suggests that a single unstable **free radical** (oxygen compounds produced in normal metabolism) can damage LDL particles. Vitamin C seems to inactivate free radicals, and vitamin E protects LDL from oxidation. **Beta-carotene** not only absorbs free radicals, keeping them from causing damage, but it also seems to increase HDL levels.

Studies on the effects of a 30%-fat diet have shown that it has little or no effect in lowering cholesterol and that CHD actually continues to progress in people who have the disease. The good news comes from a 1991 study published in the *Archives of Internal Medicine*,[10] which reported that the men and women in the study lowered their cholesterol by an average of 23% in only 3 weeks following a 10% or less fat-calorie diet combined with a regular aerobic exercise program, primarily walking. In this diet, cholesterol intake was limited to less than 25 mg/day. The author of the study concluded that the exact percent fat guideline (10% or 15%) is unknown (it also varies from individual to individual), but that 30% total fat calories is definitely too high a level when attempting to decrease cholesterol.

A daily 10% total-fat diet requires that the person limit fat intake to an absolute minimum. Some health-care professionals contend that a diet like this is difficult to follow indefinitely. People with high cholesterol levels, however, may not need to follow that diet indefinitely but should adopt the 10% fat diet while attempting to lower cholesterol. Thereafter, eating a 30%-fat-diet may be adequate to maintain recommended cholesterol levels (1991 national data indicate that current fat consumption in the United States averages 37% of total calories; see Figure 2.6 in Chapter 2).

A drawback of very low fat diets (less than 25% fat) is that they tend to lower HDL-cholesterol and increase triglycerides. If HDL-cholesterol is already low, monounsaturated fat should be added to the diet. Olive oil and nuts are sample food items that are high in monounsaturated fat. A specialized nutrition book should be consulted to determine food items that are high in monounsaturated fat.

The following dietary guidelines are recommended to lower LDL-cholesterol levels:

1. Consume fewer than three eggs per week.
2. Eat red meats (3 ounces per serving) fewer than three times per week, and no organ meats (such as liver and kidneys).
3. Do not eat commercially baked foods.
4. Drink low-fat milk (1% or less fat, preferably) and low-fat dairy products.
5. Do not use coconut oil, palm oil, or cocoa butter.
6. Eat fish instead of red meat.

Lipoproteins Complex molecules that transport cholesterol in the bloodstream.

Cholesterol A waxy substance found only in animal fats and oil.

High-density lipoproteins (HDL) Molecules that transport cholesterol. Tend to attract cholesterol, which is carried to the liver to be metabolized and excreted.

Low-density lipoproteins (LDL) Molecules that transport cholesterol. Tend to release cholesterol, which then may penetrate the lining of the arteries and speed up the process of atherosclerosis.

Atherosclerosis Plaque forming in the arteries.

Free radical Oxygen compounds produced in normal metabolism.

Beta-carotene A precursor to vitamin A.

7. Bake, broil, grill, poach, or steam food instead of frying.
8. Refrigerate cooked meat before adding to other dishes. Remove fat hardened in the refrigerator before mixing the meat with other foods.
9. Avoid fatty sauces made with butter, cream, or cheese.
10. Maintain recommended body weight.

Triglycerides, also known as free fatty acids, in combination with cholesterol, speed up the formation of plaque. Very low-density lipoproteins (VLDLs) and **chylomicrons** carry triglycerides in the bloodstream. These fatty acids are found in poultry skin, lunch meats, and shellfish, but they are manufactured mainly in the liver, from refined sugars, starches, and alcohol. High intake of alcohol and sugars (honey included) significantly raises triglyceride levels. The level can be lowered by cutting down on these foods along with reducing weight (if overweight) and doing aerobic exercise. A normal blood triglyceride level is less than 125 mg/dl (see Table 12.2).

Diabetes

The incidence of cardiovascular disease and death in the diabetic population is quite high. People with chronically elevated blood glucose levels also may have problems in metabolizing fats, which can make them more susceptible to atherosclerosis, increase the risk for coronary disease, and lead to other conditions such as vision loss and kidney damage.

Although **diabetes** has a genetic predisposition, in **adult-onset (Type II) diabetes**, approximately 70% who develop it are overweight or have a history of obesity. In most cases this condition can be corrected through a special diet, a weight-loss program, and a regular exercise program. A diet high in water-soluble fibers (found in fruits, vegetables, oats, and beans) is helpful in treating diabetes. A simple aerobic exercise program (walking, cycling, or swimming four to five times per week) often is prescribed because it increases the body's sensitivity to insulin. Individuals who have high blood glucose levels should consult a physician to decide on the best treatment.

Abnormal Electrocardiograms

Electrocardiograms are taken at rest, during the stress of exercise, and during recovery. A **stress ECG,** also known as a graded exercise stress test or a maximal exercise tolerance test, can be compared to a high-speed road test on a car. Based on the findings, ECGs may be interpreted as normal, equivocal, or abnormal. A stress ECG frequently is used to diagnose coronary heart disease. It also is administered to determine cardiorespiratory fitness levels, to screen individuals for preventive and cardiac rehabilitation programs, to detect abnormal blood pressure response during exercise, and to establish actual or functional maximal heart rate for exercise prescription purposes.

Not every adult who wishes to start or continue in an exercise program needs a stress ECG. The following guidelines can help you determine when this type of test should be conducted:

1. Men over age 40 and women over age 50.
2. A total cholesterol level above 200 mg/dl, or an HDL-cholesterol level below 35 mg/dl.
3. Hypertensive and diabetic patients.
4. Cigarette smokers.
5. Individuals with a family history of CHD, syncope, or sudden death before age 60.
6. People with an abnormal resting ECG.
7. All individuals with symptoms of chest discomfort, **arrhythmias**, syncope, or **chronotropic incompetence**.

Smoking

More than 47 million adults and 3.5 million adolescents in the United States smoke. Cigarette smoking is the single largest preventable cause of illness and premature death in the United States. When considering all related deaths, tobacco is responsible for 400,000 unnecessary deaths per year. Worldwide, smoking-related deaths account for 3 million people each year. About half of all smokers are killed by their addiction. Smoking has been linked to cardiovascular disease, cancer, bronchitis, emphysema, and peptic ulcers.

About 53,000 of the smoking-related deaths in this U.S. yearly are nonsmokers who were exposed to secondhand smoke in daily life. Both fatal and nonfatal cardiac events are increased greatly in people exposed to passive smoking. Some 37,000 yearly deaths from heart disease are attributed to secondhand smoke. Because of the slight adaptation to the harmful effects of smoking in regular smokers, adverse effects of passive smoking are much greater to the nonsmoker. Secondhand smoke is ranked behind active smoking and alcohol as the third leading preventable cause of death in the U.S.[11] Passive smoking is a significant risk factor for heart disease in children and adults alike.

In relation to coronary disease, not only does smoking speed up the process of atherosclerosis, but it also produces a threefold increase in the risk of sudden death following a **myocardial infarction.** Smoking increases heart rate and blood pressure and irritates the heart, which can trigger fatal cardiac arrhythmias. As far as the extra load on the heart is concerned, giving up one pack of cigarettes per day is the equivalent of losing between 50 and 75 pounds of excess body fat! Another harmful effect is a decrease in HDL-cholesterol, the "good" type that helps control blood lipids.

Quitting cigarette smoking enhances health, boosts energy levels, and gives people a sense of freedom, pride, and well-being.

Pipe and cigar smoking and chewing tobacco also increase the risk for heart disease. Even if no smoke is inhaled, toxic substances are absorbed through the membranes of the mouth and end up in the bloodstream. Individuals who use tobacco in any of these three forms also have a much greater risk for cancer of the oral cavity.

Cigarette smoking, a poor cholesterol profile, low fitness, and high blood pressure are the four major risk factors for coronary disease. The risk for both cardiovascular disease and cancer starts to decrease the moment you quit smoking. The risk approaches that of a lifetime nonsmoker 10 and 15 years, respectively, after cessation.

Quitting cigarette smoking is no easy task. Surveys indicate that nine of 10 smokers want to quit. Only about 20% of smokers who try to quit the first time succeed each year. The addictive properties of nicotine and smoke make quitting difficult. Smokers experience physical and psychological withdrawal symptoms when they stop smoking. Even though giving up smoking can be extremely hard, it is by no means impossible.

The most important factor in quitting cigarette smoking is the person's sincere desire to do so. More than 95% of successful ex-smokers have been able to quit on their own, either by quitting cold turkey or by using self-help kits available from organizations such as the American Cancer Society, the American Heart Association, and the American Lung Association. Only 3% of ex-smokers quit as a result of formal cessation programs. A six-step plan to help people stop smoking is contained in Figure 12.7.

Tension and Stress

Tension and stress have become a normal part of life. Everyone has to deal daily with goals, deadlines, responsibilities, pressures. Almost everything in life (whether positive or negative) can be a source of stress. The stressor itself is not what creates the health hazard but, rather, the individual's response to it.

The body's response to **stress** has been the same ever since humans were first put on the earth. Stress prepares the organism to react to **stressor.** Stressors can be biological (illness), psychological (depression, confidence), sociological (winning, losing, peer pressure), and philosophical (spiritual values). The problem is the way in which we react to stress. Many people thrive under stress, whereas others under similar circumstances are unable to handle it. An individual's reaction to a stress-causing agent determines whether stress is positive or negative.

Stress is classified into **eustress** and **distress.** Every person has an optimal level of stress that is most conducive to adequate health and performance. When stress levels reach mental, emotional, and

---

Triglycerides Fats formed by glycerol and three fatty acids.

Chylomicrons Molecules that transport triglycerides in the blood.

Diabetes mellitus A condition in which blood glucose is unable to enter the cells because the pancreas either totally stops producing insulin or does not produce enough to meet the body's needs.

Adult-onset (Type II) diabetes A form related closely to overeating, obesity, and lack of physical activity.

Electrocardiogram (ECG or EKG) A record of the electrical impulses that stimulate the heart to contract.

Stress ECG Reveals the heart's tolerance to high-intensity exercise.

Arrhythmias Irregular heart rhythms.

Chronotropic incompetence A heart rate that increases slowly during exercise and never reaches maximum.

Myocardial infarction Heart attack.

Stress The nonspecific response of the human organism to any demand placed upon it.

Stressor The stress-causing event.

Eustress Health and performance continue to improve even as stress increases (positive stress).

Distress The unpleasant or harmful stress under which health and performance begin to deteriorate.

The following six-step plan has been developed as a guide to help you quit smoking. The total program should be completed in 4 weeks or less. Steps one through four should take no longer than 2 weeks total. A maximum of 2 additional weeks are allowed for the rest of the program.

Step One Decide positively that you want to quit. Now prepare a list of the reasons why you smoke and why you want to quit.

Step Two Initiate a personal diet and exercise program. Exercise and lower body weight cause greater awareness of healthy living and increase motivation for giving up cigarettes.

Step Three Decide on the approach you will use to stop smoking. You may quit cold turkey or gradually decrease the number of cigarettes smoked daily. Many people have found that quitting cold turkey is the easiest way to do it. Although it may not work the first time, after several attempts, all of a sudden smokers are able to overcome the habit without too much difficulty. Tapering off cigarettes can be done in several ways. You may start by eliminating cigarettes you do not necessarily need, you can switch to a brand lower in nicotine or tar every couple of days, you can smoke less of each cigarette, or you can simply decrease the total number of cigarettes smoked each day.

Step Four Set the target date for quitting. In setting the target date, choosing a special date may add a little extra incentive. An upcoming birthday, anniversary, vacation, graduation, family reunion — all are examples of good dates to free yourself from smoking.

Step Five Stock up on low-calorie foods: carrots, broccoli, cauliflower, celery, popcorn (butter- and salt-free), fruits, sunflower seeds (in the shell), sugarless gum, and plenty of water. Keep these foods handy on the day you stop and the first few days following cessation. They can replace a cigarette when you want one.

Step Six This is the day that you will quit smoking. On this day and the first few days thereafter, do not keep cigarettes handy. Stay away from friends and events that trigger your desire to smoke. Drink large amounts of water and fruit juices, and eat low-calorie foods. Replace the old behavior with new behavior. You will need to replace smoking time with new, positive substitutes that will make smoking difficult or impossible. When you desire a cigarette, take a few deep breaths and then occupy yourself by doing a number of things such as talking to someone else, washing your hands, brushing your teeth, eating a healthy snack, chewing on a straw, doing dishes, playing sports, going for a walk or bike ride, going swimming, and so on.

If you have been successful and stopped smoking, a lot of events still can trigger your urge to smoke. When confronted with these events, people rationalize and think, "One won't hurt." It will not work! Before you know it, you will be back to the regular nasty habit. Be prepared to take action in those situations. Find adequate substitutes for smoking. Remind yourself of how difficult it has been and how long it has taken you to get to this point. As time goes on, it will only get easier rather than worse.

Figure 12.7 Six-step smoking cessation approach.

physiological limits, however, eustress becomes distress and the person no longer functions effectively.

Individuals who are under a lot of stress and cannot relax place a constant low-level strain on the cardiovascular system that could manifest itself in the form of heart disease. Further, chronic distress raises the risk for many other health disorders, including hypertension, eating disorders, ulcers, diabetes, asthma, depression, migraine headaches, sleep disorders, and chronic fatigue, and may even play a role in the development of certain types of cancers. Recognizing this turning point and overcoming the problem quickly and efficiently are crucial in maintaining emotional and physiological stability.

Learning to live and get ahead today is virtually impossible without practicing adequate stress management techniques. Two of the most common stress management techniques available are physical exercise and breathing exercises.

Physical Exercise

Physical exercise is one of the simplest tools to control stress. Exercise and fitness are thought to reduce the intensity of the stress response and the recovery time from a stressful event. The value of exercise in reducing stress is related to several factors, the main one being less muscular tension.

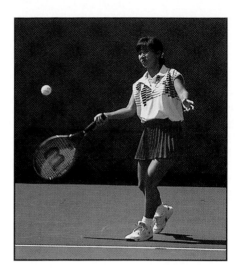

Physical activity is an excellent tool to control stress.

For example, a person may be distressed because he or she has a miserable day at work and the job requires 8 hours of work in a smoke-filled room with an intolerable boss. To make matters worse, it is late and on the way home the car in front is going much slower than the speed limit. The body's **fight or flight** mechanism is activated. No action can be initiated, however, or stress dissipated, because you just cannot hit your boss or the car in front of you. A person surely could take action, though, by "hitting" the tennis ball, the weights, the swimming pool, or the jogging trail. By engaging in physical activity, a person is able to reduce the muscular tension and eliminate the physiological changes that triggered the fight-or-flight mechanism.

Exercise has enhanced the health and quality of life of millions of people, but for a small group of individuals, exercise can become an obsessive behavior with potentially addictive properties. Compulsive exercisers often express feelings of guilt and discomfort when they miss a day's workout. Often these individuals continue to exercise even during periods of injury and sickness that require proper rest for adequate recovery. Under these circumstances, exercise becomes a biological stressor that will lead to poorer health and performance.

As a biological stressor, compulsive exercise or **overtraining** produces both physiological and psychological symptoms. Physical activity can be detrimental to a person's physical and emotional well-being if it is overdone.

Psychological symptoms of overtraining include lower motivation, depression, sleep disturbances, increased irritability, and lack of confidence. Physiological symptoms include musculoskeletal injuries, lower performance, slower recovery time, chronic fatigue, decreased appetite, loss of weight and lean tissue, fat gain, increased muscle tension, higher resting heart rate and blood pressure, and even ECG abnormalities. If you experience any of these symptoms, you need to reevaluate your exercise program and make adjustments accordingly. People who exceed the recommended guidelines for fitness development and maintenance (see Chapters 6, 8, and 10) are exercising for reasons other than health . . . and some actually may be aggravating an already stressful situation.

Breathing Exercises

Breathing techniques also can serve as an antidote to stress. These exercises have been done for centuries in Asia to improve mental, physical, and emotional stamina. Breathing exercises can be learned in only a few minutes and require considerably less time than other forms of stress management. An example of these exercises is given in Figure 12.8.

Personal and Family History

Individuals who have a family history of, or already have experienced cardiovascular problems, are at higher risk than those who never have had a problem. People with this sort of history should be encouraged strongly to keep the other risk factors as low as possible. Because most risk factors are reversible, this decreases the risk for future problems significantly.

Age and Gender

Age is a risk factor because of the greater incidence of heart disease in older people. The risk is higher in men over age 45 and women over age 55. This tendency may be induced partly by other factors stemming from changes in lifestyle as we get older (less physical activity, poor nutrition, obesity, and so on). Men are at greater risk for cardiovascular disease than women earlier in life. Following menopause,

12

Fight or flight Mechanism that prepares the body for action. Heart rate and blood pressure increase, breathing quickens and deepens, muscles tense up, and all systems say "go."

Overtraining Chronic physical activity performed at very high intensity levels or for unusually prolonged periods, leading to decrease in performance (burn out).

Breathing exercises "Breathing away" tension and inhaling fresh air to the entire body.

Breathing exercises should be done in a quiet, pleasant, well-ventilated room. Any of the three exercises listed below may be done whenever a person feels tense.

Deep breathing	Lie with your back flat against the floor, place a pillow under your knees, feet slightly separated, with toes pointing outward (the exercise also may be conducted sitting up in a chair or standing straight up). Place one hand on your abdomen and the other one on your chest. Slowly breathe in and out so the hand on your abdomen rises when you inhale and falls as you exhale. The hand on the chest should not move much at all. Repeat the exercise about 10 times. Next, scan your body for tension, and compare your present tension with the tension you felt at the beginning of the exercise. Repeat the entire process once or twice more.
Sighing	Using the abdominal breathing technique, breathe in through your nose to a specific count (4, 5, 6). Now exhale through pursed lips to double the intake count (10, 11, 12). Repeat the exercise 8 to 10 times whenever you feel tense.
Complete natural breathing:	Sit in an upright position or stand straight up. Breathing through your nose, gradually fill up your lungs from the bottom up. Hold your breath for several seconds. Now exhale slowly by allowing the chest and abdomen to relax completely. Repeat the exercise 8 to 10 times.

Figure 12.8 Breathing exercises for stress management.

women's risk increases. Based on final mortality statistics for 1991, more women (479,359) than men (446,702) died from cardiovascular disease.[12]

Young people should not think that heart disease will not affect them. The process begins early in life. It was shown clearly in American soldiers who died during the Korean and Vietnam conflicts. Autopsies conducted on soldiers killed at 22 years of age and younger revealed that approximately 70% had early stages of atherosclerosis.[13] Other studies found elevated blood cholesterol levels in children as young as 10 years old.

Even though the aging process cannot be stopped, it certainly can be slowed down. **Chronological age** versus **functional age** is an important concept in preventing disease. Some individuals in their 60s or older have the body of a 20-year-old. And 20-year-olds often are in such poor condition and health that they almost seem to have the body of a 60-year-old. Risk factor management and positive lifestyle habits are the best ways to slow down the natural aging process.

Cancer

Cell growth is controlled by **deoxyribonucleic acid (DNA)** and **ribonucleic acid (RNA)**. When nuclei lose their ability to regulate and control cell growth, cell division is disrupted and mutant cells may develop. Some of these cells may grow uncontrollably and abnormally, forming a mass of tissue called a tumor, which can be either **benign** or **malignant**.

More than 100 types of cancer can develop in any tissue or organ of the human body. Over 23% of all deaths in the United States come from cancer. An estimated 1.2 million new cases are reported, and more than half a million people die each year from cancer.

Cancer cells grow for no reason and multiply, destroying normal tissue. If the spread of cells is not controlled, death ensues. A cell may duplicate as many as 100 times. Normally, the DNA molecule is duplicated perfectly during cell division. In a few cases the DNA molecule is not replicated exactly, but repairs are made quickly by specialized enzymes. Occasionally, cells with defective DNA keep dividing and ultimately form a small tumor. As more mutations occur, the altered cells continue to divide and can become malignant. A decade or more can pass between carcinogenic exposure or mutations and the time cancer is diagnosed.

A critical turning point in the development of cancer is when a tumor reaches about one million cells. At this stage it is referred to as **carcinoma in situ**. If undetected, the tumor may go for months and years without any significant growth.

While encapsulated, a tumor does not pose a serious threat to human health. To grow, the tumor requires more oxygen and nutrients. In time, a few of the cancer cells start producing chemicals that enhance **angiogenesis**. Angiogenesis is the precursor of **metastasis**. Through these new vessels, cells now can break away from a malignant tumor and migrate to other parts of the body, where they can cause new cancer masses.

Although the immune system and the blood turbulence destroy most cancer cells, only one abnormal cell lodging elsewhere can start a new cancer. These cells also will grow and multiply uncontrollably, destroying normal tissue.

Once cancer cells metastasize, treatment becomes more difficult. Therapy can kill most cancer cells, but a few cells may become resistant to treatment. These cells then can grow into a new tumor that will not respond to the same treatment.

As with cardiovascular disease, cancer is largely preventable. As much as 80% of all human cancer is related to lifestyle or environmental factors (including diet, tobacco use, excessive use of alcohol, sexual and reproductive history, and exposure to occupational hazards).

Equally important is that more than 8 million Americans with a history of cancer were alive in 1995, nearly 5 million of whom were considered cured. For most patients, "cured" means 5 years without symptoms after treatments stop. Life expectancy for these individuals is the same as for those who never have had cancer.[14]

The most effective way to protect against cancer is by changing negative longstanding habits and behaviors. The following general recommendations have been issued in regard to cancer prevention (also see Lab 12A, page 273).

Dietary Changes

The diet should be low in fat and high in fiber and contain vitamins A and C from natural sources. Protein intake should be within the RDA guidelines. Alcohol should be consumed in moderation, and obesity should be avoided.

High fat intake has been linked primarily to breast, colon, and prostate cancers. Low intake of fiber seems to increase the risk for colon cancer. Foods high in vitamins A and C may deter larynx, esophagus, and lung cancers. Salt-cured, smoked, and nitrite-cured foods have been associated with cancer of the esophagus and stomach. Vitamin C seems to discourage the formation of nitrosamines (cancer-causing substances formed from eating cured meats).

Carrots, squash, sweet potatoes, and **cruciferous vegetables** seem to protect against cancer. These vegetables contain a lot of beta-carotene and vitamin C. Researchers believe the antioxidant effect of these vitamins protects the body from oxygen free radicals.

As discussed in Chapter 2, during normal metabolism most of the oxygen in the human body is converted into stable forms of carbon dioxide and water. A small amount, however, ends up in an unstable form known as oxygen free radicals, which are thought to attack and damage the cell membrane and DNA, leading to the formation of cancers. Antioxidants absorb free radicals before they can cause damage, and they also interrupt the sequence of reactions once damage has begun.[15]

A promising new horizon in cancer prevention is the recent discovery of phytochemicals (also see Chapter 2). These chemical compounds, found in abundance in fruits and vegetables, seem to exert a powerful effect in cancer prevention by blocking the formation of cancerous tumors and disrupting the process at almost every step of the way.[16] Phytochemicals are thought to:

- Remove carcinogens from cells
- Keep carcinogens from binding to DNA
- Prevent small tumors from accessing capillaries to get oxygen and nutrients
- Help keep cancer-causing hormones from locking onto cells

Chronological age Numerical age.

Functional age Physiological age.

Cancer A group of diseases characterized by uncontrolled growth and spread of abnormal cells into malignant tumors.

Deoxyribonucleic acid (DNA) Genetic material in the nucleus of each cell.

Ribonucleic acid (RNA) Genetic material in the nucleus of each cell.

Benign Noncancerous; can interfere with normal bodily functions but rarely cause death.

Malignant Cancerous.

Carcinoma in situ An encapsulated malignant tumor that is found at an early stage and has not spread.

Angiogenesis Capillary (blood vessel) formation into a tumor.

Metastasis The movement of bacteria or body cells from one part of the body to another.

Cruciferous vegetables Those that produce cross-shaped leaves (broccoli, cauliflower, etc.); have cancer-discouraging properties.

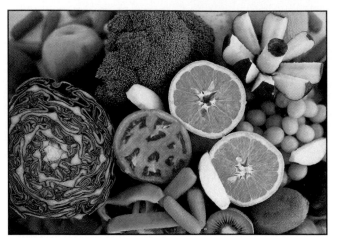

Phytochemicals found in abundance in fruits and vegetables seem to have a powerful effect in decreasing the risk for cancer.

- Disrupt the chemical combination of cell molecules that can produce carcinogens.

Nutritional guidelines also recommend avoiding excessive protein intake. Daily protein intake for some Americans is almost twice the amount the human body needs. Too much animal protein seems to decrease blood enzymes that prevent precancerous cells from developing into tumors.

Some research suggests that grilling protein (fat or lean) at high temperatures for a long time increases the formation of carcinogenic substances on the skin or surface of the meat. Microwaving the meat for a couple of minutes before barbecuing decreases the risk, as long as the fluid released by the meat is discarded. Most potential carcinogens collect in this solution. Removing the skin before serving and cooking at lower heat to a medium stage rather than well done also seems to lower the risk.

Alcohol should be consumed in moderation, as too much alcohol raises the risk for developing certain cancers, especially when it is combined with tobacco smoking or smokeless tobacco. In combination, these substances significantly increase the risk for mouth, larynx, throat, esophagus, and liver cancers. Approximately 17,000 cancer deaths yearly are attributed to excessive use of alcohol, often in combination with tobacco use. The combined action of heavy use of alcohol and tobacco can increase cancer of the oral cavity fifteenfold.

Maintaining recommended body weight also is encouraged. Obesity has been associated with cancers of the colon, rectum, breast, prostate, gallbladder, ovary, and uterus.

Cigarette Smoking

The biggest carcinogenic exposure in the workplace today is cigarette smoke. The American Cancer Society reports that 83% of lung cancers and 30% of all cancers are linked to smoking. The use of smokeless tobacco also increases the risk of mouth, larynx, throat, and esophagus cancers. About 138,600 cancer deaths annually stem from tobacco use. The average life expectancy for a chronic smoker is up to 18 years less than for a nonsmoker.

Sun Exposure

Exposure to sunlight is a major factor in the development of skin cancer. Nearly 90% of the 700,000 **nonmelanoma** skin cancer cases reported annually in the United States are related to sun exposure. People should apply sunscreen lotion when the skin is going to be exposed to sunlight for extended periods. Tanning of the skin is the body's natural reaction to cell damage from excessive sun exposure. Even brief exposures add up and can promote skin cancer and premature aging.

Sunscreen lotion should be applied about 30 minutes before lengthy exposure to the sun because the skin takes that long to absorb the protective ingredients. A sun protection factor (SPF) of at least 15 is recommended. SPF 15 means that the skin takes 15 times longer to burn than with no lotion. If you ordinarily get a mild sunburn after 20 minutes of noonday sun, an SPF 15 allows you to remain in the sun about 300 minutes before burning.

Radiation Exposure, and Potential Occupational Hazards

Although exposure to radiation increases the risk for cancer, the benefits of x-rays may outweigh the risk involved, and most medical facilities administer the lowest dose possible to keep the risk to a minimum. Occupational hazards, such as asbestos fibers, nickel and uranium dusts, chromium compounds, vinyl chloride, and bischlormethyl ether, increase cancer risk. Cigarette smoking magnifies the risk from occupational hazards.

Warning Signals for Cancer

Through early detection, many cancers can be controlled or cured. The real problem is the spreading of cancerous cells. Once that happens, the cancer becomes more difficult to wipe out. Therefore, effective prevention, or at least getting cancer when the possibility of cure is greatest, is crucial. Herein lies the importance of proper periodic screening for prevention and early detection.

Everyone should become familiar with the following seven warning signals for cancer and bring any of them to a physician's attention:

1. Change in bowel or bladder habits.
2. A sore that does not heal.
3. Unusual bleeding or discharge.
4. Thickening or lump in breast or elsewhere.
5. Indigestion or difficulty in swallowing.
6. Obvious change in wart or mole.
7. Nagging cough or hoarseness.

Scientific evidence and testing procedures for prevention and early detection of cancer do change. Studies continue to provide new information. The intent of cancer prevention programs is to educate and guide individuals toward a lifestyle that will help prevent cancer and enable early detection of malignancy. Treatment of cancer always should be left to specialized physicians and cancer clinics.

Chronic Obstructive Pulmonary Disease

Chronic obstructive pulmonary disease (COPD) encompass chronic bronchitis, emphysema, and a reactive airway component similar to that of asthma. The incidence of COPD increases proportionately with cigarette smoking (or other forms of tobacco use) and exposure to certain types of industrial pollution. In the case of emphysema, genetic factors also may play a role.

Accidents

Most people do not consider accidents a health problem, but accidents are the fourth leading cause of death in the United States, affecting the total well-being of millions of Americans each year. Accident prevention and personal safety also are part of a health enhancement program aimed at achieving a higher quality of life. Proper nutrition, exercise, abstinence from cigarette smoking, and stress management are of little help if the person is involved in a disabling or fatal accident caused by distraction, a single reckless decision, or not wearing safety seat belts properly.

Accidents do not just happen. We cause accidents, and we are victims of accidents. Although some factors in life — earthquakes, tornadoes, and airplane crashes, for example — are completely beyond our control, more often than not personal safety and accident prevention are a matter of common sense. Most accidents result from poor judgment and confused mental state. Frequently accidents happen when we are upset, not paying attention to the task with which we are involved, or abusing alcohol and other drugs.

Alcohol abuse is the number-one cause of all accidents. Alcohol intoxication is the leading cause of fatal automobile accidents. Other drugs commonly abused in society alter feelings and perceptions, cause mental confusion, and impair judgment and coordination, greatly increasing the risk for accidental morbidity and mortality.

Spiritual Well-Being

The National Interfaith Coalition on Aging has defined spiritual well-being, or spirituality as an *affirmation of life in a relationship with God, self, community, and environment that nurtures and celebrates wholeness* (see Figure 12.9). Because this definition encompasses Christians and non-Christians alike, it assumes that all people are spiritual in nature. **Spiritual health** provides a unifying power that integrates the other dimensions of wellness.

Religion has been a major part of cultures since the beginning of time. Although not everyone in the United States claims affiliation with a certain religion or denomination, surveys indicate that over 90% of the U.S. population believes in God or a universal spirit functioning as God.

People, furthermore, believe to a varying extent that (a) a relationship with God is meaningful; (b) God can grant help, guidance, and assistance in

---

Nonmelanoma Skin cancers that do not metastasize to other regions of the body.

Chronic obstructive pulmonary disease (COPD) Diseases that limit air flow.

Spirituality A sense of meaning and direction in life, a relationship to a higher being, freedom, prayer, faith, love, closeness to others, peace, joy, fulfillment, and altruism.

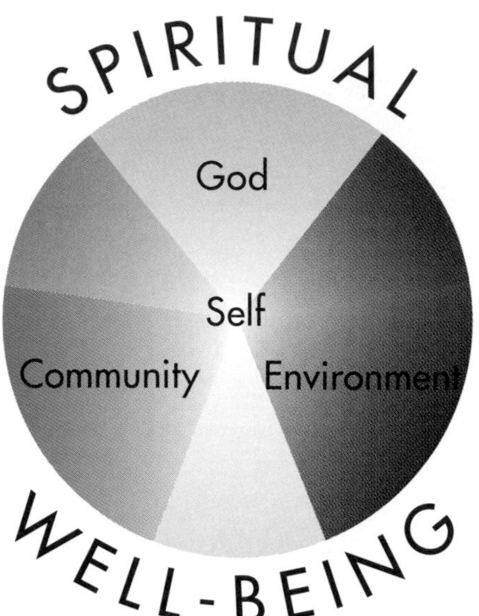

Figure 12.9 Components of spiritual well-being.

daily living; and (c) mortal existence has a purpose. If we accept any or all of these statements, attaining spirituality will have a definite effect on our happiness and well-being.

Although the reasons why religious affiliation enhances wellness are difficult to determine, possible reasons include the promotion of healthy lifestyle behaviors, social support, assistance in times of crisis and need, and counseling to overcome one's weaknesses.

Altruism, a key attribute of spiritual people, seems to enhance health and longevity. Altruism has been the focus of several studies in recent years. Researchers believe that doing good for others is good for oneself, especially for the immune system.

12

In a study of more than 2,700 people in Michigan,[17] the investigators found that people who did regular volunteer work lived longer. People who did not perform regular volunteer work (at least once a week) had a 250% greater mortality risk during the course of the study. In this same study, the authors found that the health benefits of altruism could be so powerful that even just watching films of altruistic endeavors enhances the formation of an immune system chemical that helps fight disease.

Wellness requires a balance between physical, mental, spiritual, emotional, and social well-being. The relationship between spirituality and wellness, therefore, is meaningful in our quest for a better quality of life. As with other parameters of wellness, optimum spirituality requires development of the spiritual nature to its fullest potential.

Substance Abuse Control

Chemical dependencies presently encompasses some of the most serious, self-destructive forms of addiction in our society. Abused substances include alcohol, hard drugs, and cigarettes (the latter already has been discussed in this chapter). Problems associated with substance abuse are drunken or impaired driving, mixing drug prescriptions, family difficulties, and drugs to improve athletic performance (anabolic steroids).

Recognizing that all forms of substance abuse are unhealthy, the following information focuses on three of the most self-destructive addictive substances in our society: alcohol, marijuana, and cocaine.

Alcohol

Alcohol represents one of the most significant health-related drug problems in North America today. Estimates indicate that seven in 10 adults in the United States, or more than 100 million Americans 18 years and older, are drinkers. Approximately 10 million of them will have a drinking problem, including **alcoholism**, in their lifetime. Another 3 million teenagers are thought to have a drinking problem.

Alcohol intake cuts down on peripheral vision, impairs the ability to see and hear, causes slower reactions, reduces concentration and motor performance (including swaying and poor judgment of distance and speed of moving objects), lessens fear, increases risk-taking behaviors, causes more frequent urination, and induces sleep. A single large dose of alcohol also may lower sexual function. One of the most unpleasant, dangerous, and life-threatening consequences of drinking is the **synergistic action** of alcohol when combined with other drugs, particularly central nervous system depressants.

Long-term manifestations of alcohol abuse can be serious and life-threatening. These conditions include **cirrhosis** of the liver, often fatal; greater risk for oral, esophageal, and liver cancer; **cardiomyopathy**; high blood pressure; greater risk for strokes; inflammation of the esophagus, stomach, small intestine, and pancreas; stomach ulcers; sexual impotence; malnutrition; brain cell damage and consequent loss of memory; psychosis; depression; and hallucinations.

Hard Drugs

Approximately 60% of the world's production of illegal drugs is consumed in the United States. Each year Americans spend more than $100 billion on illegal drugs, surpassing the total dollars taken in from all crops produced by U.S. farmers. According to the U.S. Department of Education, today's drugs are stronger and more addictive, posing a greater risk than ever before. Drugs lead to physical and psychological dependence. If used regularly, they integrate into the body's chemistry, raising drug tolerance and forcing the person to increase the dosage constantly for similar results. In addition to the serious health problems caused by drug abuse, more than half of all adolescent suicides are drug-related.

Marijuana

Marijuana (pot or grass) is the most widely used illegal drug in the United States. Approximately 20 million people in the country use marijuana regularly. Earlier studies in the 1960s indicated that the potential effects of marijuana were exaggerated and that the drug was relatively harmless. The drug as it is used today, however, is as much as 10 times stronger than it was when the initial studies were conducted. Long-term harmful effects of marijuana use include atrophy of the brain, leading to irreversible brain damage, less resistance to infectious diseases, chronic bronchitis, lung cancer, and possible sterility and impotence.

Cocaine

Similar to marijuana, for many years cocaine was thought to be a relatively harmless drug. This misconception came to an abrupt halt in 1986 when two well-known athletes, Len Bias (basketball) and Don Rogers (football), died suddenly following a cocaine overdose. An estimated 4 to 8 million Americans use cocaine, 96% of whom had used marijuana previously.

Sustained cocaine snorting can lead to a constant runny nose, nasal congestion and inflammation, and perforation of the nasal septum. Long-term consequences of cocaine use in general include loss of appetite, digestive disorders, weight loss, malnutrition, insomnia, confusion, anxiety, and cocaine psychosis (characterized by paranoia and hallucinations). Large overdoses of cocaine end in sudden death from respiratory paralysis, cardiac arrhythmias, and severe convulsions. Some individuals lack an enzyme used in metabolizing cocaine, and for them as few as two to three lines of cocaine may be fatal.

Recognizing the hazards of chemical use, families, teams, and communities can assist each other in preventing problems, as well as help those who have problems with chemical use. Treating chemical dependency (including alcohol) seldom is accomplished without professional guidance and support. To secure the best available assistance, people in need should contact a physician or obtain a referral from a local mental health clinic (see Yellow Pages in the phone book.)

Sexually Transmitted Diseases

The prevalence of **sexually transmitted diseases (STDs)** has reached epidemic proportions in the United States. Of the more than 25 known STDs, some are still incurable. The American Social Health Association estimated that 25% of all Americans will acquire at least one STD in their lifetime. Each year more than 12 million people are newly infected with STDs, including 4.6 million cases of chlamydia, 1.8 million of gonorrhea, 1 million of genital warts, half a million of herpes, and nearly 100,000 cases of syphilis. Attracting most of the attention because of its life-threatening potential were more than 80,691 new cases of AIDS in the United States in 1994.

Acquired immunodeficiency syndrome (AIDS) is the most frightening of all STDs because it has no known cure and none is predicted for the near future. The **human immunodeficiency virus** (HIV) is a chronic infectious disease that spreads among

---

Altruism True concern for and action on behalf of others (opposite of egoism); a sincere desire to serve others above one's personal needs.

Alcoholism Disease in which an individual loses control over drinking alcoholic-containing beverages.

Synergistic action The effect of mixing two or more drugs, which can be much greater than the sum of two or more drugs acting by themselves.

Cirrhosis Scarring of the liver; often caused by excessive intake of alcohol.

Cardiomyopathy Disease affecting the heart muscle.

Sexually transmitted diseases (STDs) Diseases spread through sexual contact.

Acquired immunodeficiency syndrome (AIDS) End stage of infection by the human immunodeficiency virus (HIV).

Human immunodeficiency virus (HIV) A viral infection marked by destruction of white blood cells, compromising the immune system.

individuals who engage in risky behavior such as unprotected sex or the sharing of hypodermic needles. When a person becomes infected with HIV, the virus multiplies and attacks and destroys white blood cells. These cells are part of the immune system, and their function is to fight off infections and diseases in the body.

As the number of white blood cells killed increases, the body's immune system breaks down gradually or may be destroyed totally. Without the immune system, a person becomes susceptible to **opportunistic** infections or cancers.

HIV is a progressive disease. At first, people who become infected with HIV may not know they are infected. An incubation period of weeks, months, or years may go by during which time no symptoms appear. The virus may live in the body 10 years or longer before symptoms emerge. As of 1994, almost 44% of the people infected with HIV in the United States did not know they were infected until they began developing AIDS-related symptoms.[18]

As the infection progresses to the point at which certain diseases develop, the person is said to have AIDS. HIV itself doesn't kill. Nor do people die of AIDS. AIDS is the final stage of HIV infection. Death is caused by a weakened immune system that is unable to fight off opportunistic diseases.

On the average, 7 to 8 years elapse after infection before the individual develops the symptoms that fit the case definition of AIDS. From that point on, the person may live another 2 to 3 years. In essence, from the point of infection, the individual may endure a chronic disease for 8 to 10 years.

No one has to become infected with HIV. Once infected with the virus, a person never will become uninfected. There is no second chance. Everyone must protect himself or herself against this chronic disease. No one should be so ignorant as to believe it can never happen to him or her!

HIV is transmitted by the exchange of cellular body fluids — blood, semen, vaginal secretions, and maternal milk. These fluids may be exchanged during sexual intercourse, by using hypodermic needles used previously by infected individuals, between a pregnant woman and her developing fetus, babies from an infected mother during childbirth, less frequently during breast feeding, and rarely from a blood transfusion or organ transplant.

AIDS is an "equal opportunity epidemic." People do not get HIV because of who they are but, rather, because of what they do. HIV and AIDS threaten anyone, anywhere: men, women, children, teenagers, young people, older adults, Whites, Blacks, Hispanics, Asians, homosexuals, heterosexuals, bisexuals, druggies, Americans, Africans, Europeans. Nobody is immune to HIV.

You cannot tell if people are infected with HIV or have AIDS simply by looking at them or taking their word. Not you, not a nurse, not even a doctor can tell, unless an HIV antibody test is done. Therefore, every time you engage in risky behavior, you run the risk of contracting HIV. The two most basic risky behaviors are: (a) having unprotected vaginal, anal, or oral sex with an HIV-infected person, and (b) sharing hypodermic needles or other drug paraphernalia with someone who is infected.

The Centers for Disease Control and Prevention estimate that 1 million Americans are infected with HIV. Because of the lengthy incubation period (7 to 8 years to develop AIDS), about 20% of the AIDS patients today are believed to have been infected as teenagers. By the end of 1995, approximately 513,000 AIDS cases had been diagnosed in the United States and about 320,000 had died from the diseases caused by HIV. Most of the people who die are in the 20- to 45-year-old age group.

Approximately 66% of all AIDS cases in the United States have occurred in gay or bisexual men. AIDS in heterosexuals, nonetheless, is on the rise and now is spreading at a faster rate in heterosexuals. Many heterosexuals practice unprotected sex because they don't believe it can happen to their segment of the population. HIV is an epidemic that does not discriminate by sexual orientation. Worldwide about 75% of the AIDS cases have been reported in heterosexuals.

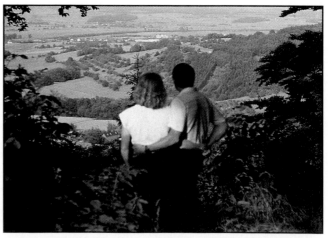

A monogamous sexual relationship almost completely removes people from risking HIV infection and the danger of developing other sexually transmitted diseases.

As with any other serious illness, AIDS patients deserve respect, understanding, and support. Rejection and discrimination are traits of immature, hateful, and ignorant people. Education, knowledge, and responsible behaviors are the best ways to minimize fear and discrimination.

The best way to prevent sexually transmitted diseases is through a mutually monogamous sexual relationship, sex with only one person who has sexual relations only with you. Risky behaviors that significantly increase the chances of contracting sexually transmitted diseases, including HIV infection, are:

1. Multiple or anonymous sexual partners such as a pickup or prostitute.
2. Anal sex with or without a condom.
3. Vaginal or oral sex with someone who shoots drugs or engages in anal sex.
4. Sex with someone you know who has several sex partners.
5. Unprotected sex (without a condom) with an infected person.
6. Sexual contact of any kind with anyone who has symptoms of AIDS or who is a member of a high-risk group for AIDS.
7. Sharing toothbrushes, razors, or other implements that could become contaminated with blood with anyone who is, or might be, infected with the HIV virus.

Avoiding risky behaviors that destroy quality of life and life itself are critical components of a healthy lifestyle. Learning the facts so you can make responsible choices can protect you and those around you from startling and unexpected conditions. Using alcohol moderately (or not at all), refraining from substance abuse, and preventing sexually transmitted diseases are keys to averting both physical and psychological damage.

Exercise and Aging

Unlike any previous time in American society, the elderly population constitutes the fastest growing segment of our population. In 1880, less than 3% of the total population, or fewer than 2 million people, were older than 65. By 1980, the elderly population had reached approximately 25 million, more than 11.3% of the population. According to estimates, the elderly will make up more than 20% of the total population by the year 2035.

Although previous research studies have documented declines in physiological functioning and motor capacity as a result of aging, no hard evidence at present proves that declines in physical work capacity are related primarily to the aging process. Lack of physical activity — a common phenomenon seen as people age — may be accompanied by decreases in physical work capacity that are greater by far than the effects of aging itself.

Unhealthy behaviors precipitate premature aging. For sedentary people, productive life ends at about age 60. Most of these people hope to live to be 65 or 70 and often must cope with serious physical ailments. These people stop living at age 60 but choose to be buried at age 70 (see Figure 12.10).

Scientists believe a healthy lifestyle allows people to live a vibrant life — a physically, intellectually, emotionally, and socially active existence — to age 95. When death comes to active people, it usually comes rather quickly and not as a result of prolonged illness. Such are the rewards of a wellness way of life.

Opportunistic Diseases Diseases arising from a compromised immune system and not seen in healthy people; associated with HIV.

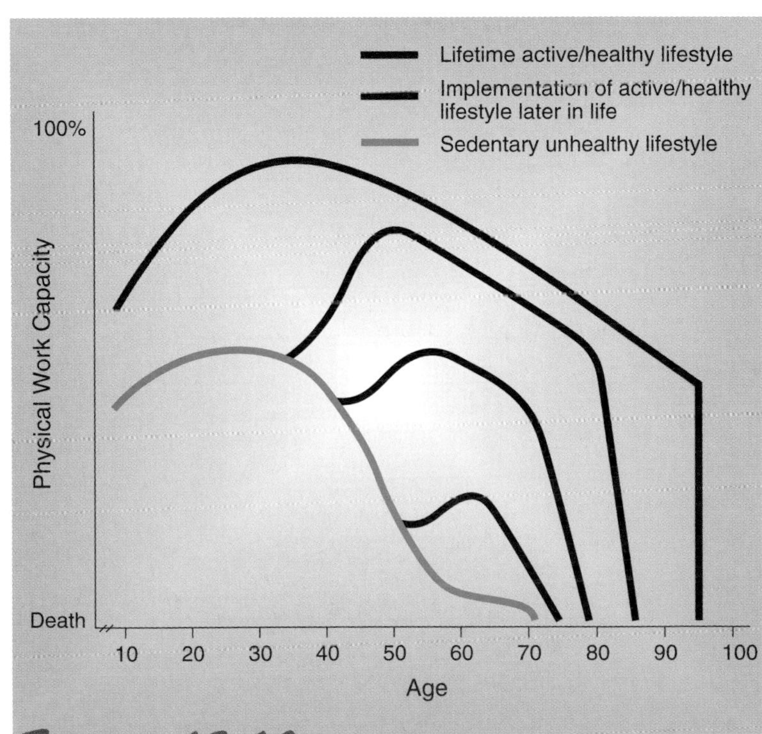

Figure 12.10 Relationship between physical work capacity, aging, and lifestyle habits.

Physical Training in the Older Adult

The trainability of older men and women and the effectiveness of physical activity as a relative modality have been demonstrated in prior research. Older adults who increase their level of physical activity experience significant changes in cardiorespiratory endurance, strength, and flexibility. The extent of the changes depends on their initial fitness level and the types of activities selected for their training (walking, cycling, strength training, and so on).

Improvements in maximal oxygen uptake in older adults are similar to those of younger people, although older people seem to require a longer training period to achieve these changes. Declines in endurance (maximal oxygen uptake) per decade of life after age 25 seem to be about 9% for sedentary adults and 5% or less in active people.

Results from a study on the effects of aging on the cardiovascular system of male exercisers versus nonexercisers showed that the maximal oxygen uptake of regular exercisers was almost twice that of the non-exercisers (see Table 12.3).[19] Between ages 50 and 68, the study revealed a decline in maximal oxygen uptake of only 13% in the active group, compared to 41% in the inactive group. These changes indicate that about one-third of the loss in maximal oxygen uptake results from aging and two-thirds of the loss comes from inactivity. Blood pressure, heart rate, and body weight also were remarkably better in the exercising group.

In strength development, older adults can increase their strength levels, but the amount of muscle hypertrophy achieved decreases with age. Strength gains as high as 200% have been found in previously inactive adults over age 90.[20] In terms of body composition, inactive adults continue to gain body fat after age 60 despite the tendency toward lower body weight.

Older adults who wish to initiate or continue an exercise program are encouraged strongly to have a complete medical exam, including a stress electrocardiogram test. Recommended activities for older adults include calisthenics, walking, jogging, swimming, cycling, and water aerobics.

Older adults should avoid isometric and other intense weight-training exercises. Activities that require all-out effort or require participants to hold their breath (valsalva maneuver) tend to lessen blood flow to the heart and cause a significant increase in blood pressure and the load placed on the heart. Older adults should participate in activities that require continuous and rhythmic muscular activity (about 50% to 70% of functional capacity). These activities do not cause large increases in blood pressure or place an intense overload on the heart.

Table 12.3 Effects of Physical Activity and Inactivity on Selected Physiological Parameters in Older Men

	Exercisers	Nonexercisers
Age (yrs)	68.0	69.8
Weight (lbs)	160.3	186.3
Resting heart rate (bpm)	55.8	66.0
Maximal heart rate (bpm)	157.0	146.0
Heart rate reserve* (bpm)	101.2	80.0
Blood pressure (mmHg)	120/78	150/90
Maximal oxygen uptake (ml/kg/min)	38.6	20.3

Data from "The Effect of Physical Activity on Aerobic Power in Older Men (a Longitudinal Study)," by F. W. Kash, J. L. Boyer, S. P. Van Camp, L. S. Verity, and J. P. Wallace. *Physician and Sports Medicine* 18(4) (1990), 73–83.

* Heart rate reserve = maximal heart rate − resting heart rate.

12

An Educated Fitness/Wellness Consumer

The rapid growth in fitness and health promotion programs during the last three decades has spurred the promotion of fraudulent products that deceive consumers into "miraculous," quick, and easy ways toward total well-being. **Quackery** and **fraud** abound.

Today's market is saturated with "special" foods, diets, supplements, pills, cures, equipment, books, and videos that promise quick, dramatic results. Advertisements for these products often are based on testimonials, unproven claims, secret research, half-truths, and quick-fix statements that the uneducated consumer wants to hear. In the meantime, the organization or enterprise making the claims stands to make a large profit from consumers' willingness to pay for astonishing and spectacular solutions to problems related to their unhealthy lifestyle.

Television, magazine, and newspaper advertisements are not necessarily reliable. For instance, one piece of equipment sold through television and newspaper advertisements promised to "bust the gut" through 5 minutes of daily exercise that appeared to include the abdominal muscle group. This piece of equipment consisted of a metal spring that attached to the feet on one end and was held in the hands on the other end. According to handling and shipping distributors, the equipment was selling like "hotcakes" and companies could barely keep up with the consumer's demands.

Three problems became apparent to the educated consumer. First, there is no such thing as spot-reducing; therefore, the claims could not be true. Second, 5 minutes of daily exercise burn hardly any calories and, therefore, have little if any effect on weight loss. Third, the intended abdominal (gut) muscles were not really involved during the exercise. The exercise engaged mostly the gluteal and lower back muscles. This piece of equipment now can be found at garage sales for about a tenth of its original cost!

Although people in the United States tend to be firm believers in the benefits, of physical activity and positive lifestyle habits as a means to promote better health, most do not reap these benefits, because they simply do not know how to put into practice a sound fitness and wellness program that will give them the results they want. Unfortunately, many uneducated wellness consumers are targets of deception by organizations making fraudulent claims for their products.

We can protect ourselves from consumer fraud. The first step, is education. You have to be an informed consumer of the product you intend to purchase. If you do not have or cannot find the answers, seek the advice of a reputable professional. Ask someone who understands the product but does not stand to profit from the transaction. As examples, a physical educator or an exercise physiologist can advise you regarding exercise equipment; a registered dietitian can provide information on nutrition and weight control programs; a physician can offer advice on nutritive supplements. Also, be alert to those who bill themselves as "experts." Look for qualifications, degrees, professional experience, certifications, reputation.

Another clue to possible fraud is that if it sounds too good to be true, it probably is. Quick-fix, miraculous, special, secret, mail orders only, money-back guarantee, and testimonials are terms often heard in advertisements of fraudulent promotions. When claims are made, ask where the claims are published. Newspapers, magazines, and trade books are apt to be unreliable sources of information. Refereed scientific journals are the most reliable sources of information. When a researcher submits information for publication in a refereed journal, at least two qualified and reputable professionals in the field conduct blind reviews of the manuscript. A blind review means the author does not know who will review the manuscript and the reviewers do not know who submitted the manuscript. Acceptance for publication is based on this input and relevant changes.*

Health/Fitness Club Memberships

As you follow a lifetime wellness program, you might consider joining a health/fitness facility. If you have mastered the contents of this book and if your choice of fitness activity is one you can pursue on your own (walking, jogging, cycling), you may not need to join a health club. Barring injuries, you may continue your exercise program outside the walls of a health club for the rest of your life. You also can conduct strength-training and stretching programs within the walls of your own home (see Chapters 8 and 10).

To stay up to date on fitness and wellness developments, you probably should buy a reputable and updated fitness/wellness book every 4 to 5 years. You also might subscribe to a credible health, fitness, nutrition, or wellness newsletter (see Table 12.4) to stay current.

If you are contemplating membership in a fitness facility:

- Examine all exercise options in your community: health clubs/spas, YMCAs, gyms, colleges, schools, community centers, senior centers, and the like.
- Check to see if the facility's atmosphere is pleasurable and nonthreatening to you. Will you feel comfortable with the instructors and other people who go there? Is it clean and well kept up? If the answer is no, this may not be the right place for you.
- Analyze costs versus facilities, equipment, and programs. Take a look at your personal budget. Will you really use the facility? Will you exercise

*If you have questions or concerns about a health product, you may write to the National Council Against Health Fraud (NCAHF), P. O. Box 1276, Loma Linda, CA 92354. The purpose of this organization is to monitor deceitful advertising, investigate complaints, and offer the public information regarding fraudulent health claims.

Quackery/Fraud The conscious promotion of unproven claims for profit.

Table 12.4 Reliable Sources of Health, Fitness, Wellness, and Nutrition Information

Newsletter	Yearly Issues	Approximate Annual Cost
Consumer Reports Health Letter P.O. Box 56356 Boulder, CO 80323-2148	12	$24
Executive Health's Good Health Report P.O. Box 8880 Chapel Hill, NC 27515	12	$34
Tufts University Diet & Nutrition Letter P.O. Box 57857 Boulder, CO 80322-7857	12	$20
University of California Berkeley *Wellness Letter* P.O. Box 420148 Palm Coast, FL 32142	12	$20

there regularly? Many people obtain memberships and permit dues to be withdrawn automatically from a local bank account, yet seldom attend the fitness center.

- Find out what types of facilities are available: running track, basketball/tennis/racquetball courts, aerobic exercise room, strength-training room, pool, locker rooms, saunas, hot tubs, handicapped access, and so on.
- Check the aerobic and strength-training equipment available. Does the facility have treadmills, bicycle ergometers, Stair Masters, cross-country skiing simulators, free weights, Universal Gym, Nautilus? Make sure the facilities and equipment meet your activity interests.
- Consider the location. Is the facility close, or do you have to travel several miles to get there? Distance often discourages participation.
- Check on times the facility is accessible. Is it open during your preferred exercise time (for example, early morning or late evening)?
- Work out at the facility several times before becoming a member. Are people standing in line to use the equipment, or is it readily available during your exercise time?
- Inquire about the instructors' qualifications. Do the fitness instructors have college degrees or professional certifications from organizations such as the American College of Sports Medicine (ACSM) or the International Dance Exercise Association (IDEA)? These organizations have rigorous standards to ensure professional preparation and quality of instruction.
- Consider the approach to fitness (including all health-related components of fitness). Is it well-rounded? Do the instructors spend time with members, or do members have to seek them out constantly for help and instruction?
- Ask about supplementary services. Does the facility provide or contract out for regular health and fitness assessments (cardiorespiratory endurance, body composition, blood pressure, blood chemistry analysis). Are wellness seminars (nutrition, weight control, stress management) offered? Do these have hidden costs?

A final consideration is that of purchasing your own exercise equipment. The first question you need to ask yourself is: Do I really need this piece of equipment? Most people buy on impulse because of television advertisements or because a salesperson convinced them it is a great piece of equipment that will do wonders for their health and fitness. With some creativity, you can implement an excellent and comprehensive exercise program with little, if any, equipment (see Chapters 6, 8, and 10).

Many people buy expensive equipment only to find they really do not enjoy that mode of activity. They do not remain regular users. Stationary bicycles (lower body only) and rowing ergometers were among the most popular pieces of equipment in the 1980s. Most of them now are seldom used and have become "fitness furniture" somewhere in the basement.

Exercise equipment does have its value for people who prefer to exercise indoors, especially during the winter months. It supports some people's motivation and adherence to exercise. The convenience of having equipment at home also allows for flexible scheduling. You can exercise before or after work or while you watch your favorite television show.

If you are going to purchase equipment, the best recommendation is to actually try it out several times before buying it. Ask yourself several questions: Did you enjoy the workout? Is the unit comfortable? Are you too short, tall, or heavy for it? Is it stable, sturdy, and strong? Do you have to assemble the machine? If so, how difficult is it to put together? How durable is it? Ask for references — people or clubs that have used the equipment extensively. Are they satisfied? Have they enjoyed the activity (the equipment)? Talk with professionals at colleges, sportsmedicine clinics, or health clubs.

Another consideration is to look at used units for signs of wear and tear. Quality is important. Cheaper brands may not be durable, so your investment would be wasted.

Finally, watch out for expensive gadgets. Monitors that provide exercise heart rate, work output, caloric expenditure, speed, grade, and distance may help motivate you, but they are expensive, need repairs, and do not enhance the actual fitness benefits of the workout. Look at maintenance costs and check for service personnel in your community.

Self-Evaluation and Behavioral Objectives for the Future

The main objective of this book is to provide the information and experiences necessary to implement your personal fitness program. If you have implemented the programs in this book, including exercise, you should be convinced that a healthy lifestyle is the only way to attain a higher quality of life.

Most people who engage in a personal fitness program experience this new quality of life after only a few weeks of training and practicing healthy lifestyle patterns. In some instances — especially individuals who have led a poor lifestyle for a long time — a few months may be required to establish positive habits and feelings of well-being. In the end, though, everyone who applies the fitness principles will reap the desired benefits.

Through various laboratory experiences, you have had an opportunity to assess fitness components and write behavioral objectives to improve your quality of life. You now should take the time to evaluate how well you have achieved your own objectives. Ideally, if time allows and facilities and technicians are available, you should reassess at least the health-related components of physical fitness. If you are unable to reassess these components, determine subjectively how well you accomplished your objectives. You will find a self-evaluation form in Lab 12B, page 279.

The Fitness Experience and a Challenge for the Future

Patty Neavill is a typical example of someone who often tried to change her life but was unable to do so because she did not know how to implement a sound exercise and weight-control program. At age 24 and at 240 pounds, she was discouraged with her weight, level of fitness, self-image, and quality of life in general. She had struggled with her weight most of her life. Like thousands of other people, she had made many unsuccessful attempts to lose weight.

Patty put her fears aside and decided to enroll in a fitness course. As part of the course requirement, a battery of fitness tests was administered at the beginning of the semester. Patty's cardiorespiratory fitness and strength ratings were poor, her flexibility classification was average, and her percent body fat was 41.

Following the initial fitness assessment, Patty met with her course instructor, who prescribed an exercise and nutrition program like the one in this book. Patty committed fully to carry out the prescription. She walked/jogged five times a week. She enrolled in a weight-training course that met twice a week. Her daily caloric intake was set in the range of 1,500 to 1,700 calories.

Determined to increase her level of activity further, Patty signed up for recreational volleyball and basketball courses. Besides fun, these classes provided 4 additional hours of activity per week.

She took care to meet the minimum required servings from the basic food groups each day, which contributed about 1,200 calories to her diet. The remainder of the calories came primarily from complex carbohydrates.

At the end of the 16-week semester, Patty's cardiorespiratory fitness, strength, and flexibility ratings all had improved to the "good" category, she had lost 50 pounds, and her percent body fat had decreased to 22.5!

Patty was tall. At 190 pounds, most people would have thought she was too heavy. Her percent body fat, however, was lower than the average for college female physical education major students (about 23% body fat).

A thank-you note from Patty to the course instructor at the end of the semester read:

> Thank you for making me a new person. I truly appreciate the time you spent with me. Without your kindness and motivation, I would have never

12

made it. It is great to be fit and trim. I've never had this feeling before, and I wish everyone could feel like this once in their life.

Thank you,

Your trim Patty

Patty never had been taught the principles governing a sound weight-loss program. In Patty's case, not only did she need this knowledge, but, like most Americans who never have experienced the process of becoming physically fit, she needed to be in a structured exercise setting to truly feel the joy of fitness.

Even more significant, Patty maintained her aerobic and strength-training programs. A year after ending her calorie-restricted diet, her weight increased by 10 pounds, but her body fat decreased from 22.5% to 21.2%. As you may recall from Chapter 4, this weight increase is related mostly to changes in lean tissue, lost during the weight-reduction phase.

In spite of only a slight drop in weight during the second year following the calorie-restricted diet, the 2-year follow-up revealed a further decrease in body fat, to 19.5%. Patty understood the new quality of life reaped through a sound fitness program, and, at the same time, she finally learned how to apply the principles that regulate weight.

If you have read and successfully completed all of the assignments set out in this book, including a regular exercise program, you should be convinced of the value of exercise and healthy lifestyle habits in achieving a new quality of life.

Perhaps this new quality of life was explained best by the late Dr. George Sheehan, when he wrote:[21]

> For every runner who tours the world running marathons, there are thousands who run to hear the leaves and listen to the rain, and look to the day when it is all suddenly as easy as a bird in flight. For them, sport is not a test but a therapy, not a trial but a reward, not a question but an answer.

The real challenge will come now: a lifetime commitment to fitness and a healthy lifestyle. To make the commitment easier, enjoy yourself and have fun along the way. Implement your program based on your interests and what you enjoy doing most. Then adhering to your new lifestyle will not be difficult.

Your activities over the last few weeks or months may have helped you develop "positive addictions" that will carry on throughout life. If you truly experience the feelings Dr. Sheehan expressed, there will be no looking back. If you don't get there, you won't know what it's like. Fitness is a process, and you need to put forth a constant and deliberate effort to achieve and maintain a higher quality of life. Improving the quality of your life, and most likely your longevity, is in your hands. Only you can take control of your lifestyle and thereby reap the benefits.

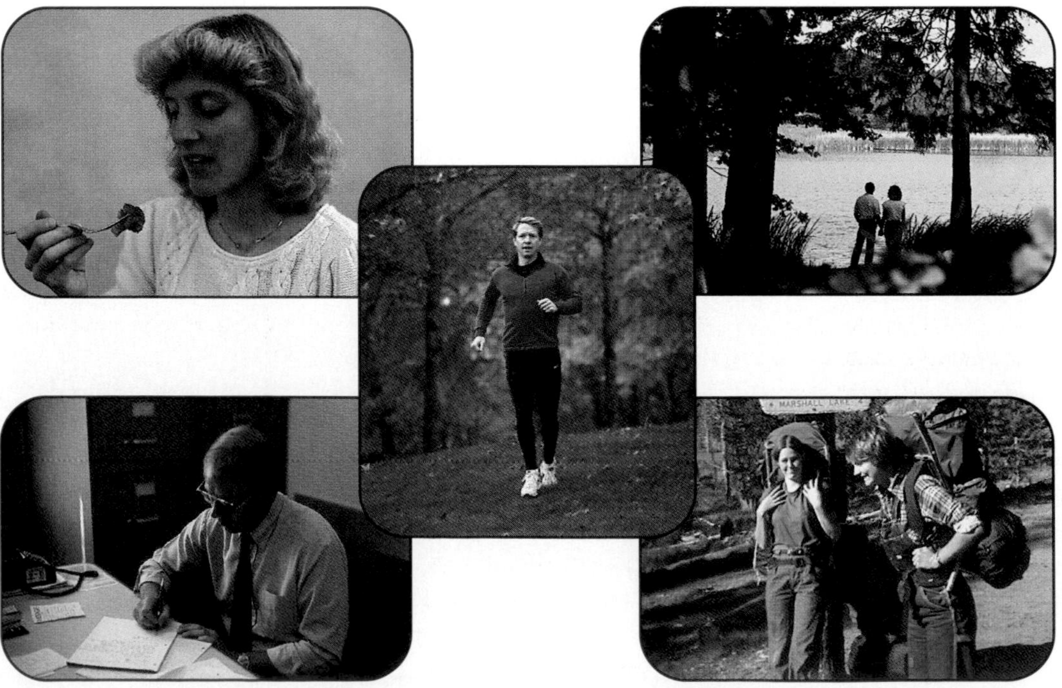

Fitness and healthy lifestyle habits lead to improved health, quality of life, longevity, and wellness.

Laboratory Experience

LAB 12A
Cardiovascular Disease and Cancer Risk Management

Lab Preparation
Review Chapter 12 prior to this lab.

LAB 12B
Self-Evaluation and Behavioral Objectives for the Future

Lab Preparation
If possible, repeat fitness testing for all health-related components.

Notes

1. U. S. Department of Health and Human Services, National Center for Health Statistics, *Monthly Vital Statistics Report: Advance Report of Final Mortality Statistics*, 43:6, Supplement (1992), March 22, 1995.
2. J. M. McGinnis and W. H. Foege, "Actual Causes of Death in the United States," *Journal of the American Medical Association* 270 (1993), 2207–2212.
3. American Heart Association, *Heart and Stroke Facts: 1995* (Statistical Supplement) (Dallas: AHA, 1994).
4. U. S. Department of Health and Human Services.
5. P. N. Hopkins and R. R. Williams, "Identification and Relative Weight of Cardiovascular Risk Factors," *Cardiology Clinics*, 4 (1986), 3–32.
6. S. N. Blair, H. W. Kohl III, R. S. Paffenbarger, Jr., D. G. Clark, K. H. Cooper, and L. W. Gibbons, "Physical Fitness and All-Cause Mortality: A Prospective Study of Healthy Men and Women," *Journal of the American Medical Association*, 262 (1989), 2395–2401.
7. American Heart Association, *Fact Sheet on Heart Attack, Stroke and Risk Factors* (Dallas: AHA, 1994).
8. W. P. Castelli and K. Anderson, "A Population at Risk. Prevalence of High Cholesterol Levels in Hypertensive Patients in the Framingham Study," *American Journal of Medicine* 80, Supplement 2A (1986), 23-32.
9. J. M. Gaziano and C. H. Hennekens, "A New Look at What Can Unclog Your Arteries," *Executive Health Report*, 27:8 (1991), 16.
10. R. J. Barnard, "Effects of Lifestyle Modification on Serum Lipids," *Archives of Internal Medicine*, 151 (1991), 1389–1394.
11. S. A. Glantz and W. W. Parmley. "Passive Smoking and Heart Disease," *Journal of the American Medical Association*, 273 (1995), 1047–1053.
12. American Heart Association.
13. P.E. Allsen, J. M. Harrison, B. Vance, *Fitness for Life* (Madison, WI: Brown & Benchmark, 1993), p. 3.
14. American Cancer Society. *1995 Cancer Facts and Figures* (New York: ACS, 1995).
15. Gaziano and Hennekens.
16. S. Begley. "Beyond Vitamins." *Newsweek*, April 25, 1994, pp. 45–49.
17. E. R. Growald and A. Lusks, "Beyond Self." *American Health*, March 1988, pp. 51–53.
18. E. Pennisi, "AIDS Becomes More of an Equal Opportunity Epidemic," *American Society for Microbiology News*, 61:5 (1995), 236–240.
19. F. W. Kash, J. L. Boyer, S. P. Van Camp, L. S. Verity, and J. P. Wallace, "The Effect of Physical Activity on Aerobic Power in Older Men (a Longitudinal Study)," *Physician and Sports Medicine*, 18:4 (1990), 73–83.
20. F. W. Kash, J. L. Boyer, S. P. Van Camp, L. S. Verity, and J. P Wallace. "The Effect of Physical Activity on Aerobic Power in Older Men: A Longitudinal Study," *The Physician and Sportsmedicine*, 18:4 (1990), 73–83.
21. Human Relations Media, "What is Fitness?" *Dynamics of Fitness: The Body in Action* (Pleasantville, NY: Author, 1980).

Suggested Readings

American Cancer Society. *Cancer Facts & Figures – 1994*. New York: ACS, 1994.

American Cancer Society. *Fifty Most Often Asked Questions About Smoking and Health and the Answers*. New York: ACS, 1982.

American Cancer Society. *Quitter's Guide: Seven-Day Plan to Help You Stop Smoking Cigarettes*. New York: ACS, 1978.

American Heart Association. *The Good Life: A Guide to Becoming a Nonsmoker*. Dallas: AHA, 1984.

American Heart Association. *Heart at Work: Smoking Reduction Program — Coordinator's Guide*. Dallas: AHA, 1984.

American Heart Association. *How to Quit*. Dallas: AHA, 1984.

American Heart Association. *Smoking and Heart Disease*. Dallas: AHA, 1981.

Carroll, C. R. *Drugs in Modern Society*. Dubuque, IA: Wm. C. Brown, 1985.

Channing L. Bete Co. *Smoking and Your Heart*. South Deerfield, MA: Author, 1982.

Girdano, D. A., D. Dusek, and G. S. Everly. *Experiencing Health*. Englewood Cliffs, NJ: Prentice Hall, 1985.

Halper, M. S. *How to Stop Smoking: A Preventive Medicine Institute/Strang Clinic Health Action Plan*. New York: Holt, Rinehart and Winston, 1980.

Hodgson, R. J., and P. Miller. *Self-Watching: Addictions, Habits, Compulsions, What to Do*. New York: Facts on File, 1982.

National Cancer Institute. *Clearing the Air: A Guide to Quitting Smoking*. Bethesda, MD: NCI, 1979.

Public Health Service. *Chronic Obstructive Lung Disease: A Report of the Surgeon General*. Rockville, MD: U.S. Department of Health and Human Services, 1984.

Public Health Service. *A Self-Test for Smokers*. Rockville, MD: U.S. Department of Health and Human Services, 1983.

Public Health Service. *Smoking Tobacco and Health: A Fact Book*. Rockville, MD: U.S. Department of Health and Human Services, 1981.

Public Health Service. *Why People Smoke Cigarettes*. Rockville, MD: U.S. Department of Health and Human Services, 1982.

U.S. Office on Smoking and Health. *Smoking and Health: A Report of the Surgeon General*. Washington, DC: U.S. Department of Health, Education and Welfare, 1979.

Labs

LAB 1A CLEARANCE FOR EXERCISE PARTICIPATION

Name: ______________________ Date: ____________ Grade: ________

Instructor: ______________________ Course: ____________ Section: ________

NECESSARY LAB EQUIPMENT None.

LAB 1A

OBJECTIVE To determine the safety of exercise participation.

INTRODUCTION Although exercise testing and exercise participation are relatively safe for most apparently healthy individuals under the age of 45, the reaction of the cardiovascular system to increased levels of physical activity cannot always be totally predicted. Consequently, there is a small but real risk of certain changes occurring during exercise testing and participation. Some of these changes may be abnormal blood pressure, irregular heart rhythm, fainting, and in rare instances a heart attack or cardiac arrest. Therefore, you must provide honest answers to this questionnaire. Exercise may be contraindicated under some of the conditions listed below; others may simply require special consideration. **If any of the conditions apply, you should consult your physician before you participate in an exercise program.** You also should promptly report to your instructor any exercise-related abnormalities that you may experience during the course of the semester.

A. Have you ever had or do you now have any of the following conditions?

- ☐ 1. A myocardial infarction.
- ☐ 2. Coronary artery disease.
- ☐ 3. Congestive heart failure.
- ☐ 4. Elevated blood lipids (cholesterol and triglycerides).
- ☐ 5. Chest pain at rest or during exertion.
- ☐ 6. Shortness of breath.
- ☐ 7. An abnormal resting or stress electrocardiogram.
- ☐ 8. Uneven, irregular, or skipped heartbeats (including a racing or fluttering heart).
- ☐ 9. A blood embolism.
- ☐ 10. Thrombophlebitis.
- ☐ 11. Rheumatic heart fever.
- ☐ 12. Elevated blood pressure.
- ☐ 13. A stroke.
- ☐ 14. Diabetes.
- ☐ 15. A family history of coronary heart disease, syncope, or sudden death before age 60.
- ☐ 16. Any other heart problem that makes exercise unsafe.

B. Do you have any of the following conditions?

- ☐ 1. Arthritis, rheumatism, or gout.
- ☐ 2. Chronic low-back pain.
- ☐ 3. Any other joint, bone, or muscle problems.
- ☐ 4. Any respiratory problems.
- ☐ 5. Obesity (more than 30% overweight).
- ☐ 6. Anorexia.
- ☐ 7. Bulimia.
- ☐ 8. Mononucleosis.
- ☐ 9. Any physical disability that could interfere with safe participation in exercise.

C. Do any of the following conditions apply?

- ☐ 1. Do you smoke cigarettes?
- ☐ 2. Are you taking any prescription drug?
- ☐ 3. Are you 45 years or older?

D. Do you have any other concern regarding your ability to safely participate in an exercise program? If so, explain:

____

____

Student's Signature: ______________________________ Date: ____________

LAB 2A

NUTRIENT ANALYSIS

Name: ______________________________ Date: ______________ Grade: ________

Instructor: ___________________________ Course: ____________ Section: ________

NECESSARY LAB EQUIPMENT List of "Nutritive Value of Selected Foods," Appendix A. An IBM-PC or Macintosh computer, if the computer software for use with this book is used. Otherwise, only a small calculator is needed.

OBJECTIVE To evaluate your present diet using the Recommended Dietary Allowances (RDA).

INSTRUCTIONS To conduct the following nutritional analysis, you need a record of all foods eaten during a 3-day period (use the list of "Nutritive Value of Selected Foods" given in Appendix A). Record this information prior to this lab session in the forms provided in Figure 2A.1. After recording the nutritive values for each day, add up the values in each column and record the totals at the bottom of the form. Also do this before the lab session. During your lab, proceed to compute an average for the 3 days. The percentages for carbohydrates, fat, saturated fat, and the protein requirements can be computed by using the instructions at the bottom of Figure 2A.2. The results can then be compared against the Recommended Dietary Allowances.

The analysis can be simplified by using the computer software for this lab. Up to 7 days may be analyzed when using the software, and Figure 2A.3 should be used instead of 2A.1. Further, you have to record only the code for each food and the amount of servings eaten (.5 for half a serving, 2 for twice the standard serving, and so forth).

LAB 2A

Date: ____________________

Foods	Amount	Calories	Protein (gm)	Fat (total) (gm)	Sat. Fat (gm)	Chol-esterol (mg)	Carbo-hydrates (gm)	Cal-cium (mg)	Iron (mg)	Sodium (mg)	Vit. A (IU)	Vit. B_1 (mg)	Vit. B_2 (mg)	Niacin (mg)	Vit. C (mg)
Totals															

Figure 2A.1 Daily nutrient intake.

Date: ____________

Foods	Amount	Calories	Protein (gm)	Fat (total) (gm)	Sat. Fat (gm)	Chol- esterol (mg)	Carbo- hydrates (gm)	Cal- cium (mg)	Iron (mg)	Sodium (mg)	Vit. A (IU)	Vit. B_1 (mg)	Vit. B_2 (mg)	Niacin (mg)	Vit. C (mg)
Totals															

Figure 2A.1 Continued.

LAB 2A

Date: ____________________

Foods	Amount	Calories	Protein (gm)	Fat (total) (gm)	Sat. Fat (gm)	Chol-esterol (mg)	Carbo-hydrates (gm)	Cal-cium (mg)	Iron (mg)	Sodium (mg)	Vit. A (IU)	Vit. B_1 (mg)	Vit. B_2 (mg)	Niacin (mg)	Vit. C (mg)
Totals															

Figure 2A.1 Continued.

Name: ____________________

Day	Calories	Protein (gm)	Fat (gm)	Sat. Fat (gm)	Chol-esterol (mg)	Carbo-hydrates (gm)	Calcium (mg)	Iron (mg)	Sodium (mg)	Vit. A (IU)	Thiamin Vit. B_1 (mg)	Riboflavin Vit. B_2 (mg)	Niacin (mg)	Vit. C (mg)
One														
Two														
Three														
Totals														
Average[a]														
Percentages[b]														
Recommended Dietary Allowances*														
Men 15–18 yrs.below[c]	See below[d]	See	<30%[e]	<10%[e]	<300[e]	50%>[e]	1,200	12	2,400[e]	5,000	1.5	1.8	20	60
Men 19–24 yrs.	↓	↓	<30%[e]	<10%[e]	<300[e]	50%>[e]	1,200	10	2,400[e]	5,000	1.5	1.7	19	60
Men 25–50 yrs.	↓	↓	<30%[e]	<10%[e]	<300[e]	50%>[e]	800	10	2,400[e]	5,000	1.5	1.7	19	60
Men 51+ yrs.	↓	↓	<30%[e]	<10%[e]	<300[e]	50%>[e]	800	10	2,400[e]	5,000	1.2	1.4	15	60
Women 15–18 yrs.	↓	↓	<30%[e]	<10%[e]	<300[e]	50%>[e]	1,200	15	2,400[e]	4,000	1.1	1.3	15	60
Women 19–24 yrs.	↓	↓	<30%[e]	<10%[e]	<300[e]	50%>[e]	1,200	15	2,400[e]	4,000	1.1	1.3	15	60
Women 25–50 yrs.	↓	↓	<30%[e]	<10%[e]	<300[e]	50%>[e]	800	15	2,400[e]	4,000	1.1	1.3	15	60
Women 51+ yrs.	↓	↓	<30%[e]	<10%[e]	<300[e]	50%>[e]	800	10	2,400[e]	4,000	1.0	1.2	13	60
Pregnant	↓	↓	<30%[e]	<10%[e]	<300[e]	50%>[e]	1,200	30	2,400[e]	4,000	1.5	1.6	17	70
Lactating	↓	↓	<30%[e]	<10%[e]	<300[e]	50%>[e]	1,200	15	2,400[e]	6,000	1.6	1.8	20	95

[a]Divide totals by 3 or number of days assessed.
[b]Percentages: Protein and Carbohydrates = multiply average by 4, divide by average calories, and multiply by 100.
Fat and Saturated Fat = multiply average by 9, divide by average calories, and multiply by 100.
[c]Use Table 4.1 (Page 84) for all categories.
[d]Protein intake should be .8 grams per kilogram of body weight. Pregnant women should consume an additional 15 grams of daily protein, while lactating women should have an extra 20 grams.
[e]Based on recommendations by nutrition experts.

*Adapted from *Recommended Dietary Allowances*, © 1989, by the National Academy of Sciences, National Academy Press, Washington, D.C.

Figure 2A.2 Three-day nutritional analysis.

Date: ______________

Name: ________________________________ Age: ______________ Weight: ______________

Sex: Male-M, Female-F (Pregnant-P, Lactating-L, Neither-N)

Activity Rating: Sedentary (limited physical activity) = 1
Moderate physical activity = 2
Hard labor (strenuous physical activity) = 3

Number of days to be analyzed: ______________ Day: ______________

No.	Code*	Food	Amount
1			
2			
3			
4			
5			
6			
7			
8			
9			
10			
11			
12			
13			
14			
15			
16			
17			
18			
19			
20			
21			
22			
23			
24			
25			
26			
27			
28			
29			
30			
31			

*When done, to advance to the next day or end, type 0 (zero).

Figure 2A.3 Daily nutrient intake form for computer software use.

LAB 2B ACHIEVING A BALANCED DIET

HOMEWORK ASSIGNMENT

Name: ______________________________ Date: ____________________ Grade: ____________

Instructor: ______________________________ Course: ____________________ Section: ____________

ASSIGNMENT This laboratory experience should be carried out as a homework assignment to be completed over the next 7 days.

LAB RESOURCES "Food Guide Pyramid" (Figure 2.1, page 24) and list of "Nutritive Value of Selected Foods" (Appendix A).

OBJECTIVE To meet the minimum daily required servings of the basic food groups and monitor total daily fat intake.

INSTRUCTIONS Keep a 7-day record of your food consumption using the Food Guide Pyramid and the form given in Figure 2B.1 (make additional copies of this form as needed — at least 3 days are recommended). Whenever you have something to eat, record the food code from the Nutritive Value of Selected Foods list contained in Appendix A, the number of calories, grams of fat, and the servings in the corresponding spaces provided for each food group. If a food item is not listed in the Nutritive Value of Selected Foods list, the information can be obtained from the food container itself or some of the references given at the end of the list of foods in Appendix A.

Record all information immediately after each meal, because it will be easier to keep track of foods and amounts eaten. If twice the amount of a particular serving is eaten, the calories and grams of fat must be doubled and two servings should be recorded under the respective food group.

At the end of the day, the diet is evaluated by checking whether the minimum required servings for each food group were met, and by the total amount of fat consumed. If you meet the required servings, you are well on your way to achieving a well-balanced diet. In addition, fat intake should not exceed 30% of the total daily caloric consumption. If you are on a diet, you may want to reduce fat intake to less than 20% of total daily calories (see Table 4.3, page 86).

LAB 2B

Name: ______________________

No.	Code*	Food	Amount	Calories	Fat (gm)	Food Groups (servings): Bread, Cereal, Rice & Pasta	Vegetable	Fruit	Milk, Yogurt & Cheese	Meat, Poultry, Fish, Dry Beans, Eggs, & Nuts
1										
2										
3										
4										
5										
6										
7										
8										
9										
10										
11										
12										
13										
14										
15										
16										
17										
18										
19										
20										
21										
22										
23										
24										
25										
26										
27										
28										
29										
30										
Totals										
Recommended Amount				**	***	6–11	3–5	2–4	2–3	2–3
Deficiencies										

*See list of nutritive value of selected foods in Appendix A.
**Compute using Table 4.1, page 84.
***Multiply the recommended amount of calories by .30 (30%) and divide by 9 to obtain the recommended amount of grams of fat (if on a diet, multiply by .20 or .10 — see Table 4.3, page 86).

Figure 2B.1 Daily diet record form.

LAB 3A HYDROSTATIC WEIGHING FOR BODY COMPOSITION ASSESSMENT

Name: ______________________________ Date: ______________ Grade: ________

Instructor: ____________________________ Course: ______________ Section: ________

NECESSARY LAB EQUIPMENT Hydrostatic or underwater weighing tank and residual volume spirometer (if no spirometer is available, predicting equations can be used to determine this volume — see Figure 3.1, page 57).

OBJECTIVE To determine body density and percent body fat.

LAB PREPARATION Bring a swimsuit and towel to this lab. A 6- to 8-hour fast and bladder and bowel movements are recommended prior to underwater weighing.

LAB 3A

INSTRUCTIONS Follow the procedure outlined in Figure 3.1, page 57. If time is a factor, assess only the body composition of one or two participants in the course, and compute the results using the form provided below. A sample of the computations is provided on the back of this page.

Name: ______________________________

Age: ________ Weight: ________ lbs Height: ________ inches × 2.54 = cm

Water Temperature: _____ °C Water Density (WD)*: _____ gr/ml

Residual Volume (RV)*: _____ lt

Body Weight (BW) in kg = weight in pounds ÷ 2.2046

BW in kg = ÷ 2.2046 = Kg

Gross Underwater Weights:

1. _____ kg	2. _____ kg	3. _____ kg	4. _____ kg	5. _____ kg
6. _____ kg	7. _____ kg	8. _____ kg	9. _____ kg	10. _____ kg

Average of Three Heaviest Underwater Weights (AUW): __________ kg

Tare Weight (TW): _____ kg

Net Underwater Weight (UW) = AUW − TW

Net Underwater Weight (UW) = − = kg

Body Density (BD):

$$BD = \frac{BW}{\frac{BW - UW}{WD} - RV - .1}$$

$$BD = \frac{\qquad}{\frac{\quad - \quad}{\qquad} - \quad - .1} =$$

Percent Body Fat (%Fat):

$$\%Fat = \frac{495}{BD} - 450$$

$$\%Fat = \frac{495}{\qquad} - 450 = \quad \%$$

*See Figure 3.1, page 57

LAB 3A

Name: Jane Doe

Age: 20 Weight: 148.5 lbs Height: 67 inches × 2.54 = 170.2 cm

Water Temperature: 33 °C Water Density (WD): .99473 gr/ml

Residual Volume (RV): 1.37 lt

Body Weight (BW) in kg = weight in pounds ÷ 2.2046

BW in kg = 148.5 ÷ 2.2046 = 67.36 kg

Gross Underwater Weights:

1. 6.15 Kg	2. 6.12 Kg	3. 6.24 Kg	4. 6.26 Kg	5. 6.21 Kg
6. 6.29 Kg	7. 6.27 Kg	8. 6.28 Kg	9. ______ Kg	10. ______ Kg

Average of Three Heaviest Underwater Weights (AUW): 6.28 Kg

Tare Weight (TW): 5.154 Kg

Net Underwater Weight (UW) = AUW − TW

Net Underwater Weight (UW) = 6.28 − 5.154 = 1.126 kg

Body Density (BD):

$$BD = \frac{BW}{\frac{BW - UW}{WD} - RV - .1} \qquad BD = \frac{67.36}{\frac{67.36 - 1.126}{.99473} - 1.37 - .1} = 1.03448$$

Percent Body Fat (%Fat):

$$\%Fat = \frac{495}{BD} - 450 \qquad \%Fat = \frac{495}{1.03448} - 450 = 28.5\%$$

Figure 3A.1 Sample computation for percent body fat according to hydrostatic weighing.

LAB 3B ANTHROPOMETRIC MEASUREMENTS FOR BODY COMPOSITION ASSESSMENT AND RECOMMENDED BODY WEIGHT DETERMINATION

Name: ______________________ Date: ______________ Grade: ________

Instructor: ______________________ Course: ______________ Section: ________

NECESSARY LAB EQUIPMENT Skinfold calipers and standard measuring tapes.

OBJECTIVE To assess percent body fat using skinfold thickness or girth measurements.

INSTRUCTIONS If skinfold calipers are available, use the skinfold thickness technique to assess your percent body fat (see Figure 3.3, page 59). If calipers are unavailable, estimate the percent fat according to the girth measurements technique (see Figure 3.4, page 63). You may wish to use both techniques and compare the results. Compute your recommended body weight according to your current and the recommended percent body fat guidelines provided in Table 3.7, page 68.

LAB 3B

I. Percent Body Fat According to Skinfold Thickness

Men		Women	
Chest (mm):	________	Triceps (mm):	________
Abdomen (mm):	________	Suprailium (mm):	________
Thigh (mm):	________	Thigh (mm):	________
Total (mm):	________	Total (mm):	________
Percent Fat:	________	Percent Fat:	________

II. Percent Fat According to Girth Measurements

Men

Waist (inches):	________
Wrist (inches):	________
Difference:	________
Body Weight:	________
Percent Fat:	________

Women

Upper Arm (cm):	________	Constant A =	________
Age:	________	Constant B =	________
Hip (cm):	________	Constant C =	________
Wrist (cm):	________	Constant D =	________

BD* = A − B − C + D

BD = ______ − ______ − ______ + ______ = ______

Percent Fat = (495 ÷ BD) − 450 = (495 ÷ ______) − 450 = ______

*Body density

III. Recommended Body Weight Determination

A. Body Weight (BW): __________

B. Current Percent Fat (%F)*: __________

C. Fat Weight (FW) = BW × %F

FW = × =

D. Lean Body Mass (LBM) = BW − FW = − =

E. Age: __________

F. Desired Fat Percent (DFP − *see* Table 3.7, page 68): __________

G. Recommended Body Weight (RBW) = LBM ÷ (1.0 − DFP*)

RBW = ÷ (1.0 −) =

*Express percentages in decimal form (for example., 25% = .25)

IV. Percent Body Fat Objective

1. Indicate what percent body fat you would like to achieve by the end of the semester: __________
2. Briefly state how you are planning to achieve this objective:

____

____

____

____

____

LAB 3C WEIGHT AND HEALTH: DISEASE RISK ASSESSMENT

Name: ______________________________ Date: ________________ Grade: __________

Instructor: ______________________________ Course: ________________ Section: __________

NECESSARY LAB EQUIPMENT Scale and standard measuring tapes.

OBJECTIVE To determine disease risk based on the waist-to-hip ratio and the body mass index (BMI)

INSTRUCTIONS Determine your height, waist, and hip measurements in inches. Record your body weight in pounds. Compute your waist-to-hip ratio and BMI as indicated below.

LAB 3C

I. Waist-to-Hip Ratio

Waist (inches): __________

Hip (inches): __________

Ratio (waist ÷ hip): __________ Disease Risk: ______________

Recommended Standards

Waist-to-Hip Ratio		
Men	**Women**	**Disease Risk**
≤0.95	≤0.80	Very Low
0.96–0.99	0.81–0.84	Low
≥1.00	≥0.85	High

II. Body Mass Index

Weight (pounds): __________

Height (inches): __________

BMI = Weight × 705 ÷ Height ÷ Height

BMI = ______ × 705 ÷ ______ ÷ ______

BMI = ______ Disease Risk: ______________

Recommended Standards

BMI	Disease Risk	Classification
<20.00	Moderate to Very High	Underweight
20.00 to 21.99	Low	Acceptable
22.00 to 24.99	Very Low	
25.00 to 29.99	Low	Overweight
30.00 to 34.99	Moderate	Obese
35.00 to 39.99	High	
≥ 40.00	Very High	

LAB 4A ESTIMATION OF DAILY CALORIC REQUIREMENT

Name: ______________________ Date: ______________ Grade: ________

Instructor: ______________________ Course: ______________ Section: ________

NECESSARY LAB EQUIPMENT Tables 4.1 (page 84) and 4.2 (page 84).

OBJECTIVE To determine an estimated daily caloric requirement with exercise for weight maintenance and or reduction.

Computation Form for Daily Caloric Requirement

A. Current body weight ________

B. Caloric requirement per pound of body weight (use Table 4.1) ________

LAB 4A

C. Typical daily caloric requirement without exercise to maintain body weight (A × B) ________

D. Selected physical activity (e.g., jogging)* ________

E. Number of exercise sessions per week ________

F. Duration of exercise session (in minutes) ________

G. Total weekly exercise time in minutes (E × F) ________

H. Average daily exercise time in minutes (G ÷ 7) ________

I. Caloric expenditure per pound per minute (cal/lb/min) of physical activity (use Table 4.2) ________

J. Total calories burned per minute of physical activity (A × I) ________

K. Average daily calories burned as a result of the exercise program (H × J) ________

L. Total daily caloric requirement with exercise to maintain body weight (C + K) ________

M. Number of calories to subtract from daily requirement to achieve a negative caloric balance** ________

N. Target caloric intake to lose weight (L – M) ________

---

* If more than one physical activity is selected, you will need to estimate the average daily calories burned as a result of each additional activity (steps D through K) and add all of these figures to L above.

** Subtract 500 calories if the total daily requirement with exercise (L) is below 3,000 calories. As many as 1,000 calories may be subtracted for daily requirements above 3,000 calories.

LAB 4B BEHAVIORAL OBJECTIVES FOR EXERCISE, NUTRITION, AND WEIGHT MANAGEMENT

Name: ______________________ Date: ______________ Grade: __________

Instructor: ______________________ Course: ______________ Section: __________

NECESSARY LAB EQUIPMENT None.

OBJECTIVE To prepare a plan to initiate a lifetime exercise, nutrition, and weight management program.

LAB PREPARATION Read Chapters 2, 3 and 4 prior to this lab.

Please answer all of the following:

1. State your own feelings regarding your current body weight.

____

____

____

2. If you suffer from an eating disorder, indicate what type of professional advice you will seek to help you overcome this condition.

____

____

____

3. Is your present diet adequate according to the nutritional analysis? _____ Yes _____ No

3A. If your answer to the previous question was "no," state what general dietary changes are necessary to achieve a balanced diet and/or lose weight (increase or decrease caloric intake, decrease fat intake, increase intake of complex carbohydrates, etc.).

____

____

____

3B. List specific foods that will help you to meet the recommended dietary allowances in areas where you may have deficiencies (*see* Figure 2.13, page 42, and the "Nutritive Value of Selected Foods" list in Appendix A).

____

____

____

3C. List foods that you should avoid to help you achieve better nutrition and/or a balanced diet.

____

____

____

4. Indicate your feelings about participating in an exercise program.

____

____

____

5. Will you commit to participate in a combined aerobic and strength-training program?* _____ Yes _____ No

   If your answer is "yes," proceed to the next question.

   If you answered "no," please review Chapters 2, 3 and 4 again and read Chapters 5, 6, 7, and 8.

6. List aerobic activities you enjoy or may enjoy doing.

____

7. Select one or two aerobic activities in which you will participate regularly.

____

8. List facilities available to you where you can carry out the aerobic and strength-training program.

____

____

____

9. Indicate days and times you will set aside for your aerobic and strength-training program (4 to 6 days should be devoted to aerobic exercise and 3 nonconsecutive days to strength-training).

   Monday: ____

   Tuesday: ____

   Wednesday: ____

   Thursday: ____

   Friday: ____

   Saturday: ____

   Sunday: A complete day of rest once a week is recommended to allow your body to fully recover from exercise.

---

* Flexibility programs are necessary for the development and maintenance of good health and adequate fitness but are not effective in the achievement of weight loss. Stretching exercises should be conducted regularly either to warm up or cool down in conjunction with your aerobic and strength-training program (*see* Chapters 9 and 10).

LAB 4C WEIGHT MANAGEMENT: BEHAVIOR MODIFICATION PROGRESS FORM

Name: ______________________________ Date: ________________ Grade: __________

Instructor: ______________________________ Course: ________________ Section: __________

NECESSARY LAB EQUIPMENT None required.

OBJECTIVE To monitor behavioral improvements for weight management.

INSTRUCTIONS Read the section on *tips for behavior modification and adherence to a weight management program* in Chapter 4, page 86. On a weekly basis, go through the list of strategies given on the back of this sheet and provide a "Yes" or "No" answer to each statement. If you are able to answer "Yes" to most questions, you have succeeded in implementing positive weight management behaviors.

Strategy Date:															
1. I made a commitment to change															
2. I set realistic goals															
3. I exercise regularly															
4. I have healthy eating patterns															
5. I avoid automatic eating															
6. I stay busy															
7. I plan meals ahead of time															
8. I cook wisely															
9. I do not serve more food than I should eat															
10. I eat slowly and at the table only															
11. I avoid social binges															
12. I avoid refrigerator and cookie-jar raids															
13. I avoid eating out. If I do, I eat low-fat meals															
14. I practice stress management															
15. I monitor behavior changes															
16. I reward my accomplishments															
17. I think positive															

LAB 5A CARDIORESPIRATORY ENDURANCE ASSESSMENT

Name: ______________________ Date: ______________ Grade: ________

Instructor: ______________________ Course: ______________ Section: ________

NECESSARY LAB EQUIPMENT

1.5 -Mile Run: School track or premeasured course and a stopwatch.

1.0-Mile Walk Test: School track or premeasured course and a stopwatch.

Step Test: A bench or gymnasium bleachers 16¼ inches high, a metronome, and a stopwatch.

Astrand-Ryhming Test: A bicycle ergometer that allows for regulation of workloads in kilopounds per meter (or watts) and a stopwatch.

12-Minute Swim Test: Swimming pool and a stopwatch.

OBJECTIVE To assess maximal oxygen uptake (VO_{2max}) and cardiorespiratory endurance classification.

LAB PREPARATION Wear appropriate exercise clothing including jogging shoes and a swimsuit if required. Be prepared to take the 1.0-Mile Walk Test, the Step Test, the Astrand-Ryhming Test, the 1.5-Mile Run Test, and/or the 12-Minute Swim Test. If more than one test will be conducted, perform them in the order just listed and allow at least 15 minutes between tests. Avoid vigorous physical activity 24 hours prior to this lab.

I. 1.5-Mile Run Test

1.5-Mile Run Time: _______ minutes and _______ seconds

VO_{2max} (see Table 5.2, page 96): ml/kg/min

Cardiorespiratory Fitness Classification (Table 5.8, page 104): _______________

II. 1.0-Mile Walk Test

Weight (W) = _______ lbs

Age (A) = _______

Gender (G) = _______ (females = 0, males = 1)

Time = _______ minutes and _______ seconds

Time in minutes (T) = min. + (sec ÷ 60)

T = + (÷ 60) = min

Heart Rate (HR) = _______ bpm

VO_{2max} = 132.853 − (.0769 × W) − (.3877 × A) + (6.315 × G) − (3.2649 × T) − (.1565 × HR)

VO_{2max} = 132.853 − (.0769 × ____) − .3877 × ____) + (6.315 × ____) − (3.2649 × ____) − (.1565 × ____)

VO_{2max} = 132.853 − ( ) − ( ) + ( ) − ( ) − ( )

VO_{2max} = ml/kg/min

Cardiorespiratory Fitness Classification (Table 5.8, page 104): _______________

III. Step Test

15 second recovery heart rate: __________ beats

VO_{2max} (Table 5.3, page 98): ml/kg/min

Cardiorespiratory Fitness Classification (Table 5.8, page 104): ________________

IV. Astrand-Ryhming Test

Weight (W) = __________ lbs

Body weight (BW) in kilograms = (W ÷ 2.2046) = __________ kg

Workload = __________ kpm

Exercise heart rates

	30-second pulse count	Heart Rate in bpm*
First minute:	__________	__________
Second minute:	__________	__________
Third minute:	__________	__________
Fourth minute:	__________	__________
Fifth minute:	__________	__________
Sixth minute:	__________	__________

*Use Table 5.4, page 100

Average heart rate for the fifth and sixth minutes = __________ bpm

Maximal oxygen uptake in liters per minute (Table 5.5, page 101) = __________ l/min

Correction factor (Table 5.6, page 102) = __________

Corrected maximal oxygen uptake in liters per minute (VO_{2max} in l/min × correction factor) = __________ l/min

Maximal oxygen uptake in milliliters per kilogram per minute (Corrected VO_{2max} in l/min × 1000 ÷ by BW in kg) = __________ × 1000

VO_{2max} = ml/kg/min

Cardiorespiratory Fitness Classification (Table 5.8, page 104): ________________

V. 12-Minute Swim Test

Distance swum in 12-minutes: __________ yards

Cardiorespiratory Fitness Classification (Table 5.7, page 103): ________________

LAB 5A

VI. University of Houston Non-Exercise Test (See sample computation in Figure 5.7, page 104)

Age (A) = ___________

Physical Activity Rating (PAR) (see Figure 5.6, page 103) = __________

Percent Fat (N-Ex % Fat) Model

Men VO_{2max} = 56.370 − (.289 × A) − (.552 × %Fat) + (1.589 × PAR)

Women VO_{2max} = 50.513 − (.289 × A) − (.552 × %Fat) + (1.589 × PAR)

VO_{2max} = − (.289 ×) − (.552 ×) + (1.589 ×)

VO_{2max} = ml/kg/min

Body Mass Index (N-Ex BMI) Model

BMI = Weight in pounds × 705 ÷ Height in inches ÷ Height in inches

BMI = × 705 ÷ ÷

BMI =

Men VO_{2max} = 67.350 − (.381 × A) − (.754 × BMI) + (1.951 × PAR)

Women VO_{2max} = 56.363 − (.381 × A) − (.754 × BMI) + (1.951 × PAR)

VO_{2max} = − (.381 ×) − (.754 ×) + (1.951 ×)

VO_{2max} = ml/kg/min

Cardiorespiratory Fitness Classification (Table 5.8, page 104): _______________

VII. Cardiorespiratory Endurance Objectives

1. Indicate what cardiorespiratory endurance classification you would like to achieve by the end of the semester:

____

2. Briefly state how you are planning to achieve this objective (also refer to Lab 4B, questions 6, 7, 8, and 9):

____

____

____

____

LAB 5A

LAB 5B HEART RATE AND BLOOD PRESSURE ASSESSMENT

Name: ______________________ Date: ______________ Grade: ________

Instructor: ______________________ Course: ______________ Section: ________

NECESSARY LAB EQUIPMENT Stopwatches, stethoscopes, and blood pressure sphygmomanometers.

OBJECTIVE To determine resting heart rate and blood pressure.

PREPARATION The instructions to determine heart rate and blood pressure are given at the end of Chapter 1. Many factors can affect heart rate and blood pressure. Factors such as excitement, nervousness, stress, food, smoking, pain, temperature, and physical exertion all can alter heart rate and blood pressure significantly. Therefore, whenever possible, readings should be taken in a quiet, comfortable room following a few minutes of rest in the recording position. Avoid any form of exercise several hours prior to the assessment. Wear exercise clothing, including a shirt with short or loose-fitting sleeves to allow for placement of the blood pressure cuff around the upper arm.

LAB 5B

Resting Heart Rate and Blood Pressure

Determine your resting heart rate and blood pressure in the right and left arms while sitting comfortably in a chair.

Resting Heart Rate: ________ bpm Rating:* ____________

Blood Pressure:	Right Arm	Risk Rating**	Left Arm	Risk Rating
Systolic	________	________	________	________
Diastolic	________	________	________	________

Standing, Walking, Jogging Heart Rate and Blood Pressure

Have one individual measure your heart rate and another individual your blood pressure immediately after standing for one minute, after walking for one minute, and after jogging in place for one minute. For blood pressure assessment use the arm with the highest reading in the sitting position.

Activity	Heart Rate (bpm)	Systolic/Diastolic Blood Pressure (mmHg)
Standing	________	________ / ________
Walking	________	________ / ________
Jogging	________	________ / ________

Conclusions. Draw conclusions based on your observed resting and activity heart rates and blood pressures.

____

____

____

____

*See Table 5.9, page 105.
**See Table 5.10, page 106.

LAB 6A ADVANTAGES AND DISADVANTAGES OF ADDING EXERCISE TO YOUR LIFESTYLE

Name: ______________________ Date: ______________ Grade: ________

Instructor: ______________________ Course: ______________ Section: ________

NECESSARY LAB EQUIPMENT None required.

OBJECTIVE To determine personal factors that may help you add exercise to your lifestyle.

INSTRUCTIONS The basic question for you is: Are you willing to give exercise a try? The first step is to decide positively that you will try. Based on your personal feelings and the information learned in this course, prepare a list of the advantages and disadvantages of adding exercise to your lifestyle. When the reasons for exercise outweigh the reasons for not exercising, it will become easier to give exercise a try.

Advantages of Starting an Exercise Program

1. ______________________
2. ______________________
3. ______________________
4. ______________________
5. ______________________
6. ______________________
7. ______________________
8. ______________________

Disadvantages of Starting an Exercise Program

1. ______________________
2. ______________________
3. ______________________
4. ______________________
5. ______________________
6. ______________________
7. ______________________
8. ______________________

LAB 6B EXERCISE READINESS QUESTIONNAIRE

Name: ______________________________ Date: __________________ Grade: __________

Instructor: ____________________________ Course: ________________ Section: __________

NECESSARY LAB EQUIPMENT None required.

OBJECTIVE To determine your preparedness to start an exercise program.

INSTRUCTIONS Read each statement carefully and circle the number that best describes your feelings in each statement. Please be completely honest with your answers.

Exercise Readiness Questionnaire

	Strongly Agree	Mildly Agree	Mildly Disagree	Strongly Disagree
1. I can walk, ride a bike (or a wheelchair), swim, or walk in a shallow pool.	4	3	2	1
2. I enjoy exercise.	4	3	2	1
3. I believe exercise can help decrease the risk for disease and premature mortality.	4	3	2	1
4. I believe exercise contributes to better health.	4	3	2	1
5. I have previously participated in an exercise program.	4	3	2	1
6. I have experienced the feeling of being physically fit.	4	3	2	1
7. I can envision myself exercising.	4	3	2	1
8. I am contemplating an exercise program.	4	3	2	1
9. I am willing to stop contemplating and give exercise a try for a few weeks.	4	3	2	1
10. I am willing to set aside time at least three times a week for exercise.	4	3	2	1
11. I can find a place to exercise (the streets, a park, a YMCA, a health club).	4	3	2	1
12. I can find other people who would like to exercise with me.	4	3	2	1
13. I will exercise when I am moody, fatigued, and even when the weather is bad.	4	3	2	1
14. I am willing to spend a small amount of money for adequate exercise clothing (shoes, shorts, leotards, swimsuit).	4	3	2	1
15. If I have any doubts about my present state of health, I will see a physician before beginning an exercise program.	4	3	2	1
16. Exercise will make me feel better and improve my quality of life.	4	3	2	1

Scoring Your Test:

This questionnaire allows you to examine your readiness for exercise. You have been evaluated in four categories: mastery (self-control), attitude, health, and commitment. Mastery indicates that you can be in control of your exercise program. Attitude examines your mental disposition toward exercise. Health provides evidence of the wellness benefits of exercise. Commitment shows dedication and resolution to carry out the exercise program. Write the number you circled after each statement in the corresponding spaces below. Add the scores on each line to get your totals. Scores can vary from 4 to 16. A score of 12 and above is a strong indicator that that factor is important to you, and 8 and below is low. If you score 12 or more points in each category, your chances of initiating and adhering to an exercise program are good. If you fail to score at least 12 points in three categories, your chances of succeeding at exercise may be slim. You need to be better informed about the benefits of exercise, and a retraining process may be required.

Mastery: 1.________ + 5. ________ + 6. ________ + 9. ________ = ________

Attitude: 2.________ + 7. ________ + 8. ________ + 13. ________ = ________

Health: 3.________ + 4. ________ + 15. ________ + 16. ________ = ________

Commitment: 10.________ + 11. ________ + 12. ________ + 14. ________ = ________

LAB 6C CARDIORESPIRATORY EXERCISE PRESCRIPTION

Name: ______________________________ Date: ______________ Grade: ________

Instructor: ______________________________ Course: ______________ Section: ________

NECESSARY LAB EQUIPMENT None required.

OBJECTIVE To write your own cardiorespiratory exercise prescription.

Intensity of Exercise

1. Estimate your own maximal heart rate (MHR)

   MHR = 220 minus age (220 − age)

   MHR = 220 − ________ = ________ bpm

2. Resting Heart Rate (RHR) = ________ bpm

3. Heart Rate Reserve (HRR) = MHR − RHR

   HRR = ________ − ________ = ________ beats

4. Training Intensities (TI) = HRR × TI + RHR

   50 Percent TI = ________ × .50 + ________ = ________ bpm

   70 percent TI = ________ × .70 + ________ = ________ bpm

   85 Percent TI = ________ × .85 + ________ = ________ bpm

5. Cardiorespiratory Training Zone. The optimum cardiorespiratory training zone is found between the 70% and 85% training intensities. Individuals who have been physically inactive or are in the poor or fair cardiorespiratory fitness categories should use a 50% training intensity during the first few weeks of the exercise program.

   Cardiorespiratory Training Zone: ________ (70% TI) to ________ (85% TI)

   Rate of Perceived Exertion (see Figure 6.2, page 110): ____________ to ____________

Mode of Exercise

Select any activity or combination of activities that you enjoy doing. The activity has to be continuous in nature and must get your heart rate up to the cardiorespiratory training zone and keep it there for as long as you exercise. Indicate your preferred mode(s) of exercise:

1. ________________ 2. ________________ 3. ________________

4. ________________ 5. ________________ 6. ________________

Cardiorespiratory Exercise Program

The following is your weekly program for development of cardiorespiratory endurance. If you are in the average, good, or excellent fitness category, you may start at week 5. After completing this 12-week program, for you to maintain your fitness level, you should exercise in the 70% to 85% training zone for about 20 to 30 minutes, a minimum of three times per week, on nonconsecutive days. You also should recompute your target zone periodically because you will experience a significant reduction in resting heart rate with aerobic training (approximately 10 to 20 beats in about 8 to 12 weeks).

Week	Duration (min.)	Frequency	Training Intensity	10-Sec. Pulse Count*
1	15	3	Approximately 50%	
2	15	4	Approximately 50%	
3	20	4	Approximately 50%	_____ beats
4	20	5	Approximately 50%	
5	20	4	About 70%	
6	20	5	About 70%	
7	30	4	About 70%	_____ beats
8	30	5	About 70%	
9	30	4	Between 70% and 85%	
10	30	5	Between 70% and 85%	
11	30–40	5	Between 70% and 85%	_____ to _____ beats
12	30–40	5	Between 70% and 85%	

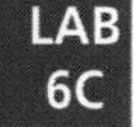

*Fill out your own 10-second pulse count under this column.

LAB 6D EXERCISE HEART RATE AND CALORIC COST OF PHYSICAL ACTIVITY

Name: ______________________________ Date: ________________ Grade: __________

Instructor: ______________________________ Course: ________________ Section: __________

NECESSARY LAB EQUIPMENT A school track (or premeasured course) and a stopwatch. Each student also should bring a watch with a second hand.

OBJECTIVE To monitor exercise heart rate and determine the caloric cost of physical activity based on exercise heart rate.

LAB PREPARATION Wear exercise clothing, including jogging shoes. Do not engage in vigorous physical activity prior to this lab. Read the information on *predicting caloric expenditure from exercise heart rates* in Chapter 6, page 128.

PROCEDURE

1. **Cardiorespiratory Training Zone.** Look up your cardiovascular training zone at 70% and 85% of heart rate reserve in Lab 6C. Record this information in beats per minute (bpm) and in 10-second pulse counts in the blank spaces provided below.

	Beats/minute	10-sec. count
70% intensity =	________	________
85% intensity =	________	________

2. **Resting Heart Rate (HR) and Body Weight (BW).** Determine your resting HR prior to exercise and your body weight in kilograms (divide pounds by 2.2046).

   Resting HR: ________ bpm

   BW: __________lbs ÷ 2.2046 = kg

3. **Walking HR, Oxygen Uptake (VO_2), and Caloric Expenditure.** Walk two laps around a 400-meter (440-yard) track at an average speed of 75 to 100 meters per minute. Try to maintain a constant speed around the track. You can monitor your speed by starting the walk at the beginning of the 100-meter straightway and making sure you have walked at least 75 meters and no more than 100 meters in one minute. As soon as you complete the two laps (800 meters), notice the time required to walk this distance and immediately check your exercise HR by taking a 10-second pulse count. Record this information in the spaces provided below. Do not record the time until after you have checked your pulse. Exercise HR will remain at the same rate for about 15 seconds following cessation of exercise. Therefore, you need to check your pulse as soon as you finish the walk, after noticing the 800-meter walk time.

   10-sec. pulse count: ______ beats

   800-meter time: ______ min. and ______ sec.

   HR in bpm = 10-sec pulse count × 6

   HR in bpm = ________ × 6 = bpm

   800-meter time in minutes = min. + (sec. ÷ 60)

   800-meter time in minutes = ________ + (________ ÷ 60) = min.

   Speed in meters per minute (mts/min.) = 800 ÷ 800-meter time in min.

   Speed in mts/min. = 800 ÷ ________ = mts/min.

   VO_2 in ml/kg/min at this walking speed (Use Table 6.3, page 129) = ml/kg/min.

LAB 6D

VO_2 in l/min = VO_2 in ml/kg/min × BW in kg ÷ 1000

VO_2 in l/min = _________ × _________ ÷ 1000 = l/min

Caloric expenditure for 800-meter walk = VO_2 in l/min × 5 × 800-meter time in min.

Caloric expenditure for 800-meter walk = _________ × 5 × _________ = calories

4. **Slow-Jogging HR, VO_2, and Caloric Expenditure.** Slowly jog 800 meters (two laps) around the track. Try to maintain the same slow-jogging pace throughout the two laps. Do NOT jog fast or sprint. This is not a speed test and is intended to be a slow jog only. As soon as you complete the 800 meters, notice the time required to complete the distance, and check your exercise HR immediately by taking another 10-second pulse count. Record this information below.

   10-sec. pulse count: _______ beats

   800-meter time: _______ min., _______ sec.

   HR in bpm = 10-sec. pulse count × 6

   HR in bpm = _________ × 6 = bpm

   800-meter time in minutes = min. + (sec. ÷ 60)

   800-meter time in minutes = _________ + (_________ ÷ 60) = min.

   Speed in mts/min. = 800 ÷ 800-meter time in min.

   Speed in mts/min. = 800 ÷ _________ = mts/min.

   VO_2 in ml/kg/min at this slow-jogging speed (Use Table 6.3, page 129) = ml/kg/min

   VO_2 in l/min = VO_2 in ml/kg/min × BW in kg ÷ 1000

   VO_2 in l/min = _________ × _________ ÷ 1000 = l/min

   Caloric expenditure for 800-meter slow jog = VO_2 in l/min × 5 × 800-meter time in min.

   Caloric expenditure for 800-meter slow jog = _________ × 5 × _________ = calories

LAB 6D

5. **Fast-Jogging HR, VO_2, Caloric Expenditure, and Recovery HR.** Jog another 800 meters at a faster speed around the track. Again try to maintain the same jogging pace throughout the two laps. Do NOT sprint. Your HR should not exceed 180 bpm on this test. As soon as you complete the 800 meters, notice your time for the two laps and check your 10-second pulse count. Record this information below. You also should check your 2- and 5-minute recovery HRs after the run and record these rates below.

   10-sec. pulse count: _______ beats

   800-meter time: _______ min. and _______ sec.

   HR in bpm = 10-sec. pulse count × 6

   HR in bpm = _________ × 6 = bpm

   800-meter time in minutes = min. + (sec. ÷ 60)

   800-meter time in minutes = _________ + (_________ ÷ 60) = min.

   Speed in mts/min. = 800 ÷ 800-meter time in min.

   Speed in mts/min. = 800 ÷ _________ = mts/min.

   VO_2 in ml/kg/min. at this fast-jogging speed (Use Table 6.3, page 129) = ml/kg/min

   VO_2 in l/min = VO_2 in ml/kg/min × BW in kg ÷ 1000

   VO_2 in l/min = _________ × _________ ÷ 1000 = l/min

   Caloric expenditure for 800-meter fast jog = VO_2 in l/min × 5 × 800-meter time in min.

   Caloric expenditure for 800-meter fast jog = _________ × 5 × _________ = calories

Recovery HRs

	10-sec. count	bpm
2 minutes	________	________
5 minutes*	________	________

6. **Resting, Exercise, and Recovery HRs.** Plot your resting, exercise, and recovery HRs on the graph provided below.

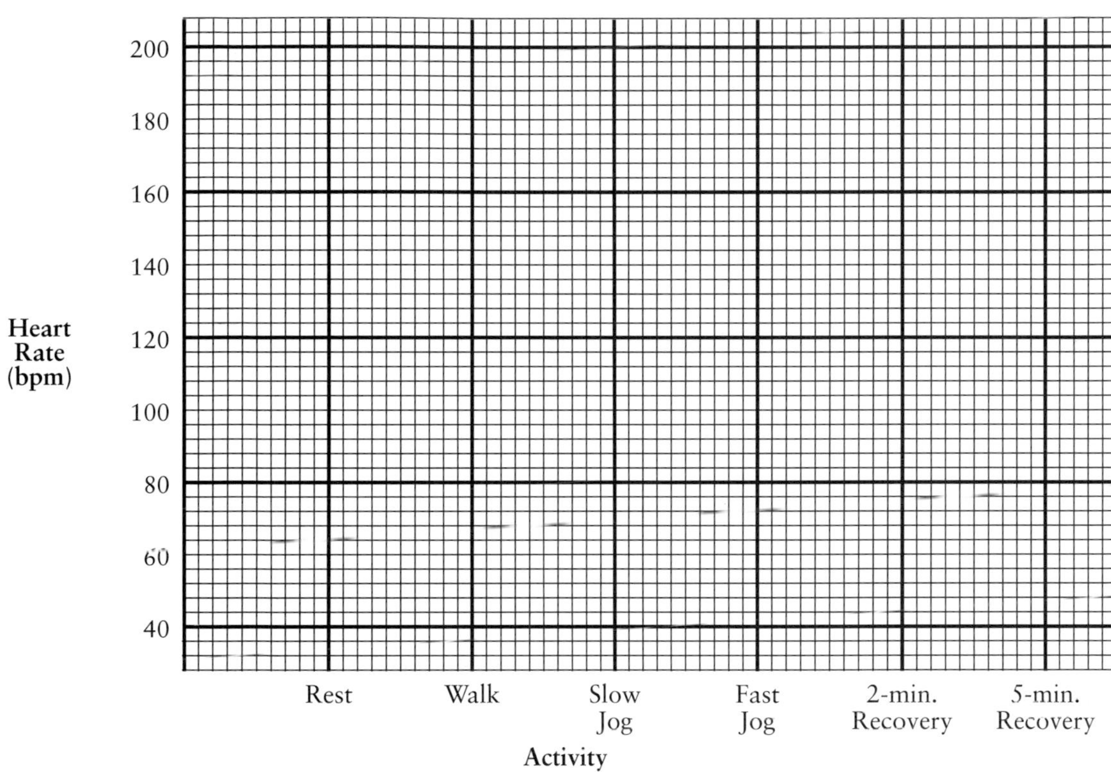

7. **Training Exercise HR and Equivalent Caloric Expenditure.** This part of the lab should be completed outside your regular lab time, during the next 2 or 3 days prior to turning in the assignment. According to the previous exercise HRs (items 3, 4, and 5), try to select a walking or jogging speed that will allow you to maintain your exercise HR in the appropriate cardiovascular training zone. Using a 400-meter track, walk or jog for 20 minutes at the selected speed and again try to maintain a constant speed throughout the exercise time. At the end of the 20 minutes, check your 10-second pulse count and estimate the distance covered in meters. Record this information below, and estimate the VO_2 and caloric expenditure.

10-sec. pulse count: _______ beats

HR in bpm = 10-sec pulse count × 6

HR in bpm = __________ × 6 = __________ bpm

Approximate distance covered in twenty minutes: __________ meters

Speed in mts/min. = distance in meters ÷ 20 minutes

Speed in mts/min. = __________ ÷ 20 = __________ mts/min.

VO_2 at this speed (see Table 6.3, page 129) = __________ ml/kg/min

VO_2 in l/min = VO_2 in ml/kg/min × BW in kg ÷ 1000

*Your 5-minute recovery HR should be below 120 bpm. If it is above 120, you most likely have overexerted yourself and, therefore, need to decrease the intensity of exercise (and/or duration when exercising for long periods of time). If your 5-minute recovery HR is still above 120 after decreasing the intensity of exercise, you should consult a physician regarding this condition.

VO_2 in l/min = __________ × __________ ÷ 1000 = l/min

Caloric expenditure for 20-min. walk/jog = VO_2 in l/min × 5 × 20 min.

Caloric expenditure for 20-min. walk/jog = __________ × 5 × 20 = calories

Using the previous information, how many calories would you have burned if you had maintained this pace for:

10 minutes (VO_2 in l/min × 5 × 10) = __________ × 5 × 10 = calories

30 minutes (VO_2 in l/min × 5 × 30) = __________ × 5 × 30 = calories

60 minutes (VO_2 in l/min × 5 × 60) = __________ × 5 × 60 = calories

PREDICTING CALORIC EXPENDITURE ACCORDING TO EXERCISE HR

Research indicates that there is a linear relationship between HR and VO_2, as long as the HR ranges from about 110 to 180 bpm. If you were able to obtain two exercise HRs in this range and the equivalent oxygen uptakes (in l/min), you can easily predict your VO_2 and caloric expenditure for any given HR in the specified range. Plot your two exercise HRs and the corresponding VO_2 values on the graph provided below. Next, draw a line between these two points on the graph and extend the line to 110 and 180 bpm. You now may look up the VO_2 for any HR by finding the desired HR on the Y axis, then going across to the reference line and straight down to the X axis, where you will find the corresponding VO_2 in l/min. To obtain the caloric expenditure in calories per minute, simply multiply the VO_2 by 5. You also may predict your maximal VO_2 (in l/min) by extending the line up to your maximal HR. The maximal HR is estimated by subtracting your age from 220. To convert the maximal VO_2 to ml/kg/min, multiply the l/min value by 1000 and divide by body weight in kilograms.

Using the results from your lab and the graph below, indicate the VO_2 in l/min and the caloric expenditure at the following HRs:

	VO_2 (l/min)	Caloric Expenditure (calories per minute)
120 bpm	__________	__________
150 bpm	__________	__________
170 bpm	__________	__________

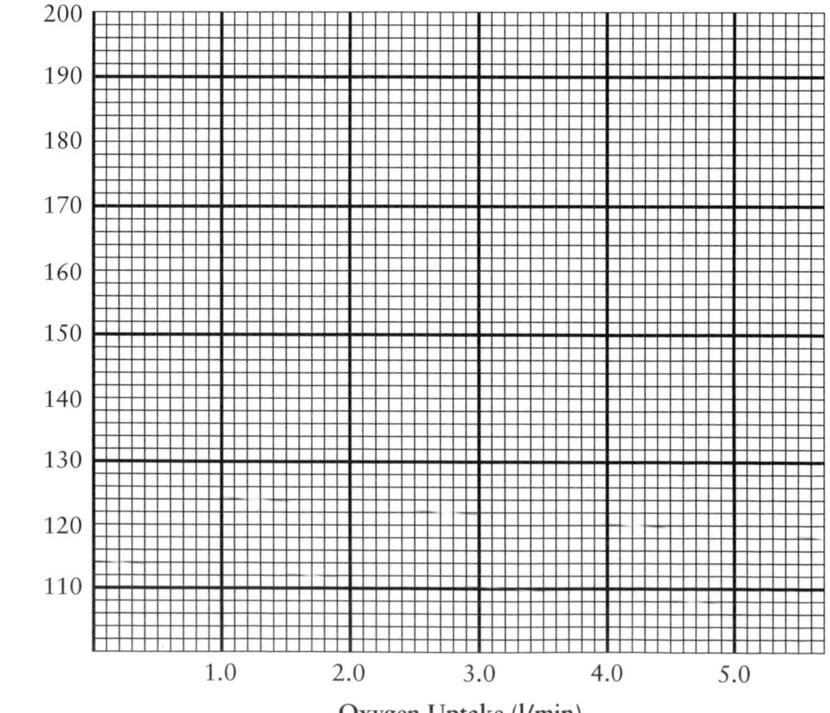

LAB 7A

MUSCULAR STRENGTH AND ENDURANCE ASSESSMENT

Name: ______________________ Date: ______________ Grade: ________

Instructor: ______________________ Course: ______________ Section: ________

NECESSARY LAB EQUIPMENT A 16-station, fixed-resistance, Universal Gym Apparatus and a metronome are required for the Muscular Strength and Endurance Test (2½ and 5-pound weights, also obtainable from Universal Gym Equipment, are recommended to get to within one pound of the actual resistance to be lifted). A metronome, gymnasium bleachers, and a stopwatch are needed for the Muscular Endurance Test. *A Lafayette hand grip dynamometer model 78010 is recommended for the Hand Grip Test.*

OBJECTIVE To determine muscular strength and/or endurance and the respective fitness classification.

LAB PREPARATION Wear exercise clothing and avoid strenuous strength training 48 hours prior to this lab.

I. Muscular Strength and Endurance Test

Perform the Muscular Strength and Endurance Test according to the procedure outlined in Figure 7.3, page 138 in Chapter 7. Record the results and percentile ranks (use Table 7.2, page 139) in the appropriate blanks provided below.

Body Weight: ____________ lbs.

Lift	Percent of Body Weight	Resistance (pounds)	Repetitions	Percentile Rank
	Men	Women		
Lat Pull-Down	.70	.45		
Leg Extension	.65	.50		
Bench Press	.75	.45		
Abdominal Crunch	NA*	NA		
Leg Curl	.32	.25		
Arm Curl	.35	.18		

*Not applicable — no resistance required. Use same test described in Figure 7.4, page 140.

Total: ________

Average Percentile Rank (divide total by 6): ________

Overall Strength/Endurance Fitness Category (*see* item 6 in Figure 7.3, page 138): ____________

LAB 7A

II. Muscular Endurance Test

Conduct this test using the guidelines provided in Figure 7.4, page 140. Record your results and percentile ranks (use Table 7.3, page 141).

Exercise	Metronome Cadence	Results (Repetitions)	Percentile Rank
Bench Jumps	none		
Modified Dips (Men)	56 bpm		
Modified Push-Ups (Women)	56 bpm		
Abdominal Crunches	60 bpm		

Total: __________

Average Percentile Rank (divide total by three): __________

Overall Muscular Endurance Fitness Category (*see* Figure 7.4): ____________________

III. Hand Grip Strength Test

The instructions for the Hand Grip Strength Test are provided in Figure 7.2, page 137. Perform the test according to the instructions and look up your results in Table 7.1, page 138.

Hand Used: ☐ Right ☐ Left

Reading: __________ lbs.

Fitness Category (*see* item 6 in Figure 7.2, page 137): __________

IV. Muscular Strength and Endurance Objectives

1. Indicate what muscular strength and endurance classification you would like to achieve by the end of the semester: ______________________________

2. Indicate what muscular endurance classification you would like to achieve by the end of the semester:

____

3. Briefly state how you are planning to achieve these objectives (also refer to Lab 4B, questions 8 and 9):

____

____

____

____

LAB 8A SAMPLE STRENGTH-TRAINING PROGRAM

Name: ________________________ Date: ______________ Grade: __________

Instructor: ________________________ Course: ______________ Section: __________

NECESSARY LAB EQUIPMENT Free weights, strength-training machines, or no equipment if the "Strength-Training Exercises Without Weights" program is selected.

OBJECTIVE To become acquainted with a sample strength-training exercise program, which may be carried out throughout life.

LAB PREPARATION Wear exercise clothing and prepare to participate in a sample strength-training exercise session. All of the strength-training exercises are illustrated at the end of Chapter 8, pages 153–162.

INSTRUCTIONS Select one of the two strength-training exercise programs. Perform all of the recommended exercises and, with the exception of the bent-leg curl-up or abdominal crunch exercises, determine the resistance required to do approximately 10 repetitions maximum (for "Strength-Training Exercises Without Weights," simply indicate the total number of repetitions performed). For the bent-leg curl-up or abdominal crunch exercises, perform or build up to about 20 repetitions.

I. Strength-Training Exercises Without Weights

Exercise	Repetitions
Step-Up or High Jumper (select and circle one)	________
Push-Up	________
Abdominal Crunch or Bent-leg Curl-Up	________
Leg Curl	________
Modified Dip	________
Pull-Up or Arm Curl (select one)	________
Heel Raise	________
Leg Abduction and Adduction	________
Reverse Crunch	________
Pelvic Tilt	________

II. Strength-Training Exercises with Weights

Exercise	Repetitions	Resistance
Bench Press, Shoulder Press, or Chest Press (select and circle one)	________	________
Leg Press or Squat (select one)	________	________
Abdominal Crunch	________	________
Rowing Torso	________	________
Arm Curl or Upright Rowing (select one)	________	________
Leg Curl or Seated Leg Curl (select one)	________	________
Seated Back	________	________
Heel Raise	________	________
Lat Pull-Down or Bent-Arm Pullover (select one)	________	________
Rotary Torso	________	________
Triceps Extension or Dip (select one)	________	________
Leg Extension	________	________

LAB 9A MUSCULAR FLEXIBILITY ASSESSMENT

Name: ______________________ Date: ______________ Grade: ________

Instructor: ______________________ Course: ______________ Section: ________

NECESSARY LAB EQUIPMENT Acuflex I, Acuflex II, and Acuflex III Flexibility Testers* or homemade flexibility testing equipment as described in Chapter 9, Figures 9.1 (page 166), 9.2 (page 167), and 9.3 (page 169).

OBJECTIVE To assess muscular flexibility and the respective fitness categories.

LAB PREPARATION The procedures for the flexibility tests* administered in this lab are explained in Chapter 9 (Figures 9.1, 9.2, and 9.3, pages 166–169). It is important that you warm up properly before you perform any of these tests. Do gentle stretching exercises specific to the tests that will be administered. Wear loose exercise clothing for this lab. Be sure to circle either inches or cm, depending on which system you use.

I. Modified Sit-and-Reach Test

Trials: 1. ________ inches ________ cm. 2. ________ inches ________ cm. (circle either inches or cm)

Average Score: ________ inches ________ cm. Percentile Rank: ________

Fitness Classification: ____________

II. Total Body Rotation Test

Right Side Left Side (circle one)

Trials: 1. ________ inches ________ cm. 2. ________ ________ inches ________ cm.

Average Score: ________ inches ________ cm. Percentile Rank: ________

Fitness Classification: ____________

III. Shoulder Rotation Test

Biacromial Width: ________ inches ________ cm. Rotation Score: ________ inches ________ cm.

Final Score = Rotation score – biacromial width

Final Score = ________ – ________ = ________ inches / cm. (circle one) Percentile Rank: ________

Fitness Classification: ____________

IV. Overall Flexibility Rating

Test	Percentile Rank
Modified Sit-and-Reach:	________
Total Body Rotation (right, left — circle one):	________
Shoulder Rotation:	________

Total: ________

Average Percentile Rank (divide total by 3): ________

Overall Flexibility Classification: ________

* The Acuflex I, II, and III Flexibility Testers can be obtained from Figure Finder Collection, Novel Products, Inc., P.O. Box 408, Rockton, IL 61072-0408, Phone (800) 323-5143.

V. Flexibility Objectives

1. Indicate what flexibility classification you would like to achieve by the end of the semester: __________
2. Briefly state how you are planning to achieve this objective.

____

____

____

____

LAB 9B POSTURE EVALUATION

Name: ______________________________ Date: ____________________ Grade: __________

Instructor: ______________________________ Course: ____________________ Section: __________

NECESSARY LAB EQUIPMENT A plumb line, two large mirrors set at about an 85° angle, and a Polaroid camera (the mirrors and the camera are optional — *see* "Evaluating Body Posture" in Chapter 9, page 170).

OBJECTIVE To determine current body alignment.

LAB PREPARATION To conduct the posture analysis, men should wear shorts only and women, shorts and a tank top. Shoes should also be removed for this test.

LAB ASSIGNMENT The class should be divided in groups of four students each. The group should carefully study the posture form given in this lab, then proceed to fill out the form for each member according to the instructions given under "Evaluating Body Posture" in Chapter 9, page 170. If no mirrors and camera are available, three members of the group are to rate the fourth person's posture while he/she first stands with the side of the body and then with the back to the plumb line. A final score is obtained by totaling the points given for each body segment and looking up the posture rating according to the total score found in the Table provided below.

Results

Total Score: ____________________

Classification: ____________________

Posture Evaluation Standards

Total Points	Classification
≥45	Excellent
40-44	Good
30-39	Average
20-29	Fair
≤19	Poor

Source: *The Complete Guide for the Development and Implementation of Health Promotion Programs*, by W. W. K. Hoeger (Englewood, CO: Morton Publishing, 1987). Reproduced by permission.

Posture Improvement

Indicate which areas of your posture should be corrected and what steps you can take to make improvements.

____

____

____

____

	Good — 5	Fair — 3	Poor — 1	Score
HEAD Left Right	head erect, gravity passes directly through center	head twisted or turned to one side slightly	head twisted or turned to one side markedly	
SHOULDERS Left Right	shoulders level horizontally	one shoulder slightly higher	one shoulder markedly higher	
SPINE Left Right	spine straight	spine slightly	spine markedly curved laterally	
HIPS Left Right	hips level horizontally	one hip slightly higher	one hip markedly higher	
KNEES and ANKLES	feet pointed straight ahead, legs vertical	feet pointed out, legs deviating outward at the knee	feet pointed out markedly, legs deviate markedly	
NECK and UPPER BACK	neck erect, head in line with shoulders, rounded upper back	neck slightly forward, chin out, slightly more rounded upper back	neck markedly forward, chin markedly out, markedly rounded upper back	
TRUNK	trunk erect	trunk inclined to rear slightly	trunk inclined to rear markedly	
ABDOMEN	abdomen flat	abdomen protruding	abdomen protruding and sagging	
LOWER BACK	lower back normally curved	lower back slightly hollow	lower back markedly hollow	
LEGS	legs straight	knees slightly hyper-extended	knees markedly hyper-extended	
			Total Score	

LAB 9B

Adapted with permission from *The New York Physical Fitness Test: A Manual for Teachers of Physical Education*, New York State Education Department (Division of HPER), 1958.

Figure 9B.1 Posture Analysis Form.

LAB 10A SAMPLE FLEXIBILITY DEVELOPMENT PROGRAM

Name: ________________________________ Date: ____________________ Grade: ___________

Instructor: ______________________________ Course: __________________ Section: ___________

NECESSARY LAB EQUIPMENT Minor implements such as a chair, a table, an elastic band (surgical tubing or a wood or aluminum stick), and a stool or steps.

OBJECTIVE To be introduced to a sample stretching exercise program that may be carried out throughout life.

LAB PREPARATION Wear exercise clothing and prepare to participate in a sample stretching exercise session. All of the flexibility exercises are illustrated in Chapter 10, page 179–182.

INSTRUCTIONS Perform all of the recommended flexibility exercises given in Chapter 10, page 179–182. Use a combination of slow-sustained and proprioceptive neuromuscular facilitation stretching techniques. Indicate the technique(s) used for each exercise, and, where applicable, the number of repetitions performed and the length of time that the final degree of stretch was held.

Stretching Exercises

Exercise	Stretching Technique	Repetitions	Length of Final Stretch
Lateral Head Tilt	____________	______	NA*
Arm Circles	____________	______	NA
Side Stretch	____________	______	______
Body Rotation	____________	______	______
Chest Stretch	____________	______	______
Shoulder Hyperextension Stretch	____________	______	______
Shoulder Rotation Stretch	____________	______	NA
Quad Stretch	____________	______	______
Heel Cord Stretch	____________	______	______
Adductor Stretch	____________	______	______
Sitting Adductor Stretch	____________	______	______
Sit-and-Reach Stretch	____________	______	______
Triceps Stretch	____________	______	______

*Not Applicable

LAB 10A

LAB 10B EXERCISES FOR THE PREVENTION AND REHABILITATION OF LOW BACK PAIN

Name: ______________________ Date: ______________ Grade: ________

Instructor: ______________________ Course: ______________ Section: ________

NECESSARY LAB EQUIPMENT Chair.

OBJECTIVE To participate in an exercise program for the prevention and rehabilitation of low-back pain.

LAB PREPARATION Wear exercise clothing and prepare to participate in the lab session. All of the exercises for this lab are illustrated in Chapter 10.

I. Stretching Exercises

Perform all of the recommended exercises for the prevention and rehabilitation of low back pain given in Chapter 10. Indicate the number of repetitions performed for each exercise.

Exercise	Repetitions
Single-Knee to Chest Stretch	________
Double-Knee to Chest Stretch	________
Upper and Lower Back Stretch	________
Sit-and-Reach Stretch	________
Gluteal Stretch	________
Back Extension Stretch	________
Trunk Rotation and Lower Back Stretch	________
Pelvic Tilt	________
Cat Stretch	________
Abdominal Crunch or Abdominal Curl-Up	________

II. Proper Body Mechanics

Perform the following tasks using the proper body mechanics given in Figure 10.3, page 177 (check off each item as you perform the task):

________ Standing (Carriage) Position

________ Sitting Position

________ Bed Posture

________ Resting Position for Tired and Painful Back

________ Lifting an Object

III. "Rules To Live By — From Now On"

Read the 18 "Rules To Live By — From Now On" given in Figure 10.3, page 178, and indicate below those rules that you need to work on to improve posture and body mechanics and prevent low back pain.

____

____

____

____

LAB 11A ASSESSMENT OF SKILL-RELATED COMPONENTS OF FITNESS

Name: ______________________ Date: ______________ Grade: ________

Instructor: ______________________ Course: ______________ Section: ________

NECESSARY LAB EQUIPMENT

Agility: Free-throw area of a basketball court (or any smooth area 12 by 19 feet with sufficient running space around it), four plastic cones, and a stopwatch.

Balance: Any flat, smooth floor (not carpeted) and a stopwatch.

Coordination: A cardboard with six circles drawn on it as explained in Chapter 11 (Figure 11.2, page 187), three full cans of soda pop (12 oz.), and a stopwatch.

Power: A flat, smooth surface, and a 10-foot-long tape measure (or two standard cloth measuring tapes, each 60 inches long).

Reaction Time: A standard yardstick with a shaded "concentration zone" drawn on the first 2 inches of the stick.

Speed: A school track or premeasured 50-yard straightway.

OBJECTIVE To assess the fitness level for each skill-related fitness component.

LAB PREPARATION Wear exercise clothing, including running shoes. Do not exercise strenuously several hours prior to this lab.

INSTRUCTIONS Perform all six tests for the fitness-related components as outlined in Chapter 11. Report the results below and answer the questions given at the end of this lab.

Skill-Related Fitness:	**Test Results**			
Agility	Trials:	1. ___ ___ . ___	2. ___ ___ . ___	
Balance	Trials:	1. ___ ___ . ___	2. ___ ___ . ___	
Coordination	Trials:	1. ___ ___ . ___	2. ___ ___ . ___	
Power	Trials:	1. ___ ___	2. ___ ___	3. ___ ___
Reaction Time	Trials:	1. ___ ___ . ___	2. ___ ___ . ___	3. ___ ___ . ___
	4. ___ ___ . ___	5. ___ ___ . ___	6. ___ ___ . ___	7. ___ ___ .
	8. ___ ___ . ___	9. ___ ___ . ___	10. ___ ___ . ___	11. ___ ___ . ___
	12. ___ ___ . ___		Average (6 middle scores) =	___ ___ . ___
Speed	Trial:	1. ___ ___ . ___		

LAB 11A

Skill-Related Fitness Classifications

Fitness Component (test)	Percentile Rank	Classification
Agility: SEMO test (Figure 11.1, page 185)	__________	______________
Balance: 1-foot stand (page 185)	__________	______________
Coordination: Soda pop test (Figure 11.2, page 187)	__________	______________
Power: Standing long jump (Figure 11.3, page 188)	__________	______________
Reaction Time:Yardstick test (page 187)	__________	______________
Speed: 50-yard dash (page 188)	__________	______________

Interpretation of Test Results

1. What conclusions can you draw from your test results?

____

____

____

____

2. Briefly state how you could improve your test results and what activities you could engage in to obtain the desired results?

____

____

____

____

3. Did you ever participate in organized sports, or have you found success in a particular game or sport?

_______ Yes _______ No

3a. If your answer is positive, list the sports, games, or events in which you enjoy(ed) success.

____

3b. Is there a relationship between the sports, games, or events in which you enjoyed particular success and your test results in this lab?

____

____

____

LAB 12A CARDIOVASCULAR DISEASE AND CANCER RISK MANAGEMENT

Name: ______________________ Date: ______________ Grade: ________

Instructor: ______________________ Course: ______________ Section: ________

NECESSARY LAB EQUIPMENT None required.

OBJECTIVE Evaluate family and lifestyle factors that may affect your risk for cardiovascular disease and cancer.

LAB PREPARATION Read Chapter 12 prior to this lab so you may become familiar with normal blood lipids, blood glucose, and blood pressure values, as well as the seven warning signals for cancer.

CARDIOVASCULAR DISEASE	Yes	No
1. I accumulate at least 30 minutes of physical activity on most days of the week?	☐	☐
2. I exercise aerobically a minimum of three times a week in the appropriate target zone for at least 20 minutes per session?	☐	☐
3. I am at or slightly below the health fitness recommended percent body fat?	☐	☐
4. My blood lipids within normal range?	☐	☐
5. I follow a healthy diet plan?	☐	☐
6. I am not a diabetic?	☐	☐
7. My blood pressure normal?	☐	☐
8. I do not smoke cigarettes or use tobacco in any other form?	☐	☐
9. I manage stress adequately in daily life?	☐	☐
10. I do not have a personal or family history of heart disease?	☐	☐

Evaluation

A "no" answer to any of the above items increases your risk for cardiovascular disease. The greater the number of "no" responses, the higher the risk for developing cardiovascular disease.

Please indicate lifestyle changes you will implement or maintain to decrease your personal risk for cardiovascular disease.

____

____

____

____

____

____

____

CANCER RISK: ARE YOU TAKING CONTROL?

	Yes	No
1. **Are you eating more cabbage-family vegetables?** They include broccoli, cauliflower, brussels sprouts, all cabbages, and kale.	☐	☐
2. **Are high-fiber foods included in your diet?** Fiber is present in whole grains, fruits and vegetables including peaches, strawberries, potatoes, spinach, tomatoes, wheat and bran cereals, rice, popcorn and whole-wheat bread.	☐	☐
3. **Do you choose foods with vitamin A?** Fresh foods with beta-carotene including carrots, peaches, apricots, squash, and broccoli are the best source, not vitamin pills.	☐	☐
4. **Is vitamin C included in your diet?** You'll find it naturally in lots of fresh fruits and vegetables including grapefruit, cantaloupe, oranges, strawberries, red and green peppers, broccoli and tomatoes.	☐	☐
5. **Do you exercise and monitor calorie intake to avoid weight gain?** Walking is ideal exercise for many people.	☐	☐
6. **Are you cutting overall fat intake?** This is done by eating lean meat, fish, skinned poultry, and low-fat dairy products.	☐	☐
7. **Do you limit salt-cured, smoked, nitrite-cured foods?** Choose bacon, ham, hot dogs or salt-cured fish only occasionally if you like them a lot.	☐	☐
8. **If you smoke, have you tried quitting?**	☐	☐
9. **If you drink alcohol, are you moderate in your intake?**	☐	☐
10. **Do you respect the sun's rays?** Protect yourself with sunscreen (at least #15), wear long sleeves and a hat, especially during midday hours (11 a.m. to 3 p.m.)	☐	☐
11. **Do you have a family history of any type of cancer? If so, have you brought this to the attention of your personal physician?**	☐	☐
12. **Are you familiar with the seven warning signals for cancer?**	☐	☐

Evaluation

If you answered yes to most of these questions, **congratulations.** You are taking control of simple lifestyle factors that will help you feel better and reduce your risk for cancer.

LAB 12A

Please indicate lifestyle changes you will implement or maintain to decrease your personal risk for cancer:

____

____

____

____

____

____

Adapted from the American Cancer Society, Texas Division.

LAB 12B SELF-EVALUATION AND BEHAVIORAL OBJECTIVES FOR THE FUTURE

Name: ______________________ Date: ______________ Grade: ________

Instructor: ______________________ Course: ______________ Section: ________

NECESSARY LAB EQUIPMENT None required, unless fitness tests are repeated.

OBJECTIVE To conduct a self-evaluation of the objectives achieved during this course and write behavioral objectives for the future.

LAB PREPARATION In this lab you will conduct a self-evaluation of the objectives you accomplished in this course. To carry out this assignment, you will need to review the objectives written in previous laboratories. If you are able to repeat the various assessments, you can indicate objectively if your objectives were met. If you are unable to conduct the reassessments, determine subjectively how well you reached your objectives (answer only the "yes" or "no" questions under item I below).

I. Did you accomplish your objective for:

Cardiorespiratory Endurance (see Lab 5A) ________ Yes ________ No

Pre-assessment VO_{2max}: ________ ml/kg/min Fitness Classification: ____________

Post-assessment VO_{2max}: ________ ml/kg/min Fitness Classification: ____________

Body Composition (see Labs 3A and 3B) ________ Yes ________ No

Pre-assessment Percent Body Fat: ________ Body Composition Classification: ________

Post-assessment Percent Body Fat: ________ Body Composition Classification: ________

Muscular Strength and Endurance (see Lab 7A) ________ Yes ________ No

Pre-assessment Percentile Rank: ________ Fitness Classification: ____________

Post-assessment Percentile Rank: ________ Fitness Classification: ____________

Muscular Flexibility (see Lab 9A) ________ Yes ________ No

Pre-assessment Percentile Rank: ________ Fitness Classification: ____________

Post-assessment Percentile Rank: ________ Fitness Classification: ____________

LAB 12B

II. Indicate nutritional and dietary changes that you were able to implement this semester (refer to Chapters 2 and 4 and Labs 2A, 2B, 4A, and 4B).

____

____

____

III. Did you implement your regular exercise program as outlined in Labs 4B, 6C, 8A, 10A, and Chapters 6, 8, and 10?

____

IV. Indicate any lifestyle changes you were able to make that will decrease your personal risk for cardiorespiratory disease and cancer, including stress management and smoking cessation.

____

____

____

V. Briefly evaluate this course and indicate whether it has had an effect on the quality of your life and your personal well-being.

____

____

____

____

VI. Behavioral Objectives for the Future

Indicate below one or two general objectives you will work on in the next couple of months, and write specific behavioral objectives that you will use to accomplish each general objective (you may not need eight specific objectives; write only as many as you need).

General Objective: ______________________________

Specific Objectives:

1. ______________________________
2. ______________________________
3. ______________________________
4. ______________________________
5. ______________________________
6. ______________________________
7. ______________________________
8. ______________________________

General Objective: ______________________________

Specific Objectives:

1. ______________________________
2. ______________________________
3. ______________________________
4. ______________________________
5. ______________________________
6. ______________________________
7. ______________________________
8. ______________________________

APPENDIX

A

Nutritive Value of Selected Foods

Code	Food	Amount	Weight gm	Calories	Protein gm	Fat gm	Sat. Fat gm	Cholesterol mg	Carbohydrate gm	Calcium mg	Iron mg	Sodium mg	Vit A I.U.	Thiamin (Vit B_1) mg	Riboflavin (Vit B_2) mg	Niacin mg	Vit C mg
1.	Almond Joy, candy bar	1.5 oz.	42	227	2.5	12	10.2	0	28	3	1.2	0	0	0.00	0.00	0.0	0
2.	Almonds, shelled	1/4 c	36	213	6.6	19	1.4	0	9	83	1.7	2	0	0.09	0.33	1.3	0
3.	Apple, raw, unpared	1 med	150	80	0.3	1	0.0	0	20	10	0.4	1	120	0.04	0.03	0.1	6
4.	Apple juice, canned or bottled	1/2 c	124	59	0.1	0	0.0	0	15	8	0.7	1	0	0.01	0.03	0.1	1
5.	Apple Pie, McDonald's	1	307	260	2	15	10.0	6	30	0	0.48	240	0	0.06	0	0	12
6.	Applesauce, canned, sweetened	1/2 c	128	116	0.3	0	0.0	0	31	5	0.7	3	50	0.02	0.01	0.0	2
7.	Apricots, canned, heavy syrup	3 halves; 1¾ tbsp liq.	85	73	0.5	0	0.0	0	19	9	0.3	1	1,480	0.02	0.02	0.3	3
8.	Apricots, dried, sulfured, uncooked	10 med halves	35	91	1.8	0	0.0	0	23	23	1.9	9	3,820	0.00	0.06	1.2	4
9.	Apricots, raw	3 (12 per lb)	114	55	1.1	0	0.0	0	14	18	0.5	1	2,890	0.06	0.04	0.6	11
10.	Arby Q, Arby's	1	190	389	18	15	5.5	29	48	84	6.1	1,268	0	0.27	0.41	9.2	0
11.	Arby Sauce, Arby's	.5 oz.	14	15	0	0	0.0	0	3	0	0.2	113	0	0.00	0.00	0.0	0
12.	Asparagus, cooked green spears	4 med	60	12	1.3	0	0.0	0	2	13	0.4	1	540	0.10	0.11	0.8	16
13.	Avocado, raw	1/2 med	120	185	2.4	19	3.2	0	7	11	0.6	4	310	0.12	0.22	1.7	15
14.	Bacon, cooked, drained	2 slices	15	86	3.8	8	2.7	30	1	2	0.5	153	0	0.08	0.05	0.8	0
15.	Bacon, lettuce, tomato sandwich	1	130	327	11.6	19	4.7	21	31	84	2.5	661	426	0.42	0.28	4.1	12
16.	Bagel	1 3½ in.	68	180	7.0	1	0.2	0	35	20	2.1	124	0	0.26	0.20	2.4	0
17.	Banana, raw	1 sm (7¼")	140	81	1.0	0	0.0	0	21	8	0.7	1	180	0.05	0.06	0.7	10
18.	Banana, nut bread	1 slice	50	169	3.0	8	1.5	33	22	18	0.9	172	49	0.09	0.09	0.8	1
19.	BBQ Sauce, McDonald's	1.12 oz.	32	50	0	0.6	0.2	0	12	0.0	0.0	350	200	0.00	0.00	0	2.4
20.	Beans, green snap, cooked	1/2 c	65	16	1.0	0	0.0	0	3	32	0.4	4	340	0.05	0.06	0.3	8
21.	Beans, lentils	1/4 c	50	53	3.9	0	0.0	0	10	12	1.0	0	10	0.03	0.04	0.4	0
22.	Beans, lima (Fordhook), froz., cooked	1/2 c	85	84	6.0	0	0.0	0	17	40	2.1	1	240	0.15	0.08	1.1	15
23.	Beans, red kidney, cooked	1 c	185	218	14.4	1	0.0	0	40	70	4.4	6	10	0.20	0.11	1.3	0
24.	Beans, refried	1/2 c	145	148	9.0	1	0.2	0	25	71	2.6	614	0	0.07	0.08	0.7	9
25.	Bean sprouts, mung, raw	1/2 c	52	18	2.0	0	0.0	0	4	10	0.7	3	10	0.07	0.07	0.4	10
26.	Beef, chuck, cooked,	3 oz.	85	212	25.0	12	7.8	80	0	11	3.1	43	20	0.05	0.19	3.8	0
27.	Beef, corned, canned	3 oz.	85	163	21.0	10	8.0	70	0	22	5.0	802	0	0.02	0.27	3.9	0
28.	Beef, ground, lean	3 oz.	85	186	23.3	10	5.0	81	0	10	3.0	57	20	0.08	0.20	5.1	0
29.	Beef, Lite Roast Deluxe, Arby's	1	182	294	18	10	3.5	42	33	156	3.0	826	200	0.27	0.52	8.4	8
30.	Beef, meatloaf	1 piece	111	246	20.0	15	6.1	125	6	37	2.4	434	181	0.08	0.23	4.1	1
491.	Beef, Meatloaf, traditional Healthy Choice	1	340	320	16.0	8	4.0	35	46	40	1.8	460	750	0.00	0.00	0.0	54
31.	Beef N' Cheddar, Arby's	1	194	508	25	27	7.7	52	43	180	4.1	1,166	0	0.42	0.67	9.8	1
32.	Beef, round steak, cooked, trimmed	3 oz.	85	222	24.3	13	6.0	77	0	10	3.0	60	20	0.07	0.20	4.8	0
33.	Beef, rump roast	3 oz.	85	177	24.7	9	4.0	80	0	10	3.1	61	10	0.06	0.19	4.4	0
34.	Beef, sirloin, cooked	3 oz.	85	329	19.6	27	13.0	77	0	9	2.5	48	50	0.05	0.15	4.0	0
493.	Beef, Sirloin tips, Healthy Choice	1	334	280	23.0	8	0.0	65	30	20	2.7	370	3,500	0.15	0.17	5.0	42
500.	Beef stroganoff, Weight Watchers	1	238	290	22.0	9	4.0	25	26	8	2.7	600	300	0.23	0.26	4.0	4
35.	Beef, T-bone steak	3 oz.	85	403	16.7	37	15.6	66	0	7	2.2	40	23	0.07	0.14	3.5	0
36.	Beef, thin, sliced	3 oz.	85	105	18.5	3	1.4	36	0	11	1.8	1,409	0	0.07	0.16	4.5	0
37.	Beer	12 fl. oz.	360	151	1.1	0	1.1	0	14	18	0.0	25	0	0.01	0.11	2.2	0
38.	Beer, light	12 fl. oz.	354	96	0.7	0	0.0	0	4	17	0.1	10	0	0.03	0.10	1.3	0
39.	Beets, red, canned, drained	1/2 c	80	32	0.8	0	0.0	0	8	15	0.6	164	15	0.01	0.02	0.1	2
40.	Beet greens, cooked	1/2 c	73	13	1.3	0	0.0	0	2	72	1.4	55	3,700	0.05	0.11	0.2	11
41.	Biscuits, baking powder	1 med	35	114	2.5	6	1.1	0	18	60	0.8	272	0	0.06	0.06	0.7	0
42.	Blueberries, fresh cultivated	1/2 c	73	45	0.5	0	0.0	0	11	10	0.8	1	75	0.02	0.05	0.4	10
43.	Bologna	1 slice (1 oz.)	28	86	3.4	8	3.0	15	0	2	0.5	369	0	0.05	0.06	0.7	0

44.	Bologna, turkey	2 slices	57	113	7.8	9	3.0	56	1	47	0.9	498	0	0.03	0.09	2.1	0
45.	Bouillon, broth	1 cube	4	5	0.8	0	0.0	0	0	0	0.0	960	0	0.00	0.00	0.0	0
46.	Brandy	1 oz.	28	69	0.0	0	0.0	0	11	0	0.0	1	0	0.00	0.00	0.0	0
47.	Bread, Corn	1 slice	78	161	5.8	6	0.1	0	23	94	0.9	490	120	0.10	0.15	0.5	1
48.	Bread, Cracked wheat	1 slice	25	65	2.3	1	0.2	0	12	16	0.7	106	0	0.10	0.10	0.8	0
49.	Bread, French enriched	1 slice	35	102	3.2	1	0.2	0	19	15	0.8	203	0	0.10	0.08	0.9	0
50.	Bread, Oatmeal	1 slice	25	65	2.1	1	0.2	0	12	15	0.7	124	0	0.12	0.07	0.9	0
51.	Bread, Pita pocket	1 piece	60	165	6.2	1	0.1	0	33	49	1.5	339	0	0.27	0.13	2.3	0
52.	Bread, Pumpernickel	1 slice	32	80	2.9	1	0.2	0	15	23	0.9	277	0	0.11	0.17	1.1	0
53.	Bread, Rye (American)	1 slice	25	61	2.3	0	0.0	0	13	19	0.4	139	0	0.05	0.02	0.4	0
54.	Bread, white enriched	1 slice	25	68	2.2	1	0.2	0	13	21	0.6	127	0	0.06	0.05	0.6	0
55.	Bread, whole wheat	1 slice	25	61	2.6	1	0.6	0	12	25	0.8	132	0	0.06	0.03	0.7	0
56.	Broccoli, cooked drained	1 sm stalk	140	36	4.3	0	0.0	0	6	123	1.1	14	3,500	0.13	0.28	1.1	126
57.	Broccoli, raw	1 sm stalk	114	38	4.1	0	0.0	0	7	117	1.3	17	2,835	0.10	0.23	0.9	125
58.	Brownies, with nuts	1	20	95	1.3	6	2.3	18	11	9	0.4	51	20	0.05	0.05	0.3	0
59.	Brussels sprouts, froz., cooked, drained	1/2 c	78	28	3.2	0	0.0	0	5	25	0.8	8	405	0.06	0.11	0.5	63
60.	Bulgur, wheat	1 c	135	227	8.4	1	0.0	0	47	27	1.8	809	0	0.07	0.04	3.2	0
61.	Burrito, bean	1	166	307	12.5	9.5	3.6	14	45	173	2.4	983	283	0.15	0.22	2.3	5
62.	Burrito, combination, Taco Bell	1	175	404	21.0	16	0.0	0	43	91	3.7	300	1,666	0.34	0.31	4.6	15
482.	Burrito, 7 Layer, Taco Bell	1	234	458	14.0	20	5.9	17	55	85	2.3	983	1,485	0.00	0.00	0.0	5
483.	Burrito, 7 Layer Light, Taco Bell	1	276	440	19.0	9	3.5	8	67	250	4.5	1,430	1,750	0.00	0.00	0.0	5
63.	Butter	1 tsp	5	36	0.0	4	0.4	12	0	1	0.0	46	160	0.00	0.00	0.0	0
64.	Buttermilk, cultured	1 c	245	88	8.8	0	1.3	5	12	296	0.1	319	10	0.10	0.44	0.2	2
65.	Cabbage, boiled, drained wedge	1/2 c	85	16	0.9	0	0.0	0	3	36	0.3	10	100	0.02	0.02	0.1	21
66.	Cabbage, raw chopped	1/2 c	45	11	0.6	0	0.0	0	3	22	0.2	9	60	0.03	0.03	0.2	21
67.	Cake, Angel food, plain	1 piece	60	161	4.3	0	0.0	0	36	5	0.1	170	0	0.01	0.08	0.1	0
68.	Cake, Carrot	1 piece	96	385	4.2	21	4.1	74	48	44	1.3	279	75	0.11	0.12	0.9	1
69.	Cake, Cheesecake	1 piece (3½")	85	257	4.6	16	9.0	150	24	48	0.4	189	216	0.03	0.11	0.4	4
70.	Cake, Chocolate, w/icing	1 piece	69	235	3.0	8	3.6	37	40	41	1.4	181	100	0.07	0.10	0.6	0
71.	Cake, Coffee	1 piece	72	230	4.5	7	2.5	47	38	44	1.2	310	120	0.14	0.15	1.3	0
72.	Cake, Devil's food, iced	1 piece	99	365	4.5	16	5.0	68	55	69	1.0	233	160	0.02	0.10	0.2	0
73.	Cake, Pound	1 piece	30	120	2.0	5	1.0	32	15	20	0.5	98	200	0.05	0.06	0.5	0
74.	Cake, White, choc. icing	1 piece	71	268	3.5	11	3.7	2	48	35	0.3	162	40	0.19	0.14	1.6	0
75.	Candy, hard	1 oz.	28	109	0.0	0	0.0	0	28	6	0.5	9	0	0.00	0.00	0.0	0
76.	Cantaloupe	1/4 melon 5" diam.	239	35	2.0	0	0.0	0	10	20	0.8	17	4,620	0.06	0.04	0.6	45
77.	Caramel (candy, plain or choc.)	1 oz.	28	113	1.1	3	1.6	0	22	42	0.4	64	0	0.01	0.05	0.1	0
78.	Carrots, cooked, drained	1/2 c	73	23	0.7	0	0.0	0	5	24	0.5	10	7,615	0.04	0.04	0.4	5
79.	Carrots, raw	1 carrot 7½" long	81	30	0.8	0	0.0	0	7	27	0.5	34	7,930	0.04	0.04	0.4	6
80.	Cashew, roasted, unsalted	2 oz.	57	326	9.2	27	5.4	0	16	23	2.3	10	0	0.24	0.10	1.0	0
81.	Cauliflower, cooked, drained	1/2 c	63	14	1.5	0	0.0	0	3	13	0.5	6	40	0.06	0.05	0.4	35
82.	Celery, green, raw, long	1 outer stalk 8"	40	7	0.4	0	0.0	0	2	16	0.1	50	110	0.01	0.01	0.1	4
83.	Cereal, All-Bran	1/4 c	21	53	3.0	0	0.1	0	16	17	3.4	242	947	0.28	0.33	3.8	11
84.	Cereal, Alpha Bits	1 c	28	111	2.2	1	0.0	0	25	8	1.8	219	1,875	0.40	0.40	5.0	0
85.	Cereal, Bran	1/2 c	30	72	3.8	1	0.0	0	22	25	3.0	247	2,000	1.00	0.80	3.0	20
86.	Cereal, Cheerios	1 c	23	89	3.4	1	1.2	0	16	38	3.6	246	949	0.32	0.32	4.0	12
87.	Cereal, Corn Chex	1 c	28	111	2.0	0	0.1	0	25	3	1.8	271	75	0.40	0.07	5.0	15
88.	Cereal, Corn Flakes	1 c	25	97	2.0	0	0.0	0	21	3	0.6	251	180	0.29	0.55	2.9	9
89.	Cereal, Cream of Wheat	1 c	244	140	3.6	1	0.1	0	29	54	10.9	5	0	0.24	0.07	1.5	0
90.	Cereal, Frosted Mini-Wheats	4 biscuits	31	111	3.2	0	0.0	0	26	10	2.0	9	2,050	0.40	0.50	5.5	16
91.	Cereal, Fruit & Fibre w/dates	1 c	56	180	6.0	2	0.3	0	42	20	9.0	340	3,780	0.75	0.85	10.0	0
92.	Cereal, Granola, Nature Valley	1/2 c	57	252	5.8	10	7.0	0	38	36	1.9	116	41	0.20	0.10	0.4	0
93.	Cereal, Grape Nuts	1/2 c	57	202	6.6	0	0.0	0	47	22	2.5	394	3,815	0.80	0.80	10.0	0
94.	Cereal, Life	1 c	44	162	8.1	1	0.1	0	32	154	11.6	229	0	0.95	1.00	11.6	0

Code	Food	Amount	Weight gm	Calories	Protein gm	Fat gm	Sat. Fat gm	Cholesterol mg	Carbohydrate gm	Calcium mg	Iron mg	Sodium mg	Vit A I.U.	Thiamin (Vit B_1) mg	Riboflavin (Vit B_2) mg	Niacin mg	Vit C mg
95.	Cereal, Nutri-Grain Wheat	1 c	44	158	3.8	1	0.1	0	37	12	1.2	299	2,915	0.60	0.70	7.7	23
96.	Cereal, Oatmeal, quick, cooked	1/2 c	120	66	2.4	1	0.2	0	12	11	0.7	262	0	0.10	0.03	0.1	0
97.	Cereal, Raisin Bran	1 c	49	160	4.0	1	0.2	0	40	25	24.0	293	2,500	0.51	0.57	6.7	0
98.	Cereal, Rice Krispies	3/4 c	22	85	1.4	0	0.0	0	19	3	1.4	255	971	0.30	0.30	3.8	11
99.	Cereal, Shredded Wheat	1 c	19	65	2.1	0	0.0	0	11	8	0.6	1	0	0.06	0.05	0.9	0
100.	Cereal, Special K	1 c	21	83	4.2	0	0.0	0	16	6	3.4	199	1,430	0.30	0.30	3.8	11
101.	Cereal, Sugar Corn Pops	1 c	28	108	1.4	0	0.0	0	26	1	1.8	103	1,875	0.40	0.40	5.0	15
102.	Cereal, Sugar Frosted Flakes	1 c	35	133	1.8	0	0.0	0	32	1	2.2	284	2,315	0.50	0.50	6.2	19
103.	Cereal, Sugar Smacks	1 c	37	141	2.7	1	0.1	0	32	4	2.4	100	2,500	0.49	0.57	6.7	20
104.	Cereal, Total	1 c	33	116	3.3	1	0.1	0	26	56	21.0	409	8,845	1.70	2.00	23.3	70
105.	Cereal, Wheat Chex	1 c	46	169	4.5	1	0.2	0	38	18	7.3	308	0	0.60	0.17	8.1	24
106.	Cereal, whole wheat, cooked	1/2 c	123	55	2.2	0	0.0	0	12	9	0.06	260	0	0.08	0.03	0.8	0
107.	Cereal, whole wheat flakes, ready-to-eat	1 c	30	106	3.1	1	0.0	0	24	12	2.0	310	1,410	0.35	0.42	3.5	11
108.	Cereal, 40% Bran Flakes	1 c	39	125	4.9	1	0.1	0	31	19	11.2	363	2,610	0.51	0.59	6.9	0
109.	Cereal, 100% Bran	1/2 c	33	89	4.2	2	0.3	0	24	23	4.1	229	0	0.80	0.90	10.4	31
110.	Champagne	4 oz.	113	87	0.2	0	0.1	0	2	6	0.4	7	0	0.00	0.01	0.1	0
111.	Cheese, American	1 oz. slice	28	100	6.0	8	5.6	27	0	188	0.1	307	343	0.01	0.10	0.0	0
112.	Cheese, Bleu	1 oz.	28	100	6.0	8	5.3	25	1	89	0.1	510	204	0.01	0.11	0.3	0
113.	Cheese, Cheddar	1 oz.	28	114	7.0	9	6.0	30	0	204	0.2	171	300	0.01	0.11	0.0	0
114.	Cheese, Cottage, 2%	1/2 c	113	103	15.5	2	1.4	10	4	78	0.2	459	79	0.03	0.21	0.2	0
115.	Cheese, Cottage, creamed	1/2 c	105	112	14.0	5	6.4	15	3	99	0.3	241	180	0.03	0.26	0.1	0
116.	Cheese, Creamed	1 oz.	28	99	6.0	8	3.0	31	1	167	0.3	71	320	0.02	0.14	0.0	0
117.	Cheese, Feta	1 oz.	28	75	4.5	6	4.2	25	1	140	0.2	316	180	0.04	0.23	0.3	0
118.	Cheese, Monterey jack	1 oz.	28	106	6.9	9	5.4	26	0	212	0.2	152	405	0.00	0.11	0.0	0
119.	Cheese, Mozzarella, skim	1 oz.	28	80	7.6	5	3.1	15	1	207	0.1	150	216	0.01	0.10	0.0	0
120.	Cheese, Parmesan	1 tbsp	5	23	2.1	2	1.0	4	0	69	0.1	93	45	0.00	0.02	0.0	0
121.	Cheese, Ricotta, part skim	1 oz.	28	39	3.2	2	1.4	9	1	77	0.1	35	160	0.01	0.05	0.0	0
122.	Cheese, Souffle	1 portion	110	240	10.9	19	9.5	189	7	221	1.1	400	880	0.06	0.26	0.2	0
123.	Cheese, Swiss	1 oz.	28	107	8.0	8	5.0	26	1	272	0.1	74	360	0.01	0.10	0.0	0
124.	Cheese puffs, Cheetos	1 oz.	28	158	2.2	10	4.8	5	14	17	0.4	344	130	0.01	0.03	0.2	0
125.	Cheeseburger, McDonald's	1	115	321	15.2	16	6.7	40	29	170	2.9	736	353	0.30	0.24	4.4	2
126.	Cherries	10	75	47	0.9	0	0.0	0	12	15	0.3	8	450	0.20	0.24	1.6	41
127.	Chicken, BK Broiler sandwich, Burger King	1 sandwich	168	379	24.0	18	3.0	53	31	48	2.3	764	350	0.42	0.22	9.2	5
128.	Chicken Breast Filet, Arby's	1	204	445	22	23.0	3.0	45	52	72	1.9	958	0	0.23	0.58	9.0	5
129.	Chicken breast, roast w/skin	1	98	193	29.2	8	2.1	83	0	14	1.0	69	91	0.07	0.12	12.5	0
501.	Chicken burrito w/vegetables Weight Watchers	1	216	330	15.0	14	4.0	65	36	56	2.3	800	190	0.52	0.39	5.9	3
484.	Chicken cacciatore, Budget Gourmet	1	312	300	20.0	13	0.0	60	27	150	1.8	810	200	0.23	0.51	5.0	21
496.	Chicken cacciatore, Lean Cuisine	1	308	280	22.0	7	2.0	45	31	40	1.4	570	500	0.22	0.17	6.0	9
130.	Chicken chow mein	1 c	250	255	31.0	11	3.6	75	10	58	2.5	718	250	0.08	0.23	4.3	10
488.	Chicken chow mein, Healthy Choice	1	241	220	18.0	3	0.8	45	31	20	1.4	440	405	0.15	0.14	4.0	4
497.	Chicken chow mein, Lean Cuisine	1	255	240	14.0	5	1.0	30	34	40	1.1	530	300	0.15	0.17	5.0	6
502.	Chicken chow mein Weight Watchers	1	255	200	12.0	2	0.5	25	34	40	0.7	430	1,500	0.00	0.00	0.0	36
131.	Chicken club sandwich, Wendy's	1	220	520	30	25	6.0	75	44	120	9.6	980	100	0.60	0.45	16.0	9
132.	Chicken Cordon Bleu, Arby's	1	225	518	30	27	5.3	92	52	204	2.1	1,463	0	0.42	0.68	10.2	5
133.	Chicken, drumstick Kentucky Fried	1	54	136	14.0	8	2.2	73	2	20	0.9	320	30	0.04	0.12	2.7	0

134. Chicken, drumstick, roasted	1	52	112	14.1	6	1.6	48	0	6	0.7	47	52	0.04	0.11	3.1	0
135. Chicken McNuggets	6	111	329	19.5	21	5.2	64	15	11	1.3	521	92	0.16	0.14	7.7	2
136. Chicken Nuggets, Wendy's	6 pc.	94	280	14	20	5.0	50	12	48	0.48	600	0	0.09	0.11	6.0	0
137. Chicken, patty sandwich	1	157	436	24.8	23	6.1	68	34	44	1.9	2,732	47	0.13	0.26	9.2	4
138. Chicken, wing, Kentucky Fried	1	45	151	11.0	10	2.9	70	4	0	0.6	300	0	0.03	0.07	0.0	0
139. Chicken, roast, light meat without skin	3 oz.	85	141	27.0	3	0.4	45	0	10	1.2	54	51	0.03	0.09	9.9	0
140. Chicken, roast, dark meat without skin	3 oz.	85	149	24.0	5	0.8	50	0	11	1.5	54	127	0.06	0.19	4.7	0
141. Chicken, Roast Deluxe, Arby's	1	195	276	24	7	1.7	33	33	156	1.9	777	200	0.44	0.80	9.4	7
510. Chicken, Rotisserie, dark w/skin Kentucky Fried	1/4 chicken	146	333	30.0	24	6.6	163	1	10	0.2	980	75	0.00	0.00	0.0	1
511. Chicken, Rotisserie, light w/skin Kentucky Fried	1/4 chicken	176	335	40.0	19	5.4	157	1	10	0.2	1,100	75	0.00	0.00	0.0	1
142. Chicken Sandwich, breaded Wendy's	1	208	450	26	20	4.0	60	44	120	9.6	740	100	0.45	0.36	14.0	6
143. Chicken Sandwich, Grilled, Wendy's	1	177	290	24	7	1.0	60	35	120	2.4	670	100	0.38	0.27	10.0	6
144. Chicken Sandwich, McChicken	1	187	415	19	19	9.0	50	39	180	1.8	830	100	0.90	0.18	9.0	2.4
485. Chicken, Teriyaki, Budget Gourmet	1	340	360	20.0	12	0.0	55	44	80	1.4	610	1,500	0.15	0.34	6.0	12
145. Chili con carne	1 c	255	339	19.1	16	5.8	28	31	82	4.3	1,354	150	0.08	0.18	3.3	8
146. Chocolate fudge	1 oz.	28	115	0.6	3	2.1	1	21	22	0.3	54	0	0.01	0.03	0.1	0
147. Chocolate, milk	1 oz.	28	147	2.0	9	3.6	5	16	65	0.3	27	80	0.02	0.10	0.1	0
148. Chocolate, milk w/almonds	1 oz.	28	150	2.9	10	4.4	5	15	61	0.6	23	30	0.03	0.13	0.3	0
149. Clam, canned, drained	3 oz.	85	83	13.0	2	0.2	50	2	46	3.5	750	93	0.01	0.09	0.9	9
150. Cocoa, hot, with whole milk	1 c	250	218	9.1	9	6.1	33	26	298	0.8	123	318	0.10	0.44	0.4	2
151. Cocoa, plain, dry	1 tbsp	5	14	0.9	1	0.0	0	3	7	0.6	0	0	0.01	0.02	0.1	0
152. Coconut, shredded, packed	1/2 c	65	225	2.3	23	20.0	0	6	8	1.1	165	0	0.03	0.01	0.3	2
153. Cod, batter fried	3.5 oz.	100	199	19.6	10	3.9	55	8	80	0.5	100	2	0.02	0.02	1.8	0
154. Cod, cooked	3 oz.	85	144	24.3	4	1.5	60	0	27	0.9	63	150	0.06	0.09	2.7	0
155. Cod, poached	3.5 oz.	100	94	20.9	1	0.3	60	0	29	0.5	110	2	0.08	0.08	3.0	0
156. Coffee	3/4 cup	180	1	0.0	0	0.0	0	0	1	0.2	2	0	0.00	0.00	0.1	0
157. Coleslaw	1 c	120	173	1.6	17	1.0	5	6	53	0.5	144	190	0.06	0.06	0.4	35
158. Collards, leaves without stems, cooked, drained	1/2 c	95	32	3.4	1	2.0	0	5	178	0.8	28	7,410	0.01	0.19	1.2	72
159. Cookies, Chocolate chip homemade	2 2¼" diam.	20	103	1.0	6	1.7	14	12	7	0.4	70	20	0.02	0.02	0.2	0
160. Cookies, Fig bars	4 bars	56	210	2.0	4	1.0	27	42	40	1.4	180	31	0.08	0.07	0.7	0
161. Cookies, Oatmeal raisin	2 2" diam.	26	122	1.5	5	1.3	1	18	9	0.6	74	20	0.04	0.04	0.5	0
162. Cookies, Peanut butter, homemade	2 cookies	24	123	2.0	7	2.0	11	14	10	0.5	71	12	0.03	0.03	0.9	0
163. Cookies, sandwich, all	4 cookies	40	195	2.0	8	2.0	0	29	12	1.4	189	0	0.90	0.07	0.8	0
164. Cookies, Shortbread	4 cookies	32	155	2.0	8	2.9	27	20	13	0.8	123	40	0.10	0.09	0.9	0
165. Cookies, Vanilla	5 1¾" diam.	20	93	1.0	3	0.8	10	15	8	0.1	50	25	0.00	0.01	0.0	0
166 Cookies, Vanilla wafers	10 wafers	40	185	2.0	7	1.8	25	29	16	0.8	150	70	0.07	0.10	1.0	0
167. Corn, boiled on cob	1 ear 5" long	140	70	2.5	1	0.0	0	16	2	0.5	1	310	0.09	0.08	1.1	7
168. Corn, canned, drained	1/2 c	83	70	2.2	1	0.0	0	16	4	0.4	195	290	0.03	0.04	0.8	4
169. Corn chips	1 oz.	28	155	2.0	9	1.8	0	16	35	0.5	233	110	0.04	0.05	0.4	1
170. Cornmeal, degermed, yellow, enriched, cooked	1/2 c	120	60	1.3	0	0.0	0	13	1	0.5	264	70	0.07	0.05	0.6	0
171. Crab, canned	1 c	135	135	23.0	3	0.5	135	1	61	1.1	1,350	70	0.11	0.11	2.6	0
172. Crackers, Cheese	10 crackers	10	50	1.0	3	0.9	6	5	11	0.4	112	25	0.05	0.04	0.4	0
173. Crackers, Graham	2 squares	14	55	1.1	1	0.3	0	10	6	0.2	95	0	0.01	0.03	0.2	0
174. Crackers, Ritz	1 cracker	3	15	0.2	1	0.2	0	2	3	0.1	30	0	0.01	0.01	0.1	0
175. Crackers, Ryewafers, whole grain	2 crackers	14	55	1.0	1	0.3	0	10	7	0.5	115	0	0.06	0.03	0.5	0

Code	Food	Amount	Weight gm	Calories	Protein gm	Fat gm	Sat. Fat gm	Cholesterol mg	Carbohydrate gm	Calcium mg	Iron mg	Sodium mg	Vit A I.U.	Thiamin (Vit B_1) mg	Riboflavin (Vit B_2) mg	Niacin mg	Vit C mg
176.	Crackers, Saltines	4 squares	11	48	1.0	1	0.3	0	8	2	0.1	123	0	0.00	0.00	0.1	0
177.	Crackers, Soda	1	3	13	0.3	0	0.1	0	2	1	0.1	39	0	0.02	0.01	0.1	0
178.	Crackers, Triscuits	1	5	23	0.4	1	0.3	0	3	0	0.0	0	0	0.00	0.00	0.0	0
179.	Crackers, Wheat Thins	1	2	9	0.2	0	0.1	0	1	1	0.1	17	0	0.01	0.01	0.1	0
180.	Cranberry juice	1 c	253	145	0.1	0	0.0	0	36	8	0.4	5	5	0.02	0.02	0.1	90
181.	Cream, light coffee or table	1 tbsp	15	20	0.5	2	0.5	5	1	16	0.0	7	70	0.00	0.02	0.0	0
182.	Cream, heavy whipping	1 tbsp	15	53	0.3	6	1.3	12	1	11	0.0	5	230	0.00	0.02	0.0	0
183.	Croissant	1	57	235	4.7	12	4.0	13	27	20	2.1	452	50	0.17	0.13	1.3	0
184.	Croissants (Sara Lee)	1 roll	18	59	1.6	2	0.3	0	8	22	0.6	105	0	0.14	0.09	0.8	0
185.	Croissan'wich, egg, cheese Burger King	1 sandwich	110	315	13.0	20	7.0	222	19	112	1.8	607	500	0.22	0.37	1.4	0
186.	Cucumbers, raw pared	9 sm slices	28	4	0.3	0	0.0	0	1	7	0.3	2	70	0.01	0.01	0.1	3
187.	Danish, Apple, McDonald's	1	115	390	6	17	11.0	25	51	0	1.0	370	0	0.30	0.18	2.0	15
188.	Danish, Cinnamon Raisin	1	110	440	6	21	13.0	34	58	48	0.12	430	0	0.30	0.27	3.0	4
189.	Dates hydrated	5	46	110	0.9	0	0.0	0	29	24	1.2	1	20	0.04	0.04	0.9	0
190.	Doughnut, plain	1	42	164	1.9	8	2.0	19	22	17	0.6	210	30	0.07	0.07	0.5	0
191.	Doughnut, yeast raised	1	27	235	4.0	13	5.2	21	26	17	1.4	222	2	0.28	0.12	1.8	0
192.	Dressing, Bleu cheese	1 tbsp	15	77	0.7	8	1.9	4	1	12	0.0	8	32	0.00	0.02	0.0	0
193.	Dressing, French	1 tbsp	16	83	0.1	9	1.4	0	1	2	0.1	184	0	0.00	0.00	0.0	0
194.	Dressing, French, low cal	1 tbsp.	15	24	0.0	2	0.2	0	2	6	0.1	306	0	0.00	0.00	0.0	0
195.	Dressing, Italian	1 tbsp.	15	69	0.1	9	1.3	0	2	1	0.0	73	29	0.00	0.00	0.0	0
196.	Dressing, Italian, low cal	1 tbsp.	15	10	0.0	1	0.0	0	1	1	0.0	136	1	0.00	0.00	0.0	0
197.	Dressing, Ranch style	1 tbsp.	15	54	0.4	6	0.9	6	1	15	0.0	65	36	0.01	0.02	0.0	0
198.	Dressing, Thousand island	1 tbsp.	15	60	0.2	6	1.0	4	2	2	0.1	110	75	0.00	0.01	0.0	1
199.	Dressing, Thousand island, low cal	1 tbsp.	15	25	0.1	2	0.2	2	3	2	0.1	153	70	0.00	0.00	0.0	0
200.	Egg, hard cooked	1 large	50	72	6.0	5	1.6	212	1	24	1.0	113	520	0.05	0.13	0.0	0
201.	Egg, fried with butter	1	46	95	5.4	7	2.4	240	1	28	0.9	162	320	0.04	0.13	0.0	0
202.	Egg McMuffin	1	138	327	18.5	15	5.9	259	31	226	2.9	885	591	0.47	0.44	3.8	1
203.	Egg salad sandwich	1	111	325	10.0	19	3.9	215	28	95	2.5	461	242	0.29	0.29	2.1	0
204.	Egg, scrambled, with milk, butter	1 egg	64	95	6.0	7	3.0	244	1	54	0.9	176	510	0.04	0.18	0.0	0
205.	Egg, white	1 large	33	17	3.6	0	0.0	0	0	3	0.0	48	0	0.00	0.09	0.0	0
206.	Egg, yolk, raw	1 yolk	17	63	2.8	5	1.6	212	0	26	1.0	8	390	0.04	0.07	0.0	0
207.	Enchilada, beef	1	200	487	21.8	23	8.8	63	26	425	2.9	262	595	0.02	0.27	3.5	5
208.	Enchilada, cheese	1	230	632	25.3	34	17.6	82	31	876	2.6	596	1,672	0.13	0.40	1.2	15
209.	Figs, dried	1 large	21	60	1.0	0	0.0	0	15	26	0.6	1	20	0.16	0.17	3.9	0
210.	Filet of Fish, McDonald's	1	131	402	15.0	23	7.9	43	34	105	1.8	709	152	0.28	0.28	3.9	4
489.	Fish, fillet, florentine, Healthy Choice	1	273	220	26.0	7	3.0	65	13	150	0.7	590	2,500	0.15	0.34	2.0	1
211.	Fish sandwich, Wendy's	1	182	460	16	25	5.0	55	42	120	1.8	780	0	0.60	0.45	4.0	1
494.	Fish, Sole Au Gratin, Healthy Choice	1	312	270	16.0	5	0.0	55	40	80	1.1	470	0	0.23	0.17	1.6	6
212.	Fish, sticks	2	56	140	12.0	6	1.6	52	8	22	0.6	106	40	0.06	0.10	1.2	0
213.	Flounder	3 oz.	85	171	25.5	7	1.0	60	0	21	1.2	201	0	0.06	0.06	2.1	3
214.	Flour, all purpose enriched	1 c	125	455	13.0	1	0.0	0	95	20	3.6	3	0	0.55	0.33	4.4	0
215.	Flour, whole wheat	1 c	120	400	16.0	2	0.0	0	85	49	4.0	4	0	0.66	0.14	5.2	0
216.	Frankfurter, cooked	1	57	176	7.0	16	5.6	45	1	4	1.1	627	0	0.09	0.11	1.5	0
217.	Frankfurter, turkey, cooked	1	45	102	6.4	8	2.7	39	1	58	0.8	454	60	0.04	0.08	1.7	0
218.	French Dip, Arby's	1	154	368	22	15	5.6	43	35	60	2.8	1,018	0	0.20	0.50	8.4	0
219.	French toast	1 piece	65	123	4.9	4	1.1	73	15	79	1.1	189	285	0.15	0.17	1.1	0
220.	Fries, Curly, Arby's	1 small	99	337	4	18	7.4	0	43	24	1.0	167	0	0.06	0.07	2.0	0
221.	Fruit cocktail	1 c	245	91	1.0	0	0.0	0	24	22	1.0	12	370	0.05	0.02	1.2	5
222.	Fruit cocktail, juice pack	1 c	248	115	1.1	0	0.0	0	29	20	0.5	10	380	0.03	0.04	1.0	7
223.	Grapefruit, raw white	1/2 med	301	56	1.0	0	0.0	0	15	22	0.5	1	10	0.05	0.03	0.3	52

224. Grapefruit juice, unsweet. canned	1/2 c	124	50	0.6	0	0.0	0	12	11	0.2	2	10	0.05	0.03	0.3	46
225. Grapes, seedless, European	10 grapes	50	34	0.3	0	0.0	0	9	6	0.2	2	50	0.03	0.03	0.2	2
226. Grape juice, unsweetened bottled	1/2 c	127	84	0.3	0	0.0	0	21	14	0.4	3	0	0.05	0.03	0.3	0
227. Gravy, beef, homemade	1 tbsp	17	19	0.3	2	1.0	1	1	1	0.1	49	0	0.01	0.01	0.2	0
228. Haddock, fried (dipped in egg, milk, bread crumbs)	3 oz.	85	141	17.0	5	1.0	54	5	33	0.9	150	0	0.03	0.06	2.7	3
229. Halibut, broiled with butter or margarine	3 oz.	85	144	21.0	6	2.1	55	0	15	0.6	114	570	0.03	0.06	7.2	1
230. Ham (cured pork)	3 oz.	85	318	20.0	26	9.4	77	0	9	2.6	48	0	0.43	0.20	3.8	0
231. Ham, lunch meat	1 slice	28	37	5.5	1	0.5	13	.3	2	0.2	405	0	0.26	0.06	1.4	7
508. Hamburger, Arch Deluxe, McDonalds	1	242	560	27.0	32	11.0	90	42	120	3.0	960	650	0.40	0.43	7.5	3
509. Hamburger, Arch Deluxe w/bacon, McDonalds	1	253	610	31.0	36	13.0	105	42	120	3.7	1,190	650	0.40	0.43	7.5	3
232. Hamburger, Big Classic, Wendy's	1	251	480	27	23	7.0	75	44	180	4.2	850	300	0.45	0.27	7.0	12
233. Hamburger, Big Mac	1	204	581	25.1	36	12.0	85	40	207	5.0	999	388	0.49	0.39	7.3	3
234. Hamburger bun	1 bun	40	129	3.7	2	1.0	0	23	61	1.3	271	2	0.22	0.15	1.8	0
235. Hamburger, Jr. Bacon Cheeseburger, Wendy's	1	170	440	22	25	8.0	65	33	240	3.0	870	300	0.45	0.27	6.0	9
236. Hamburger, McDonald's	1	99	257	13.0	9	3.7	26	30	63	3.0	526	231	0.23	0.23	5.1	2
237. Hamburger, McLean Deluxe	1	206	320	22	10	5.0	60	35	180	2.4	670	500	0.38	0.36	7.0	6
238. Hamburger, McLean Deluxe, w/cheese	1	219	370	24	14	8.0	75	35	240	2.4	890	750	0.38	0.36	7.0	6
239. Hamburger, Quarter pounder	1 burger	160	427	24.6	24	9.1	80	29	98	4.3	718	115	0.35	0.32	7.2	3
240. Hamburger, Quarter pounder, with cheese	1 burger	186	525	29.6	32	12.8	107	31	255	4.8	1,195	640	0.37	0.41	7.1	3
241. Hamburger, Wendy's	1	219	440	26	23	7.0	75	36	120	3.6	850	300	0.38	0.18	7.0	9
242. Ham N' Cheese, Arby's	1	169	355	25	14	5.1	55	35	204	1.8	1400	0	0.83	0.40	7.8	0
243. Honey	1 tbsp	21	64	0.0	0	0.0	0	17	1	0.1	1	0	0.00	0.01	0.1	0
244. Honeydew melon	1 slice (1/10 melon)	129	45	0.6	0	0.0	0	12	8	0.1	13	25	0.10	0.02	0.8	32
245. Horsey Sauce, Arby's	.5 oz.	14	55	0	5	2.0	0	3	24	0.0	105	0	0.00	0.00	0.0	0
246. Hotcakes w/Margarine & Syrup, McDonald's	1 serving	174	440	8	12	5.0	8	74	120	1.2	685	200	0.30	0.36	3.0	0
247. Hotdog bun	1 bun	40	115	3.3	2	1.0	0	20	54	1.2	241	2	0.20	0.13	1.6	0
248. Ice cream, vanilla	1/2 c	67	135	3.0	7	4.4	27	14	97	0.1	42	295	0.03	0.14	0.1	1
249. Ice cream cone	1 small	115	185	4.3	5	2.2	24	30	183	0.1	109	218	0.06	0.36	0.4	1
250. Ice cream cone, Dairy Queen	medium	142	230	6.0	7	4.6	15	35	200	0.0	150	300	0.09	0.26	0.0	0
251. Ice cream, hot fudge sundae	1	164	357	7.0	11	5.4	27	58	215	0.6	170	233	0.07	0.31	1.1	2
252. Ice milk, vanilla	1/2 c	61	100	3.0	3	1.8	13	15	102	0.1	45	140	0.04	0.15	0.1	1
253. Instant breakfast, whole milk	1 c	281	280	15.0	8	5.1	33	34	301	8.0	286	2,057	0.39	0.46	5.2	29
254. Instant breakfast, skim milk	1 c	282	216	15.4	0	0.0	4	35	312	8.0	292	1,635	0.39	0.41	5.2	29
255. Jams or preserves	1 tbsp	7	18	0.0	0	0.0	0	5	1	0.1	1	1	0.00	0.00	0.0	0
256. Jelly	1 tbsp	18	49	0.0	0	0.0	0	13	4	0.3	3	0	0.00	0.01	0.0	1
257. Kale, fresh cooked, drained	1/2 c	55	22	2.5	0	0.0	0	3	103	0.9	24	4,565	0.06	0.10	0.9	51
258. Kiwi fruit, raw	1 med	76	46	1.0	0	0.0	0	11	20	0.3	4	65	0.02	0.04	0.4	75
259. Kool Aid, with sugar	1 c	240	100	0.0	0	0.0	0	25	0	0.0	0	0	0.00	0.00	0.0	6
260. Lamb leg, roast, trimmed	3 oz	85	237	22.0	16	7.3	60	0	9	1.4	53	0	0.13	0.23	4.7	0
261. Lamb loin chop, broiled, lean	3 oz	84	183	25.0	8	3.4	78	0	16	1.7	70	7	0.10	0.23	5.7	0
490. Lasagna, Healthy Choice	1	284	260	18.0	5	0.0	20	37	100	2.7	420	750	0.30	0.26	2.0	2
262. Lasagna, homemade	1 piece	220	357	23.6	18	8.3	50	27	413	2.8	703	1,008	0.19	0.30	3.3	6
498. Lasagna, Lean Cuisine	1	291	260	19.0	5	2.0	25	34	150	1.8	590	500	0.15	0.25	3.0	6
263. Lemon juice, fresh	1 tbsp	15	4	0.1	0	0.0	0	1	1	0.0	0	0	0.00	0.00	0.0	7
264. Lemonade (concentrate)	12 oz.	340	137	0.2	0	0.1	0	36	11	0.6	11	73	0.02	0.07	0.1	13
265. Lentils, cooked	1/2 c	100	106	8.0	0	0.0	0	19	25	2.1	0	20	0.07	0.06	0.6	0
266. Lettuce, crisp head	1 c sm chunks	75	10	0.7	0	0.0	0	2	15	0.4	7	250	0.05	0.05	0.2	5
267. Lettuce, cos or romaine	1 c chopped	55	10	0.7	0	0.0	0	2	37	0.8	5	1,050	0.08	0.04	0.2	10
268. Liver, beef, fried	1 slice 3 oz.	85	195	22.0	9	2.5	345	5	9	7.5	156	45,390	0.22	3.56	14.0	23
269. Liverwurst, fresh	1 slice 1 oz.	28	87	5.0	7	3.5	50	1	3	1.5	0	1,800	0.06	0.37	1.6	0

Code	Food	Amount	Weight gm	Calories	Protein gm	Fat gm	Sat. Fat gm	Cholesterol mg	Carbohydrate gm	Calcium mg	Iron mg	Sodium mg	Vit A I.U.	Thiamin (Vit B_1) mg	Riboflavin (Vit B_2) mg	Niacin mg	Vit C mg
270.	Lobster	1 c	145	138	27.0	2	1.0	293	0	94	1.2	305	0	0.15	0.10	0.0	0
271.	M&M's, Chocolate, plain	1 oz.	28	140	1.9	6	3.3	0	19	47	0.5	24	30	0.01	0.07	0.2	0
272.	M&M's, Chocolate, w/peanuts	1 oz.	28	145	3.2	7	3.2	0	17	36	0.4	17	15	0.02	0.05	0.9	0
273.	Macaroni, enriched, cooked	1/2 c	70	78	2.4	0	0.0	0	16	6	0.7	1	0	0.10	0.06	0.8	0
274.	Macaroni and cheese	1/2 c	100	215	8.2	11	4.0	21	20	181	0.9	543	430	0.10	0.20	0.9	0
275.	Margarine	1 tsp	5	34	0.0	4	0.7	2	0	1	0.0	46	160	0.00	0.00	0.0	0
276.	Mars bar	1 bar	50	240	4.0	11	4.8	0	30	85	0.6	85	1	0.02	0.16	0.5	0
277.	Matzo	1 piece	30	117	3.0	0	0.0	0	25	*	*	0	*	*	*	*	*
278.	Mayonnaise	1 tsp	5	36	0.0	4	0.7	3	0	1	0.0	28	13	0.00	0.00	0.0	0
507.	Milk, 1% fat	1 c	244	102	8.0	3	1.6	10	12	300	0.1	123	720	0.09	0.41	0.2	2
279.	Milk, chocolate, 2%	1 c	250	180	8.0	5	3.1	17	26	284	0.6	151	143	0.09	0.41	0.3	2
280.	Milk, evaporated whole	1/2 c	126	172	9.0	10	5.8	40	13	329	0.2	149	405	0.05	0.43	0.2	2
281.	Milk, lowfat 2% fat	1 c	244	121	8.0	5	2.9	18	12	295	0.1	121	695	0.09	0.40	0.2	2
282.	Milk shake, chocolate	1 (10 fluid oz.)	340	433	11.5	13	7.8	45	70	383	1.1	328	312	0.20	0.83	0.5	0
283.	Milk shake, Frosty, Wendy's	16 oz.	324	460	13	13	7.0	55	76	480	1.0	260	500	0.15	1.08	0.8	0
284.	Milk shake, strawberry	1 (10 fluid oz.)	340	383	11.4	10	6.0	37	64	384	0.4	281	418	0.14	0.61	0.5	4
285.	Milk shake, vanilla, McDonald's	1	289	323	10	8	5.1	29	52	346	0.2	250	346	0.12	0.66	0.6	3
286.	Milk, skim	1 c	245	85	8.0	1	0.3	4	12	301	0.1	126	745	0.09	0.34	0.2	2
287.	Milk, whole 3.5% fat	1 c	244	149	8.0	8	5.1	33	11	290	0.1	119	380	0.09	0.39	0.2	2
288.	Milky Way bar	1 bar	60	260	3.2	9	5.4	14	43	86	0.5	140	125	0.03	0.15	0.2	1
289.	Molasses, medium	1 tbsp	20	50	0.0	0	0.0	0	13	33	0.9	3	0	0.01	0.01	0.0	0
290.	Muffin, apple bran, fat free, McDonald's	1	75	180	5	0	0.0	0	40	48	0.7	200	0	0.15	0.18	2.0	0
291.	Muffin, blueberry	1	45	135	3.0	5	1.5	19	20	54	0.9	198	40	0.10	0.11	0.9	1
292.	Muffin, bran	1	45	125	3.0	6	1.4	24	19	60	1.4	189	230	0.11	0.13	1.3	3
293.	Muffin, cornmeal	1	45	145	3.0	5	1.5	23	21	66	0.9	169	80	0.11	0.11	0.9	0
294.	Muffin, English, plain	1	57	140	4.5	1	0.3	0	26	96	1.7	378	0	0.26	0.18	2.1	0
295.	Muffin, English w/butter	1	63	186	5.0	5	2.3	15	30	117	1.5	310	164	0.28	0.49	2.6	1
296.	Mushrooms, fresh cultivated	1/2 c sliced	35	12	1.0	0	0.0	0	2	4	0.5	4	0	0.04	0.12	2.4	1
297.	Mustard greens, cooked drained	1/2 c	70	16	1.7	0	0.0	0	3	96	1.2	13	4,060	0.05	0.10	0.4	33
298.	Noodles, egg, enriched cooked	1/2 c	80	100	3.3	1	0.0	0	19	8	0.7	2	55	0.11	0.07	1.0	0
299.	Nuts, Brazil	1 oz. (6-8 nuts)	28	185	4.1	19	4.8	0	3	53	1.0	0	0	0.27	0.03	0.5	0
300.	Nuts, Pecans	1 oz.	28	195	2.6	20	1.4	0	4	21	0.7	0	40	0.24	0.04	0.3	1
301.	Nuts, Walnuts	1 oz. (14 halves)	28	185	4.2	18	1.0	0	5	28	0.9	1	10	0.09	0.04	0.3	1
302.	Oil, Corn	1 tbsp.	15	125	0.0	14	1.8	0	0	0	0.0	0	0	0.00	0.00	0.0	0
303.	Oil, Olive	1 tbsp.	15	125	0.0	14	1.9	0	0	0	0.0	0	0	0.00	0.00	0.0	0
304.	Oil, Safflower	1 tbsp.	15	125	0.0	14	1.3	0	0	0	0.0	0	0	0.00	0.00	0.0	0
305.	Oil, Soybean	1 tsp.	5	44	0.0	5	2.0	0	0	0	0.0	0	0	0.00	0.00	0.0	0
306.	Okra, cooked, drained	1/2 c	80	23	1.6	0	0.0	0	5	74	0.4	2	390	0.11	0.15	0.7	16
307.	Olives, black, ripe	10 extra large	55	61	0.5	7	1.0	0	1	40	0.8	385	30	0.00	0.00	0.0	0
308. 309.	Onions, mature, cooked, drained	1/2 c sliced	105	31	1.3	0	0.0	0	7	25	0.4	8	40	0.03	0.03	0.2	8
310.	Onion rings, fried	3	30	122	1.6	8	2.3	0	11	9	0.5	113	68	0.08	0.04	1.1	0
311.	Onion rings (Brazier) Dairy Queen	1 serving	85	360	6.0	17	6.0	15	33	20	0.4	125	0	0.09	0.00	0.4	2
312.	Orange juice, froz. reconstituted	1/2 c	125	61	0.9	0	0.0	0	15	13	0.1	1	270	0.12	0.02	0.5	60
313.	Orange, raw (medium skin)	1 med	180	64	1.3	0	0.0	0	16	54	0.5	1	260	0.13	0.05	0.5	66
314.	Oysters, Eastern, breaded, fried	1 oyster	45	90	5.0	5	1.4	35	5	49	3.0	70	220	0.07	0.10	1.3	4
315.	Oysters, raw, Eastern	1/2 c (6-9 med)	120	79	10.0	2	1.3	60	4	113	6.6	145	370	0.17	0.22	3.0	0

Food	Amount															
316. Pancakes	1 6" diam x 1/2" thick	73	169	5.2	5	1.0	36	25	74	0.9	310	90	0.12	0.16	0.9	0
317. Pancakes, buckwheat	1 4 in. diam.	27	55	2.0	2	0.9	20	6	59	0.4	125	17	0.04	0.05	0.2	0
318. Pancakes w/butter, syrup	1 large	100	250	4.0	5	1.9	24	47	1	1.1	535	160	0.13	0.18	1.1	2
319. Papaya, raw	1/2 med	227	60	0.9	0	0.0	0	15	31	0.5	5	2,660	0.06	0.06	0.5	85
320. Parsnips, cooked	1 large 9" long	160	106	2.4	1	0.0	0	24	72	1.0	13	50	0.11	0.13	0.2	16
503. Pasta primavera, Weight Watchers	1	238	260	15.0	11	0.8	5	22	300	1.8	800	1,750	0.23	0.26	3.0	18
321. Peaches, canned, heavy syrup	1 half 2⅛ tbsp liq.	96	75	0.4	0	0.0	0	19	4	0.3	2	410	0.01	0.02	0.6	3
322. Peaches, canned, juice pack	1 half	77	34	0.5	0	0.0	0	9	5	0.2	3	147	0.01	0.01	0.5	3
323. Peaches, raw, peeled	1 2¾" diam.	175	58	0.9	0	0.0	0	15	14	0.8	2	2,030	0.03	0.08	1.5	11
324. Peanut butter	2 tbsp	32	188	8.0	16	1.0	0	6	18	0.6	194	0	0.04	0.04	4.8	0
325. Peanut butter, jam sandwich	1	100	340	11.4	14	2.6	0	45	87	2.3	414	1	0.32	0.22	5.3	0
326. Peanuts, roasted	1 oz.	28	166	7.0	14	1.0	0	5	21	0.6	119	0	0.09	0.04	4.9	0
327. Pears, canned, heavy syrup	1 half 2¼ tbsp liq.	103	78	0.2	0	0.0	0	20	5	0.2	1	0	0.01	0.02	0.1	1
328. Pears, canned, juice pack	1 half	77	38	0.3	0	0.0	0	10	7	0.2	3	3	0.01	0.01	0.2	1
329. Pears, raw	1 pear	180	100	1.1	1	0.0	0	25	13	0.5	2	30	0.03	0.07	0.2	7
330. Peas, canned, drained	1/2 c	85	75	4.0	0	0.0	0	14	22	1.6	200	585	0.08	0.05	0.7	7
331. Peas, frozen, cooked drained	1/2 c	80	55	4.1	0	0.0	0	10	15	1.5	92	480	0.22	0.07	1.4	11
332. Peppers, sweet, raw	1 pepper 3¼" x 3" diam.	200	36	2.0	0	0.0	0	8	15	1.1	21	690	0.13	0.13	0.8	210
333. Pickles, dill	1 large 4" long	135	15	0.9	0	0.0	0	3	35	1.4	1,928	140	0.00	0.03	0.0	8
334. Pickles, sweet	1 large 3" long	35	51	0.2	0	0.0	0	13	4	0.4	0	30	0.00	0.01	0.0	2
335. Pie, Apple	1 piece (3½")	118	302	2.6	13	3.5	120	45	9	0.4	355	40	0.02	0.02	0.5	1
336. Pie, Apple, fried	1 pie	85	255	2.2	14	5.8	14	32	12	0.9	326	15	0.09	0.06	1.0	1
337. Pie, Blueberry	1 piece (3½")	158	380	4.0	17	4.0	0	55	26	2.1	423	140	0.17	0.14	1.7	6
338. Pie, Cherry	1 piece (3½")	118	308	3.1	13	5.0	137	45	17	0.4	355	40	0.02	0.02	0.5	1
339. Pie, Cherry, fried	1 pie	85	250	2.0	14	5.8	13	32	11	0.7	371	95	0.06	0.06	0.6	1
340. Pie, Chocolate cream	1 piece (1/6 pie)	175	311	7.4	13	4.5	15	42	160	1.1	427	170	0.15	0.30	1.1	1
341. Pie, Lemon meringue	1 piece (1/6 pie)	140	355	4.7	14	3.5	137	53	25	1.4	395	330	0.10	0.14	0.8	4
342. Pie, Pecan	1 piece (1/6 pie)	138	583	6.3	24	3.9	13	92	35	1.9	304	206	0.22	0.17	1.1	0
343. Pie, Pumpkin	1 (3½")	114	241	4.6	13	3.0	70	28	58	0.6	244	2,810	0.03	0.11	0.6	0
344. Pineapple, canned, heavy syrup	1/2 c	128	95	0.4	0	0.0	0	25	14	0.4	2	65	0.10	0.03	0.3	9
345. Pineapple, canned, juice pack	1/2 c	125	75	0.5	0	0.0	0	20	17	0.3	1	24	0.12	0.24	0.3	12
346. Pineapple, raw	1/2 c diced	78	41	0.3	0	0.0	0	11	13	0.4	1	55	0.07	0.03	0.2	13
347. Pizza, Cheese, Thin 'n Crispy, Pizza Hut	1/2 10" pie	*	450	25.0	15	7.0	125	54	450	4.5	1,200	750	0.30	0.51	5.0	1
348. Pizza, Cheese, Thick 'n Chewy, Pizza Hut	1/2 10" pie	*	560	34.0	14	6.0	110	71	500	5.4	1,100	1,000	0.68	0.68	7.0	1
504. Pizza, Cheese, Weight Watchers	1	164	300	22.0	7	3.0	35	37	450	1.4	630	1,000	0.30	0.51	3.0	12
505. Pizza, Deluxe Comb. Weight Watchers	1	203	330	26.0	10	3.0	25	35	350	1.8	650	1,750	0.30	0.51	3.0	21
506. Pizza, Pepperoni, Weight Watchers	1	171	320	26.0	10	3.0	35	31	400	1.8	710	1,000	0.23	0.51	3.0	15
480. Pizza, Pepperoni, Pan, Pizza Hut	2 pieces	211	540	29.0	22	9.2	42	62	520	6.3	1,127	500	0.63	0.49	5.4	8
481. Pizza, Supreme, Pan, Pizza Hut	2 pieces	255	589	32.0	30	13.8	48	53	500	5.0	1,363	600	0.81	0.80	6.0	10
349. Plums, Japanese and hybrid, raw	1 plum 2⅛" diam.	70	32	0.3	0	0.0	0	8	8	0.3	1	160	0.02	0.02	0.3	4
350. Popcorn, cooked, oil	1 c	11	55	0.9	3	0.5	0	6	3	0.3	86	20	0.01	0.02	0.1	0
351. Popcorn, popped, plain, large kernel	1 c	6	12	0.8	0	0.0	0	5	1	0.2	0	0	0.00	0.01	0.1	0
352. Pork, roast, trimmed	2 slices 3 oz.	85	179	24.0	8	2.2	65	0	11	3.1	863	0	0.55	0.22	4.3	0
353. Pork, sausage, cooked	1 sm link	17	72	2.8	6	2.1	13	1	0	0.3	221	0	0.00	0.00	0.0	0
354. Potato, au gratin	1 c	245	228	5.6	10	6.3	12	32	203	0.8	1,076	380	0.05	0.20	2.3	8
355. Potato, baked in skin	1 potato 2⅓ x 4¼"	202	145	4.0	0	0.0	0	33	14	1.1	6	0	0.15	0.07	2.7	31
356. Potato chips	10 chips	20	114	1.1	8	2.1	0	10	8	0.4	150	0	0.04	0.01	1.0	3
357. Potato, French fried long	10 strips 3½-4"	78	214	3.4	10	1.7	0	28	12	1.0	5	0	0.10	0.06	2.4	16

Code	Food	Amount	Weight gm	Calories	Protein gm	Fat gm	Sat. Fat gm	Cholesterol mg	Carbohydrate gm	Calcium mg	Iron mg	Sodium mg	Vit A I.U.	Thiamin (Vit B_1) mg	Riboflavin (Vit B_2) mg	Niacin mg	Vit C mg
358.	Potato, Hashbrowns, McDonald's	1 patty	55	144	1.4	9	3.0	4	15	5	0.4	325	6	0.06	0.01	0.8	4
359.	Potato, mashed, milk added	1/2 c	105	69	2.2	1	0.4	8	14	25	0.4	316	20	0.09	0.06	1.1	11
360.	Potato salad w/eggs, mayo	1/2 c	125	179	3.4	10	7.8	85	14	24	0.8	662	262	0.10	0.08	1.1	12
361.	Potato, hash brown	1/2 c	78	170	2.5	9	3.5	0	22	12	1.2	27	0	0.09	0.02	1.9	5
362.	Pretzel, thin, twists	1 oz.	28	113	2.8	1	0.3	0	23	8	0.6	456	0	0.09	0.07	1.2	0
363.	Prunes, dried "softenized" without pits	5 prunes	61	137	1.1	0	0.0	0	36	26	0.1	4	860	0.05	0.09	0.9	2
364.	Prune juice, canned or bottled	1/2 c	128	99	0.5	0	0.0	0	24	18	5.3	3	0	0.02	0.02	0.5	3
365.	Pudding, Chocolate, canned	5 oz.	142	205	3	11	9.5	1	30	74	1.2	285	155	0.04	0.17	0.6	0
366.	Pudding, Tapioca, canned	5 oz.	142	160	3	5	4.8	1	28	119	0.3	252	5	0.03	0.14	0.4	0
367.	Pudding, Vanilla, canned	5 oz.	142	220	2	10	9.5	1	33	79	0.2	305	1	0.03	0.12	0.6	0
368.	Quiche, Lorraine	1 piece	242	825	18	66	31.9	392	40	290	1.9	898	2,250	0.15	0.44	1.7	1
369.	Raisins, unbleached, seedless	1 oz.	28	82	0.7	0	0.0	0	22	18	1.0	8	10	0.03	0.02	0.1	0
370.	Raspberries, fresh	1 c	123	60	1.1	1	0.0	0	14	27	0.7	0	80	0.04	0.11	1.1	31
371.	Raspberries, frozen	1 c	250	255	1.7	1	0.0	0	62	38	1.6	3	75	0.05	0.11	1.5	41
495.	Ravioli, Baked cheese, Lean Cuisine	1	241	240	13.0	8	3.0	55	30	200	1.4	590	300	0.06	0.25	1.2	36
372.	Rice, brown, cooked	1/2 c	96	116	2.5	1	0.0	0	25	12	0.5	275	0	0.09	0.02	1.3	0
373.	Rice, white enriched, cooked	1/2 c	103	113	2.1	0	0.0	0	25	11	0.9	384	0	0.12	0.01	1.1	0
374.	Rice, wild, cooked	1/2 c	100	92	3.6	0	0.0	0	19	5	1.1	2	0	0.11	0.16	1.6	0
375.	Roast Beef sand., Regular, Arby's	1	155	383	22	18	7.0	43	35	72	3.2	936	0	0.28	0.50	11.0	0
376.	Roast Beef Sub, Arby's	1	305	623	38	32	11.5	73	47	492	5.2	1,847	500	0.56	0.76	14.2	9
377.	Roll, hard, white	1 roll	50	155	5	2	0.0	0	30	24	1.4	313	0	0.20	0.12	1.7	0
378.	Reuben sandwich	1	237	488	28.7	28	10.4	85	30	364	5.3	1,685	461	0.25	0.44	3.9	12
379.	Salad, Caesar side, Wendy's	1	130	160	10	6	1.0	10	18	96	1.2	700	1,250	0.23	0.27	2.0	24
380.	Salad, Chef, Burger King	1 serving	273	178	17	9	4.0	103	7	128	1.6	568	4,750	0.35	0.26	3.6	15
381.	Salad, Chef, McDonald's	1	265	170	17	9	4.0	111	8	180	1.0	400	5,000	0.30	0.27	4.0	21
382.	Salad, Chicken, Burger King	1 serving	258	142	20	4	1.0	49	8	32	1.3	443	4,600	0.14	0.17	8.5	20
383.	Salad, Chicken w/celery	1/2 c	78	266	10.5	25	4.1	48	1	16	0.7	199	153	0.03	0.08	3.3	1
384.	Salad, Deluxe Garden, Wendy's	1	271	110	7	5	1.0	0	9	240	1.0	380	3,000	0.15	0.36	1.2	36
385.	Salad, Garden, Arby's	1	330	117	7	5	2.7	12	11	192	1.1	134	4,900	0.17	0.20	1.2	52
386.	Salad, Grilled Chicken, Wendy's	1	338	200	25	8	1.0	55	9	240	1.8	690	3,000	0.23	0.36	8.0	36
387.	Salad, Tuna	1 c	205	375	33	19	3.3	80	19	31	2.5	877	53	0.06	0.14	13.3	6
388.	Salami, dry	1 oz.	28	128	7.0	11	1.6	24	0	4	1.0	349	0	0.10	0.07	1.5	0
389.	Salmon, broiled with butter or margarine	3 oz.	85	156	23.0	6	2.2	53	0	0	0.9	99	150	0.15	0.06	8.4	0
390.	Salmon, canned Chinook	3 oz.	85	179	16.6	12	0.8	30	0	131	0.7	105	197	0.03	0.01	6.2	0
391.	Sardines, canned drained	1 oz.	28	58	7.0	3	1.0	20	0	124	0.8	233	60	0.01	0.06	1.5	0
392.	Sauerkraut, canned	1/2 c	118	21	1.2	0	0.0	0	5	43	0.6	878	60	0.04	0.05	0.3	17
393.	Sausage Biscuit w/Egg, McDonald's	1	175	505	19	33	20.0	260	33	120	2.4	1,210	300	0.45	0.36	4.0	0
394.	Sausage McMuffin, McDonald's	1	135	345	15	20	11.0	57	27	240	1.8	770	200	0.53	0.27	5.0	0
395.	Sausage McMuffin, w/Egg	1	159	430	21	25	14.0	270	27	300	2.4	920	500	0.53	0.45	5.0	0
396.	Sausage, smoked link, pork	1	68	265	15	22	7.7	46	1	20	0.8	1,020	0	1.04	0.29	5.0	14
397.	Scallops, breaded, cooked	6 pieces	90	195	15	10	2.5	70	10	39	2.0	298	105	0.11	0.11	1.6	0
398.	Sherbet	1/2 c	97	135	1.1	2	1.3	7	29	52	0.2	44	92	0.02	0.04	0.1	2
399.	Shrimp, boiled	3 oz.	85	99	18.0	1	0.1	128	1	99	2.7	0	60	0.00	0.03	1.5	0
400.	Shrimp, fried	7 medium	85	200	16.0	10	2.5	168	11	61	2.0	384	130	0.06	0.09	2.8	0
487.	Shrimp, Linguini, Budget Gourmet	1	284	330	15.0	15	0.0	75	33	10	3.6	1,250	1,000	0.30	0.17	3.0	2
401.	Snickers bar	1 bar	61	290	6.6	4	5.4	0	37	70	0.5	170	25	0.03	0.11	1.8	0
402.	Soda pop, cola	12 oz.	369	144	0.0	0	0.0	0	37	27	0.0	30	0	0.00	0.00	0.0	0
403.	Soda pop, diet	12 oz.	340	2	0.1	0	0.0	0	0	13	0.1	31	0	0.00	0.00	0.0	0
404.	Soda pop, Ginger ale	12 oz.	366	113	0.0	0	0.0	0	29	0	0.0	45	0	0.00	0.00	0.0	0

405.	Soda pop, Lemon-lime	12 oz.	340	138	0.0	0	0.0	0	35	8	0.2	38	0	0.00	0.00	0.0	0
406.	Soda pop, Root beer	12 oz.	340	140	0.0	0	0.0	0	36	17	0.2	45	0	0.00	0.00	0.0	0
407.	Soup, Chicken, cream	1 c	248	191	7.5	12	4.6	27	15	180	0.7	1,046	710	0.07	0.26	0.9	1
408.	Soup, Chicken noodle	1 c	241	75	4.0	2	0.7	7	9	17	0.8	900	711	0.05	0.06	1.4	0
409.	Soup, Clam chowder, Manhattan	1 c	244	78	4.2	2	0.4	2	12	34	1.9	1,808	460	0.06	0.05	1.3	3
410.	Soup, Clam chowder, north east	1 c	248	163	9.5	7	3.0	22	16	187	1.5	992	160	0.07	0.24	1.0	4
411.	Soup, Cream of mushroom condensed, prepared with equal volume of milk	1 c	245	216	7.0	14	5.4	15	16	191	0.5	955	250	0.05	0.34	0.7	1
412.	Soup, Minestrone	1 c	241	80	4.3	3	0.5	2	11	34	0.9	911	1,170	0.05	0.04	0.9	1
413.	Soup, Split pea, condensed, prepared with equal volume of water	1 c	245	145	9.0	3	1.1	0	21	29	1.5	941	440	0.25	0.15	1.5	1
414.	Soup, Tomato, condensed, prepared with equal volume of water	1 c	245	88	2.0	3	0.5	0	16	15	0.7	970	1,000	0.05	0.05	1.2	12
415.	Soup, Tomato with milk	1 c	248	160	6.0	6	2.9	17	22	159	1.8	932	850	0.13	0.25	1.5	68
416.	Soup, vegetable beef, condensed, prepared with equal volume of water	1 c	245	78	5.0	2	0.0	0	10	12	0.7	1,046	2,700	0.05	0.05	1.0	0
417.	Soup, Vegetarian vegetable	1 c	250	70	2.1	2	0.3	0	12	21	1.1	823	1,505	0.05	0.05	0.9	1
418.	Sour cream	1 tbsp	14	30	0.4	3	1.8	6	1	16	0.0	8	135	0.01	0.02	0.0	0
419.	Soup cream, imitation	1 tbsp.	14	29	0.3	3	2.5	0	1	0	0.0	14	0	0.00	0.00	0.0	0
492.	Spaghetti, Healthy Choice	1	284	280	14.0	6	0.0	20	42	6	3.6	480	1,250	0.38	0.26	2.0	5
420.	Spaghetti, in tomato sauce with cheese	1 c	250	260	8.8	9	2.0	10	37	80	2.3	955	1,080	0.25	0.18	2.3	13
421.	Spaghetti, plain, cooked	1 c	140	155	5.0	1	0.1	0	32	11	1.7	1	0	0.20	0.11	1.5	0
422.	Spaghetti, whole wheat, cooked	1 c	125	151	6.6	1	0.1	0	32	19	1.1	16	0	0.21	0.09	1.5	0
423.	Spaghetti, with meatballs and tomato sauce	1 c	243	332	18.6	11.7	3.0	75	39	124	3.7	1,009	1,590	0.25	0.30	4.0	22
499.	Spaghetti w/meatballs, Lean Cuisine	1	290	280	19.0	7	2.0	35	35	100	1.8	490	300	0.15	0.25	3.0	4
424.	Spareribs, cooked	3 oz.	85	377	17.8	33	12.0	73	0	8	2.2	31	0	0.37	0.18	2.9	0
425.	Spinach, canned, drained	1/2 c	103	25	2.3	1	0.0	0	4	121	2.6	242	8,200	0.02	0.12	0.3	15
426.	Spinach, frozen, cooked, drained	1/2 c	103	24	3.1	0	0.0	0	4	116	2.2	54	8,100	0.07	0.16	0.4	20
427.	Spinach, raw, chopped	1 c	55	14	1.8	0	0.0	0	2	51	1.7	39	4,460	0.06	0.11	0.3	28
428.	Squash, summer, cooked	1/2 c	90	13	0.8	0	0.0	0	3	23	0.4	1	350	0.05	0.07	0.7	9
429.	Squash, winter, baked mashed	1/2 c	103	70	1.9	0	0.0	0	18	41	1.0	1	6,560	0.05	0.14	0.7	8
430.	Strawberries, frozen, sweetened	1 c	250	245	1.4	0	0.0	0	66	28	1.5	8	31	0.04	0.13	1.0	106
431.	Strawberries, raw	1 c	149	55	1.0	1	0.0	0	13	31	1.5	1	90	0.04	0.10	0.9	88
432.	Stuffing, bread, prepared	1/2 c	70	250	4.6	15	3.1	0	25	46	1.1	627	455	0.09	0.10	1.3	0
433.	Sundae, choc. Dairy Queen	medium	184	300	6.0	7	4.9	79	53	200	1.1	175	300	0.06	0.26	0.0	0
434.	Sugar, brown granulated	1 tsp	5	17	0.0	0	0.0	0	5	4	0.1	0	0	0.00	0.00	0.1	0
435.	Sugar, white granulated	1 tsp	4	15	0.0	0	0.0	0	4	0	0.0	0	0	0.00	0.00	0.0	0
436.	Super Roast Beef, Arby's	1	254	552	24	28	7.6	43	54	108	4.3	1,174	150	0.39	0.61	12.4	9
437.	Sweet N' Sour Sauce, McDonald's	1.12 oz.	32	60	0	0.2	0.1	0	14	0	0	190	300	0.00	0.00	0.0	0
438.	Sweet potato, baked	1 pctato 5" long	146	161	2.4	1	0.0	0	37	46	1.0	14	9,230	0.10	0.08	0.8	25
439.	Syrup (maple)	1 tbsp	20	50	0.0	0	0.0	0	13	33	0.2	3	0	0.00	0.00	0.0	0
440.	Taco Salad, Wendy's	1	510	640	34	30	12.0	80	70	540	5.4	960	1,750	0.23	0.45	3.0	27
441.	Taco shell	1 shell	10	60	1.1	3	0.3	0	9	26	0.3	62	36	0.00	0.01	0.3	0
512.	Taco, soft, Taco Bell	1	92	225	12.0	12	5.4	32	18	116	2.3	550	150	0.39	0.22	2.7	1
442.	Taco, Taco Bell	1	83	186	15.0	8	0.0	0	14	120	2.4	79	120	0.09	0.16	2.9	0
443.	Tangerine	1 med 2⅛" diam.	116	39	0.7	0	0.0	0	10	34	0.3	2	360	0.05	0.02	0.1	27
444.	Tartar sauce	1 tbsp.	14	74	0.2	8	1.2	4	1	3	0.1	182	54	0.00	0.00	0.0	0
445.	Tea, brewed	1/4 c	180	0	0.0	0	0.0	0	0	0	0.0	0	0	0.00	0.00	0.0	0
446.	Tomato juice, canned	1 c	244	42	1.9	0	0.1	0	10	22	1.4	881	1,357	0.12	0.08	1.6	45

Code	Food	Amount	Weight gm	Calories	Protein gm	Fat gm	Sat. Fat gm	Cholesterol mg	Carbohydrate gm	Calcium mg	Iron mg	Sodium mg	Vit A I.U.	Thiamin (Vit B_1) mg	Riboflavin (Vit B_2) mg	Niacin mg	Vit C mg
447.	Tomato sauce (catsup)	1 tbsp	15	16	0.3	0	0.0	0	4	3	0.1	156	105	0.01	0.01	0.2	2
448.	Tomato, canned	1/2 c	121	26	1.2	0	0.0	0	5	7	0.6	157	1,085	0.06	0.04	0.9	21
449.	Tomato, raw	1 tomato 3½ oz.	100	20	1.0	0	0.0	0	4	12	0.5	3	820	0.05	0.04	0.6	21
450.	Tortilla chips	1 oz.	28	139	2.2	8	1.1	0	7	82	1.0	140	7	0.01	0.02	0.2	0
451.	Tortilla, corn, lime	1 6" diam.	30	63	1.5	1	0.0	0	14	60	0.9	0	6	0.04	0.02	0.3	0
452.	Tortilla, flour	1	35	105	2.6	3	0.4	0	19	21	0.5	134	0	0.13	0.08	1.2	0
453.	Tostada	1	148	206	9.2	18	3.0	14	25	167	1.8	200	445	0.06	0.13	0.8	6
454.	Trout, broiled w/butter, lemon	3 oz.	85	175	21.0	9	4.1	71	0	26	1.0	122	300	0.07	0.07	2.3	1
455.	Tuna, canned, oil pack, drained	3 oz.	85	167	25.0	7	1.7	60	0	7	1.6	0	70	0.04	0.10	10.1	0
456.	Tuna, canned, water pack, solids and liquid	3½ oz.	99	126	27.7	1	0.0	55	0	16	1.6	161	0	0.00	0.10	13.2	0
457.	Turkey, Lite Roast Deluxe, Arby'	1	195	260	20	6	1.6	33	33	156	2.3	1,262	200	0.29	0.43	15.4	12
458.	Turkey, roast (light and dark mixed)	3 oz.	85	162	27.0	5	1.5	73	0	7	1.5	111	0	0.04	0.15	6.5	0
459.	Turnip, cooked, drained	1/2 c cubed	78	18	0.6	0	0.0	0	4	27	0.3	27	0	0.03	0.04	0.3	17
460.	Turnip greens, cooked drained	1/2 c	73	19	2.1	0	0.0	0	3	98	1.3	14	5,695	0.04	0.08	0.4	16
461.	Veal, cooked loin	3 oz.	85	199	22.0	11	4.0	90	0	9	2.7	55	0	0.06	0.21	4.6	0
462.	Veal cutlet, braised, broiled	3 oz.	85	185	23.0	9	4.0	109	0	9	0.8	56	5	0.06	0.21	4.6	0
486.	Veal parmigiana, Budget Gourmet	1	340	440	26.0	20	0.0	165	39	30	4.5	1,160	5,000	0.45	0.60	6.0	6
463.	Vegetables, mixed, cooked	1 c	182	116	5.8	0	0.0	0	24	46	2.4	348	4,505	0.02	0.13	2.0	15
464.	Waffles	1 waffle	75	205	6.9	8	2.7	59	27	179	1.2	515	49	0.14	0.23	0.9	0
465.	Watermelon	1 c diced	160	42	0.8	0	0.0	0	10	11	0.8	2	940	0.05	0.05	0.3	11
466.	Wheat germ, plain toasted	1 tbsp	6	23	1.8	1	0.0	0	3	3	0.5	0	10	0.11	0.05	0.3	1
467.	Whiskey, gin, rum, vodka 90 proof	1/2 11 oz (jigger)	42	110	0	0	0.0	0	0	0	0.0	0	0	0.00	0.00	0.0	0
468.	Whopper, Burger King	1 sandwich	270	614	27.0	36	12.0	90	45	64	4.9	865	550	0.34	0.41	6.1	12
469.	Whopper with cheese, Burger King	1 sandwich	294	706	32.0	44	16.0	115	47	176	4.9	1,177	950	0.34	0.48	6.1	12
470.	Whopper, double, Burger King	1 sandwich	351	844	46.0	53	19.0	169	45	72	7.2	933	550	0.35	0.56	9.4	12
471.	Wine, dry table 12% alc.	3½ fl. oz.	102	87	0.1	0	0.0	0	4	9	0.4	5	0	0.00	0.01	0.1	0
472.	Wine, red dry 18.8% alc.	2 oz.	59	81	0.1	0	0.0	0	5	5	0.0	4	0	0.01	0.02	0.2	0
473.	Yeast, brewers	1 tbsp	8	23	3.1	0	0.0	0	3	17	1.4	10	0	1.25	0.34	3.0	0
474.	Yogurt, fruit	1 c	227	231	9.9	2	1.6	10	43	345	0.2	125	104	0.08	0.40	0.2	2
475.	Yogurt, nonfat, TCBY	4 oz.	113	110	4	0	0	0	23	96	0	45	0	0.03	0.14	0	0
476.	Yogurt, plain low fat	1 8-oz. container	226	113	7.7	4	2.3	15	12	271	0.1	115	150	0.09	0.41	0.2	2
477.	Yogurt, regular, TCBY	4 oz.	113	120	4	3	2.0	13	23	180	0.5	60	0	0.06	0.18	0	0
478.	Yogurt, sugar free, TCBY	4 oz.	113	80	4	0	0	0	18	96	0	40	200	0.06	0.18	0	0
479.	Yogurt, vanilla lowfat, McDonald's	3 oz.	85	105	4	1	0.3	3	22	120	0	80	100	0.03	0.18	0.4	0

"0" represents both less than 1 and 0

Sources:

Nutritive Value of American Foods in Common Units. *Agriculture Handbook No. 456*. U.S. Dept. of Agriculture. Washington, D.C. 1988.

Young, E. A., E. H. Brennan, and C. L. Irving, Guest Eds. Perspectives on Fast Foods. *Public Health Currents*, 19(1), 1979, Published by Ross Laboratories, Columbus, OH.

Dennison, D. *The Dine System: the Nutrition Plan For Better Health*. C. V. Mosby Company St. Louis, Missouri, 1982.

Pennington, S. A. T. and H. N. Church. *Food Values of Portions Commonly Used*. Harper and Row Publishers, New York, 1985.

Kullman, D. A. *ABC Milligram Cholesterol Diet Guide*. Merit Publications, Inc. North Miami Beach, Florida 1978.

Food Processor nutrient analysis software by Esha Corporation, P.O. Box 13028, Salem, Oregon, 97309. With permission.

APPENDIX

B

Computer Data Form

Preliminary Information

Data Disk Drive A B C (circle drive)

Pre-test ________ Post-test ________

Date (mm-dd-year) ________-________-________

Course name ____________________

Section number ____________________

Instructor ____________________

General Information

Name ____________________

I.D. (9 digits or less) ____________________

Age ________

Male or female (circle one) M F

Body weight (pounds) ________

Resting heart rate ________

Systolic blood pressure ________

Diastolic blood pressure ________

Cardiorespiratory Endurance (circle one)

1. 1.5-mile run Time _______:_______
2. 1.0-mile walk Time _______:_______ HR _______
3. Step test Recov. HR _______
4. Astrand test WLoad _______
   5th min HR _____ 6th min HR _____ Avg. HR _______
5. 12-min swim test Distance _______

Muscular Strength (circle 1 or 2)

1. Muscular strength and endurance

Exercise	BW	×	%BW Men	%BW Women	=	Resist.	Reps
Lat pull down	_____:_____	×	.70	.45	=	_____	_____
Leg extension	_____:_____	×	.65	.50	=	_____	_____
Bench press	_____:_____	×	.75	.45	=	_____	_____
Abd crunch	_____:_____					NA	_____
Leg curl	_____:_____	×	.32	.25	=	_____	_____
Arm curl	_____:_____	×	.35	.18	=	_____	_____

2. Muscular endurance

Men		Women	
Bench jumps	_______	Bench jumps	_______
Chair dips	_______	Mod. push-ups	_______
Abd crunches	_______	Abd crunches	_______

Muscular Flexibility

Sit and reach _______:_______

Right or left body rotation (circle one) R L

Right body rotation _______:_______

Left body rotation _______:_______

Shoulder width _______:_______

Shoulder rotation _______:_______

Body Composition (circle 1 2 or 3)

1. Skinfolds

Men		Women	
Chest	_______	Triceps	_______
Abdomen	_______	Suprailium	_______
Thigh	_______	Thigh	_______

2. Girth measurements

Men (use inches)		Women (use cm)	
Waist	_______	Upper arm	_______
Wrist	_______	Hip	_______
		Wrist	_______

3. Other technique

   Indicate percent body fat _________

Skill Fitness

Agility	_______	Power	_____ ft. _____ in.
Balance	_______	Reaction time	_______
Coordination	_______	Speed	_______

NUTRIENT ANALYSIS DATA

Use the computer form provided on page 227 and follow the instructions on page 34 of the book.

CARDIORESPIRATORY EXERCISE PRESCRIPTION DATA

Date (mm-dd-year) ________-________-________

Name ____________________

Age ________

Resting heart rate ________

Male or female (circle one) M F

Current cardiorespiratory fitness (circle one)

Excellent	= 1	Fair	= 4
Good	= 2	Poor	= 5
Average	= 3		

EXERCISE LOG DATA

Use the activity list provided on page 84. Keep track of the exercise date, body weight, mode of exercise (activity), duration of exercise and exercise heart rate. Then simply follow the computer instructions.

Preliminary Information

Data Disk Drive A B C (circle drive)

Pre-test ________ Post-test ________

Date (mm-dd-year) ________-________-________

Course name ______________________

Section number ______________________

Instructor ______________________

General Information

Name ______________________

I.D. (9 digits or less) ______________________

Age ____________

Male or female (circle one) M F

Body weight (pounds) ____________

Resting heart rate ____________

Systolic blood pressure ____________

Diastolic blood pressure ____________

Cardiorespiratory Endurance (circle one)

1. 1.5-mile run Time _______:_______
2. 1.0-mile walk Time _______:_______ HR _______
3. Step test Recov. HR _______
4. Astrand test WLoad _______
   5th min HR _____ 6th min HR _____ Avg. HR _______
5. 12-min swim test Distance _______

Muscular Strength (circle 1 or 2)

1. Muscular strength and endurance

Exercise	BW	× %BW (Men)	%BW (Women)	= Resist.	Reps
Lat pull down	_____:_____	× .70	.45	= _____	_____
Leg extension	_____:_____	× .65	.50	= _____	_____
Bench press	_____:_____	× .75	.45	= _____	_____
Abd crunch	_____:_____			NA	_____
Leg curl	_____:_____	× .32	.25	= _____	_____
Arm curl	_____:_____	× .35	.18	= _____	_____

2. Muscular endurance

Men		Women	
Bench jumps	_______	Bench jumps	_______
Chair dips	_______	Mod. push-ups	_______
Abd crunches	_______	Abd crunches	_______

Muscular Flexibility

Sit and reach _______:_______

Right or left body rotation (circle one) R L

Right body rotation _______:_______

Left body rotation _______:_______

Shoulder width _______:_______

Shoulder rotation _______:_______

Body Composition (circle 1 2 or 3)

1. Skinfolds

Men		Women	
Chest	_______	Triceps	_______
Abdomen	_______	Suprailium	_______
Thigh	_______	Thigh	_______

2. Girth measurements

Men (use inches)		Women (use cm)	
Waist	_______	Upper arm	_______
Wrist	_______	Hip	_______
		Wrist	_______

3. Other technique

   Indicate percent body fat _________

Skill Fitness

Agility	_______	Power _____ ft. _____ in.	
Balance	_______	Reaction time	_______
Coordination	_______	Speed	_______

NUTRIENT ANALYSIS DATA

Use the computer form provided on page 227 and follow the instructions on page 34 of the book.

CARDIORESPIRATORY EXERCISE PRESCRIPTION DATA

Date (mm-dd-year) ________-________-________

Name ______________________

Age ____________

Resting heart rate ____________

Male or female (circle one) M F

Current cardiorespiratory fitness (circle one)

Excellent	= 1	Fair	= 4
Good	= 2	Poor	= 5
Average	= 3		

EXERCISE LOG DATA

Use the activity list provided on page 84. Keep track of the exercise date, body weight, mode of exercise (activity), duration of exercise and exercise heart rate. Then simply follow the computer instructions.

The Recommended Quality and Quantity of Exercise for Developing and Maintaining Cardiorespiratory and Muscular Fitness in Healthy adults*

APPENDIX

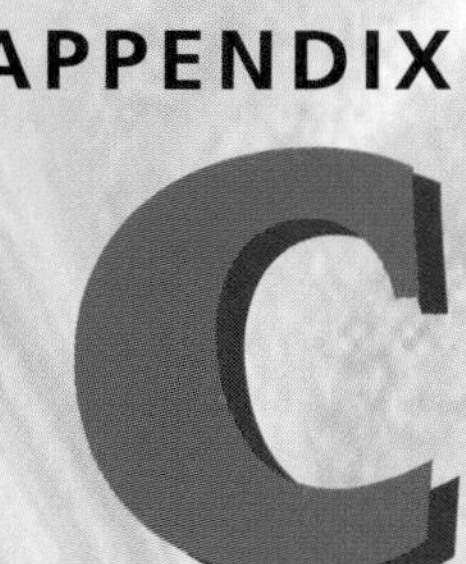

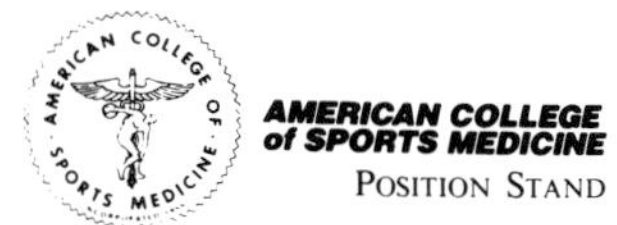

POSITION STAND

This Position Stand replaces the 1978 ACSM position paper, "The Recommended Quantity and Quality of Exercise for Developing and Maintaining Fitness in Healthy Adults."

Increasing numbers of persons are becoming involved in endurance training and other forms of physical activity, and, thus, the need for guidelines for exercise prescription is apparent. Based on the existing evidence concerning exercise prescription for healthy adults and the need for guidelines, the American College of Sports Medicine (ACSM) makes the following recommendations for the quantity and quality of training for developing and maintaining cardiorespiratory fitness, body composition, and muscular strength and endurance in the healthy adult:

1. Frequency of training: 3–5 $d \cdot wk^{-1}$.
2. Intensity of training: 60–90% of maximum heart rate (HR_{max}), or 50–85% of maximum oxygen uptake ($\dot{V}O_{2max}$) or HR_{max} reserve.[1]
3. Duration of training: 20–60 min of continuous aerobic activity. Duration is dependent on the intensity of the activity; thus, lower intensity activity should be conducted over a longer period of time. Because of the importance of "total fitness" and the fact that it is more readily attained in longer duration programs, and because of the potential hazards and compliance problems associated with high intensity activity, lower to moderate intensity activity of longer duration is recommended for the nonathletic adult.
4. Mode of activity: any activity that uses large muscle groups, can be maintained continuously, and is rhythmical and aerobic in nature, e.g., walking-hiking, running-jogging, cycling-bicycling, cross-country skiing, dancing, rope skipping, rowing, stair climbing, swimming, skating, and various endurance game activities.
5. Resistance training: Strength training of a moderate intensity, sufficient to develop and maintain fat-free weight (FFW), should be an integral part of an adult fitness program. One set of 8–12 repetitions of eight to ten exercises that condition the major muscle groups at least 2 $d \cdot wk^{-1}$ is the recommended minimum.

[1] Maximum heart rate reserve is calculated from the difference between resting and maximum heart rate. To estimate training intensity, a percentage of this value is added to the resting heart rate and is expressed as a percentage of HR_{max} reserve (85).

RATIONALE AND RESEARCH BACKGROUND

Introduction

The questions "How much exercise is enough," and "What type of exercise is best for developing and maintaining fitness?" are frequently asked. It is recognized that the term "physical fitness" is composed of a variety of characteristics included in the broad categories of cardiovascular-respiratory fitness, body composition, muscular strength and endurance, and flexibility. In this context fitness is defined as the ability to perform moderate to vigorous levels of physical activity without undue fatigue and the capability of maintaining such ability throughout life (167). It is also recognized that the adaptive response to training is complex and includes peripheral, central, structural, and functional factors (5,172). Although many such variables and their adaptive response to training have been documented, the lack of sufficient in-depth and comparative data relative to frequency, intensity, and duration of training makes them inadequate to use as comparative models. Thus, in respect to the above questions, fitness is limited mainly to changes in $\dot{V}O_{2max}$, muscular strength and endurance, and body composition, which includes total body mass, fat weight (FW), and FFW. Further, the rationale and research background used for this position stand will be divided into programs for cardiorespiratory fitness and weight control and programs for muscular strength and endurance.

Fitness versus health benefits of exercise. Since the original position statement was published in 1978, an important distinction has been made between physical activity as it relates to health versus fitness. It has been pointed out that the quantity and quality of exercise needed to attain health-related benefits may differ from what is recommended for fitness benefits. It is now clear that lower levels of physical activity than recommended by this position statement may reduce the risk for certain chronic degenerative diseases and yet may not be of sufficient quantity or quality to improve $\dot{V}O_{2max}$ (71,72,98,167). ACSM recognizes the potential health benefits of regular exercise performed more frequently and for a longer duration, but at lower intensities than prescribed in this position statement (13A,71,100,120,160). ACSM will address the issue concerning the proper amount of physical activity necessary to derive health benefits in another statement.

Need for standardization of procedures and reporting results. Despite an abundance of information available concerning the training of the human organism, the lack of standardization of testing protocols and procedures, of methodology in relation to training procedures and experimental design, and of a preciseness in the documentation and reporting of the quantity and quality of training prescribed make interpretation difficult (123,133,139,164,167). Interpretation and comparison of results are also dependent on the initial level of fitness (42,43,58,114,148,151,156), length of time of the training experiment (17,45,125,128,139, 145,150), and specificity of the testing and training (5,43,130,139,145A,172). For example, data from training studies using subjects with varied levels of $\dot{V}O_{2max}$, total body mass, and FW have found changes to occur in relation to their initial values (14,33,109, 112,113,148,151); i.e., the lower the initial $\dot{V}O_{2max}$ the larger the percentage of improvement found, and the higher the FW the greater the reduction. Also, data evaluating trainability with age, comparison of the different magnitudes and quantities of effort, and comparison of the trainability of men and women may have been influenced by the initial fitness levels.

In view of the fact that improvement in the fitness variables discussed in this position statement continues over many months of training (27,86,139,145,150), it is reasonable to believe that short-term studies conducted over a few weeks have certain limitations. Middle-aged sedentary and older participants may take several weeks to adapt to the initial rigors of training, and thus need a longer adaptation period to get the full benefit from a program. For example, Seals et al. (150) exercise trained 60–69-yr-olds for 12 months. Their subjects showed a 12% improvement in $\dot{V}O_{2max}$ after 6 months of moderate intensity walking training. A further 18% increase in $\dot{V}O_{2max}$ occurred during the next 6 months of training when jogging was introduced. How long a training experiment should be conducted is difficult to determine, but 15–20 wk may be a good minimum standard. Although it is difficult to control exercise training experiments for more than 1 yr, there is a need to study this effect. As stated earlier, lower doses of exercise may improve $\dot{V}O_{2max}$ and control or maintain body composition, but at a slower rate.

Although most of the information concerning training described in this position statement has been conducted on men, the available evidence indicates that women tend to adapt to endurance training in the same manner as men (19,38,46,47,49,62,65,68,90,92,122, 166).

Exercise Prescription for Cardiorespiratory Fitness and Weight Control

Exercise prescription is based upon the frequency, intensity, and duration of training, the mode of activity (aerobic in nature, e.g., listed under No. 4 above), and the initial level of fitness. In evaluating these factors, the following observations have been derived from studies conducted for up to 6–12 months with endurance training programs.

Improvement in $\dot{V}O_{2max}$ is directly related to frequency (3,6,50,75–77,125,126,152,154,164), intensity (3,6,26,29,58,61,75–77,80,85,93,118,152,164), and duration (3,29,60,61,70,75–77,101,109,118,152,162, 164,168) of training. Depending upon the quantity and quality of training, improvement in $\dot{V}O_{2max}$ ranges from 5 to 30% (8,29,30,48,59,61,65,67,69,75–77,82,84,96, 99,101,102,111,115,119,123,127,139,141,143,149, 150,152,153,158,164,168,173). These studies show that a minimum increase in $\dot{V}O_{2max}$ of 15% is generally attained in programs that meet the above stated guidelines. Although changes in $\dot{V}O_{2max}$ greater than 30% have been shown, they are usually associated with large total body mass and FW loss, in cardiac patients, or in persons with a very low initial level of fitness. Also, as a result of leg fatigue or a lack of motivation, persons with low initial fitness may have spuriously low initial $\dot{V}O_{2max}$ values. Klissouras (94A) and Bouchard (16A) have shown that human variation in the trainability of $\dot{V}O_{2max}$ is important and related to current phenotype level. That is, there is a genetically determined pretraining status of the trait and capacity to adapt to physical training. Thus, physiological results should be interpreted with respect to both genetic variation and the quality and quantity of training performed.

Intensity-duration. Intensity and duration of training are interrelated, with total amount of work accomplished being an important factor in improvement in fitness (12,20,27,48,90,92,123,127,128,136,149,151,164). Although more comprehensive inquiry is necessary, present evidence suggests that, when exercise is performed above the minimum intensity threshold, the total amount of work accomplished is an important factor in fitness development (19,27,126,127,149,151) and maintenance (134). That is, improvement will be similar for activities performed at a lower intensity-longer duration compared to higher intensity-shorter duration if the total energy costs of the activities are equal. Higher intensity exercise is associated with greater cardiovascular risk (156A), orthopedic injury (124,139) and lower compliance to training than lower intensity exercise (36,105,124,146). Therefore, programs emphasizing low to moderate intensity training with longer duration are recommended for most adults.

The minimal training intensity threshold for improvement in $\dot{V}O_{2max}$ is approximately 60% of the HR_{max} (50% of $\dot{V}O_{2max}$ or HR_{max} reserve) (80,85). The 50% of HR_{max} reserve represents a heart rate of approximately 130–135 beats·min^{-1} for young persons. As a result of the age-related change in maximum heart rate, the absolute heart rate to achieve this threshold is inversely related to age and can be as low as 105–115 beats·min^{-1} for older persons (35,65,150). Patients who are taking beta-adrenergic blocking drugs may have significantly lower heart rate values (171). Initial level of fitness is another important consideration in prescribing exercise (26,90,104,148,151). The person with a low fitness level can achieve a significant training effect with a sustained training heart rate as low as 40–50% of HR_{max} reserve, while persons with higher fitness levels require a higher training stimulus (35,58,152,164).

Classification of exercise intensity. The classification of exercise intensity and its standardization for exercise prescription based on a 20–60 min training session has been confusing, misinterpreted, and often taken out of context. The most quoted exercise classification system is based on the energy expenditure (kcal·min^{-1}·kg^{-1}) of industrial tasks (40,89). The original data for this classification system were published by Christensen (24) in 1953 and were based on the energy expenditure of working in the steel mill for an 8-h day. The classification of industrial and leisure-time tasks by using absolute values of energy expenditure have been valuable for use in the occupational and nutritional setting. Although this classification system has broad application in medicine and, in particular, making recommendations for weight control and job placement, it has little or no meaning for preventive and rehabilitation exercise training programs. To extrapolate absolute values of energy expenditure for completing an industrial task based on an 8-h work day to 20–60 min regimens of exercise training does not make sense. For example, walking and jogging/running can be accomplished at a wide range of speeds; thus, the relative intensity becomes important under these conditions. Because the endurance training regimens recommended by ACSM for nonathletic adults are geared for 60 min or less of physical activity, the system of classification of exercise training intensity shown in Table 1 is recommended (139). The use of a realistic time period for training and an individual's relative exercise intensity makes this system amenable to young, middle-aged, and elderly participants, as well as patients with a limited exercise capacity (3,137,139).

TABLE 1. Classification of intensity of exercise based on 20–60 min of endurance training.

Relative Intensity (%)		Rating of Perceived Exertion	Classification of Intensity
HR_{max}*	$\dot{V}O_{2max}$* or HR_{max} reserve		
<35%	<30%	<10	Very light
35–59%	30–49%	10–11	Light
60–79%	50–74%	12–13	Moderate (somewhat hard)
80–89%	75–84%	14–16	Heavy
≥90%	≥85%	>16	Very heavy

Table from Pollock, M. L. and J. H. Wilmore. *Exercise in Health and Disease: Evaluation and Prescription for Prevention and Rehabilitation*, 2nd Ed. Philadelphia: W.B. Saunders, 1990. Published with permission.

* HR_{max} = maximum heart rate; $\dot{V}O_{2max}$ = maximum oxygen uptake.

Table 1 also describes the relationship between relative intensity based on percent HR_{max}, percentage of HR_{max} reserve or percentage of $\dot{V}O_{2max}$, and the rating of perceived exertion (RPE) (15,16,137). The use of heart rate as an estimate of intensity of training is the common standard (3,139).

The use of RPE has become a valid tool in the monitoring of intensity in exercise training programs (11,37,137,139). It is generally considered an adjunct to heart rate in monitoring relative exercise intensity, but once the relationship between heart rate and RPE is known, RPE can be used in place of heart rate (23,139). This would not be the case in certain patient populations where a more precise knowledge of heart rate may be critical to the safety of the program.

Frequency. The amount of improvement in $\dot{V}O_{2max}$ tends to plateau when frequency of training is increased above 3 d·wk^{-1} (50,123,139). The value of the added improvement found with training more than 5 d·wk^{-1} is small to not apparent in regard to improvement in $\dot{V}O_{2max}$ (75–77,106,123). Training of less than 2 d·wk^{-1} does not generally show a meaningful change in $\dot{V}O_{2max}$ (29,50,118,123,152,164).

Mode. If frequency, intensity, and duration of training are similar (total kcal expenditure), the training adaptations appear to be independent of the mode of aerobic activity (101A,118,130). Therefore, a variety of endurance activities, e.g., those listed above, may be used to derive the same training effect.

Endurance activities that require running and jumping are considered high impact types of activity and generally cause significantly more debilitating injuries to beginning as well as long-term exercisers than do low impact and non-weight bearing type activities (13,93, 117,124,127,135,140,142). This is particularly evident in the elderly (139). Beginning joggers have increased foot, leg, and knee injuries when training is performed more than 3 d·wk^{-1} and longer than 30 min duration per exercise session (135). High intensity interval training (run-walk) compared to continuous jogging training was also associated with a higher incidence of injury (124,136). Thus, caution should be taken when recommending the type of activity and exercise prescription for the beginning exerciser. Orthopedic injuries as related to overuse increase linearly in runners/joggers when performing these activities (13,140). Thus, there is a need for more inquiry into the effect that different types of activities and the quantity and quality of training has on injuries over short-term and long-term participation.

An activity such as weight training should not be considered as a means of training for developing $\dot{V}O_{2max}$, but it has significant value for increasing muscular strength and endurance and FFW (32,54,107, 110,165). Studies evaluating circuit weight training (weight training conducted almost continuously with moderate weights, using 10–15 repetitions per exercise session with 15–30 s rest between bouts of activity) show an average improvement in $\dot{V}O_{2max}$ of 6% (1,51–54,83,94,108,170). Thus, circuit weight training is not recommended as the only activity used in exercise programs for developing $\dot{V}O_{2max}$.

Age. Age in itself does not appear to be a deterrent to endurance training. Although some earlier studies showed a lower training effect with middle-aged or elderly participants (9,34,79,157,168), more recent studies show the relative change in $\dot{V}O_{2max}$ to be similar to younger age groups (7,8,65,132,150,161,163). Although more investigation is necessary concerning the rate of improvement in $\dot{V}O_{2max}$ with training at various ages, at present it appears that elderly participants need longer periods of time to adapt (34,132,150). Earlier studies showing moderate to no improvement in $\dot{V}O_{2max}$ were conducted over a short time span (9), or exercise was conducted at a moderate to low intensity (34), thus making the interpretation of the results difficult.

Although $\dot{V}O_{2max}$ decreases with age and total body mass and FW increase with age, evidence suggests that this trend can be altered with endurance training (22,27,86–88,139). A 9% reduction in $\dot{V}O_{2max}$ per decade for sedentary adults after age 25 has been shown (31,73), but for active individuals the reduction may be less than 5% per decade (21,31,39,73). Ten or more yr follow-up studies where participants continued training at a similar level showed maintenance of cardiorespiratory fitness (4,87,88,138). A cross-sectional study of older competitive runners showed progressively lower values in $\dot{V}O_{2max}$ from the fourth to seventh decades of life, but also showed less training in the older groups (129). More recent 10-yr follow-up data on these same athletes (50–82 yr of age) showed $\dot{V}O_{2max}$ to be unchanged when training quantity and quality remained unchanged (138). Thus, lifestyle plays a significant role in the maintenance of fitness. More inquiry into the relationship of long-term training (quantity and quality), for both competitors and noncompetitors, and physiological function with increasing age is necessary before more definitive statements can be made.

Maintenance of training effect. In order to maintain the training effect, exercise must be continued on a regular basis (18,25,28,47,97,111,144,147). A significant reduction in cardiorespiratory fitness occurs after 2 wk of detraining (25,144), with participants returning to near pretraining levels of fitness after 10 wk (47) to 8 months of detraining (97). A loss of 50% of their initial improvement in $\dot{V}O_{2max}$ has been shown after 4–12 wk of detraining (47,91,144). Those individuals who have undergone years of continuous training maintain some benefits for longer periods of detraining than subjects from short-term training studies (25). While stopping training shows dramatic reductions in $\dot{V}O_{2max}$, reduced training shows modest to no reductions for periods of 5–15 wk (18,75–77,144). Hickson et al., in a series of experiments where frequency (75), duration (76), or intensity (77) of training were manipulated, found that, if intensity of training remained unchanged, $\dot{V}O_{2max}$ was maintained for up to 15 wk when frequency and duration of training were reduced by as much as ⅔. When frequency and duration of training remained constant and intensity of training was reduced by ⅓ or ⅔, $\dot{V}O_{2max}$ was significantly reduced. Similar findings were found in regards to reduced strength training exercise. When strength training exercise was reduced from 3 or 2 $d \cdot wk^{-1}$ to at least 1 $d \cdot wk^{-1}$, strength was maintained for 12 wk of reduced training (62). Thus, it appears that missing an exercise session periodically or reducing training for up to 15 wk will not adversely effect $\dot{V}O_{2max}$ or muscular strength and endurance as long as training intensity is maintained.

Even though many new studies have given added insight into the proper amount of exercise, investigation is necessary to evaluate the rate of increase and decrease of fitness when varying training loads and reduction in training in relation to level of fitness, age, and length of time in training. Also, more information is needed to better identify the minimal level of exercise necessary to maintain fitness.

Weight control and body composition. Although there is variability in human response to body composition change with exercise, total body mass and FW are generally reduced with endurance training programs (133,139,171A), while FFW remains constant (123,133,139,169) or increases slightly (116,174). For example, Wilmore (171A) reported the results of 32 studies that met the criteria for developing cardiorespiratory fitness that are outlined in this position stand and found an average loss in total body mass of 1.5 kg and percent fat of 2.2%. Weight loss programs using dietary manipulation that result in a more dramatic decrease in total body mass show reductions in both FW and FFW (2,78,174). When these programs are conducted in conjunction with exercise training, FFW loss is more modest than in programs using diet alone (78,121). Programs that are conducted at least 3 d·wk^{-1} (123,125,126,128,169), of at least 20 min duration (109,123,169), and of sufficient intensity to expend approximately 300 kcal per exercise session (75 kg person)[2] are suggested as a threshold level for total body mass and FW loss (27,64,77,123,133,139). An expenditure of 200 kcal per session has also been shown to be useful in weight reduction if the exercise frequency is at least 4 d·wk^{-1} (155). If the primary purpose of the training program is for weight loss, then regimens of greater frequency and duration of training and low to moderate intensity are recommended (2,139). Programs with less participation generally show little or no change in body composition (44,57,93,123,133,159, 162,169). Significant increases in $\dot{V}O_{2max}$ have been shown with 10–15 min of high intensity training (6,79,109,118,123,152,153); thus, if total body mass and FW reduction are not considerations, then shorter duration, higher intensity programs may be recommended for healthy individuals at low risk for cardiovascular disease and orthopedic injury.

Exercise Prescription for Muscular Strength and Endurance

The addition of resistance/strength training to the position statement results from the need for a well-rounded program that exercises all the major muscle groups of the body. Thus, the inclusion of resistance training in adult fitness programs should be effective in the development and maintenance of FFW. The effect of exercise training is specific to the area of the body being trained (5,43,145A,172). For example, training the legs will have little or no effect on the arms, shoulders, and trunk muscles. A 10-yr follow-up of master runners who continued their training regimen, but did no upper body exercise, showed maintenance of $\dot{V}O_{2max}$ and a 2-kg reduction in FFW (138). Their leg circumference remained unchanged, but arm circumference was significantly lower. These data indicate a loss of muscle mass in the untrained areas. Three of the athletes who practiced weight training exercise for the upper body and trunk muscles maintained their FFW. A comprehensive review by Sale (145A) carefully documents available information on specificity of training.

Specificity of training was further addressed by Graves et al. (63). Using a bilateral knee extension exercise, they trained four groups: group A, first ½ of the range of motion; group B, second ½ of the range of motion; group AB, full range of motion; and a control group that did not train. The results clearly showed that the training result was specific to the range of motion trained, with group AB getting the best full range effect. Thus, resistance training should be performed through a full range of motion for maximum benefit (63,95).

Muscular strength and endurance are developed by the overload principle, i.e., by increasing more than normal the resistance to movement or frequency and duration of activity (32,41,43,74,145). Muscular strength is best developed by using heavy weights (that require maximum or nearly maximum tension development) with few repetitions, and muscular endurance is best developed by using lighter weights with a greater number of repetitions (10,41,43,145). To some extent, both muscular strength and endurance are developed under each condition, but each system favors a more specific type of development (43,145). Thus, to elicit improvement in both muscular strength and endurance, most experts recommend 8–12 repetitions per bout of exercise.

Any magnitude of overload will result in strength development, but higher intensity effort at or near maximal effort will give a significantly greater effect (43,74,101B,103,145,172). The intensity of resistance training can be manipulated by varying the weight load, repetitions, rest interval between exercises, and number of sets completed (43). Caution is advised for training that emphasizes lengthening (eccentric) contractions, compared to shortening (concentric) or isometric contractions, as the potential for skeletal muscle soreness and injury is accentuated (3A,84A).

Muscular strength and endurance can be developed by means of static (isometric) or dynamic (isotonic or isokinetic) exercises. Although each type of training has its favorable and weak points, for healthy adults, dynamic resistance exercises are recommended. Resistance training for the average participant should be rhythmical, performed at a moderate to slow speed, move through a full range of motion, and not impede normal forced breathing. Heavy resistance exercise can cause a dramatic acute increase in both systolic and diastolic blood pressure (100A,101C).

The expected improvement in strength from resistance training is difficult to assess because increases in strength are affected by the participants' initial level of strength and their potential for improvement (43,66,74,114,172). For example, Mueller and Rohmert (114) found increases in strength ranging from 2 to 9% per week depending on initial strength levels. Although the literature reflects a wide range of improvement in strength with resistance training programs, the average improvement for sedentary young and middle-aged men and women for up to 6 months of training is 25–30%. Fleck and Kraemer (43), in a review of 13 studies representing various forms of isotonic training, showed an average improvement in bench press strength of 23.3% when subjects were tested on the

[2] Haskell and Haskell et al. (71,72) have suggested the use of 4 kcal·kg^{-1} of body weight of energy expenditure per day for a minimum standard for use in exercise programs.

equipment with which they were trained and 16.5% when tested on special isotonic or isokinetic ergometers (six studies). Fleck and Kraemer (43) also reported an average increase in leg strength of 26.6% when subjects were tested with the equipment that they trained on (six studies) and 21.2% when tested with special isotonic or isokinetic ergometers (five studies). Results of improvement in strength resulting from isometric training have been of the same magnitude as found with isotonic training (17,43,62,63).

In light of the information reported above, the following guidelines for resistance training are recommended for the average healthy adult. A minimum of 8–10 exercises involving the major muscle groups should be performed a minimum of two times per week. A minimum of one set of 8–12 repetitions to near fatigue should be completed. These minimal standards for resistance training are based on two factors. First, the time it takes to complete a comprehensive, well-rounded exercise program is important. Programs lasting more than 60 min per session are associated with higher dropout rates (124). Second, although greater frequencies of training (17,43,56) and additional sets or combinations of sets and repetitions elicit larger strength gains (10,32,43,74,145,172), the magnitude of difference is usually small. For example, Braith et al. (17) compared training 2 $d \cdot wk^{-1}$ with 3 $d \cdot wk^{-1}$ for 18 wk. The subjects performed one set of 7–10 repetitions to fatigue. The 2 $d \cdot wk^{-1}$ group showed a 21% increase in strength compared to 28% in the 3 $d \cdot wk^{-1}$ group. In other words, 75% of what could be attained in a 3 $d \cdot wk^{-1}$ program was attained in 2 $d \cdot wk^{-1}$. Also, the 21% improvement in strength found by the 2 $d \cdot wk^{-1}$ regimen is 70–80% of the improvement reported by other programs using additional frequencies of training and combinations of sets and repetitions (43). Graves et al. (62,63), Gettman et al. (55), Hurley et al. (83) and Braith et al. (17) found that programs using one set to fatigue showed a greater than 25% increase in strength. Although resistance training equipment may provide a better graduated and quantitative stimulus for overload than traditional calisthenic exercises, calisthenics and other resistance types of exercise can still be effective in improving and maintaining strength.

SUMMARY

The combination of frequency, intensity, and duration of chronic exercise has been found to be effective for producing a training effect. The interaction of these factors provide the overload stimulus. In general, the lower the stimulus the lower the training effect, and the greater the stimulus the greater the effect. As a result of specificity of training and the need for maintaining muscular strength and endurance, and flexibility of the major muscle groups, a well-rounded training program including resistance training and flexibility exercises is recommended. Although age in itself is not a limiting factor to exercise training, a more gradual approach in applying the prescription at older ages seems prudent. It has also been shown that endurance training of fewer than 2 $d \cdot wk^{-1}$, at less than 50% of maximum oxygen uptake and for less than 10 $min \cdot d^{-1}$, is inadequate for developing and maintaining fitness for healthy adults.

In the interpretation of this position statement, it must be recognized that the recommendations should be used in the context of participants' needs, goals, and initial abilities. In this regard, a sliding scale as to the amount of time allotted and intensity of effort should be carefully gauged for both the cardiorespiratory and muscular strength and endurance components of the program. An appropriate warm-up and cool-down, which would include flexibility exercises, is also recommended. The important factor is to design a program for the individual to provide the proper amount of physical activity to attain maximal benefit at the lowest risk. Emphasis should be placed on factors that result in permanent lifestyle change and encourage a lifetime of physical activity.

REFERENCES

1. Allen, T. E., R. J. Byrd, and D. P. Smith. Hemodynamic consequences of circuit weight training. *Res. Q.* 43:299–306, 1976.
2. American College of Sports Medicine. Proper and improper weight loss programs. *Med. Sci. Sports Exerc.* 15:ix–xiii, 1983.
3. American College of Sports Medicine. *Guidelines for Graded Exercise Testing and Exercise Prescription*, 3rd Ed. Philadelphia: Lea and Febiger, 1986.

3A. Armstrong, R. B. Mechanisms of exercise-induced delayed onset muscular soreness: a brief review. *Med. Sci. Sports Exerc.* 16:529–538, 1984.

4. Åstrand, P. O. Exercise physiology of the mature athlete. In: *Sports Medicine for the Mature Athlete*, J. R. Sutton and R. M. Brock (Eds.). Indianapolis, IN: Benchmark Press, Inc., 1986, pp. 3–16.
5. Åstrand, P. O. and K. Rodahl. *Textbook of Work Physiology*, 3rd Ed. New York: McGraw-Hill, 1986, pp. 412–485.
6. Atomi, Y., K. Ito, H. Iwasaski, and M. Miyashita. Effects of intensity and frequency of training on aerobic work capacity of young females. *J. Sports Med.* 18:3–9, 1978.
7. Badenhop, D. T., P. A. Cleary, S. F. Schaal, E. L. Fox, and R. L. Bartels. Physiological adjustments to higher- or lower-intensity exercise in elders. *Med. Sci. Sports Exerc.* 15:496–502, 1983.
8. Barry, A. J., J. W. Daly, E. D. R. Pruett, et al. The effects of physical conditioning on older individuals. I. Work capacity, circulatory-respiratory function, and work electrocardiogram. *J. Gerontol.* 21:182–191, 1966.
9. Benestad, A. M. Trainability of old men. *Acta Med. Scand.* 178:321–327, 1965.
10. Berger, R. A. Effect of varied weight training programs on strength. *Res. Q.* 33:168–181, 1962.

11. BIRK, T. J. and C. A. BIRK. Use of ratings of perceived exertion for exercise prescription. *Sports Med.* 4:1–8, 1987.
12. BLAIR, S. N., J. V. CHANDLER, D. B. ELLISOR, and J. LANGLEY. Improving physical fitness by exercise training programs. *South. Med. J.* 73:1594–1596, 1980.
13. BLAIR, S. N., H. W. KOHL, and N. N. GOODYEAR. Rates and risks for running and exercise injuries: studies in three populations. *Res. Q. Exerc. Sports* 58:221–228, 1987.
13A. BLAIR, S. N., H. W. KOHL, III, R. S. PAFFENBARGER, D. G. CLARK, K. H. COOPER, and L. H. GIBBONS. Physical fitness and all-cause mortality. A prospective study of healthy men and women. *J.A.M.A.* 262:2395–2401, 1989.
14. BOILEAU, R. A., E. R. BUSKIRK, D. H. HORSTMAN, J. MENDEZ, and W. NICHOLAS. Body composition changes in obese and lean men during physical conditioning. *Med. Sci. Sports* 3:183–189, 1971.
15. BORG, G. A. V. Psychophysical bases of perceived exertion. *Med. Sci. Sports Exerc.* 14:377–381, 1982.
16. BORG, G. and D. OTTOSON (Eds.). *The Perception of Exertion in Physical Work.* London, England: The MacMillan Press, Ltd., 1986, pp. 4–7.
16A. BOUCHARD, C. Gene-environment interaction in human adaptability. In: *The Academy Papers,* R. B. Malina and H. M. Eckert (Eds.). Champaign, IL: Human Kinetics Publishers, 1988, pp. 56–66.
17. BRAITH, R. W., J. E. GRAVES, M. L. POLLOCK, S. L. LEGGETT, D. M. CARPENTER, and A. B. COLVIN. Comparison of two versus three days per week of variable resistance training during 10 and 18 week programs. *Int. J. Sports Med.* 10:450–454, 1989.
18. BRYNTESON, P. and W. E. SINNING. The effects of training frequencies on the retention of cardiovascular fitness. *Med. Sci. Sports* 5:29–33, 1973.
19. BURKE, E. J. Physiological effects of similar training programs in males and females. *Res. Q.* 48:510–517, 1977.
20. BURKE, E. J. and B. D. FRANKS. Changes in $\dot{V}O_{2max}$ resulting from bicycle training at different intensities holding total mechanical work constant. *Res. Q.* 46:31–37, 1975.
21. BUSKIRK, E. R. and J. L. HODGSON. Age and aerobic power: the rate of change in men and women. *Fed. Proc.* 46:1824–1829, 1987.
22. CARTER, J. E. L. and W. H. PHILLIPS. Structural changes in exercising middle-aged males during a 2-year period. *J. Appl. Physiol* 27:787–794, 1969.
23. CHOW, J. R. and J. H. WILMORE. The regulation of exercise intensity by ratings of perceived exertion. *J. Cardiac Rehabil.* 4:382–387, 1984.
24. CHRISTENSEN, E. H. Physiological evaluation of work in the Nykroppa iron works. In: *Ergonomics Society Symposium on Fatigue,* W. F. Floyd and A. T. Welford (Eds.). London, England: Lewis, 1953, pp. 93–108.
25. COYLE, E. F., W. H. MARTIN, D. R. SINACORE, M. J. JOYNER, J. M. HAGBERG, and J. O. HOLLOSZY. Time course of loss of adaptation after stopping prolonged intense endurance training. *J. Appl. Physiol.* 57:1857–1864, 1984.
26. CREWS, T. R. and J. A. ROBERTS. Effects of interaction of frequency and intensity of training. *Res. Q.* 47:48–55, 1976.
27. CURETON, T. K. *The Physiological Effects of Exercise Programs upon Adults.* Springfield, IL: Charles C. Thomas Co., 1969, pp. 3–6, 33–77.
28. CURETON, T. K. and E. E. PHILLIPS. Physical fitness changes in middle-aged men attributable to equal eight-week periods of training, non-training and retraining. *J. Sports Med. Phys. Fitness* 4:1–7, 1964.
29. DAVIES, C. T. M. and A. V. KNIBBS. The training stimulus, the effects of intensity, duration and frequency of effort on maximum aerobic power output. *Int. Z. Angew. Physiol.* 29:299–305, 1971.
30. DAVIS, J. A., M. H. FRANK, B. J. WHIPP, and K. WASSERMAN. Anaerobic threshold alterations caused by endurance training in middle-aged men. *J. Appl. Physiol.* 46:1039–1049, 1979.
31. DEHN, M. M. and R. A. BRUCE. Longitudinal variations in maximal oxygen intake with age and activity. *J. Appl. Physiol.* 33:805–807, 1972.
32. DELORME, T. L. Restoration of muscle power by heavy resistance exercise. *J. Bone Joint Surg.* 27:645–667, 1945.
33. DEMPSEY, J. A. Anthropometrical observations on obese and nonobese young men undergoing a program of vigorous physical exercise. *Res. Q.* 35:275–287, 1964.
34. DEVRIES, H. A. Physiological effects of an exercise training regimen upon men aged 52 to 88. *J. Gerontol.* 24:325–336, 1970.
35. DEVRIES, H. A. Exercise intensity threshold for improvement of cardiovascular-respiratory function in older men. *Geriatrics* 26:94–101, 1971.
36. DISHMAN, R. K., J. SALLIS, and D. ORENSTEIN. The determinants of physical activity and exercise. *Public Health Rep.* 100:158–180, 1985.
37. DISHMAN, R. K., R. W. PATTON, J. SMITH, R. WEINBERG, and A. JACKSON. Using perceived exertion to prescribe and monitor exercise training heart rate. *Int. J. Sports Med.* 8:208–213, 1987.
38. DRINKWATER, B. L. Physiological responses of women to exercise. In: *Exercise and Sports Sciences Reviews,* Vol. 1, J. H. Wilmore (Ed.). New York: Academic Press, 1973, pp. 126–154.
39. DRINKWATER, B. L., S. M. HORVATH, and C. L. WELLS. Aerobic power of females, ages 10 to 68. *J. Gerontol.* 30:385–394, 1975.
40. DURNIN, J. V. G. A. and R. PASSMORE. *Energy, Work and Leisure.* London, England: Heinemann Educational Books, Ltd., 1967, pp. 47–82.
41. EDSTROM, L. and L. GRIMBY. Effect of exercise on the motor unit. *Muscle Nerve* 9:104–126, 1986.
42. EKBLOM, B., P. O. ÅSTRAND, B. SALTIN, J. STENBERG, and B. WALLSTROM. Effect of training on circulatory response to exercise. *J. Appl. Physiol.* 24:518–528, 1968.
43. FLECK, S. J. and W. J. KRAEMER. *Designing Resistance Training Programs.* Champaign, IL: Human Kinetics Books, 1987, pp. 15–46, 161–162.
44. FLINT, M. M., B. L. DRINKWATER, and S. M. HORVATH. Effects of training on women's response to submaximal exercise. *Med. Sci. Sports* 6:89–94, 1974.
45. FOX, E. L., R. L. BARTELS, C. E. BILLINGS, R. O'BRIEN, R. BASON, and D. K. MATHEWS. Frequency and duration of interval training programs and changes in aerobic power. *J. Appl. Physiol.* 38:481–484, 1975.
46. FRANKLIN, B., E. BUSKIRK, J. HODGSON, H. GAHAGAN, J. KOLLIAS, and J. MENDEZ. Effects of physical conditioning on cardiorespiratory function, body composition and serum lipids in relatively normal weight and obese middle-age women. *Int. J. Obes.* 3:97–109, 1979.
47. FRINGER, M. N. and A. G. STULL. Changes in cardiorespiratory parameters during periods of training and detraining in young female adults. *Med. Sci. Sports* 6:20–25, 1974.
48. GAESSER, G. A. and R. G. RICH. Effects of high- and low-intensity exercise training on aerobic capacity and blood lipids. *Med. Sci. Sports Exerc.* 16:269–274, 1984.
49. GETCHELL, L. H. and J. C. MOORE. Physical training: comparative responses of middle-aged adults. *Arch. Phys. Med. Rehabil.* 56:250–254, 1975.
50. GETTMAN, L. R., M. L. POLLOCK, J. L. DURSTINE, A. WARD, J. AYRES, and A. C. LINNERUD. Physiological responses of men to 1,3, and 5 day per week training programs. *Res. Q.* 47:638–646, 1976.
51. GETTMAN, L. R., J. J. AYRES, M. L. POLLOCK, and A. JACKSON. The effect of circuit weight training on strength, cardiorespiratory function, and body composition of adult men. *Med. Sci. Sports* 10:171–176, 1978.
52. GETTMAN, L. R., J. AYRES, M. L. POLLOCK, J. L. DURSTINE, and W. GRANTHAM. Physiological effects of circuit strength training and jogging. *Arch. Phys. Med. Rehabil.* 60:115–120, 1979.
53. GETTMAN, L. R., L. A. CULTER, and T. STRATHMAN. Physiologic changes after 20 weeks of isotonic vs. isokinetic circuit training. *J. Sports Med. Phys. Fitness* 20:265–274, 1980.
54. GETTMAN, L. R. and M. L. POLLOCK. Circuit weight training: a critical review of its physiological benefits. *Phys. Sports Med.* 9:44–60, 1981.
55. GETTMAN, L. R., P. WARD, and R. D. HAGMAN. A comparison of combined running and weight training with circuit weight

training. *Med. Sci. Sports Exerc.* 14:229–234, 1982.
56. Gillam, G. M. Effects of frequency of weight training on muscle strength enhancement. *J. Sports Med.* 21:432–436, 1981.
57. Girandola, R. N. Body composition changes in women: effects of high and low exercise intensity. *Arch. Phys. Med. Rehabil.* 57:297–300, 1976.
58. Gledhill, N. and R. B. Eynon. The intensity of training. In: *Training Scientific Basis and Application*, A. W. Taylor and M. L. Howell (Eds.). Springfield, IL: Charles C Thomas Co., 1972, pp. 97–102.
59. Golding, L. Effects of physical training upon total serum cholesterol levels. *Res. Q.* 32:499–505, 1961.
60. Goode, R. C., A. Virgin, T. T. Romet, et al. Effects of a short period of physical activity in adolescent boys and girls. *Can. J. Appl. Sports Sci.* 1:241–250, 1976.
61. Gossard, D., W. L. Haskell, B. Taylor, et al. Effects of low- and high-intensity home-based exercise training on functional capacity in healthy middle-age men. *Am. J. Cardiol.* 57:446–449, 1986.
62. Graves, J. E., M. L. Pollock, S. H. Leggett, R. W. Braith, D. M. Carpenter, and L. E. Bishop. Effect of reduced training frequency on muscular strength. *Int. J. Sports Med.* 9:316–319, 1988.
63. Graves, J. E., M. L. Pollock, A. E. Jones, A. B. Colvin, and S. H. Leggett. Specificity of limited range of motion variable resistance training. *Med. Sci. Sports Exerc.* 21:84–89, 1989.
64. Gwinup, G. Effect of exercise alone on the weight of obese women. *Arch. Int. Med.* 135:676–680, 1975.
65. Hagberg, J. M., J. E. Graves, M. Limacher, et al. Cardiovascular responses of 70–79 year old men and women to exercise training. *J. Appl. Physiol.* 66:2589–2594,1989.
66. Hakkinen, K. Factors influencing trainability of muscular strength during short term and prolonged training. *Natl. Strength Cond. Assoc. J.* 7:32–34, 1985.
67. Hanson, J. S., B. S. Tabakin, A. M. Levy, and W. Nedde. Long-term physical training and cardiovascular dynamics in middle-aged men. *Circulation* 38:783–799, 1968.
68. Hanson, J. S. and W. H. Nedde. Long-term physical training effect in sedentary females. *J. Appl. Physiol.* 37:112–116, 1974.
69. Hartley, L. H., G. Grimby, A. Kilbom, et al. Physical training in sedentary middle-aged and older men. *Scand. J. Clin. Lab. Invest.* 24:335–344, 1969.
70. Hartung, G. H., M. H. Smolensky, R. B. Harrist, and R. Runge. Effects of varied durations of training on improvement in cardiorespiratory endurance. *J. Hum. Ergol.* 6:61–68, 1977.
71. Haskell, W. L. Physical activity and health: need to define the required stimulus. *Am. J. Cardiol.* 55:4D–9D, 1985.
72. Haskell, W. L., H. J. Montoye, and D. Orenstein. Physical activity and exercise to achieve health-related physical fitness components. *Public Health Rep.* 100:202–212, 1985.
73. Heath, G. W., J. M. Hagberg, A. A. Ehsani, and J. O. Holloszy. A physiological comparison of young and older endurance athletes. *J. Appl. Physiol.* 51:634–640, 1981.
74. Hettinger, T. *Physiology of Strength.* Springfield, IL: C. C Thomas Publisher, 1961, pp. 18–40.
75. Hickson, R. C. and M. A. Rosenkoetter. Reduced training frequencies and maintenance of increased aerobic power. *Med. Sci. Sports Exerc.* 13:13–16, 1981.
76. Hickson, R. C., C. Kanakis, J. R. Davis, A. M. Moore, and S. Rich. Reduced training duration effects on aerobic power, endurance, and cardiac growth. *J. Appl. Physiol.* 53:225–229, 1982.
77. Hickson, R. C., C. Foster, M. L. Pollock, T. M. Galassi, and S. Rich. Reduced training intensities and loss of aerobic power, endurance, and cardiac growth. *J. Appl. Physiol.* 58:492–499, 1985.
78. Hill, J. O., P. B. Sparling, T. W. Shields, and P. A. Heller. Effects of exercise and food restriction on body composition and metabolic rate in obese women. *Am. J. Clin. Nutr.* 46:622–630, 1987.
79. Hollmann, W. *Changes in the Capacity for Maximal and Continuous Effort in Relation to Age. Int. Res. Sports Phys. Ed.*, E. Jokl and E. Simon (Eds.). Springfield, IL: Charles C Thomas Co., 1964, pp. 369–371.
80. Hollmann, W. and H. Venrath. Die Beinflussung von Herzgrösse, maximaler O_2—Aufnahme und Ausdauergranze durch ein Ausdauertraining mittlerer und hoher Intensität. *Der Sportarzt* 9:189–193, 1963.
81. No reference 81 due to renumbering in proof.
82. Huibregtse, W. H., H. H. Hartley, L. R. Jones, W. D. Doolittle, and T. L. Criblez. Improvement of aerobic work capacity following non-strenuous exercise. *Arch. Environ. Health* 27:12–15, 1973.
83. Hurley, B. F., D. R. Seals, A. A. Ehsani, et al. Effects of high-intensity strength training on cardiovascular function. *Med. Sci. Sports Exerc.* 16:483–488, 1984.
84. Ismail, A. H., D. Corrigan, and D. F. McLeod. Effect of an eight-month exercise program on selected physiological, biochemical, and audiological variables in adult men. *Br. J. Sports Med.* 7:230–240, 1973.
84A. Jones, D. A., D. J. Newman, J. M. Round, and S. E. L. Tolfree. Experimental human muscle damage: morphological changes in relation to other indices of damage. *J. Physiol. (Lond.)* 375:435–438, 1986.
85. Karvonen, M., K. Kentala, and O. Mustala. The effects of training heart rate: a longitudinal study. *Ann. Med. Exp. Biol. Fenn* 35:307–315, 1957.
86. Kasch, F. W., W. H. Phillips, J. E. L. Carter, and J. L. Boyer. Cardiovascular changes in middle-aged men during two years of training. *J. Appl. Physiol.* 314:53–57, 1972.
87. Kasch, F. W. and J. P. Wallace. Physiological variables during 10 years of endurance exercise. *Med. Sci. Sports* 8:5–8, 1976.
88. Kasch, F. W., J. P. Wallace, and S. P. Van Camp. Effects of 18 years of endurance exercise on physical work capacity of older men. *J. Cardiopulmonary Rehabil.* 5:308–312, 1985.
89. Katch, F. I. and W. D. McArdle. *Nutrition, Weight Control and Exercise*, 3rd Ed. Philadelphia: Lea and Febiger, 1988, pp. 110–112.
90. Kearney, J. T., A. G. Stull, J. L. Ewing, and J. W. Strein. Cardiorespiratory responses of sedentary college women as a function of training intensity. *J. Appl. Physiol.* 41:822–825, 1976.
91. Kendrick, Z. B., M. L. Pollock, T. N. Hickman, and H. S. Miller. Effects of training and detraining on cardiovascular efficiency. *Am. Corr. Ther. J.* 25:79–83, 1971.
92. Kilbom, A. Physical training in women. *Scand. J. Clin. Lab. Invest.* 119 (Suppl.):1–34, 1971.
93. Kilbom, A., L. Hartley, B. Saltin, J. Bjure, G. Grimby, and I. Åstrand. Physical training in sedentary middle-aged and older men. *Scand. J. Clin. Lab. Invest.* 24:315–322, 1969.
94. Kimura, Y., H. Itow, and S. Yamazakie. The effects of circuit weight training on VO_{2max} and body composition of trained and untrained college men. *J. Physiol. Soc. Jpn.* 43:593–596, 1981.
94A. Klissouras, V., F. Pirnay, and J. Petit. Adaptation to maximal effort: genetics and age. *J. Appl. Physiol.* 35:288–293, 1973.
95. Knapik, J. J., R. H. Maudsley, and N. V. Rammos. Angular specificity and test mode specificity of isometric and isokinetic strength training. *J. Orthop. Sports Phys. Ther.* 5:58–65, 1983.
96. Knehr, C. A., D. B. Dill, and W. Neufeld. Training and its effect on man at rest and at work. *Am. J. Physiol.* 136:148–156, 1942.
97. Knuttgen, H. G., L. O. Nordesjo, B. Ollander, and B. Saltin. Physical conditioning through interval training with young male adults. *Med. Sci. Sports* 5:220–226, 1973.
98. Laporte, R. E., L. L. Adams, D. D. Savage, G. Brenes, S. Dearwater, and T. Cook. The spectrum of physical activity, cardiovascular disease and health: an epidemiologic perspective. *Am. J. Epidemiol.* 120:507–517, 1984.
99. Leon, A. S., J. Conrad, D. B. Hunninghake, and R. Serfass. Effects of a vigorous walking program on body composition, and carbohydrate and lipid metabolism of obese young men. *Am. J. Clin. Nutr.* 32:1776–1787, 1979.
100. Leon, A. S., J. Connett, D. R. Jacobs, and R. Rauramaa. Leisure-time physical activity levels and risk of coronary heart disease and death: the multiple risk of coronary heart disease and death: the multiple risk factor intervention trial. *J.A.M.A.* 258:2388–2395, 1987.
100A. Lewis, S. F., W. F. Taylor, R. M. Graham, W. A. Pettinger,

J. E. SHUTTE, and C. G. BLOMQVIST. Cardiovascular responses to exercise as functions of absolute and relative work load. *J. Appl. Physiol.* 54:1314–1323, 1983.

101. LIANG, M. T., J. F. ALEXANDER, H. L. TAYLOR, R. C. SERFRASS, A. S. LEON, and G. A. STULL. Aerobic training threshold, intensity duration, and frequency of exercise. *Scand. J. Sports Sci.* 4:5–8, 1982.

101A. LIEBER, D. C., R. L. LIEBER, and W. C. ADAMS. Effects of run-training and swim-training at similar absolute intensities on treadmill $\dot{V}O_{2max}$. *Med. Sci. Sports Exerc.* 21:655–661, 1989.

101B. MACDOUGALL, J. D., G. R. WARD, D. G. SALE, and J. R. SUTTON. Biochemical adaptation of human skeletal muscle to heavy resistance training and immobilization. *J. Appl. Physiol.* 43:700–703, 1977.

101C. MACDOUGALL, J. D., D. TUXEN, D. G. SALE, J. R. MOROZ, and J. R. SUTTON. Arterial blood pressure response to heavy resistance training. *J. Appl. Physiol.* 58:785–790, 1985.

102. MANN, G. V., L. H. GARRETT, A. FARHI, et al. Exercise to prevent coronary heart disease. *Am. J. Med.* 46:12–27, 1969.

103. MARCINIK, E. J., J. A. HODGDON, U. MITTLEMAN, and J. J. O'BRIEN. Aerobic/calisthenic and aerobic/circuit weight training programs for Navy men: a comparative study. *Med. Sci. Sports Exerc.* 17:482–487, 1985.

104. MARIGOLD, E. A. The effect of training at predetermined heart rate levels for sedentary college women. *Med. Sci. Sports* 6:14–19, 1974.

105. MARTIN, J. E. and P. M. DUBBERT. Adherence to exercise. In: *Exercise and Sports Sciences Reviews*, Vol. 13, R. L. Terjung (Ed.). New York: MacMillan Publishing Co., 1985, pp. 137–167.

106. MARTIN, W. H., J. MONTGOMERY, P. G. SNELL, et al. Cardiovascular adaptations to intense swim training in sedentary middle-aged men and women. *Circulation* 75:323–330, 1987.

107. MAYHEW, J. L. and P. M. GROSS. Body composition changes in young women with high resistance weight training. *Res. Q.* 45:433–439, 1974.

108. MESSIER, J. P. and M. DILL. Alterations in strength and maximal oxygen uptake consequent to Nautilus circuit weight training. *Res. Q. Exerc. Sport* 56:345–351, 1985.

109. MILESIS, C. A., M. L. POLLOCK, M. D. BAH, J. J. AYRES, A. WARD, and A. C. Linnerud. Effects of different durations of training on cardiorespiratory function, body composition and serum lipids. *Res Q.* 47:716–725, 1976.

110. MISNER, J. E., R. A. BOILEAU, B. H. MASSEY, and J. H. MAYHEW. Alterations in body composition of adult men during selected physical training programs. *J. Am. Geriatr. Soc.* 22:33–38, 1974.

111. MIYASHITA, M., S. HAGA, and T. MITZUTA. Training and detraining effects on aerobic power in middle-aged and older men. *J. Sports Med.* 18:131–137, 1978.

112. MOODY, D. L., J. KOLLIAS, and E. R. BUSKIRK. The effect of a moderate exercise program on body weight and skinfold thickness in overweight college women. *Med. Sci. Sports* 1:75–80, 1969.

113. MOODY, D. L., J. H. WILMORE, R. N. GIRANDOLA, and J. P. ROYCE. The effects of a jogging program on the body composition of normal and obese high school girls. *Med. Sci. Sports* 4:210–213, 1972.

114. MUELLER, E. A. and W. ROHMERT. Die geschwindigkeit der muskelkraft zunahme bein isometrischen training. *Int. Z. Angew. Physiol.* 19:403–419, 1963.

115. NAUGHTON, J. and F. NAGLE. Peak oxygen intake during physical fitness program for middle-aged men. *J.A.M.A.* 191:899–901, 1965.

116. O'HARA, W., C. ALLEN, and R. J. SHEPHARD. Loss of body weight and fat during exercise in a cold chamber. *Eur. J. Appl. Physiol.* 37:205–218, 1977.

117. OJA, P., P. TERASLINNA, T. PARTANEN, and R. KARAVA. Feasibility of an 18 months' physical training program for middle-aged men and its effect on physical fitness. *Am. J. Public Health* 64:459–465, 1975.

118. OLREE, H. D., B. CORBIN, J. PENROD, and C. SMITH. Methods of achieving and maintaining physical fitness for prolonged space flight. Final Progress Rep. to NASA, Grant No. NGR-04-002-004, 1969.

119. OSCAI, L. B., T. WILLIAMS, and B. HERTIG. Effects of exercise on blood volume. *J. Appl. Physiol.* 24:622–624, 1968.

120. PAFFENBARGER, R. S., R. T. HYDE, A. L. WING, and C. HSIEH. Physical activity and all-cause mortality, and longevity of college alumni. *N. Engl. J. Med.* 314:605–613, 1986.

121. PAVLOU, K. N., W. P. STEFFEE, R. H. LEARMAN, and B. A. BURROWS. Effects of dieting and exercise on lean body mass, oxygen uptake, and strength. *Med. Sci. Sports Exerc.* 17:466–471, 1985.

122. PELS, A. E., M. L. POLLOCK, T. E. DOHMEIER, K. A. LEMBERGER, and B. F. OEHRLEIN. Effects of leg press training on cycling, leg press, and running peak cardiorespiratory measures. *Med. Sci. Sports Exerc.* 19:66–70, 1987.

123. POLLOCK, M. L. The quantification of endurance training programs. In: *Exercise and Sport Sciences Reviews*, J. H. Wilmore (Ed.). New York: Academic Press, 1973, pp. 155–188.

124. POLLOCK, M. L. Prescribing exercise for fitness and adherence. In: *Exercise Adherence: Its Impact on Public Health*, R. K. Dishman (Ed.). Champaign, IL: Human Kinetics Books, 1988, pp. 259–277

125. POLLOCK, M. L., T. K. CURETON, and L. GRENINGER. Effects of frequency of training on working capacity, cardiovascular function, and body composition of adult men. *Med. Sci. Sports* 1:70–74, 1969.

126. POLLOCK, M. L., J. TIFFANY, L. GETTMAN, R. JANEWAY, and H. LOFLAND. Effects of frequency of training on serum lipids, cardiovascular function, and body composition. In: *Exercise and Fitness*, B. D. Franks (Ed.). Chicago: Athletic Institute, 1969, pp. 161–178.

127. POLLOCK, M. L., H. MILLER, R. JANEWAY, A. C. LINNERUD, B. ROBERTSON, and R. VALENTINO. Effects of walking on body composition and cardiovascular function of middle-aged men. *J. Appl. Physiol.* 30:126–130, 1971.

128. POLLOCK, M. L., J. BROIDA, Z. KENDRICK, H. S. MILLER, R. JANEWAY, and A. C. LINNERUD. Effects of training two days per week at different intensities on middle-aged men. *Med. Sci. Sports* 4:192–197, 1972.

129. POLLOCK, M. L., H. S. MILLER, JR., and J. WILMORE. Physiological characteristics of champion American track athletes 40 to 70 years of age. *J. Gerontol.* 29:645–649, 1974.

130. POLLOCK, M. L., J. DIMMICK, H. S. MILLER, Z. KENDRICK, and A. C. LINNERUD. Effects of mode of training on cardiovascular function and body composition of middle-aged men. *Med. Sci. Sports* 7:139–145, 1975.

131. No reference 131 due to renumbering in proof.

132. POLLOCK, M. L., G. A. DAWSON, H. S. MILLER, JR., et al. Physiologic response of men 49 to 65 years of age to endurance training. *J. Am. Geriatr. Soc.* 24:97–104, 1976.

133. POLLOCK, M. L. and A. JACKSON. Body composition: measurement and changes resulting from physical training. Proceedings National College Physical Education Association for Men and Women, January, 1977, pp. 125–137.

134. POLLOCK, M. L., J. AYRES, and A. WARD. Cardiorespiratory fitness: response to differing intensities and durations of training. *Arch. Phys. Med. Rehabil.* 58:467–473, 1977.

135. POLLOCK, M. L., R. GETTMAN, C. A. MILESIS, M. D. BAH, J. L. DURSTINE, and R. B. JOHNSON. Effects of frequency and duration of training on attrition and incidence of injury. *Med. Sci. Sports* 9:31–36, 1977.

136. POLLOCK, M. L., L. R. GETTMAN, P. B. RAVEN, J. AYRES, M. BAH, and A. WARD. Physiological comparison of the effects of aerobic and anaerobic training. In: *Physical Fitness Programs for Law Enforcement Officers: A Manual for Police Administrators*, C. S. Price, M. L. Pollock, L. R. Gettman, and D. A. KENT (Eds.). Washington, D. C.: U. S. Government Printing Office, No. 027-000-00671-0, 1978, pp. 89–96.

137. POLLOCK, M. L., A. S. JACKSON, and C. FOSTER. The use of the perception scale for exercise prescription. In: *The Perception of Exertion in Physical Work*, G. Borg and D. Ottoson (Eds.). London, England: The MacMillan Press, Ltd., 1986, pp. 161–176.

138. POLLOCK, M. L., C. FOSTER, D. KNAPP, J. S. ROD, and D. H. SCHMIDT. Effect of age and training on aerobic capacity and

body composition of master athletes. *J. Appl. Physiol.* 62:725–731, 1987.

139. POLLOCK, M. L. and J. H. WILMORE. *Exercise in Health and Disease: Evaluation and Prescription for Prevention and Rehabilitation*, 2nd Ed. Philadelphia: W. B. Saunders, Co., 1990.
140. POWELL, K. E., H. W. KOHL, C. J. CASPERSEN, and S. N. BLAIR. An epidemiological perspective of the causes of running injuries. *Phys. Sportsmed.* 14:100–114, 1986.
141. RIBISL, P. M. Effects of training upon the maximal oxygen uptake of middle-aged men. *Int. Z. Angew. Physiol.* 26:272–278, 1969.
142. RICHIE, D. H., S. F. KELSO, and P. A. BELLUCCI. Aerobic dance injuries: a retrospective study of instructors and participants. *Phys. Sportsmed.* 13:130–140, 1985.
143. ROBINSON, S. and P. M. HARMON. Lactic acid mechanism and certain properties of blood in relation to training. *Am. J. Physiol.* 132:757–769, 1941.
144. ROSKAMM, H. Optimum patterns of exercise for healthy adults. *Can. Med. Assoc. J.* 96:895–899, 1967.
145. SALE, D. G. Influence of exercise and training on motor unit activation. In: *Exercise and Sport Sciences Reviews*, K. B. Pandolf (Ed.). New York: MacMillan Publishing Co., 1987, pp. 95–152.

145A. SALE, D. G. Neural adaptation to resistance training. *Med. Sci. Sports Exerc.* 20:S135–S145, 1988.

146. SALLIS, J. F., W. L. HASKELL, S. P. FORTMAN, K. M. VRANIZAN, C. B. TAYLOR, and D. S. SOLOMAN. Predictors of adoption and maintenance of physical activity in a community sample. *Prev. Med.* 15:131–141, 1986.
147. SALTIN, B., G. BLOMQVIST, J. MITCHELL, R. L. JOHNSON, K. WILDENTHAL, and C. B. CHAPMAN. Response to exercise after bed rest and after training. *Circulation* 37, 38(Suppl. 7):1–78, 1968.
148. SALTIN, B., L. HARTLEY, A. KILBOM, and I. ÅSTRAND. Physical training in sedentary middle-aged and older men. *Scand. J. Clin. Lab. Invest.* 24:323–334, 1969.
149. SANTIGO, M. C., J. F. ALEXANDER, G. A. STULL, R. C. SERFRASS, A. M. HAYDAY, and A. S. LEON. Physiological responses of sedentary women to a 20-week conditioning program of walking or jogging. *Scand. J. Sports Sci.* 9:33–39, 1987.
150. SEALS, D. R., J. M. HAGBERG, B. F. HURLEY, A. A. EHSANI, and J. O. HOLLOSZY. Endurance training in older men and women. I. Cardiovascular responses to exercise. *J. Appl. Physiol.* 57:1024–1029, 1984.
151. SHARKEY, B. J. Intensity and duration of training and the development of cardiorespiratory endurance. *Med. Sci. Sports* 2:197–202, 1970.
152. SHEPHARD, R. J. Intensity, duration, and frequency of exercise as determinants of the response to a training regime. *Int. Z. Angew. Physiol.* 26:272–278, 1969.
153. SHEPHARD, R. J. Future research on the quantifying of endurance training. *J. Hum. Ergol.* 3:163–181, 1975.
154. SIDNEY, K. H., R. B. EYNON, and D. A. CUNNINGHAM. Effect of frequency of training of exercise upon physical working performance and selected variables representative of cardiorespiratory fitness. In: *Training Scientific Basis and Application*, A. W. Taylor (Ed.). Springfield, IL: Charles C Thomas Co., 1972, pp. 144–188.
155. SIDNEY, K. H., R. J. SHEPHARD, and J. HARRISON. Endurance training and body composition of the elderly. *Am. J. Clin. Nutr.* 30:326–333, 1977.
156. SIEGEL, W., G. BLOMQVIST, and J. H. MITCHELL. Effects of a quantitated physical training program on middle-aged sedentary males. *Circulation* 41:19–29, 1970.

156A. SISCOVICK, D. S., N. S. WEISS, R. H. FLETCHER, and T. LASKY. The incidence of primary cardiac arrest during vigorous exercise. *N. Engl. J. Med.* 311:874–877, 1984.

157. SKINNER, J. The cardiovascular system with aging and exercise. In: *Physical Activity and Aging*, D. Brunner and E. Jokl (Eds.). Baltimore: University Park Press, 1970, pp. 100–108.
158. SKINNER, J., J. HOLLOSZY, and T. CURETON. Effects of a program of endurance exercise on physical work capacity and anthropometric measurements of fifteen middle-aged men. *Am. J. Cardiol.* 14:747–752, 1964.
159. SMITH, D. P. and F. W. STRANSKY. The effect of training and detraining on the body composition and cardiovascular response of young women to exercise. *J. Sports Med.* 16:112–120, 1976.
160. SMITH, E. L., W. REDDAN, and P. E. SMITH. Physical activity and calcium modalities for bone mineral increase in aged women. *Med. Sci. Sports Exerc.* 13:60–64, 1981.
161. SUOMINEN, H., E. HEIKKINEN, and T. TARKATTI. Effect of eight weeks physical training on muscle and connective tissue of the m. vastus lateralis in 69-year-old men and women. *J. Gerontol.* 32:33–37, 1977.
162. TERJUNG, R. L., K. M. BALDWIN, J. COOKSEY, B. SAMSON, and R. A. SUTTER. Cardiovascular adaptation to twelve minutes of mild daily exercise in middle-aged sedentary men. *J. Am. Geriatr. Soc.* 21:164–168, 1973.
163. THOMAS, S. G., D. A. CUNNINGHAM, P. A. RECHNITZER, A. P. DONNER, and J. H. HOWARD. Determinants of the training response in elderly men. *Med. Sci. Sports Exerc.* 17:667–672, 1985.
164. WENGER, H. A. and G. J. BELL. The interactions of intensity, frequency, and duration of exercise training in altering cardiorespiratory fitness. *Sports Med.* 3:346–356, 1986.
165. WILMORE, J. H. Alterations in strength, body composition, and anthropometric measurements consequent to a 10-week weight training program. *Med. Sci. Sports* 6:133–138, 1974.
166. WILMORE, J. Inferiority of female athletes: myth or reality. *J. Sports Med.* 3:1–6, 1974.
167. WILMORE, J. H. Design issues and alternatives in assessing physical fitness among apparently healthy adults in a health examination survey of the general population. In: *Assessing Physical Fitness and Activity in General Population Studies*, T. F. Drury (Ed.). Washington, D.C.: U.S. Public Health Service, National Center for Health Statistics, 1988 (in press).
168. WILMORE, J. H., J. ROYCE, R. N. GIRANDOLA, F. I. KATCH, and V. L. KATCH. Physiological alternatives resulting from a 10-week jogging program. *Med. Sci. Sports* 2:7–14, 1970.
169. WILMORE, J. H., J. ROYCE, R. N. GIRANDOLA, F. I. KATCH, and V. L. KATCH. Body composition changes with a 10-week jogging program. *Med. Sci. Sports* 2:113–117, 1970.
170. WILMORE, J., R. B. PARR, P. A. VODAK, et al. Strength, endurance, BMR, and body composition changes with circuit weight training. *Med. Sci. Sports* 8:58–60, 1976.
171. WILMORE, J. H., G. A. EWY, A. R. MORTAN, et al. The effect of beta-adrenergic blockade on submaximal and maximal exercise performance. *J. Cardiac Rehabil.* 3:30–36, 1983.

171A. WILMORE, J. H. Body composition in sport and exercise: directions for future research. *Med. Sci. Sports Exerc.* 15:21–31, 1983.

172. WILMORE, J. H. and D. L. COSTILL. *Training for Sport and Activity. The Physiological Basis of the Conditioning Process*, 3rd Ed. Dubuque, IA: Wm. C. Brown, 1988, pp. 113–212.
173. WOOD, P. D., W. L. HASKELL, S. N. BLAIR, et al. Increased exercise level and plasma lipoprotein concentrations: a one-year, randomized, controlled study in sedentary, middle-aged men. *Metabolism* 32:31–39, 1983.
174. ZUTI, W. B. and L. A. GOLDING. Comparing diet and exercise as weight reduction tools. *Phys. Sports Med.* 4:49–53, 1976.

Glossary

A

AIDS *See* Acquired immunodeficiency syndrome.

ATP *See* Adenosine triphosphate.

Acquired immunodeficiency syndrome (AIDS) Any of a number of diseases that arise when the body's immune system is compromised by HIV.

Addiction Compulsive and uncontrollable behavior(s) or use of substance(s).

Adenosine triphosphate (ATP) A high-energy chemical compound used for immediate energy by the body.

Adipose tissue Fat cells.

Adult-onset diabetes (Type II) A condition in which insulin is not processed correctly.

Aerobic exercise Exercise that requires oxygen to produce the necessary energy (ATP) to carry out the activity.

Agility Ability to change body position and direction quickly and efficiently.

Alcohol (ethyl alcohol) A depressant drug that affects the brain and slows down central nervous system activity; has strong addictive properties.

Alcoholism Disease in which an individual loses control over drinking alcoholic beverages.

Altruism True concern for the welfare of others

Alveoli Air sacs in the lungs where gas exchange (oxy gen and carbon dioxide) takes place.

Amenorrhea Cessation of regular menstrual flow.

Amino acids Chemical compounds that contain nitrogen, carbon, hydrogen, and oxygen; the basic building blocks the body uses to build different types of protein.

Amotivational syndrome A condition characterized by loss of motivation, dullness, apathy, and no interest in the future.

Anabolic steroids Synthetic versions of the male sex hormone testosterone, which promotes muscle development and hypertrophy.

Anaerobic exercise Exercise that does not require oxygen to produce the necessary energy (ATP) to carry out the activity.

Angina pectoris Chest pain due to coronary heart disease.

Angiogenesis Formation of blood vessels, or capillaries.

Angioplasty A procedure in which a balloon-tipped catheter is inserted to widen the inner lumen of one or more arteries.

Anorexia nervosa An eating disorder characterized by self-imposed starvation to lose and maintain very low body weight.

Anthropometric measurement techniques Measurement of body girths at different sites.

Anticoagulant Any substance that inhibits blood clotting.

Antioxidants Compounds such as vitamins C, E, beta-carotene, and selenium that prevent oxygen from combining with other substances to which it may cause damage.

Aquaphobic Having a fear of water.

Arrhythmias Irregular heart rhythms.

Atherosclerosis Fatty/cholesterol deposits in the walls of the arteries leading to plaque formation.

Atrophy Decrease in the size of a cell.

Autogenic training Stress management technique. It is a form of self-suggestion where an individual is able to place him/herself in an autohypnotic state by repeating and concentrating on feelings of heaviness and warmth in the extremities.

B

Balance Ability to maintain the body in proper equilibrium.

Ballistic or dynamic stretching (flexibility) Movements performed using jerky, rapid, and bouncy movements.

Basal metabolic rate The lowest level of oxygen consumption necessary to sustain life.

Behavior modification The process of replacing destructive or negative behaviors permanently with positive behaviors that will lead to better health and well-being.

Benign Noncancerous.

Beta-carotene A precursor to vitamin A.

Bioelectrical impedance Technique to assess body composition, including percent body fat, by running a weak electrical current through the body.

Biofeedback Stress management technique. A process in which a person learns to reliably influence physiological responses of two kinds: either responses which are not ordinarily under voluntary control or responses which ordinarily are easily regulated but for which regulation has broken down due to trauma or disease.

Blood lipids (fat) Cholesterol and triglycerides.

Blood pressure A measure of the force exerted against the walls of the vessels by the blood flowing through them.

Body composition Refers to the fat and nonfat components of the human body. Important in assessing recommended body weight.

Body mass index (BMI) Ratio of weight to height, used to determine thinness and fatness and risk for disease.

Bradycardia Slower heart rate than normal.

Breathing exercises Stress management technique where the individual concentrates on "breathing away" the tension and inhaling fresh air to the entire body.

Bulimia An eating disorder characterized by a pattern of binge eating and purging to attempt to lose and maintain low body weight.

C

Calorie The amount of heat necessary to raise the temperature of one gram of water one degree Centigrade. Used to measure the energy value of food and cost of physical activity.

Cancer Group of diseases characterized by uncontrolled growth and spread of abnormal cells into malignant tumors.

Capillaries Smallest blood vessels carrying oxygenated blood to the tissues in the body.

Carbohydrates Compounds containing carbon, hydrogen, and oxygen; the major source of energy for the human body.

Carbohydrate loading Increasing intake of carbohydrates during heavy aerobic training or prior to aerobic endurance events lasting longer than 90 minutes.

Carcinogens Substances that contribute to the formation of cancers.

Carcinoma in situ Encapsulated malignant tumor that is found at an early stage and has not spread.

Cardiac output Amount of blood pumped by the heart in one minute.

Cardiomyopathy A disease affecting the heart muscle.

Cardiorespiratory endurance The ability of the lungs, heart, and blood vessels to deliver adequate amounts of oxygen to the cells to meet the demands of prolonged physical activity.

Cardiovascular disease The array of conditions that affect the heart and the blood vessels.

Catecholamines Hormones, including epinephrine and norepinephrine.

Cellulite Term frequently used in reference to fat deposits that "bulge out." These deposits are nothing but enlarged fat cells from excessive accumulation of body fat.

Chlamydia A sexually transmitted disease caused by a bacterial infection that can cause significant damage to the reproductive system.

Cholesterol A waxy substance, technically a steroid alcohol, found only in animal fats and oil; used in making cell membranes, as a building block for some hormones, in the fatty sheath around nerve fibers, and in other necessary substances.

Chronic diseases Illnesses that develop and last over a long time.

Circuit training Alternating exercises by performing them in sequence of three to six or more.

Cirrhosis A disease characterized by scarring of the liver.

Cocaine 2-beta-carbomethoxy-3-betabenozoxytropane, the primary psychoactive ingredient derived from coca plant leaves.

Cold turkey Complete elimination of a negative behavior all at once.

Complex carbohydrates Carbohydrates formed by three or more simple sugar molecules linked together; also referred to as polysaccharides.

Cool-down Tapering off an exercise session slowly.

Coordination Integration of the nervous and the muscular systems to produce correct, graceful, and harmonious body movements.

Coronary heart disease (CHD) Condition in which the arteries that supply the heart muscle with oxygen and nutrients are narrowed by fatty deposits such as cholesterol and triglycerides.

Cross-training Combining two or more activities to achieve a similar training effect.

Cruciferous vegetables Plants that produce cross-shaped leaves (cauliflower, broccoli, cabbage, Brussels sprouts, and kohlrabi); these vegetables seem to have a protective effect against cancer.

D

DNA *See* deoxyribonucleic acid.

Daily values A set of standard nutritive values developed by the FDA (replaces the U.S. RDA).

Dehydration Loss of body water below normal volume.

Deoxyribonucleic acid (DNA) Genetic substance of which genes are made; molecule that bears cell's genetic code.

Diabetes mellitus A disease in which the body doesn't produce or properly utilize insulin.

Diastolic blood pressure Pressure exerted by the blood against the walls of the arteries during the relaxation phase (diastole) of the heart.

Dietary fiber A complex carbohydrate in plant foods that cannot be digested by the human body but is essential in the digestion process.

Disaccharides Simple carbohydrates formed by two monosaccharide units linked together, one of which is glucose. The major disaccharides are sucrose, lactose, and maltose.

Distress Negative stress. Refers to unpleasant or harmful stress under which health and performance begin to deteriorate.

Duration How long a person exercises.

Dynamic strength training Strength training method referring to a muscle contraction with movement.

Dynamic Stretching *See* Ballistic.

Dysmenorrhea Painful menstruation.

E

ECG *See* electrocardiogram

EKG *See* electrocardiogram

Elastic elongation Temporary lengthening of soft tissue (muscles, tendons, ligaments).

Electrocardiogram (ECG or EKG) A recording of the electrical activity of the heart.

Endorphines Morphine-like substances released from the pituitary gland in the brain during prolonged aerobic exercise. They are thought to induce feelings of euphoria and natural well-being.

Endurance *See* Cardiovascular endurance; Muscular endurance.

Energy The ability to do work.

Energy-balancing equation A principle holding that as long as caloric input equals caloric out put, the person will not gain or lose weight. If caloric intake exceeds output, the person gains weight; when output exceeds input, the person loses weight.

Enzymes Catalysts that facilitate chemical reactions in the body.

Epidemiology Science that studies the relationship between diverse factors (lifestyle and environmental) and the occurrence of disease.

Essential fat Minimal amount of body fat needed for normal physiological functions; constitutes about 3% of the total weight in men and 12% in women.

Estrogen Female sex hormone; essential for bone formation and bone density conservation.

Eustress Positive stress: health and performance continue to improve, even as stress increases.

Exercise A type of physical activity that requires "planned, structured, and repetitive bodily movement done to improve or maintain one or more components of physical fitness."

F

Fast-twitch fibers Muscle fibers with greater anaerobic potential and fast speed of contraction.

Fats Compounds made by a combination of triglycerides.

Ferritin Iron stored in the body.

Fiber *See* Dietary fiber.

Fight or flight Physiological response of the body to stress which prepares the individual to take action by stimulating the vital defense systems.

Fitness *See* Physical Fitness.

Fixed resistance Type of exercise in which a constant resistance is moved through a joint's full range of motion.

Flexibility The ability of a joint to move freely through its full range of motion.

Fraud The conscious promotion of unproven claims for profit.

Free fatty acids (FFA) *See* Triglycerides.

Free radicals *See* Oxygen free radicals

Free weights Barbells and dumbbells.

Frequency How often a person engages in an exercise session.

G

Genital warts Sexually transmitted disease caused by a viral infection.

Girth measurements Technique to assess body composition, including percent body fat, by measuring circumferences at various body sites.

Glucose Blood sugar, type of carbohydrate (monosaccharide), a primary source of energy for the human body.

Glycogen Form in which glucose is stored in muscle.

Gonorrhea Sexually transmitted disease caused by a bacterial infection.

H

HDL *See* high density lipoprotein.

Health fitness standards The lowest fitness requirements for maintaining good health, decreasing the risk for chronic diseases, and lowering the incidence of muscular-skeletal injuries.

Heart rate reserve (HRR) The difference between the maximal heart rate and the resting heart rate.

Heat cramps Muscle spasms caused by heat-induced changes in electrolyte balance in muscle cells.

Heat exhaustion Heat-related fatigue.

Heat stroke Heat-related emergency.

Hemoglobin Protein-iron compound in red blood cells that transports oxygen in the blood.

Herpes A sexually transmitted disease caused by a viral infection (herpes simplex virus types I and II).

High density lipoprotein (HDL) Cholesterol-transporting molecules in the blood (good cholesterol).

Human immunodeficiency virus (HIV) Virus that leads to acquired immunodeficiency syndrome (AIDS).

Hydrostatic weighing Underwater technique to assess body composition, including percent body fat.

Hyperglycemia Elevated blood sugar (glucose).

Hypertension Chronically elevated blood pressure.

Hypertrophy An increase in the size of the cell (for example, muscle hypertrophy).

Hypoglycemia Low blood sugar (glucose).

Hypokinetic diseases Diseases associated with a lack of physical activity.

Hypotension Low blood pressure.

Hypothermia A breakdown in the body's ability to generate heat with a drop in temperature below 95°F.

I

IU International units, for measuring nutrients.

Insulin Hormone secreted by the pancreas used in the absorption and utilization of glucose by the body.

Intensity In cardiorespiratory exercise, how hard a person has to exercise to improve or maintain fitness.

Isokinetic Strength-training method in which the speed of the muscle contraction is kept constant because the equipment (machine) provides an accommodating resistance to match the user's force (maximal) through the range of motion.

Isometric Strength training method referring to a muscle contraction that produces little or no movement, such as pushing or pulling against an immovable object.

J

Juvenile diabetes (Type I) Insulin-dependent diabetes. *See also* Diabetes mellitus.

L

LDL *See* low density lipoprotein

Lactic acid End product of anaerobic glycolysis (metabolism).

Lactovegetarians Vegetarians who eat foods from the milk group.

Lean body mass Body weight without body fat.

Leisure-time physical activity Any activity undertaken during an individual's discretionary time that helps to increase resting energy or caloric expenditure.

Life experiences survey Questionnaire used to assess sources of stress in life.

Lipoproteins Lipids covered by proteins; transport fats in the blood.

Locus of control A concept examining the extent to which a person believes he or she can influence the external environment.

Low-density lipoprotein (LDL) Cholesterol-transporting molecules in the blood (bad cholesterol).

M

MET Represents the rate of resting energy expenditure at rest; one MET is the equivalent of 3.5 ml/kg/min.

Malignant Cancerous.

Marijuana A psychoactive drug, prepared from a mixture of crushed leaves, flowers, small branches, stems, and seeds from the hemp plant *cannabis sativa*.

Maximal heart rate (MHR) Highest heart rate for a person, primarily related to age.

Maximal oxygen uptake (VO_{2max}) The maximum amount of oxygen the body is able to utilize per minute of physical activity, commonly expressed in ml/kg/min. The best indicator of cardiorespiratory or aerobic fitness.

Meditation Stress management technique used to gain control over one's attention, clearing the mind and blocking out the stressor(s) responsible for the increased tension.

Megadoses For most vitamins, 10 times the RDA or more. For A and D, five and two times the RDA, respectively.

Melanoma The most virulent, rapidly spreading form of skin cancer.

Metabolism All energy and material transformations that occur within living cells necessary to sustain life.

Metastasis The movement of cells from one part of the body to another.

Minerals Inorganic elements found in the body and in food; essential for normal body functions.

Mitochondria Structures within the cells where energy transformations take place.

Mode Form of exercise.

Monogamous A sexual relationship in which two people have sexual relations only with each other.

Monosaccharides The simplest carbohydrates (sugars) formed by five- or six-carbon skeletons. The three most common are glucose, fructose, and galactose

Motivation The desire and will to do something.

Motor neurons Nerves traveling from the central nervous system to the muscle.

Muscular endurance The ability of a muscle to exert submaximal force repeatedly over time.

Muscular strength The ability of a muscle to exert maximum force against resistance (for example, 1 repetition maximum or 1 RM on the bench press exercise).

Myocardial infarction Heart attack; damaging or death of an area of the heart muscle as a result of an obstructed artery to that area.

Myocardium Heart muscle.

N

Neuron A nerve cell.

Nicotine Poisonous compound found in tobacco leaves.

Nitrosamines Potentially cancer-causing compounds formed when nitrites and nitrates, which are used to prevent the growth of harmful bacteria in processed meats, combine with other chemicals in the stomach.

Nonmelanoma skin cancer Spreads or grows directly from the original site but does not metastasize to other regions of the body.

Nutrients Substances found in food that provide energy, regulate metabolism, and help with growth and repair of body tissues.

Nutrition Science that studies the relationship of foods to optimal health and performance.

O

Obesity A chronic disease characterized by an excessively high amount of body fat in relation to lean body mass.

Olestra Fat substitute made from sugar and fatty acids; provides no calories to the body because it passes through the digestive system without being absorbed.

Omega-3 fatty acids Polyunsaturated fatty acids found primarily in cold-water seafood; thought to be effective in lowering blood cholesterol and triglycerides.

Oncogenes Initiate cell division.

One repetition maximum (1 RM) The maximum amount of resistance an individual is able to lift in a single effort.

Opportunistic infections Diseases that arise in the absence of a healthy immune system that would fight them off in healthy people.

Osteoporosis The softening, deterioration, or loss of total body bone.

Overload principle Training concept stating that the demands placed on a system (cardiorespiratory, muscular) must be increased systematically and progressively over a period of time to cause physiologic adaptation (development or improvement).

Overweight An excess amount of weight against a given standard such as height or recommended percent body fat.

Ovolactovegetarians Vegetarians who include eggs and milk products in the diet.

Ovovegetarians Vegetarians who allow eggs in the diet.

Oxygen free radicals Substances formed during metabolism which attack and damage proteins and lipids, in particular the cell membrane and DNA, leading to the development of diseases such as heart disease, cancer, and emphysema.

P

PNF *See* Proprioceptive neuromuscular facilitation.

Pelvic inflammatory disease (PID) An overall designation referring to the effects of chlamydia and gonorrhea.

Percent body fat Total amount of fat in the body based on the person's weight, includes both essential and storage fat.

Peripheral vascular disease Narrowing of the peripheral blood vessels (it excludes the cerebral and coronary arteries).

Physical activity Bodily movement produced by skeletal muscles that requires energy expenditure and produces progressive health benefits.

Physical fitness The ability to meet the ordinary as well as the unusual demands of daily life safely and effectively without being overly fatigued, and still have energy left for leisure and recreational activities.

Physical fitness standards A fitness level that allows a person to sustain moderate to vigorous physical activity without undue fatigue and the ability to closely maintain this level throughout life.

Phytochemicals Compounds, found in fruits and vegetables, that block the formation of cancerous tumors and disrupt the process.

Plastic elongation Permanent lengthening of soft tissue (capsules, tendons, ligaments).

Plyometric training Explosive jump training, incorporating speed and strength training to enhance explosiveness.

Power The ability to produce maximum force in the shortest time.

Progressive muscle relaxation Stress management technique. It involves progressive contraction and relaxation of muscle groups throughout the body.

Progressive resistance training *See* Strength Training

Proprioceptive neuromuscular facilitation (PNF) Stretching technique in which muscles are stretched out progressively with intermittent isometric contractions.

Proteins Complex organic compounds containing nitrogen and formed by combinations of amino acids; the main substances used in the body to build and repair tissues.

Q

Quackery The conscious promotion of unproven claims for profit.

R

RNA *See* ribonucleic acid.

RPE *See* rate of perceived exertion.

Range of motion Range of movement of a given joint.

Rate of perceived exertion (RPE) A perception scale to monitor or interpret the intensity of aerobic exercise.

Reaction time The time required to initiate a response to a given stimulus.

Recommended body weight Body weight at which there seems to be no harm to human health.

Recommended dietary allowances (RDA) Daily suggested intakes of nutrients for normal, healthy people, as developed by National Academy of Sciences.

Recovery time Amount of time the heart takes to return to resting heart rate after exercise.

Red muscle fibers Slow-twitch or slow contracting muscle fiber. (*Also see* slow-twitch fibers.)

Repetition The number of times a given action is performed (for example, 12 repetitions on the bench press exercise).

Repetition maximum (in strength training) The maximum number of repetitions (RM) that can performed with a specific resistance or weight (for example, 10 RM with 150).

Resistance Amount of weight that is lifted.

Resting heart rate (RHR) Rate after a person has been sitting quietly for 15–20 minutes.

Resting metabolism The amount of energy (expressed in milliliters of oxygen per minute or total calories per day) an individual requires during resting conditions to sustain proper body function.

Reverse cholesterol transport A process in which HDL molecules attract cholesterol and carry it to the liver, where it is changed to bile and eventually excreted in the stool.

Ribonucleic acid (RNA) Genetic material involved in the formation of cell proteins.

Risk factor Lifestyle and genetic variables that may lead to disease.

S

STDs *See* sexually transmitted diseases.

Serum cholesterol *See* cholesterol.

Set Number of repetitions performed for a given exercise.

Setpoint The weight control theory that indicates the body has an established weight and strongly attempts to maintain that weight.

Sexually transmitted diseases (STDs) Communicable diseases spread through sexual contact.

Shin splints Injury to the lower leg characterized by pain and irritation in the shin region or front of the leg.

Side stitch A sharp pain in the side of the abdomen.

Simple carbohydrates Formed by simple or double sugar units with little nutritive value; divided into monosaccharides and disaccharides.

Skill-related fitness Fitness components important for success in skillful activities and athletic events; encompasses agility, balance, coordination, power, reaction time, and speed.

Skinfold thickness Technique to assess body composition, including percent body fat, by measuring the thickness of a double fold of skin at different body sites.

Slow-sustained or static stretching Technique in which the muscles are lengthened gradually through a joint's complete range of motion and the final position is held for a few seconds.

Slow-twitch fibers Muscle fibers with greater aerobic potential and slow speed of contraction.

Specificity of training A principle stating that training must be done with the specific muscle the body is attempting to improve.

Speed The ability to propel the body or a part of the body rapidly from one point to another.

Spirituality An affirmation of life that recognizes a higher being and integrates the dimensions of wellness.

Sphygmomanometer An inflatable bladder contained within a cuff and a mercury gravity manometer (or an aneroid manometer) from which the pressure is read.

Spot reducing Fallacious theory that claims that exercising a specific body part will result in significant fat reduction in that area.

Steroids *See* Anabolic steroids.

Sterols Derived fats, of which cholesterol is the best known example.

Static *See* Isometric

Storage fat Body fat in excess of the essential fat; stored in adipose tissue.

Strength *See* Muscular strength.

Strength training A conditioning program that requires the use of weight to help increase muscular strength, endurance, power, and/or body size.

Stress The mental, emotional, and physical response of the body to any situation that is new, threatening, frightening, or exciting.

Stress electrocardiogram (ECG) An exercise test during which the workload is gradually increased (until the subject reaches maximal fatigue) with blood pressure and 12-lead electrocardiographic monitoring throughout the test.

Stressor Stress-causing agent.

Stretching Moving the joints beyond the accustomed range of motion.

Stress Vulnerability Scale Questionnaire used to identify a number of factors that can help people decrease their vulnerability to stress.

Stroke volume Amount of blood pumped by the heart in one beat.

Structured interview Assessment tool used in determining behavioral patterns (Type A and B personality).

Subluxation Partial dislocation of a joint.

Substrate Substance acted upon by an enzyme (examples: carbohydrates and fats).

Sun protection factor (SPF) Degree of protection offered by ingredients in sunscreen lotion; at least SPF 15 is recommended.

Synergistic action The effect of mixing two or more drugs which can be much greater than the sum of two or more drugs acting by themselves.

Synergy A reaction in which the result is greater than the sum of its two parts.

Syphilis A sexually transmitted disease caused by a bacterial infection.

Systolic blood pressure Pressure exerted by the blood against the walls of the arteries during the forceful contraction (systole) of the heart.

T

Tachycardia Faster than normal heart rate.

Tar Chemical compound that forms during the burning of tobacco leaves.

Telomerase An enzyme that allows cells to reproduce indefinitely.

Telomeres A strand of molecules at both ends of a chromosome.

Testosterone Male sex hormone.

Thermogenic response The amount of energy required to digest food.

Transfatty acid Solidified fat formed by adding hydrogen to monosaturated and polyunsaturated fats to increase shelf life.

Triglycerides Fats formed by glycerol and three fatty acids.

Tumor suppressor genes Deactivate the process of cell division.

Type A Behavior pattern characteristic of a hard-driving, overambitious, aggressive, at times hostile, and overly competitive person.

Type B Behavior pattern characteristic of a calmed, casual, relaxed, and easy-going individual.

Type C Behavior pattern of individuals who are just as highly stressed as the Type A but do not seem to be at higher risk for disease than the Type B.

U

Ultraviolet B rays (UVB) Sun rays that cause sunburn and encourage skin cancers.

V

VLDL *See* very low density lipoprotein.

VO_{2max} *See* Maximal oxygen uptake.

Variable resistance Training using special machines equipped with mechanical devices that provide differing amounts of resistance through the range of motion.

Vegans Vegetarians who eat no animal products at all.

Vegetarians Individuals whose diet is of vegetable or plant origin.

Very low-density lipoproteins (VLDLs) Triglyceride, cholesterol and phospholipid-transporting molecules in the blood. Only a small amount of cholesterol is carried by the VLDL molecules.

Vitamins Organic substances essential for normal metabolism, growth, and development of the body.

W

Waist-to-hip ratio A test to assess potential risk for diseases associated with obesity.

Warm-up Starting a workout slowly.

Weight-regulating mechanism (WRM) A feature of the hypothalamus of the brain that controls how much the body should weigh (*also see* Setpoint theory).

Wellness The constant and deliberate effort to stay healthy and achieve the highest potential for well-being.

White muscle fibers *See* Fast-twitch fibers.

Work The ability to utilize energy.

Workload Load (or intensity) placed on the body during physical activity.

Y

Yo-yo dieting Constantly losing and gaining weight.

Index